# Medical Radiology

## Radiation Oncology

*Series editors*

Luther W. Brady
Stephanie E. Combs
Jiade J. Lu

*Honorary editors*

Hans-Peter Heilmann
Michael Molls

For further volumes:
http://www.springer.com/series/4353

Nancy Y. Lee • Nadeem Riaz • Jiade J. Lu
Editors

# Target Volume Delineation for Conformal and Intensity-Modulated Radiation Therapy

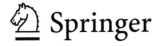 Springer

*Editors*
Nancy Y. Lee
Department of Radiation Oncology
Memorial Sloan Kettering Cancer Center
NY
USA

Nadeem Riaz
Department of Radiation Oncology
Memorial Sloan Kettering Cancer Center
NY
USA

Jiade J. Lu
Shanghai Proton and Heavy Ion Center
Shanghai
China

ISSN 0942-5373
ISBN 978-3-319-05725-5          ISBN 978-3-319-05726-2   (eBook)
DOI 10.1007/978-3-319-05726-2
Springer Cham Heidelberg New York Dordrecht London

Library of Congress Control Number: 2014957720

# Preface

Historically, radiation oncologists relied on bony landmarks to determine radiation portals and approximate areas that could be at risk for harboring gross and/or microscopic disease. The introduction of cross-axial imaging with CT scans in the 1970s and MRIs in the 1980s allowed us to more precisely visualize areas at risk for disease. The subsequent development of 3D conformal radiotherapy (3DCRT) and intensity-modulated radiotherapy (IMRT) allowed us to take advantage of more precise target definitions by sculpting the dose of radiation to avoid critical structures. These advances afforded us the possibility to improve outcomes while simultaneously decreasing toxicity from treatment.

However, these more precise techniques of radiotherapy pose a unique set of risks. Conformal radiotherapy requires significantly more attention to target volume delineation (CTV) than was previously needed. For conventional 2D treatments, knowledge of bony landmarks was sufficient. Comparatively, the interpretation of cross-axial imaging requires significantly more anatomic knowledge to accurately delineate target volumes (CTV). Further, IMRT can be very unforgiving if used inappropriately. If a region is not included in the target volume (CTV), it will receive a subtherapeutic dose and is at risk for recurrence.

Randomized trials over the past decade have demonstrated that conformal techniques can improve outcomes in patients. These trials have also uncovered significant risks from these conformal techniques. In multiple disease sites, the quality of radiotherapy is consistently associated with outcomes. Central review of treatment plans has demonstrated that inadequate target volumes (PTVs and CTVs), leads to inadequate treatment, and subsequently poorer outcomes.

Although there are many textbooks in the field, most focus on the natural history of disease and the evidence for radiotherapy, rather than on the technical details required for target delineation. We saw an urgent need for a resource that focuses on how to delineate target volumes (CTVs) for radiotherapy. The best way to understand what to target is to see cases, and so, each chapter provides slice-by-slice illustrations of target volumes on planning CT scans. We hope this book can serve as the equivalent of the radiologist's atlas. The text in each chapter is focused on knowledge that is important for accurately delineating target volumes and the reasons behind the volumes. The text is not sufficient to understand all the important oncologic aspects of a particular cancer, but it is sufficient to understand the radiotherapy technique for a particular disease.

We hope this will serve as a valuable resource to physicians in the community, residents in training, and others looking to understand the anatomic underpinnings of radiotherapy.

New York                                         Nadeem Riaz
Shanghai                                             Jiade Lu
New York                                            Nancy Lee

# Contents

**Part III   Thorax**

**Part IV   Gastrointestinal Tract**

**Part V   Gynecological Tract**

**Part VI   Genitourinary System**

# Contributors

**Matthew Abramowitz** Department of Radiation Oncology, University of Miami, Miami, FL, USA

**Bret Adams** Department of Radiation Oncology, University of Miami, Miami, FL, USA

**Harold Agbahiwe** Department of Radiation Oncology and Molecular Radiation Sciences, The Johns Hopkins Hospital, Baltimore, MD, USA

**Sara Alcorn** Department of Radiation Oncology and Molecular Radiation Sciences, The Johns Hopkins Hospital, Baltimore, MD, USA

**Ase Ballangrud** Department of Radiation Oncology, MD Anderson Cancer Center, Houston, TX, USA

**Peter Balter** Division of Radiation Oncology, University of Texas MD Anderson Cancer Center, Houston, TX, USA

**Christopher A. Barker** Department of Radiation Oncology, Memorial Sloan Kettering Cancer Center, New York, NY, USA

**Jose G. Bazan** Department of Radiation Oncology, Stanford University, Stanford, CA, USA; Department of Radiation Oncology, Arthur G. James Cancer Hospital & Solove Research Institute, The Ohio State University, Columbus, OH, USA

**Sushil Beriwal** Department of Radiation Oncology, University of Pittsburgh Cancer Institute, Pittsburgh, PA, USA

**Nicholas S. Boehling** Department of Radiation Oncology, M.D. Anderson Cancer Center, Houston, TX, USA

**Jeffrey Buchsbaum** Department of Radiation Oncology, Indiana University, Bloomington, IN, USA

**Ruben Cabanillas** Department of Radiation Oncology, Tufts Medical Center, New York, NY, USA

**Oren Cahlon** Department of Radiation Oncology, Memorial Sloan Kettering, New York, NY, USA

**Daniel T. Chang** Department of Radiation Oncology, Stanford University, Stanford, CA, USA

**Eric L. Chang** Department of Radiation Oncology, M.D. Anderson Cancer Center, Houston, TX, USA

**Samuel T. Chao** Department of Radiation Oncology, Cleveland Clinic Foundation, Cleveland, OH, USA; Taussig Cancer Institute, Cleveland Clinic Foundation, Cleveland, OH, USA; Burkhardt Brain Tumor and Neuro-Oncology Center, Cleveland Clinic Foundation, Cleveland, OH, USA

**Jason Chia-Hsien Cheng** Graduate Institute of Oncology, National Taiwan University College of Medicine, Taipei, Taiwan; Division of Radiation Oncology, Department of Oncology, National Taiwan University Hospital, Taipei, Taiwan

**Bhisham Chera** Department of Radiation Oncology, University of North Carolina, Chapel Hill, NC, USA

**John Cuaron** Department of Radiation Oncology, Memorial Sloan Kettering, New York, NY, USA

**Laura A. Dawson** Department of Radiation Oncology, Princess Margaret Cancer Centre, University of Toronto, Toronto, ON, Canada

**Neil B. Desai** Department of Radiation Oncology, Memorial Sloan Kettering Cancer Center, New York, NY, USA

**Dayssy A. Diaz** Department of Radiation Oncology, University of Miami, Miami, FL, USA

**Colleen Dickie** Radiation Medicine Department, Princess Margaret Hospital, University of Toronto, Toronto, ON, USA

**Michael R. Folker** Department of Radiation Oncology, Memorial Sloan Kettering Cancer Center, New York, NY, USA

**Daniel Gomez** Division of Radiation Oncology, University of Texas MD Anderson Cancer Center, Houston, TX, USA

**Karyn A. Goodman** Department of Radiation Oncology, Memorial Sloan Kettering Cancer Center, New York, NY, USA

**Gaorav P. Gupta** Department of Radiation Oncology, Memorial Sloan Kettering Cancer Center, New York, NY, USA

**Daniel Higginson** Department of Radiation Oncology, Memorial Sloan Kettering, New York, NY, USA

**Alice Ho** Department of Radiation Oncology, Memorial Sloan-Kettering Cancer Center, New York, NY, USA

**Bradford S. Hoppe** Department of Radiation Oncology, University of Florida, Jacksonville, FL, USA

**Richard T. Hoppe** Department of Radiation Oncology, Stanford University, Palo Alto, Stanford, CA, USA

**Feng-Ming Hsu** Division of Radiation Oncology, Department of Oncology, National Taiwan University Hospital, Taipei, Taiwan

**Lisa A. Kachnic** Department of Radiation Oncology, Boston Medical Center, Boston University School of Medicine, Boston, MA, USA

**Zachary Kohutek** Department of Radiation Oncology, Memorial Sloan-Kettering, New York, NY, USA

**Albert C. Koong** Department of Radiation Oncology, Stanford University, Stanford, CA, USA

**Rupesh Kotecha** Department of Radiation Oncology, Cleveland Clinic Foundation, Cleveland, OH, USA

**Kate Krause** Department of Radiation Oncology, Memorial Sloan Kettering Cancer Center, New York, NY, USA

**Ryan Lanning** Department of Radiation Oncology, Memorial Sloan Kettering Cancer Center, New York, NY, USA

**Nancy Y. Lee** Department of Radiation Oncology, Memorial Sloan Kettering Cancer Center, New York, NY, USA; Department of Radiation Oncology, Institute of Molecular and Oncological Medicine of Asturias (IMOMA), Oviedo, Spain

**Yiat Horng Leong** National University Health System, Singapore, Singapore

**Guang Li** Department of Medical Physics, Memorial Sloan Kettering Cancer Center, New York, NY, USA

**Zhongxing Liao** Department of Radiation Oncology, University of Texas MD Anderson Cancer Center, Houston, TX, USA

**Arthur K. Liu** Department of Radiation Oncology, University of Colorado Denver, Aurora, CO, USA

**Benjamin H. Lok** Department of Radiation Oncology, Memorial Sloan Kettering Cancer Center, New York, NY, USA

**Jiade J. Lu** Shanghai Proton and Heavy Ion Center (SPHIC), Shanghai, China

**Shannon M. MacDonald** Harvard Radiation Oncology Program, Department of Radiation Oncology, Massachusetts General Hospital, Boston, MA, USA

**Sean M. McBride** Department of Radiation Oncology, Memorial Sloan-Kettering Cancer Center, New York, NY, USA

**Minesh P. Mehta** Department of Radiation Oncology, University of Maryland School of Medicine, Baltimore, MD, USA

**Loren K. Mell** Department of Radiation Medicine and Applied Sciences, University of California San Diego, La Jolla, CA, USA

**Inigo San Miguel** Department of Radiation Oncology, Princess Margaret Cancer Centre, University of Toronto, Toronto, ON, Canada

**I. S. Miguel** Division of Radiation Oncology, Department of Oncology, National Taiwan University Hospital, Taipei, Taiwan

**Arno J. Mundt** Department of Radiation Medicine and Applied Sciences, University of California, San Diego, La Jolla, CA, USA

**Erin S. Murphy** Department of Radiation Oncology, Cleveland Clinic Foundation, Cleveland, OH, USA; Taussig Cancer Institute, Cleveland Clinic Foundation, Cleveland, OH, USA; Burkhardt Brain Tumor and Neuro-Oncology Center, Cleveland Clinic Foundation, Cleveland, OH, USA

**Brian Napolitano** Harvard Radiation Oncology Program, Department of Radiation Oncology, Massachusetts General Hospital, Boston, MA, USA

**Brian O'Sullivan** Department of Radiation Oncology, Princess Margaret Hospital, University of Toronto, Toronto, ON, USA

**Anthony J. Paravati** Department of Radiation Medicine and Applied Sciences, University of California, San Diego, La Jolla, CA, USA

**Kruti Patel** Department of Radiation Oncology, University of Maryland Medical Center, Baltimore, MD, USA

**Sagar Patel** Harvard Radiation Oncology Program, Department of Radiation Oncology, Massachusetts General Hospital, Boston, MA, USA

**Arnold C. Paulino** Department of Radiation Oncology, MD Anderson Cancer Center, Houston, TX, USA

**Alan Pollack** Department of Radiation Oncology, University of Miami, Miami, FL, USA

**Ian Poon** Department of Radiation Oncology, University of Toronto/Sunnybrook Health Sciences Centre, Toronto, ON, Canada

**Simon N. Powell** Department of Radiation Oncology, Memorial Sloan-Kettering Cancer Center, New York, NY, USA

**Nadeem Riaz** Department of Radiation Oncology, Memorial Sloan-Kettering Cancer Center, New York, NY, USA

**Paul B. Romesser** Department of Radiation Oncology, Memorial Sloan Kettering Cancer Center, New York, NY, USA

**Eli Scher** Department of Radiation Oncology, Tufts Medical Center, Memorial Sloan Kettering Cancer Center, New York, NY, USA

**Jeremy Setton** Department of Radiation Oncology, Memorial Sloan Kettering Cancer Center, New York, NY, USA

**Daniel R. Simpson** Department of Radiation Medicine and Applied Sciences, University of California, San Diego, La Jolla, CA, USA

**Chun Siu** Department of Radiation Oncology, Memorial Sloan Kettering Cancer Center, New York, NY, USA

**Daniel E. Spratt** Department of Radiation Oncology, Memorial Sloan Kettering Cancer Center, New York, NY, USA; Department of Radiation Oncology, Institute of Molecular and Oncological Medicine of Asturias (IMOMA), Oviedo, Spain

**John H. Suh** Department of Radiation Oncology, Cleveland Clinic Foundation, Cleveland, OH, USA; Taussig Cancer Institute, Cleveland Clinic Foundation, Cleveland, OH, USA; Burkhardt Brain Tumor and Neuro-Oncology Center, Cleveland Clinic Foundation, Cleveland, OH, USA

**Moses Tam** Department of Radiation Oncology, Memorial Sloan-Kettering Cancer Center, New York, NY, USA

**Stephanie Terezakis** Department of Radiation Oncology and Molecular Radiation Sciences, The Johns Hopkins Hospital, Baltimore, MD, USA

**Jeremy Tey** Department of Radiation Oncology, National University Cancer Institute, Singapore, Singapore

**Ivan W.K. Tham** National University Health System, Singapore, Singapore

**Keith Unger** Department of Radiation Oncology, Georgetown University Hospital, Washington, DC, USA

**John A. Vargo** Department of Radiation Oncology, University of Pittsburgh Cancer Institute, Pittsburgh, PA, USA

**Chia-Chun Wang** Division of Radiation Oncology, Department of Oncology, National Taiwan University Hospital, Taipei, Taiwan

**Wang** Department of Radiation Oncology, Princess Margaret Cancer Centre, University of Toronto, Toronto, ON, Canada

**David C. Weksberg** Department of Radiation Oncology, M.D. Anderson Cancer Center, Houston, TX, USA

**Abraham J. Wu** Department of Radiation Oncology, Memorial Sloan-Kettering Cancer Center, New York, NY, USA

**Catheryn M. Yashar** Department of Radiation Medicine and Applied Sciences, University of California, San Diego, La Jolla, CA, USA

**Robert Young** Department of Radiation Oncology, Memorial Sloan Kettering Cancer Center, New York, NY, USA

**Michael J. Zelefsky** Department of Radiation Oncology, Memorial Sloan Kettering Cancer Center, New York, NY, USA

**Joanne Zhung** Department of Radiation Oncology, Tufts Medical Center, New York, NY, USA

**Zachary S. Zumsteg** Department of Radiation Oncology, Memorial Sloan Kettering Cancer Center, New York, NY, USA

# Part I

# Head and Neck

# Nasopharyngeal Carcinoma

Nadeem Riaz, Moses Tam, and Nancy Lee

## Contents

N. Riaz • M. Tam • N. Lee (✉)
Department of Radiation Oncology, Memorial Sloan-Kettering
Cancer Center, New York, 10065 NY
email: leen2@mskcc.org

## 1 Anatomy and Patterns of Spread

- The nasopharynx is a cubodial chamber that is posteriorly bound by the C1–C2 vertebral body and sphenoid bone. Anteriorly, it connects with the nasal cavity and begins at the posterior choanae. Inferiorly, it connects with the oropharynx and the superior surface of the soft palate forms the floor of the cavity (Fig. 1a).

- The eustachian tube is located in the lateral wall and bounded by a prominence known as the torus tubarius. Posterior to the torus is the fossa of *Rosenmüller*, which is the most common site for nasopharyngeal malignancies. In advanced cases, the tumor can invade the middle ear through the eustachian tube (Fig. 1b).

- Anteriorly, the tumor can extend into the nasal fossa (87 %) (Fig. 7) and result in destruction of the pterygoid plates (27 %). Less commonly, the tumor can invade the ethmoid and maxillary sinus or infiltrate the orbital apex.

- Laterally, the tumor can extend into the parapharyngeal space (68 %), which is an important part of T staging for a tumor (Figs. 7 and 8b). Extension into this space can occasionally lead to invasion of cranial nerves IX to XII in advanced disease.

- Superiorly, nasopharyngeal carcinoma can directly invade the base of the skull, the sphenoid sinus, and the clivus (41 %). The foramen lacerum is a vulnerable spot through which the tumor may enter the cavernous sinus (16 %) and the middle cranial fossa to invade cranial nerves III to VI. The foramen ovale also allows access for the tumor to invade the middle cranial fossa, in addition to the petrous portion of the temporal bone (19 %), and the cavernous sinus.

- The posterior extension of NPC is less common and can include invasion of prevertebral muscles (19 %) and inferior invasion of the oropharynx (21 %).

N.Y. Lee et al. (eds.), *Target Volume Delineation for Conformal and Intensity-Modulated Radiation Therapy*,
Medical Radiology. Radiation Oncology, DOI: 10.1007/174_2014_1005, © Springer International Publishing Switzerland 2014
Published Online: 20 September 2014

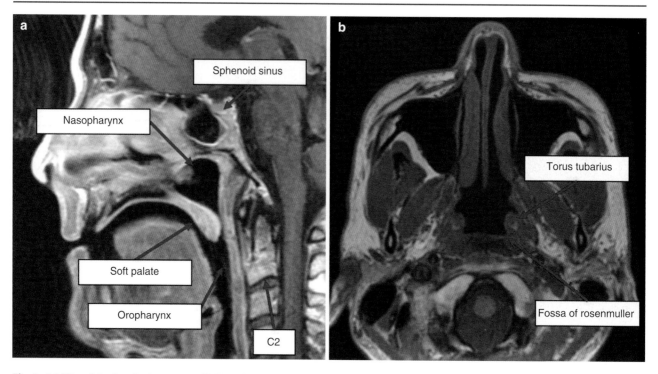

**Fig. 1** (**a**) T1-weighted sagittal sequence. (**b**) T1-weighted axial sequence

- Ipsilateral lymphadenopathy is appreciable in 85–90 % of NPC cases, and bilateral disease is present in approximately 50 % of cases.
- Retropharyngeal lymph nodes are commonly involved in nasopharyngeal cancer (Fig. 3b).
- Lypmh node chains routinely involved include levels II–V. Level IA is rarely invovled with the disease. Figure 2 shows the frequency of detection of lymph nodes at various levels in NPC based on an MR study (Ng et al. 2007).

## 2 Diagnostic Workup Relevant for Target Volume Delineation

- Fiber-optic examination provides the best means to assess the mucosal spread of disease. Typically, lesions are exophytic in nature; however, 10 % may be submucosal and not visible on endoscopic examination.
- Cranial nerve deficits can occur in 10 % of patients with NPC, and their detection will result in alterations to target volumes (most commonly CN VI, V, XII, IX, and X).
  - For CN IX and X: Cover jugular foramen
  - For CN V: Cover pterygopalatine fossa, cavernous sinus, foramen rotundum, and foramen ovale
  - For CN VI: Cover cavernous sinus
- MRI provides superior assessment of skull base involvement and tumor invasion into soft tissue structures compared to CT scan (Abdel Khalek Abdel Razek & King 2012), in particular.

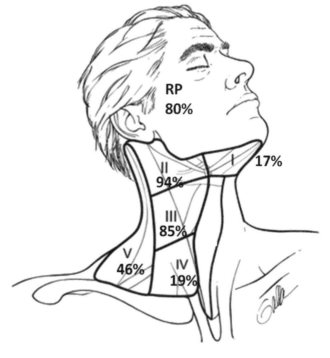

**Fig. 2** Distribution of positive nodes at different neck levels based on magnetic resonance imaging in 202 patients (Ng et al. 2007) (Adapted from Jack Baskin et al. (2013) Fig. 8.1 (with permission))

  - T2-weighted fast spin echo: Depict involvement of parapharyngeal space, paranasal sinus, and retropharyngeal lymph node involvement (Fig. 3b).

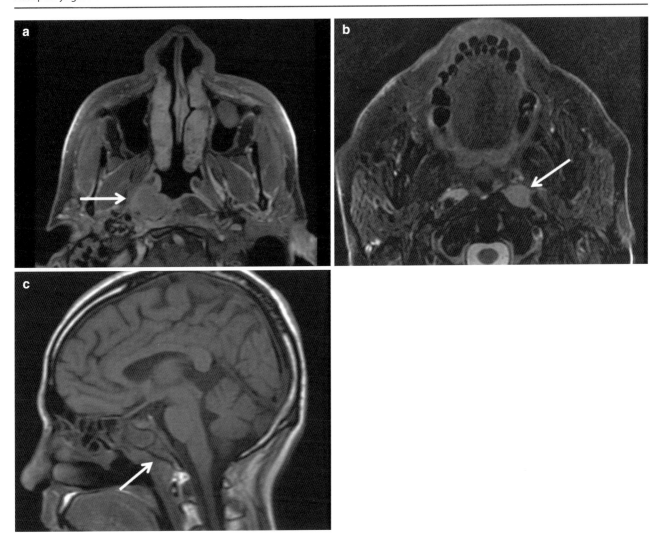

**Fig. 3** MR imaging of the nasopharynx: (**a**) T1-weighted post-contrast sequence demonstrates a right-sided nasopharyngeal primary invading the prevertebral musculature. Note that the fascial plane demarcating the parapharyngeal space is intact (*arrow*). (**b**) T2-weighted fat-saturated sequence demonstrating a left-sided retropharyngeal lymph node (*arrow*). Often on CT, these can be difficult to distinguish clearly from the primary. (**c**) Sagittal T1-weighted sequence demonstrates diffuse infiltration of the marrow of the clivus (*arrow*)

- – T1 non-contrast: Determine involvement of clivus (sagittal cuts) and skull base involvement (Fig. 3c). Tumor invasion of marrow is typically hypointense relative to normal marrow.
- – T1 post-contrast: Determine perineural invasion and intracranial involvement (Fig. 8).
- Fusion of the skull base portion of the MRI can aid in the delineation of the GTV. CT still provides superior assessment of cortical bone involvement.
- MRI is better able to differentiate retropharyngeal lymph nodes from the primary tumor compared to CT.
- Any evidence of enlarged retropharyngeal lymph nodes should be considered gross disease. For other lymph node beds, the presence of central necrosis, extracapsular spread, or a short-axis diameter of 10 mm suggests possible involvement with the disease. PET/CT may also help clarify whether borderline nodes are involved with

the disease. As a general rule, given that NPC has a high likelihood of nodal spread, any suspicious nodes should be considered as gross disease.

## 3    Simulation and Daily Localization

- Set up the patient in supine position with the head extended. The immobilization device should include at least the head and neck. If possible, shoulders should also be immobilized to ensure accurate patient setup on a daily basis especially when an extended-field IMRT plan is used. A bite block can be placed during simulation and throughout radiation to push the tongue away from the high-dose nasopharynx region.
- CT simulation using 3 mm thickness with IV contrast should be performed to help guide the GTV target,

particularly for the lymph nodes. We typically recommend a simulation scan from the top of the head including the brain to the carina. 5 mm thickness can be reconstructed below the clavicle to the level of the carina. The isocenter is typically placed just above the arytenoids.

- Image registration and fusion applications with MRI and PET scans should be used to help in the delineation of target volumes, especially for regions of interest encompassing the GTV, skull base, brainstem, and optic chiasm. The GTV and CTV and normal tissues should be outlined on all CT slices in which the structures exist.
- Daily image-guided setup with KV images can allow for reduced margins near critical structures (brainstem), and we often utilize this in our own clinical practice.

## 4    Target Volume Delineation and Treatment Planning

- Suggested target volumes at the GTV and high-risk CTV are detailed in Tables 1 and 2 and are based on guidelines from RTOG Nasopharyngeal Cancer Trials (Lee et al. 2009). Alternative volume delineation strategies and dose

**Table 1**  Suggested target volumes at the gross disease region

| Target volumes | Definition and description |
|---|---|
| $GTV_{70}^{a}$ (the subscript 70 denotes the radiation dose delivered) | Primary: all gross disease on physical examination and imaging (see above regarding the importance of MRI)<br>Neck nodes: all nodes $\geq 1$ cm or those with necrotic center |
| $CTV_{70}^{a}$ | $GTV_{70}+3$ mm margin or less around critical structures like the brainstem, a 1 mm margin is acceptable (Figs. 5 and 7) |
| $PTV_{70}^{a}$ | $CTV_{70}+3–5$ mm, depending on the comfort level of daily patient positioning. Around critical structures like the brainstem, a 1 mm margin is acceptable (Fig. 10) |

[a]$PTV_{70}$ receives 2.12 Gy/fraction to 70 Gy over 33 fractions. For the treatment of nodes that are small (i.e., ~1 cm), a lower dose of 63 Gy ($PTV_{63}$) can be considered at the discretion of the treating physician

fractionation schemes are thoroughly discussed in a review article by Wang et. al (Wang et al. 2012). Selected fractionation schemes are briefly reviewed in Table 3.

**Table 2**  Suggested target volumes at the high-risk subclinical region

| Target volumes | Definition and description |
|---|---|
| $CTV_{59.4}^{a}$ | $CTV_{59.4}$ (Figs. 4, 5, 6, 7, 8, 9, 10, and 11) should encompass $CTV_{70}$ with a 5 mm margin and regions at risk for microscopic disease which include: |
| | Entire nasopharynx |
| | Anterior 1/3 of the clivus (entire clivus, if involved) |
| | Skull base (ensuring coverage of the foramen ovale where V3 resides and the foramen rotundum) |
| | Pterygoid fossa |
| | Parapharyngeal space |
| | Inferior sphenoid sinus (entire sphenoid sinus in T3–T4 disease) |
| | Posterior 1/4 of the nasal cavity/maxillary sinuses (ensuring coverage of the pterygopalatine fossa where V2 resides) |
| | Inferior soft palate |
| | Retropharyngeal lymph nodes |
| | Retrostyloid space |
| | Bilateral nodal levels IB through V[b] |
| | Include cavernous sinus for advanced T3–T4 lesions (Fig. 7) |
| | Importance of reviewing bone window while contouring on CT scan to ensure coverage of skull base foramens (Fig. 6) |
| $PTV_{59.4}^{a}$ | $CTV_{59.4}+3–5$ mm, depending on the comfort of the physician, but around critical structures like the brainstem, a 1 mm margin is acceptable (Fig. 5) |

[a]High-risk subclinical dose ($PTV_{59.4}$): 1.8 Gy/fraction to 59.4 Gy. For lower-risk subclinical regions *excluding the nasopharynx/skull base regions where they are always considered high risk*, 1.64 Gy/fraction to 54 Gy ($PTV_{54}$), i.e., N0 neck or low neck (levels IV and VB), can be considered at the discretion of the treating physician

[b]Level IB can be omitted in node-negative disease. At the discretion of the physician, level 1B may also be spared in low-risk node-positive patients (e.g., isolated retropharyngeal nodes or isolated level IV nodes are considered low risk for level 1B involvement). At the same time, the treatment of level 1B should be considered in node-negative patients with certain features (e.g., involvement of hard palate or nasal cavity)

**Table 3** Selected IMRT dose fractionation schemes used for nasopharyngeal cancer

|  | RTOG (Lee et al. 2012) | Fujan (Lin et al. 2009) | SKL (Su et al. 2012) | PWH (Kam et al. 2004) |
|---|---|---|---|---|
| Gross Dz dose (Gy) | 69.96 | 66.0–69.75 | 68.0 | 66–74 |
| Gross Dz (dose/fraction) | 2.12 | 2.2–2.25 | 2.27 | 2.0 |
| High-risk region dose | 59.40 | 60–60.45 | 60.0 | 60 |
| High-risk region dose/Fx | 1.80 | 1.95–2 | 2.0 | 1.82 |
| Low-risk region dose | 50–54.12 | 54–55.8 | 50–54 | 54–60 |
| Low-risk region dose/Fx | 1.64–2.0 | 1.8 | 1.8–2.0 | 2 |
| Margin around GTV (mm)[a] | 10 | 8–13 | NA | 13 |

*SKL* State Key Laboratory of Oncology in Southern China (Guangzhou); *PWH* Prince of Wales Hospital (Hong Kong)
[a]Margin is for primary tumor GTV70, including CTV expansion on GTV and PTV expansion

- The gross tumor volume (GTV) is defined as all known gross disease deteremined from CT, MRI, clinical information, and endoscopic findings. Grossly positive lymph nodes are defined as any lymph nodes > 1 cm or nodes with a necrotic center.
- CTV59.4 is defined as regions at high risk for microscopic disease, which include all potential routes of spread for primary (CTV59.4-P) and nodal disease (CTV59.4-N). See Table 2 for full details.
- CTV59.4-N for microscopic nodal disease includes high-risk lymph node regions. These include the bilateral upper deep jugular, retropharyngeal, and level II, III, IV, and V lymph nodes. Level IB can be spared in selected patients (see Table 2 for full details).
- The low anterior neck can be separately treated with conventional AP or AP/PA portals. This volume is defined as a low-risk subclinical region and can receive a lower dose, 50.4 Gy in 1.8 Gy per fraction.
- At the discretion of the treating physician, an additional CTV can be used, CTV63. A lower dose of 63 Gy can be used for small-volume lymph node disease. An example of the appropriate application of this intermediate dose is when there are small lymph nodes close to the mandible or in the lower neck close to the brachial plexus.
- High-risk CTV 59.4 coverage in this case begins at the inferior extent of the sphenoid sinus, which is a common route of superior extension for NPC.
- Note that the high-risk CTV covers the posterior portion of the nasal cavity.

- The coverage of the pterygoid plates by CTV59.4 in Fig. 4 is designed to ensure adequate coverage of the pterygopalatine fossa, which is a common route of spread for NPC. The pterygoid plates serve as an easily identifiable landmark on CT.
- The CTV 59.4 contour includes several muscles that are not part of the parapharyngeal space or at high risk for microscopic spread – but, however, are included to provide a smooth volume for treatment planning purposes (see Fig. 4 annotation with parapharyngeal space and Fig. 6b).
- When the clivus is involved with the disease as in Fig. 3, the entire clivus should be included in the high-risk CTV (see also Fig. 6b).
- Note that adequate coverage of the base of the skull and foramen at high risk of microscopic disease requires bone windows for appropriate visualization (see Fig. 6a).
- Gross disease in the sphenoid sinus as in Fig. 7 requires coverage of the entire sphenoid sinus in the high-risk CTV (see MR correlate, Fig. 8). Note that in these cases, high-risk CTV will abut optic structures and may need to compromise coverage in the region to stay within the tolerance of normal tissue.
- Note that in this case, the disease invades into the infratemporal fossa and the masticator space; see Fig. 8 for MR correlates.
- Gross disease in the base of the skull is covered with very tight CTV expansion (≤1 mm) to protect the brainstem. In cases like this, daily KV imaging is recommended to ensure accurate setup.

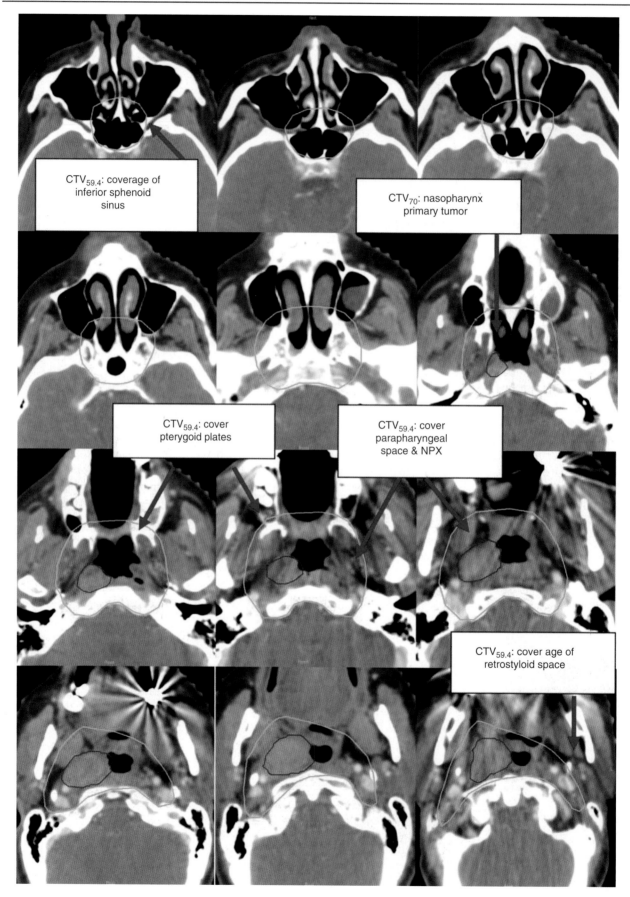

**Fig. 4** Target delineation GTV$_{70}$ (*red*) and CTV$_{59.4}$ (*green*) in a patient with T1N1 nasopharyngeal carcinoma with retropharyngeal and level II nodes in a cranial-to-caudal direction. Notice the inclusion/exclusion of nodal level 1B of the N+ (*green*) versus N0 (*blue*) neck. Please note that these are representative slices and not all slices are included

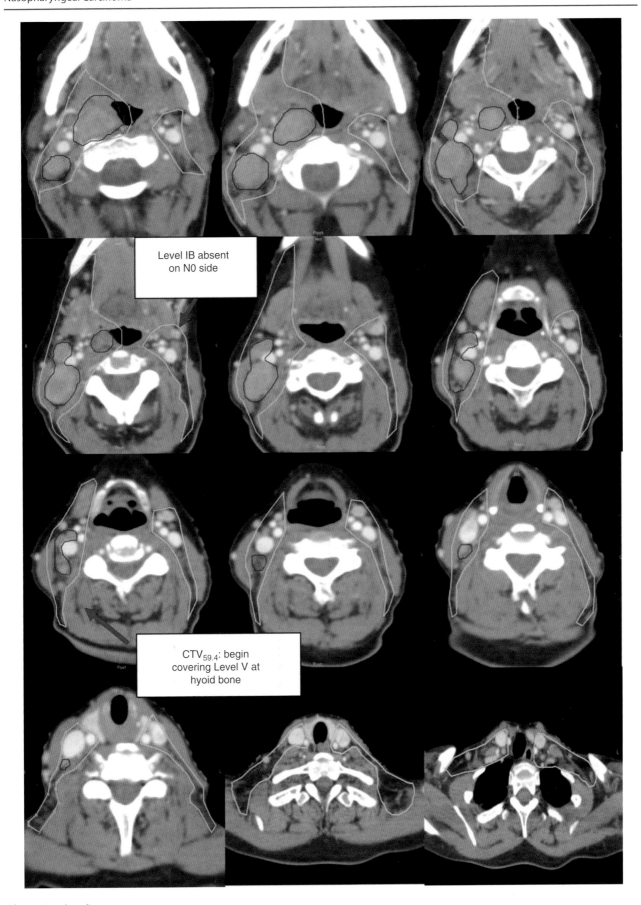

**Fig. 4** (continued)

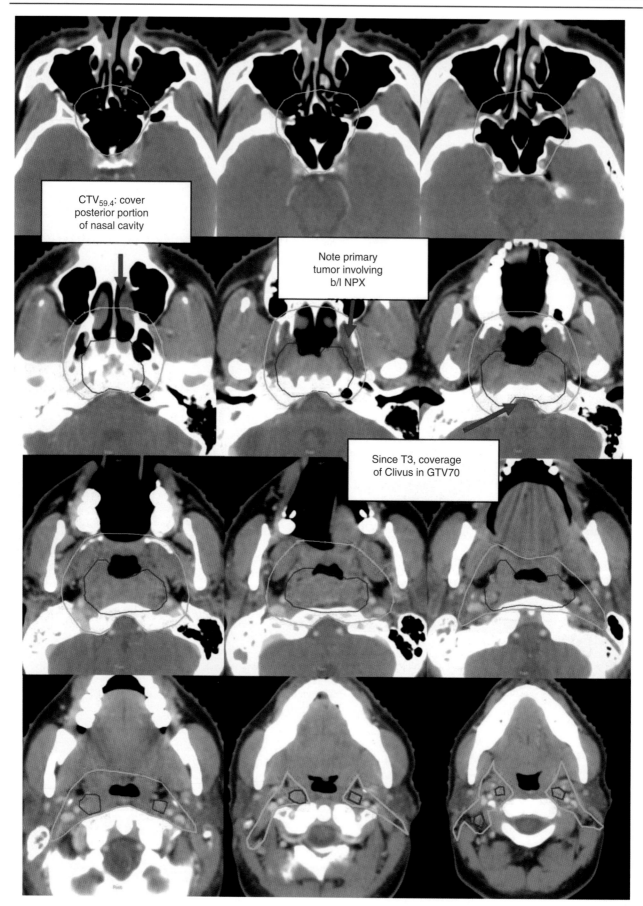

**Fig. 5** Target delineation GTV$_{70}$ (*red*) and CTV$_{59.4}$ (*green*) in a patient with T3N2 nasopharyngeal carcinoma. Please note that these are representative slices and not all slices are included

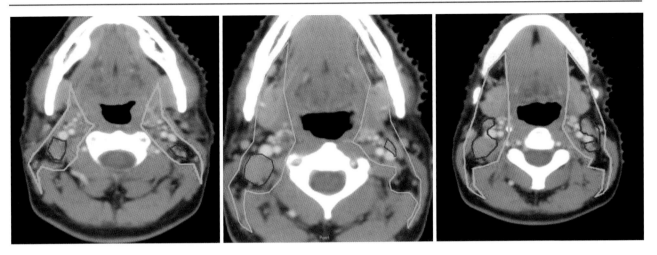

**Fig. 5** (continued)

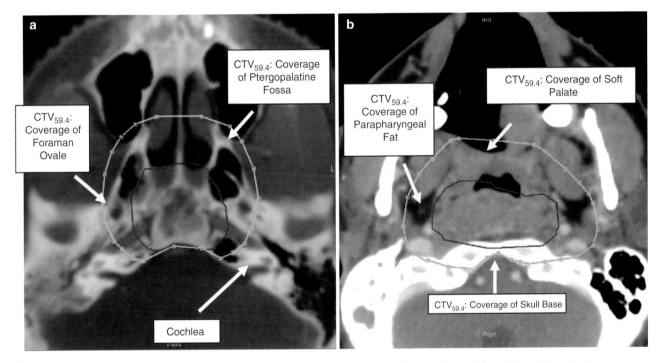

**Fig. 6** An example of $GTV_{70}$ (*red*) and $CTV_{59.4}$ (*green*) in T3N2 nasopharyngeal carcinoma: (**a**) bone window; (**b**) soft tissue window

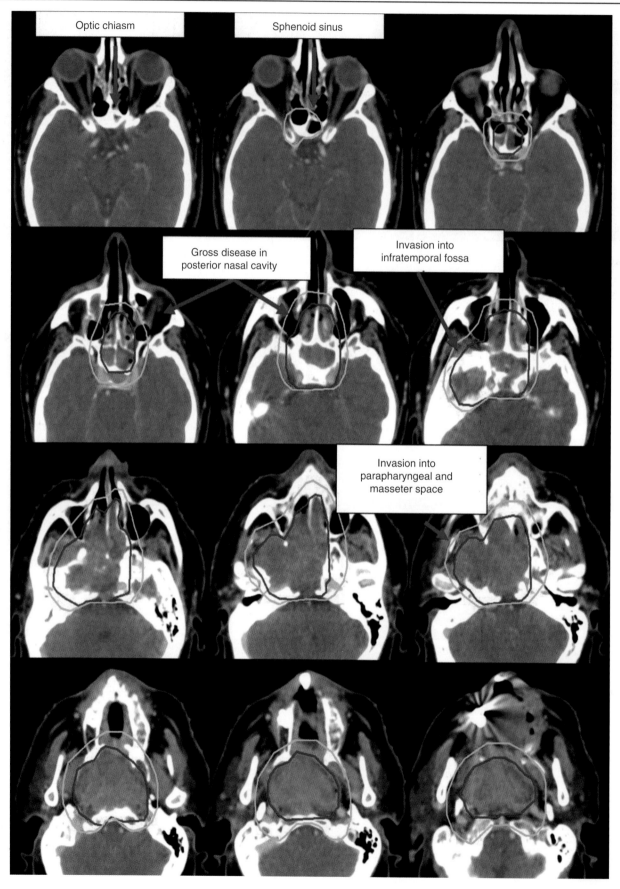

**Fig. 7** Target delineation GTV$_{70}$ (*red*) and CTV$_{59.4}$ (*green*) in a patient with T4N2 nasopharyngeal carcinoma with focus at the primary site. Please note that these are representative slices and not all slices are included

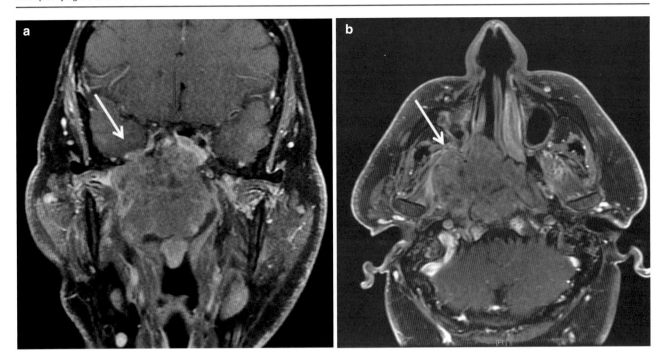

**Fig. 8** MRI for the patient in Fig. 7. (**a**) Coronal T1 post-contrast sequence demonstrating infratemporal invasion (*white arrow*) and involvement of sphenoid sinus (*red arrow*). (**b**) Axial T1 post-contrast sequence demonstrating parapharyngeal involvement and V3 involvement (*white arrow*)

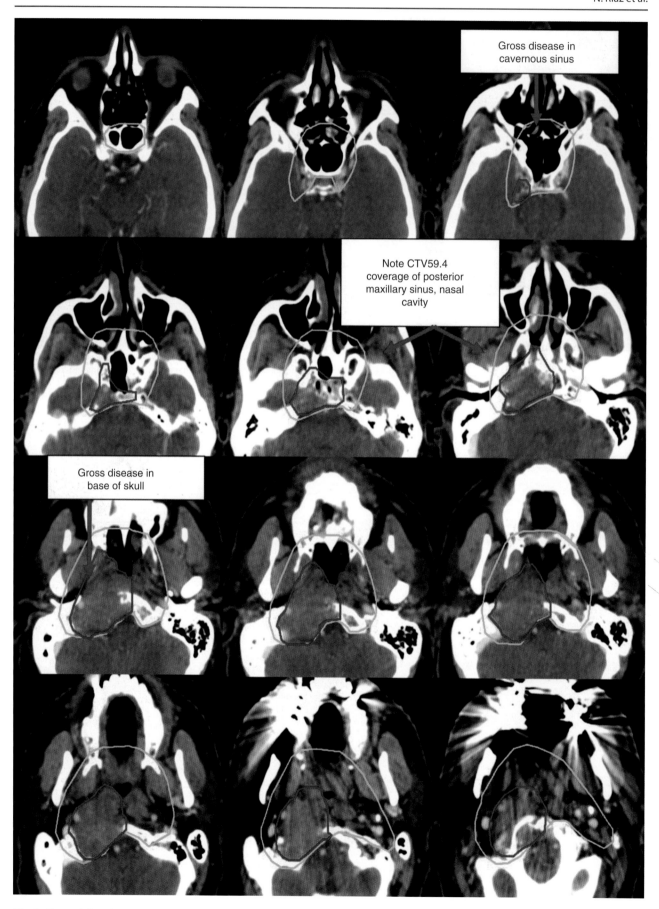

**Fig. 9** Target delineation GTV$_{70}$ (*red*) and CTV$_{59.4}$ (*green*) in another patient with T4N2 nasopharyngeal carcinoma focusing at the primary site. Please note that these are representative slices and not all slices are included

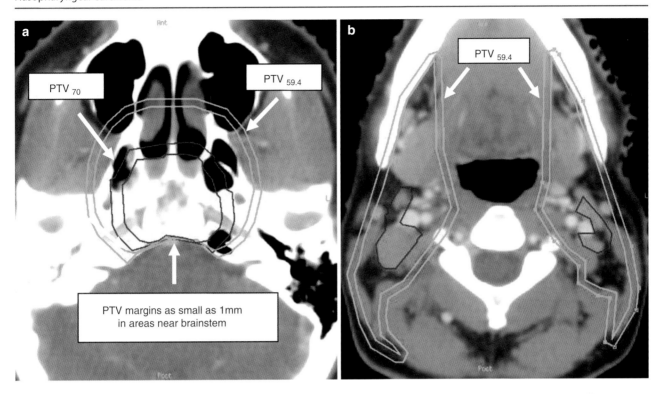

**Fig. 10** (**a**) Red: GTV70 and PTV70 (inner and outer). Green CTV and PTV 59.4. (**b**) Same coloring as (**a**)

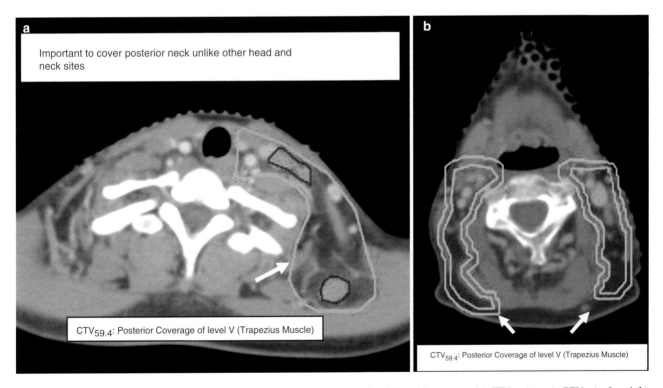

**Fig. 11** An example of level V nodal disease. Therefore, it is important to have level V nodal coverage: (**a**) CTV$_{59.4}$ (*green*), GTV$_{70}$ (*red*) and (**b**) CTV$_{59.4}$ and PTV$_{59.4}$ (inner and outer contours, respectively)

## 5    Plan Assessment

- In advanced cases, we typically prioritize normal structure constraints, specifically the brainstem, spinal cord, and optic chaism over full coverage of the tumor.
- Ideally, at least 95 % of the volume of $PTV_{70}$ should receive 70 Gy. In addition, the minimum dose to 99 % of $CTV_{70}$ should be $>65.1$ Gy. The maximum dose received by 0.03 cc of $PTV_{70}$ should be $<80.5$ Gy.
- For $PTV_{59.4}$, 95 % of the volume should receive the prescribed dose. The minimum dose to 99 % of $CTV_{59.4}$ is $>55.2$ Gy. The maxiumum dose to 0.03 cc of $PTV_{59.4}$ should be 68.3 Gy.
- Many critical normal structures surround the nasopharynx and therefore need to be outlined for dose constraints (Table 4). These structures include the brainstem, spinal cord, optic nerves, chiasm, parotid glands, pituitary, temporomandibular (T-M) joints and middle and inner ears, skin (in the region of the target volumes), oral cavity, mandible, eyes, lens, temporal lobe, brachial plexus, and esophagus (including the postcricoid pharynx), and the glottic larynx should be outlined.

## Suggested Reading

INT 00-99 (Al-Sarraf et al. 1998): Established role of chemotherapy in locally advanced NPC

RTOG 06-15 (Lee et al. 2012): Describes RTOG treatment guidelines for NPC

Wang et al. (2012): Reviews differences in treatment volumes amongst published IMRT studies in NPC

RTOG neck contouring atlas (Gregoire et al. 2003)

MRI and CT anatomy reference (Abdel Khalek Abdel Razek and King 2012): MRI and CT nasopharyngeal carcinoma anatomy

**Table 4** Intensity-modulated radiation therapy: normal tissue dose constraints

| Critical structures | Constraints |
|---|---|
| Brainstem | Max < 54 Gy or 1 % of the PTV cannot exceed 60 Gy |
| Optic nerves | Max < 54 Gy or 1 % of the PTV cannot exceed 60 Gy |
| Optic chiasm | Max < 54 Gy or 1 % of the PTV cannot exceed 60 Gy |
| Spinal cord | Max < 45 Gy or 1 cc of the PTV cannot exceed 50 Gy |
| Mandible and TMJ | Max < 70 Gy or 1 cc of the PTV cannot exceed 75 Gy |
| Brachial plexus | Max < 66 Gy |
| Temporal lobes | Max < 60 Gy or 1 % of the PTV cannot exceed 65 Gy |
| Other normal structures | Constraints |
| Oral cavity | Mean < 40 Gy |
| Parotid gland | (a) Mean ≤ 26 Gy in one gland |
| | (b) Or at least 20 cc of the combined volume of both parotid glands will receive < 20 Gy |
| | (c) Or at least 50 % of one gland will receive < 30 Gy |
| Cochlea | V55 < 5 % |
| Eyes | Mean < 35 Gy, max < 50 Gy |
| Lens | Max < 25 Gy |
| Glottic larynx | Mean < 45 Gy |
| Esophagus, postcricoid pharynx | Mean < 45 Gy |

*PTV* planning target volume

Based on guidelines presently used at Memorial Sloan-Kettering Cancer Center

## References

Abdel Khalek Abdel Razek A, King A (2012) MRI and CT of nasopharyngeal carcinoma. AJR Am J Roentgenol 198:11–18

Al-Sarraf M, LeBlanc M, Giri PG et al (1998) Chemoradiotherapy versus radiotherapy in patients with advanced nasopharyngeal cancer: phase III randomized Intergroup study 0099. J Clin Oncol 16: 1310–1317

Gregoire V, Levendag P, Ang KK et al (2003) CT-based delineation of lymph node levels and related CTVs in the node-negative neck: DAHANCA, EORTC, GORTEC, NCIC, RTOG consensus guidelines. Radiother Oncol 69:227–236

Jack Baskin H Sr, Duick DS, Levine RA (2013) Thyroid ultrasound and ultrasound-guided FNA, 3rd edn. Springer, New York

Kam MK, Teo PM, Chau RM et al (2004) Treatment of nasopharyngeal carcinoma with intensity-modulated radiotherapy: the Hong Kong experience. Int J Radiat Oncol Biol Phys 60:1440–1450

Lee N, Harris J, Garden AS et al (2009) Intensity-modulated radiation therapy with or without chemotherapy for nasopharyngeal carcinoma: radiation therapy oncology group phase II trial 0225. J Clin Oncol 27:3684–3690

Lee NY, Zhang Q, Pfister DG et al (2012) Addition of bevacizumab to standard chemoradiation for locoregionally advanced nasopharyngeal carcinoma (RTOG 0615): a phase 2 multi-institutional trial. Lancet Oncol 13:172–180

Lin S, Pan J, Han L, Zhang X, Liao X, Lu JJ (2009) Nasopharyngeal carcinoma treated with reduced-volume intensity-modulated radiation therapy: report on the 3-year outcome of a prospective series. Int J Radiat Oncol Biol Phys 75:1071–1078

Ng WT, Lee AW, Kan WK et al (2007) N-staging by magnetic resonance imaging for patients with nasopharyngeal carcinoma: pattern of nodal involvement by radiological levels. Radiother Oncol 82:70–75

Su SF, Han F, Zhao C et al (2012) Long-term outcomes of early-stage nasopharyngeal carcinoma patients treated with intensity-modulated radiotherapy alone. Int J Radiat Oncol Biol Phys 82:327–333

Wang T, Riaz N, Cheng S, Lu J, Lee N (2012) Intensity-modulated radiation therapy for nasopharyngeal carcinoma: a review. J Radiat Oncol 1:129–146

# Oropharyngeal Carcinoma

Jeremy Setton, Ian Poon, Nadeem Riaz, Eli Scher, and Nancy Lee

## Contents

## 1    Anatomy and Patterns of Spread

- The oropharynx is contiguous with the oral cavity anteriorly, the larynx and hypopharynx inferiorly, and the nasopharynx superiorly. It is commonly divided into four subsites: the tonsillar region, base of the tongue, soft palate, and pharyngeal wall (Fig. 1).
- The anterior and posterior tonsillar pillars are mucosal folds produced by the underlying palatoglossal muscle and palatopharyngeal muscle, respectively. These pillars define the borders of the tonsillar fossa, which contains the palatine tonsil. Tonsillar cancers most commonly arise on the anterior pillar and may extend superiorly along this structure towards the soft palate or inferiorly towards the base of the tongue. Anterolateral spread along the pharyngeal constrictor muscle to the pterygomandibular

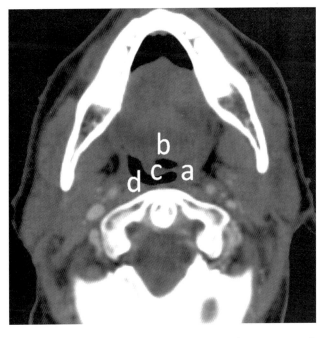

**Fig. 1** Subsites of the oropharynx: *a* tonsil, *b* base of the tongue, *c* soft palate, *d* pharyngeal wall

J. Setton • N. Riaz • E. Scher • N. Lee (✉)
Department of Radiation Oncology, Memorial Sloan Kettering Cancer Center, New York, NY

I. Poon
Department of Radiation Oncology, University of Toronto/ Sunnybrook Health Sciences Centre, Toronto, ON

N.Y. Lee et al. (eds.), *Target Volume Delineation for Conformal and Intensity-Modulated Radiation Therapy*,
Medical Radiology. Radiation Oncology, DOI: 10.1007/174_2014_1024, © Springer International Publishing Switzerland 2014
Published Online: 4 November 2014

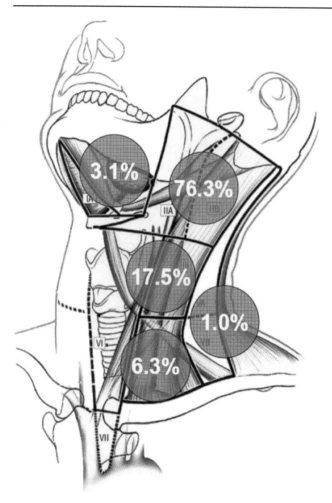

**Fig. 2** Estimated risk of pathologic nodal involvement by level when negative by CT imaging for T1–T2 oropharyngeal primary tumors (Sanguineti et al. 2009) (Figure printed with permission from publisher- Elsevier)

raphe and retromolar trigone may occur. Superolateral spread to the infratemporal space can be seen in advanced cases.

- The base of the tongue is bounded anteriorly by the circumvallate papillae. Inferiorly, the vallecula is considered part of the base of the tongue, while the epiglottis belongs to the supraglottic larynx. Cancers of the tongue base may spread anteriorly into the oral tongue and/or floor of the mouth or posteriorly/inferiorly via the vallecula into the preepiglottic space.
- The inferior surface of the soft palate and uvula belong to the oropharynx, while the superior surface is a nasopharyngeal structure. Tumors of the soft palate may spread laterally/inferiorly to the tonsil via the anterior tonsillar pillar or superiorly towards the nasopharynx.

- The superior pharyngeal constrictor muscle forms the posterior and lateral walls of the oropharynx. Cancers of the lateral and posterior pharyngeal walls may spread via the mucosa or submucosa towards the hypopharynx and/or nasopharynx. Skip lesions are not uncommon.
- Lymphatic spread is predictable. Ipsilateral level II is the most common location for lymph node metastasis. Next echelon lymphatic drainage includes levels III and IV and the retropharyngeal lymph nodes. Involvement levels I and V is uncommon (Fig. 2).
- The incidence of retropharyngeal nodal involvement varies by subsite. Bussels et al. reported a significantly higher incidence in those with primary tumors of the posterior pharyngeal wall (38 %) and soft palate (44 %) than those with primary tumors of the base of the tongue (13 %) or tonsil (14 %) (Bussels et al. 2006).

## 2    Diagnostic Workup Relevant for Target Volume Delineation

- Both physical examination and imaging should be used for delineation of the gross tumor volume.
- Visual inspection, palpation, and fiber-optic examination are critical for accurate delineation of mucosal extension. The true extent of mucosal extension may be missed on imaging but appreciated on clinical examination (Fig. 3).
- MRI has distinct advantages in soft tissue discrimination and reduced dental amalgam interference. It provides complementary information to CT and PET and may allow for improved GTV and normal tissue delineation.
  - T2-weighted with fat saturation: assessment of retropharyngeal lymph nodes, parapharyngeal space, and preepiglottic space
  - T1-weighted pre-contrast: used primarily for evaluation of fate planes, especially parapharyngeal fat space for asymmetry. Additional utility for assessment of bone marrow
  - T1-weighted post-contrast: assessment of perineural invasion
- The use of MRI requires co-registration or fusion with the CT simulation scan. The use of immobilization mask during MRI allows for improved fusion accuracy but may preclude the use of a dedicated head and neck coil.
- Diffusion-weighted (DWI) MRI provides apparent diffusion coefficients (ADC), which are inversely correlated with tissue cellularity. DW-MRI has a high negative predictive value for the assessment of lymph node metastases (Vandecaveye et al. 2009).

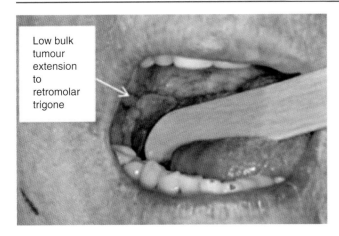

Low bulk tumour extension to retromolar trigone

**Fig. 3** Direct visualization of anterior mucosal spread to retromolar trigone

- CT remains superior to MRI for the assessment of cortical bone invasion. Administration of iodinated contrast is recommended for enhanced tumor discrimination.
- FDG-PET provides metabolic information that is complementary to CT and MRI. It has been shown to reduce interobserver variability in tumor delineation and may aid in the identification of tumor extension missed by CT or MRI (Syed et al. 2005).
- FDG-PET has been shown to provide metabolic information that is of prognostic value independent of tumor size and T-category (Romesser et al. 2012).
- Limitations of FDG-PET include poor spatial resolution and low sensitivity for small-volume lymph node metastases. The absence of FDG uptake in an otherwise suspicious lymph node should not be considered reassuring.

## 3 Simulation and Daily Localization

- The patient should be set up in the supine position with the neck extended. The immobilization device (Aquaplast mask) should provide adequate shoulder immobilization. Bite-block and/or mouth guard may be inserted.
- CT simulation using 2.5–3 mm slice thickness with IV contrast. Isocenter is typically placed just above the arytenoid cartilages.
- MRI and PET images, if available, may then be registered or fused to the CT simulation scan.
- At MSKCC, image guidance is achieved with daily linear-accelerator-mounted 2D kV imaging and weekly kV conebeam CT. Alternative methods for image guidance include orthogonal kV imaging ("ExacTrac") or linear-accelerator-mounted MV CT images ("TomoTherapy").

- CTV to PTV expansion of 3–5 mm, depending on the accuracy of daily patient positioning and image guidance.

## 4 Target Volume Delineation and Treatment Planning

### 4.1 Selected IMRT Dose Fractionation Schemes for Oropharyngeal Cancer

- Standard fractionation (33 fractions) with integrated boost. Gross disease dose: 69.96 Gy in 33 fractions. High-risk subclinical disease dose: 59.4 Gy in 33 fractions. Low-risk subclinical disease dose: 54.12 Gy in 33 fractions. Single phase (simultaneous integrated boost), with 5 fractions weekly (Garden et al. 2013; Setton et al. 2012).
- Standard fractionation (35 fractions) with cone-down. Gross disease dose: 70 Gy in 35 fractions. Subclinical disease dose: 54 Gy in 30 fractions. Initial phase (simultaneous integrated boost): 2 Gy per fraction to gross disease, 1.8 Gy per fraction to subclinical disease (30 fractions). Boost: 2 Gy per fraction to gross disease.
- RTOG 00–22. Gross disease dose: 66 Gy in 30 fractions. Subclinical disease dose: 54 Gy in 30 fractions. Optional high-risk subclinical disease dose: 60 Gy in 30 fractions. Single phase with one plan (simultaneous integrated boost), with 5 fractions weekly (Eisbruch et al. 2010).
- RTOG 10–16. Gross disease dose: 70 Gy in 35 fractions. High-risk subclinical disease dose: 56 Gy in 35 fractions. Low-risk subclinical disease dose: 50–52.5 Gy in 35 fractions. LAN field dose: 44 Gy in 22 fractions. Single phase with one plan (simultaneous integrated boost), six fractions weekly.
- Concomitant boost (RTOG 90–03, 01–29): two phases, twice daily treatment for the last 12 days. Total duration of 6 weeks. 54 Gy in 30 fractions to gross and subclinical disease. For the last 12 fractions, a second daily fraction to gross disease of 1.5 Gy is delivered (at least 6-h interval) (Ang et al. 2010; Beitler et al. 2014).

### 4.2 Split-Field Versus Whole-Field IMRT

- For patients without low neck disease, a low anterior AP field with larynx block is matched to the IMRT field at the isocenter just above the arytenoids. Dose is 45–50 Gy in 20–25 fractions, prescribed to 3 cm depth. In cases of gross involvement of the low neck or near the match-line, whole neck IMRT is preferred.

## 4.3    Suggested Target Volumes

**Table 1**  Suggested target volumes for gross disease

| Target volumes | Definition and description |
|---|---|
| GTV$_{70}$ | Primary: all gross disease as defined by clinical examination (e.g., base of tongue tumors that are superficial and not apparent on imaging) and imaging |
| | Neck nodes: all suspicious (>1 cm, necrotic, enhancing, or FDG avid) lymph nodes. Borderline suspicious lymph nodes may be treated to an intermediate dose (66 Gy in 33 fractions) |
| CTV$_{70}$ | Typically same as GTV$_{70}$ (no added margin). Margin of 5 mm may be added if there is uncertainty in extent of gross tumor so that GTV$_{70}$+5 mm=CTV$_{70}$ |
| PTV$_{70}$ | CTV$_{70}$+3–5 mm, depending on accuracy of daily patient positioning and image guidance |

**Table 2**  Suggested target volumes for subclinical disease: general guidelines

| Target volumes | Definition and description |
|---|---|
| CTV$_{59.4}$ | Primary: generally the primary CTV$_{59.4}$ should encompass GTV+minimum 1 cm margin while respecting anatomical barriers to spread, including bone, air, and skin |
| | Neck nodes – should include the at-risk lymphatic areas in the *node-positive neck*: |
| |    Levels II–IV |
| |    Lateral retropharyngeal lymph nodes up to skull base/jugular foramen |
| |    High level II/retrostyloid space (see Fig. 7) |
| | Although sparing of ipsilateral IB is controversial, at MSKCC, it is routinely spared unless there is gross involvement or extension of the primary GTV into the oral cavity (Tam et al. 2013) |
| CTV$_{54}$ | Neck nodes – should include the at-risk lymphatic areas in the *node-negative* neck: |
| |    Levels II–IV |
| |    Lateral retropharyngeal lymph nodes up to C1 |
| |    High level II/retrostyloid space is excluded |

**Table 3**  Suggested target volumes for subclinical disease: subsite-specific guidelines

| Target volumes | Definition and description |
|---|---|
| *Tonsil* | |
| Primary CTV$_{59.4}$ | Ipsilateral soft palate, ipsilateral base of the tongue, ipsilateral glossotonsillar sulcus. Superiorly, ipsilateral pharynx superiorly to pterygoid plate (Figs. 4 and 5). Inferiorly, at least 1 cm below GTV, down to level of the hyoid for advanced tumors. Consider coverage of ipsilateral retromolar trigone if anterolateral spread along pharyngeal constrictor to the pterygomandibular raphe is suspected |
| Nodal CTV$_{59.4}$ or CTV$_{54}$ | In patients with well-lateralized T1-2, N0-1 primary tumors (at least 1cm from central structures) without base of tongue or soft palate involvement, treatment of the ipsilateral neck may be considered. In such cases, the nodal CTV can be limited to ipsilateral levels II–IV, ipsilateral lateral retropharyngeal lymph nodes (Figs. 4 and 5). In node-positive patients, treat level II–IV bilaterally and lateral retropharyngeal nodes. At MSKCC, we do not routinely treat level Ib or V, unless involved or considered at high risk |
| *Base of the tongue* | |
| Primary CTV$_{59.4}$ | Glossotonsillar sulcus, vallecula, preepiglottic space (Figs. 6 and 7). Superiorly cover to level of the tip of the uvula. Consider inclusion of entire supraglottic larynx with epiglottic involvement (Fig. 7). Anteriorly, ensure the entire base of the tongue is covered; often this may require 1 cm of coverage of oral tongue (use signal differences in lymphoid tissue to help delineate as one cannot see circumvallate papillae) |
| Nodal CTV$_{59.4}$ or CTV$_{54}$ | Bilateral levels II–IV, lateral retropharyngeal LN. IB only with significant extension of the primary GTV into the oral cavity. At MSKCC, we do not routinely treat level Ib or V, unless involved or considered at high risk |
| *Soft palate* | |
| Primary CTV$_{59.4}$ | Entire soft palate, superior aspect of tonsillar pillars+fossa, adjacent nasopharynx superiorly to pterygoid plate. For advanced primaries, consider inclusion of pterygopalatine fossa. Ensure adequate coverage anteriorly, which may require coverage of portion of the hard palate. If pterygopalatine fossa is involved, assessment of the base of skull with MRI is required. |
| Nodal CTV$_{59.4}$ or CTV$_{54}$ | Bilateral levels II–IV, lateral retropharyngeal LN to skull base given propensity for involvement (Fig. 9). At MSKCC, we do not routinely treat level Ib or V, unless involved or considered at high risk |
| *Pharyngeal wall* | |
| Primary CTV$_{59.4}$ | Generous superior-inferior margins given the possibility of skip lesions. In patients with advanced primary tumors, consider extending CTV cranially to include nasopharynx and caudally to include hypopharynx (Fig. 8) |
| Nodal CTV$_{59.4}$ or CTV$_{54}$ | Bilateral levels II–IV, lateral retropharyngeal LN. Consider inclusion of lateral retropharyngeal lymph nodes to skull base given propensity for involvement. At MSKCC, we do not routinely treat level Ib or V, unless involved or considered at high risk |

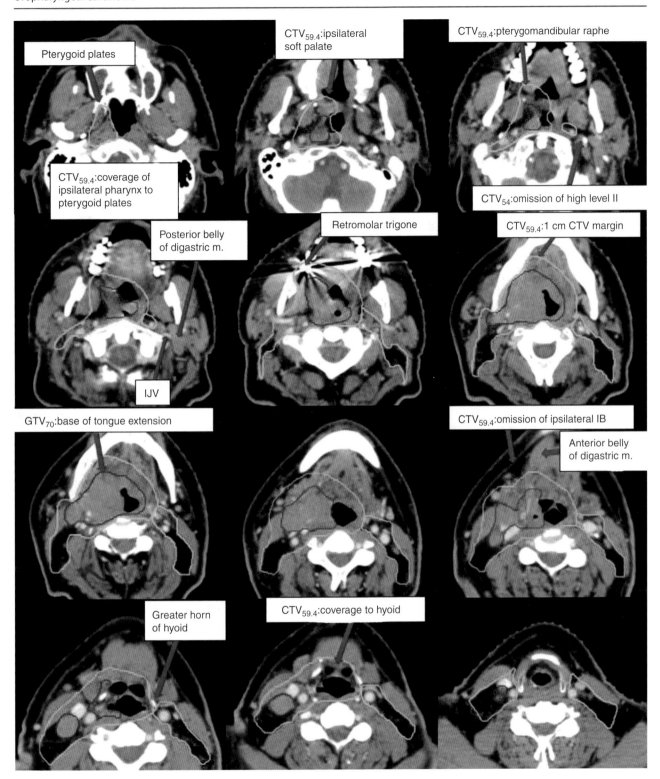

**Fig. 4** Representative slices of target delineation in a patient with cT4aN2b squamous cell carcinoma of the right tonsil. GTV$_{70}$ (*red*), CTV$_{59.4}$ (*green*), CTV$_{54}$ (*blue*)

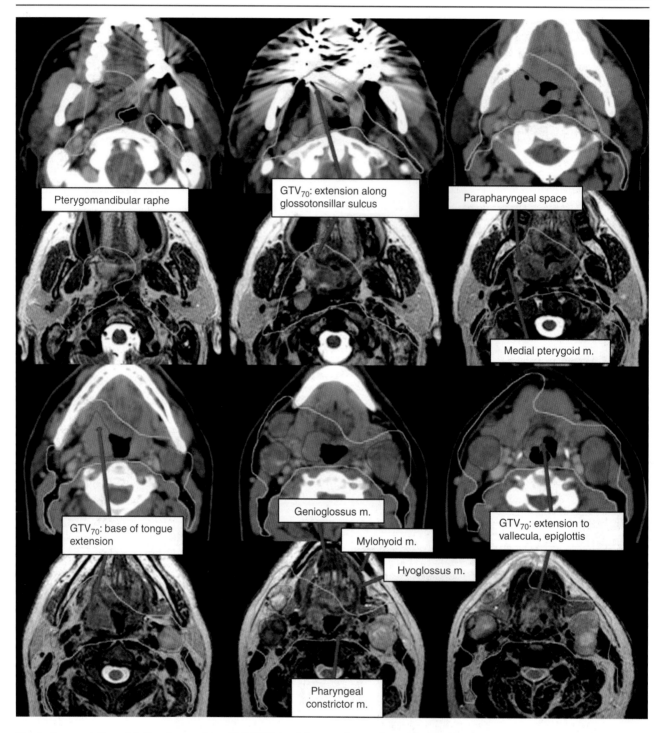

**Fig. 5** Representative axial slices from registered MRI/CT simulation scan for a patient with cT3N2c squamous cell carcinoma of the right tonsil (GTV$_{70}$: *red*, CTV$_{59.4}$: *green*)

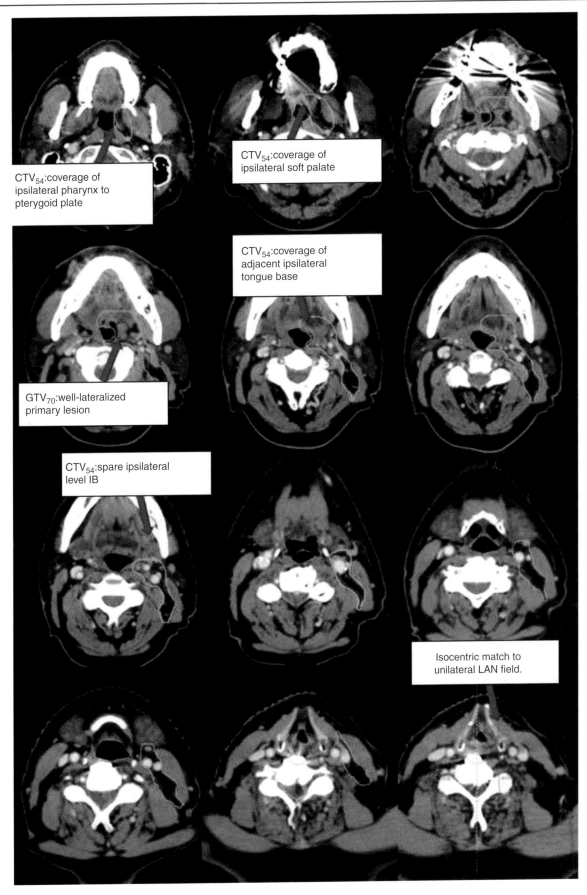

CTV$_{54}$:coverage of
ipsilateral pharynx to
pterygoid plate

CTV$_{54}$:coverage of
ipsilateral soft palate

CTV$_{54}$:coverage of
adjacent ipsilateral
tongue base

GTV$_{70}$:well-lateralized
primary lesion

CTV$_{54}$:spare ipsilateral
level IB

Isocentric match to
unilateral LAN field.

**Fig. 6** Representative slices of target delineation in a patient with cT1N0 well-lateralized squamous cell carcinoma of the left tonsil. GTV$_{70}$ (*red*),
CTV$_{54}$ (*green*)

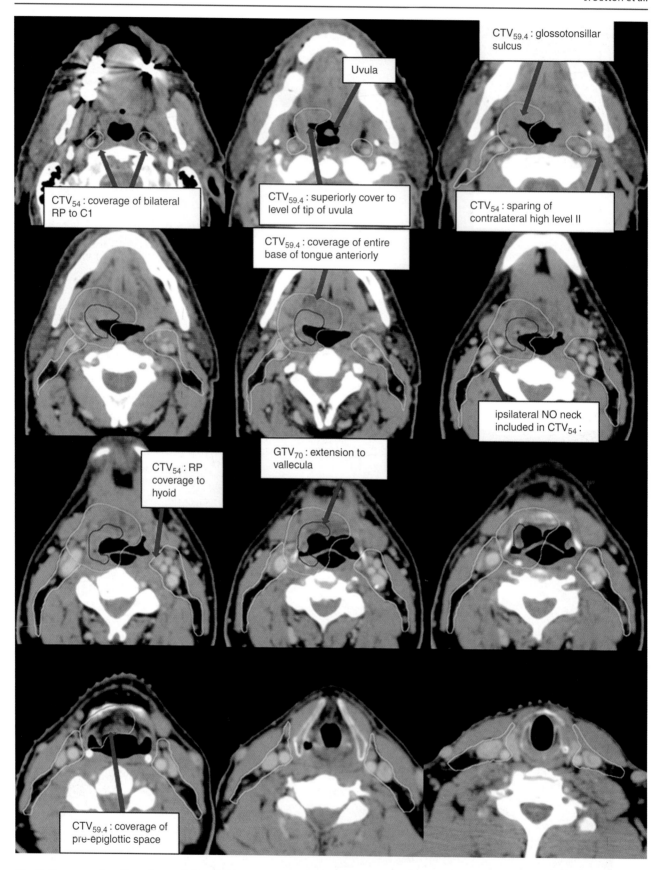

**Fig. 7** Representative slices of target delineation in a patient with cT2N0 squamous cell carcinoma of the right base of the tongue and vallecula. GTV$_{70}$ (*red*), CTV$_{59.4}$ (*green*), CTV$_{54}$ (*blue*)

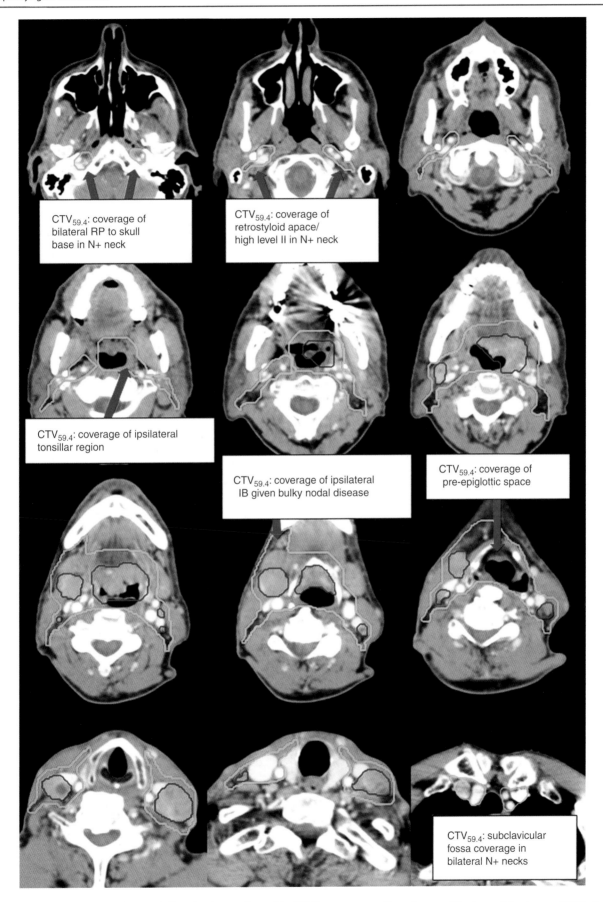

CTV$_{59.4}$: coverage of bilateral RP to skull base in N+ neck

CTV$_{59.4}$: coverage of retrostyloid apace/ high level II in N+ neck

CTV$_{59.4}$: coverage of ipsilateral tonsillar region

CTV$_{59.4}$: coverage of ipsilateral IB given bulky nodal disease

CTV$_{59.4}$: coverage of pre-epiglottic space

CTV$_{59.4}$: subclavicular fossa coverage in bilateral N+ necks

**Fig. 8** Representative slices of target delineation in a patient with cT3N2c squamous cell carcinoma of the base of the tongue. GTV$_{70}$ (*red*), CTV$_{59.4}$ (*green*)

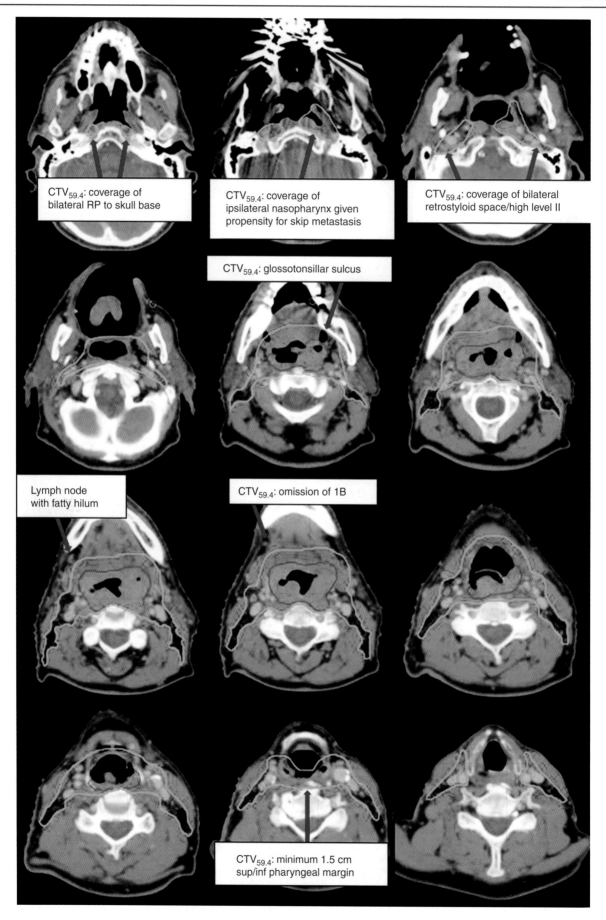

**Fig. 9** Representative slices of target delineation in a patient with cT3N2c squamous cell carcinoma arising from posterior pharyngeal wall. $GTV_{70}$ (*red*), $CTV_{59.4}$ (*green*)

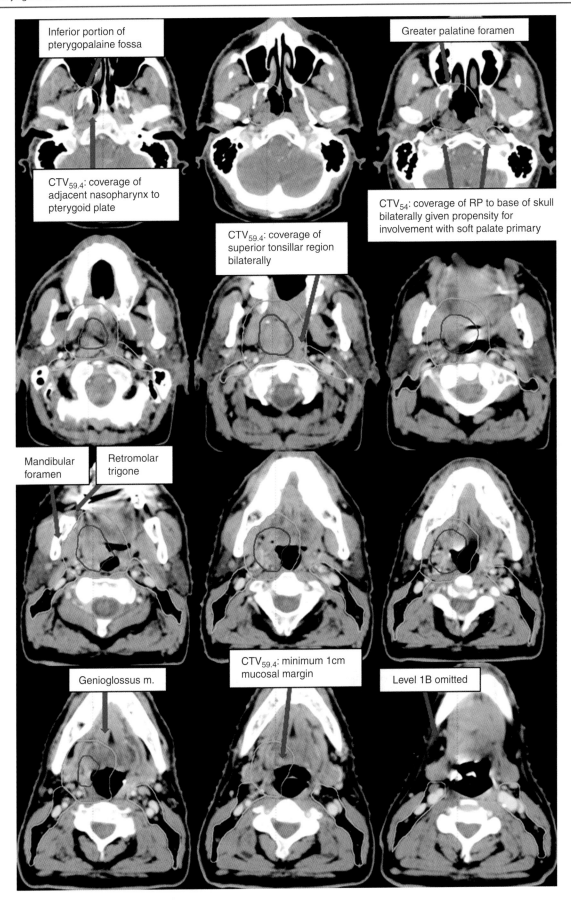

**Fig. 10** Representative slices of target delineation in a patient with cT3N0 squamous cell carcinoma of the soft palate. GTV$_{70}$ (*red*), CTV$_{54}$ (*blue*)

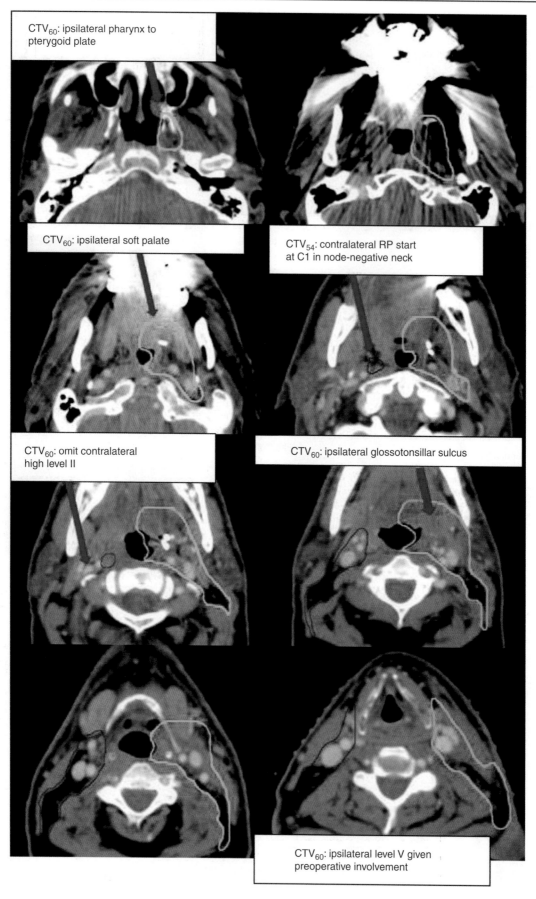

**Fig. 11** Representative axial slices from postoperative CT simulation scan of patient with pT2N2b squamous cell carcinoma of the left tonsil treated with transoral robotic radical tonsillectomy and left modified radical neck dissection yielding negative surgical margins and no evidence of extracapsular extension ($CTV_{60}$: *green*, $CTV_{54}$: *blue*)

# 5    Plan Assessment

- Prioritization for IMRT planning is as follows: critical structures>planning target volumes>other normal structures.
- PTV coverage and dose homogeneity criteria are listed in Table 4. A 3-D isodose surface display is reviewed to ensure that hot spots are located inside the PTV.

**Table 4** Intensity-modulated radiation therapy: target criteria

| PTV coverage | D95 ≥ prescription dose |
|---|---|
| Dose homogeneity | D05 $PTV_{70}$ ≤ 108 % of prescription dose (75.6 Gy) |
| | D05 of $PTV_{59.4}$ and $PTV_{54}$ ≤ prescription of next higher-dose volume (70 Gy) |

Based on guidelines presently used at Memorial Sloan-Kettering Cancer Center

*PTV* planning target volume

**Table 5** Intensity-modulated radiation therapy: normal tissue dose constraints

| Critical structures | Constraints |
|---|---|
| Brain stem | Max < 54 Gy (guideline), < 60 Gy (limit) |
| Optic nerves | Max < 54 Gy (limit) |
| Optic chiasm | Max < 54 Gy (guideline), < 60 Gy (limit) |
| Spinal cord | Max < 45 Gy (guideline), < 50 Gy (limit) |
| Brachial plexus | Max < 65 Gy (limit) |
| *Other normal structures* | *Constraints* |
| Oral cavity | Mean < 40 Gy |
| Submandibular gland | Mean < 39 Gy |
| Parotid gland | (a) Mean ≤ 26 Gy in one gland |
| | (b) Or at least 20 cc of the combined volume of both parotid glands will receive < 20 Gy |
| | (c) Or at least 50 % of one gland will receive < 30 Gy |
| Cochlea | Mean < 45 Gy, V55 < 5% |
| Eyes | Mean < 35 Gy, Max < 50 Gy |
| Lens | Max < 25 Gy |
| Glottic larynx | Mean < 45 Gy |
| Mandible not PTV | Max < 70 Gy |
| Mandible | No hot spots |
| Esophagus | Mean < 45 Gy |

Based on guidelines presently used at Memorial Sloan-Kettering Cancer Center

*PTV* planning target volume

# References

Ang KK, Harris J, Wheeler R et al (2010) Human papillomavirus and survival of patients with oropharyngeal cancer. N Engl J Med 363:24–35

Beitler JJ, Zhang Q, Fu KK et al (2014) Final results of local-regional control and late toxicity of RTOG 9003: a randomized trial of altered fractionation radiation for locally advanced head and neck cancer. Int J Radiat Oncol Biol Phys 89:13–20

Bussels B, Hermans R, Reijnders A et al (2006) Retropharyngeal nodes in squamous cell carcinoma of oropharynx: incidence, localization, and implications for target volume. Int J Radiat Oncol Biol Phys 65:733–738

Eisbruch A, Harris J, Garden AS et al (2010) Multi-institutional trial of accelerated hypofractionated intensity-modulated radiation therapy for early-stage oropharyngeal cancer (RTOG 00–22). Int J Radiat Oncol Biol Phys 76:1333–1338

Garden AS, Dong L, Morrison WH et al (2013) Patterns of disease recurrence following treatment of oropharyngeal cancer with intensity modulated radiation therapy. Int J Radiat Oncol Biol Phys 85:941–947

Romesser PB, Qureshi MM, Shah BA et al (2012) Superior prognostic utility of gross and metabolic tumor volume compared to standardized uptake value using PET/CT in head and neck squamous cell carcinoma patients treated with intensity-modulated radiotherapy. Ann Nucl Med 26:527–534

Sanguineti G, Califano J, Stafford E et al (2009) Defining the risk of involvement for each neck nodal level in patients with early T-stage node-positive oropharyngeal carcinoma. Int J Radiat Oncol Biol Phys 74:1356–1364

Setton J, Caria N, Romanyshyn J et al (2012) Intensity-modulated radiotherapy in the treatment of oropharyngeal cancer: an update of the Memorial Sloan-Kettering Cancer Center experience. Int J Radiat Oncol Biol Phys 82:291–298

Syed R, Bomanji JB, Nagabhushan N et al (2005) Impact of combined (18)F-FDG PET/CT in head and neck tumours. Br J Cancer 92:1046–1050

Tam M, Riaz N, Schupak K et al (2013) Sparing Bilateral Ib and Contralateral High Level II Nodes in Node-Positive (n+) Oropharyngeal Carcinoma (OPC) Improves Quality of Life on a Prospective Self-Reported Xerostomia Questionnaire. Int J Radiat Oncol Biol Phys 87:S437–S438

Vandecaveye V, De Keyzer F, Verslype C et al (2009) Diffusion-weighted MRI provides additional value to conventional dynamic contrast-enhanced MRI for detection of hepatocellular carcinoma. Eur Radiol 19:2456–2466

# Further Reading

Adelstein DJ, Ridge JA, Brizel DM et al (2012) Transoral resection of pharyngeal cancer: summary of a National Cancer Institute Head and Neck Cancer Steering Committee Clinical Trials Planning Meeting, November 6–7, 2011, Arlington, Virginia. Head Neck 34:1681–1703

Denis F, Garaud P, Bardet E et al (2004) Final results of the 94–01 French Head and Neck Oncology and Radiotherapy Group randomized trial comparing radiotherapy alone with concomitant radiochemotherapy in advanced-stage oropharynx carcinoma. J Clin Oncol 22:69–76

Eisbruch A, Kim HM, Feng FY et al (2011) Chemo-IMRT of oropharyngeal cancer aiming to reduce dysphagia: swallowing organs late complication probabilities and dosimetric correlates. Int J Radiat Oncol Biol Phys 81:e93–e99

O'Sullivan B, Warde P, Grice B et al (2001) The benefits and pitfalls of ipsilateral radiotherapy in carcinoma of the tonsillar region. Int J Radiat Oncol Biol Phys 51:332–343

O'Sullivan B, Huang SH, Siu LL et al (2013) Deintensification candidate subgroups in human papillomavirus related oropharyngeal cancer according to minimal risk of distant metastasis. J Clin Oncol 31:543–550

# Oral Cavity Cancer

Zachary Kohutek, Keith Unger, Nadeem Riaz, and Nancy Lee

## Contents

Z. Kohutek • N. Riaz • N. Lee (✉)
Department of Radiation Oncology, Memorial Sloan-Kettering,
New York, NY 10065, USA
e-mail: leen2@mskcc.org

K. Unger
Department of Radiation Oncology,
Georgetown University Hospital, Washington, DC, USA

## 1 Anatomy and Patterns of Spread

- The oral cavity is the most anterior head and neck site. It is separated from the oropharynx by an imaginary line extending from the anterior tonsillar pillars to the junction of hard and soft palate to the circumvallate papillae.

- The oral cavity is divided into several subsites including the oral tongue, floor of the mouth, retromolar trigone, alveolar ridge, hard palate, buccal mucosa, gingiva and lips (Fig. 1).

- *Oral tongue*: The oral tongue is the most common site of carcinoma within the oral cavity. It consists of the anterior two-thirds of the tongue and extends posteriorly to the circumvallate papillae, which separate it from the base of the tongue. Squamous cell tumors often arise along the lateral borders of the tongue. Oral tongue tumors may spread to involve the intrinsic and extrinsic musculature, floor of the mouth, neurovascular bundle or mandible.

- *Floor of the mouth*: The floor of the mouth is the second most common subsite. This semilunar space is formed by the mylohyoid, geniohyoid and genioglossus muscles inferiorly. Due to the lack of substantial fascial barriers to spread, floor of the mouth tumors tend to be locally invasive and spread to regional lymph nodes early in their course. The majority of tumors originate near the midline. These can spread laterally into the mandible, superiorly into the ventral tongue and lingual neurovascular bundle, or posteriorly into the base of the tongue. Invasion of the mylohyoid signifies involvement of the submandibular gland, which surrounds the posterior free edge of the muscle. Sublingual spread can obstruct the Wharton duct, leading to duct dilation and submandibular sialadenitis.

- *Retromolar trigone*: The retromolar trigone is a small mucosal region behind the posterior molars. Tumors of this region are associated with a high rate of occult lymph node metastases. Tumors can invade the buccinator,

N.Y. Lee et al. (eds.), *Target Volume Delineation for Conformal and Intensity-Modulated Radiation Therapy*,
Medical Radiology. Radiation Oncology, DOI: 10.1007/174_2014_1016, © Springer International Publishing Switzerland 2014
Published Online: 11 October 2014

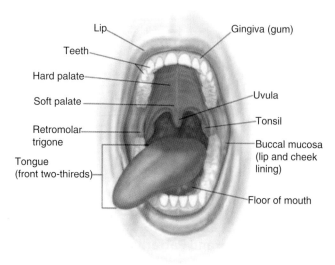

**Fig. 1** Diagram illustrating oral cavity subsites

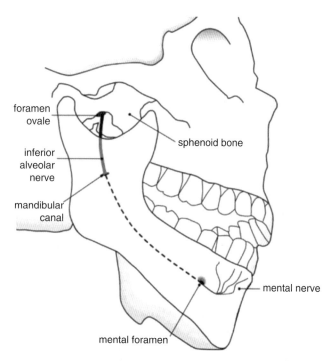

**Fig. 2** Anatomy of the inferior alveolar nerve

orbicularis oris, or superior constrictor muscles, which insert in this region. They can also spread along the ptery-gomandibular raphe, reaching the pterygoid plate and base of skull superiorly, or the floor of the mouth inferiorly. They tend to invade bone early. Perineural spread can occur along the inferior alveolar nerve, a branch of CN $V_3$ (Yao et al. 2007) (Fig. 2).

- *Alveolar ridge*: The alveolar ridges include the maxillary and mandibular alveolar processes and their overlying mucosae. The upper alveolar ridge extends from the upper gingival buccal gutter to the junction of the hard palate and is bordered posteriorly by the upper end of the ptery-

gopalatine arch. The lower alveolar ridge extends from the lower buccal gutter to the line of free mucosa along the floor of the mouth. It is bordered posteriorly by the ascending mandibular ramus. Like tumors of the retromolar trigone, carcinomas of the alveolar ridge tend to invade bone early. Carcinomas of the lower ridge may spread via the mandibular canal and inferior alveolar nerve (Fig. 2). Those of the upper alveolar ridge may invade the maxillary antrum or the base of the nose.

- *Hard palate*: The hard palate is a semilunar space encompassing the inner surface of the superior alveolar ridge to the posterior edge of the maxillary palatine bone. Tumors of the hard palate tend to be confined by the dense muco-periosteum surrounding it. However, they may invade through exposed areas at the greater palatine foramina or between the primary and secondary palates at the incisive fossa where they can access the nasal cavity. Perineural invasion is most common along the greater palatine nerves, leading to spread along CN $V_2$ from the pterygo-palatine fossa through the foramen rotundum to the cavernous sinus and Meckel's cave (Ginsberg and DeMonte 1998) (Fig. 3).
- *Buccal mucosa and gingiva*: Tumors of the buccal mucosa are rare but tend to be highly aggressive. The buccal mucosa includes the mucosal surfaces of the cheek and lips. This extends to the pterygomandibular raphe posteriorly and to the line of attachment of the mucosa of the upper and lower alveolar ridges superiorly and inferiorly. Tumors may invade the buccinator muscle, the buccal fat pad, or adjacent subcutaneous tissue.
- *Lip*: Most tumors in this region arise at the vermillion border and can spread to adjacent skin or underlying musculature. Lesions located along the gingivobuccal sulcus may erode into the mandibular or maxillary alveolar ridges. Upper lip cancers tend to be more aggressive than those originating in the lower lip.
- Lymph node involvement is dependent on several factors, including the subsite and the size of the primary tumor. Retropharyngeal lymph nodes are rarely involved in oral cavity cancer. Lymph node chains routinely involved include levels I–IV (Shah 1990) (Fig. 4).

## 2    Diagnostic Workup Relevant for Target Volume Delineation

- Initial evaluation of suspected oral cavity tumors should involve a thorough history. History taking should focus on risk factors such as tobacco and alcohol use, as well as specific symptoms that may indicate involvement of surrounding structures. Otalgia suggests involvement of branches of CN $V_3$, which innervates the ear via the auriculotemporal branch. Facial numbness can suggest CN V involvement. Trismus can indicate invasion of the pterygoid or masseter muscles.

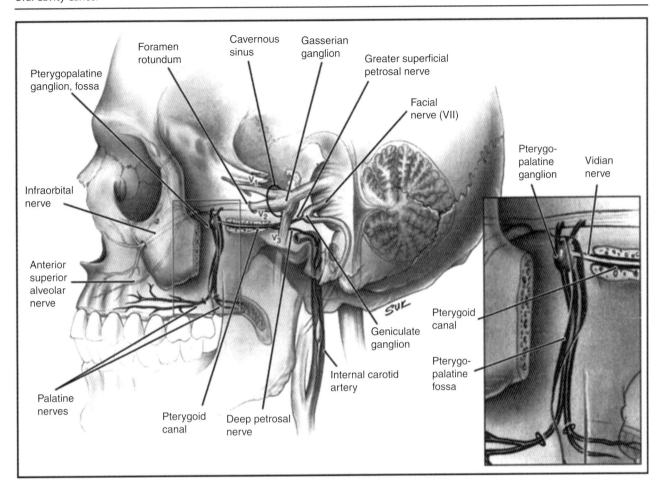

**Fig. 3** Innervation of the hard palate

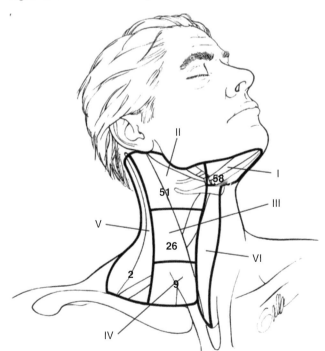

**Fig. 4** Distribution of positive lymph nodes in clinically node negative oral cavity cancer. Shah characterized 65 clinically node negative patients with pathologically positive lymph nodes at the time of radical neck dissection. Numbers indicate the percentage of patients with positive lymph nodes at each anatomic level (Shah 1990)

- Physical examination should be performed to help delineate the extent of tumor, which may be beyond what is identified on imaging. Mucosal extent of tumor is often best appreciated on physical examination. This should include inspection and palpation of the oral cavity and neck. Patients should also be referred to a dentist for a complete dental evaluation prior to treatment.
- CT can be used as an initial modality to determine the extent of soft tissue destruction and bony involvement, including the pterygopalatine fossa, mandible and hard palate. If CT cannot be obtained, dental panoramas can be used to visualize mandibular involvement.
- MRI is critical in the evaluation of perineural spread and is useful in the delineation of the extent of primary tumors. It may also be more helpful than CT if dental artifact makes visualization difficult. T1-weighted images can provide contrast between hypointense tumor and hyperintense bone marrow and fat. However, squamous cell carcinomas are often isointense to muscle on pre-contrast T1-weighted images, making delineation of tumor more difficult in regions such as the oral tongue (Fig. 5). Tumor appears more hyperintense on post-gadolinium T1-weighted images, which can help characterize true bone invasion by tumor (hyperintense) and

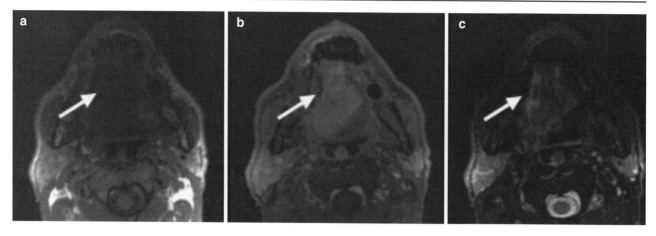

**Fig. 5** Axial T1-weighted (**a**), post-gadolinium T1-weighted (**b**) and T2- weighted (**c**) MR images, which demonstrate evaluation of a primary oral tongue squamous cell carcinoma. Arrows indicate the location of the primary tumor

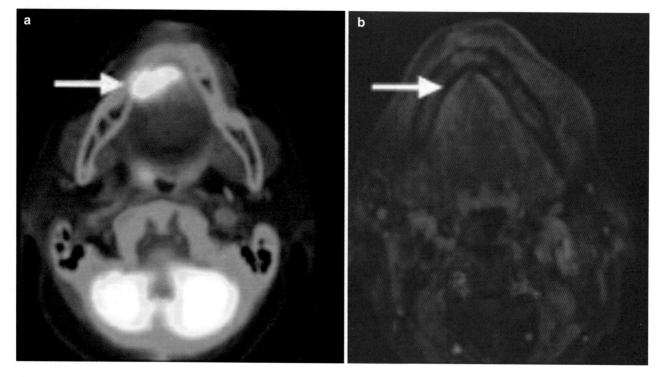

**Fig. 6** PET-CT (**a**) and post-gadolinium T1-weighted MR (**b**) imaging of a stage T1 floor of mouth squamous cell carcinoma. The tumor is FDG avid on PET but not clearly visible on MRI. Arrows indicate the location of the primary tumor

edema (hypointense) (Hermans 2012). Tumor also appears slightly hyperintense to muscle on T2-weighted images.

- PET imaging is an emerging modality for the evaluation of oral cavity cancers. PET has been shown to be superior to CT and MRI in detecting occult nodal metastasis in oral cavity cancers (Ng et al. 2006). It can also occasionally detect flat tumors that may not be visible on MRI (Fig. 6). PET remains limited, however, in the detection of small metastases and should not be used in isolation.
- In the postoperative setting, MRI and PET imaging can be employed to rule out the presence of gross recurrence prior to initiation of treatment. Any suspicious lesions on

postoperative imaging should be biopsied, and if positive, surgical re-excision should be considered prior to any course of radiation therapy. Preoperative imaging can help define those regions that should be encompassed in the high-risk CTV.

## 3 Simulation and Daily Localization

- The patient should be simulated in the supine position with the neck in slight hyperextension. A five-point mask should be utilized to immobilize the head, neck, and shoulders. For oral tongue cancers, a bite block can be used during simulation and throughout the course of treatment to elevate the hard palate and decrease dose to the superior oral cavity. For cases in which the hard palate is target, a bite block can be employed to limit dose to the tongue and inferior oral cavity.

- CT simulation should be performed using a slice thickness of 3 mm or less. IV contrast is useful in target delineation, particularly with respect to identification of cervical lymph nodes. The patient should be scanned from the top of the head to the carina. The isocenter is typically placed just superior to the arytenoids.
- If available, MRI or PET scans obtained at the time of simulation can often be helpful in defining target volumes.
- The tumor volumes and normal tissue volumes should be outlined on all CT slices on which the structures exist. Image guidance should be used to verify patient positioning during treatment. We favor daily kV imaging, which can minimize setup error and allow for smaller PTV margins. Setup uncertainty is typically greatest in the mental region, which is farthest from the pivot point for neck rotation.

## 4 Target Volume Delineation and Treatment Planning

- The $GTV_{70}$ is defined as all known gross disease, as determined by CT, MRI, PET and physical examination. This volume includes all grossly positive lymph nodes, which are those measuring >1 cm, containing a necrotic center or FDG avid on PET imaging. The high-risk $CTV_{70}$ is typically identical to the $GTV_{70}$, although a margin of 5 mm can be added if uncertainty exists regarding the extent of gross disease.
- For definitive cases, an intermediate-risk volume ($CTV_{59.4}$) encompasses an additional margin around the primary tumor, including potential sites of spread. Nodal levels at high risk for microscopic disease are also included in the $CTV_{59.4}$. Those nodal levels at lower risk are encompassed by the $CTV_{54}$. See Tables 1 and 3 for details.
- In the postoperative setting, the intermediate-risk volume ($CTV_{60}$) should encompass the preoperative gross disease, the entire operative bed, and nodal regions at greatest risk for microscopic involvement. A high-risk volume ($CTV_{66}$) should include any regions of bone invasion, positive margins, or extracapsular extension. As in the definitive setting, low-risk nodal levels within the nonsurgically violated side of the neck are encompassed by the $CTV_{54}$. See Tables 2 and 3 for details.
- Planning target volumes (PTV) should be defined at each dose level. An expansion of 3–5 mm is typically

**Table 1** Suggested target volumes for definitive treatment of oral cavity cancers

| Target volumes[a] | Definition and description |
|---|---|
| $GTV_{70}$ | Primary: all gross disease on physical examination and imaging |
| | Neck nodes: all gross disease and physical examination and imaging |
| $CTV_{70}$ | Same as $GTV_{70}$, although a 5 mm margin can be added if uncertainty exists regarding the extent of gross disease |
| $CTV_{59.4}$ | Primary: encompass the entire $CTV_{70}$ with an additional margin of up to 10 mm |
| | Neck nodes: nodal levels with pathologic involvement and adjacent ipsilateral or contralateral nodal regions at high risk for subclinical disease (site-specific recommendations given in Table 3) |
| $CTV_{54}$ | Ipsilateral and/or contralateral uninvolved nodal levels at low risk for subclinical disease (site-specific recommendations given in Table 3) |

[a]Subscript numbers represent suggested prescribed doses. $CTV_{70}$ is 2.12 Gy/fraction to 69.96 Gy in 33 fractions. $PTV_{59.4}$ is 1.8 Gy/fraction, and $PTV_{54}$ is 1.64 Gy/fraction

**Table 2** Suggested target volumes for postoperative treatment of oral cavity cancers

| Target volumes[a] | Definition and description |
|---|---|
| $CTV_{66}$ | Primary: preoperative tumor volume can guide the targeting of CTV66. Regions of soft tissue invasion, bone invasion, or microscopically positive margins should be included in this volume |
| | Neck nodes: regions of extracapsular extension |
| $CTV_{60}$ | Primary: preoperative gross disease and the entire operative bed |
| | Neck nodes: preoperative gross disease and adjacent ipsilateral or contralateral nodal regions at high risk for subclinical disease (site-specific recommendations given in Table 3) |
| $CTV_{54}$ | Ipsilateral and/or contralateral uninvolved nodal levels at low risk for subclinical disease (site-specific recommendations given in Table 3) |

[a]Subscript numbers represent suggested prescribed doses. $CTV_{66}$ is 2.0–2.2 Gy/fraction, $CTV_{60}$ is 2.0 Gy/fraction, and $CTV_{54}$ is 1.8 Gy/fraction

used around each CTV. The margin necessary will depend on setup uncertainty, as determined by immobilization and imaging techniques utilized during treatment.

- In the absence of any grossly positive low-lying cervical lymph nodes, the low anterior neck can be separately treated with conventional AP or AP/PA portals. This volume is defined as a low-risk subclinical region and can receive a lower dose of 50.4 Gy in 1.8 Gy fractions. (Figs. 7, 8, 9, 10, 11, 12, 13, 14, 15, 16, 17, and 18).

**Table 3** Site-specific guidelines for clinical target delineation of oral cavity cancers

| Tumor site | Stage | Clinical treatment volume |
|---|---|---|
| Oral tongue, floor of the mouth | T1–T4N0 | Include the tumor bed, the entire oral tongue and the base of the tongue. For floor of the mouth lesions, consider including the alveolar ridge, due to its proximity to the floor of the mouth. Both sides of the neck should be treated with radiotherapy (even for well-lateralized T1–T2N0 lesions, if the depth of invasion is >4 mm), although physician discretion can be used to determine if these should be in the low- or high-risk CTV. Consider ipsilateral and/or contralateral levels I–IV |
| | T1–T4N1–3 | Include the tumor bed, the entire oral tongue and the base of the tongue. For floor of the mouth lesions, consider including the alveolar ridge, due to its proximity to the floor of the mouth. Both sides of the neck should be treated with radiotherapy, although physician discretion can be used to determine if these should be in the low- or high-risk CTV. Consider ipsilateral and/or contralateral levels I–V |
| Buccal mucosa | T1–T4N0 | It is important to be generous with target volumes when treating the inner cheek. Include the tumor bed and the entire buccal mucosa. Posteriorly, this should extend to retromolar trigone. Superiorly, this should extend to near the inferior orbital rim. If the tumor is well lateralized, ipsilateral levels I-IV alone can be treated. Otherwise, consider treating bilateral cervical lymph nodes |
| | T1–T4N1–3 | It is important to be generous with target volumes when treating the inner cheek. Include the tumor bed and the entire buccal mucosa. Posteriorly, this should extend to retromolar trigone. Superiorly, this should extend to near the inferior orbital rim. Ipsilateral levels I-IV should be treated within the neck. Depending on pathologic findings and discussions with the surgeon, consideration can be given to treating the contralateral neck as well |
| Retromolar trigone, hard palate, gingiva | T1–T4N0 | Include the preoperative tumor volume and postoperative tumor bed. Consider covering ipsilateral levels I–IV for all cases. Treatment of the contralateral neck is at the physician's discretion. Hard palate tumors are generally minor salivary gland tumors, and treatment guidelines from "Chapter 8: Major Salivary Glands" should be used to guide treatment of lymph node regions |
| | T1–T4N1–3 | Include the preoperative tumor volume and postoperative tumor bed. Treat the ipsilateral levels I–IV for all cases and consider treatment of the contralateral neck. Hard palate tumors are generally minor salivary gland tumors, and treatment guidelines from "Chapter 8: Major Salivary Glands" should be used to guide treatment of lymph node regions |

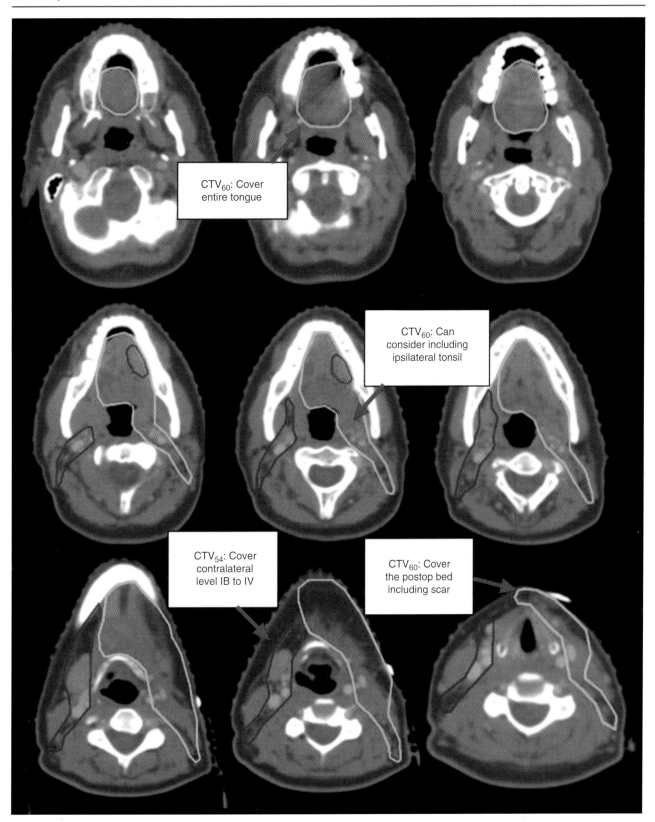

**Fig. 7** A patient with squamous cell carcinoma of the left lateral tongue, pathologic stage T1N0 with 4 mm tumor thickness, perineural invasion, and dysplasia in multiple surgical margins. The patient was randomized to radiation alone on protocol RTOG 0920. The patient was unable to tolerate a bite block at the time of simulation. The high-risk $CTV_{66}$ is shown in *red* and includes the region where dysplasia was present at the margin. The high-risk $CTV_{60}$ is shown in *green* and covers the entire tongue and ipsilateral levels I–IV. Even with small, well-lateralized tumors, the entire tongue is at risk of microscopic tumor involvement, especially when there is evidence of invasive islands. If the tumor is located posteriorly, coverage of the ipsilateral tonsil can be considered. The low-risk $CTV_{54}$, shown in *blue*, encompasses the contralateral levels IB–IV. A low anterior neck field was used to treat below the level of the arytenoids

**Fig. 8** CT image demonstrating recurrent tumor in a level IA lymph node after postoperative radiation for a T1N1 squamous cell carcinoma of the oral tongue. At our institution, we routinely cover level IA lymph nodes when treating tumors of the oral tongue, whether or not the tumors involve the anterior third of the tongue. Level IA can be omitted at the physician's discretion when tumors do not involve the floor of the mouth or the anterior third of the oral tongue

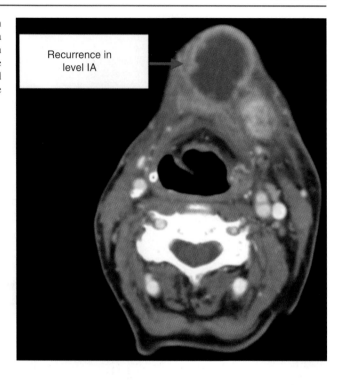

Recurrence in
level IA

**Fig. 9** A patient with squamous cell carcinoma of the oral tongue, pathologic stage T2N1, status post partial glossectomy and left neck dissection, with one positive lymph node and multiple close margins. A bite block was used at the time of simulation. The high-risk $CTV_{66}$ is shown in *red* and includes the region where close margins were identified. The high-risk $CTV_{60}$ is shown in *green* and covers the entire tongue and all postoperative changes, including the flap reconstruction. In the absence of bone invasion, the mandible can be excluded from the $CTV_{60}$. Note that the region near the ipsilateral parotid gland is well covered. The high-risk $CTV_{60}$ within the neck includes the ipsilateral levels I–V, including level IA. We utilize bolus and flash anteriorly to adequately dose level IA. The low-risk $CTV_{54}$, shown in blue, again encompasses the contralateral levels IB–IV

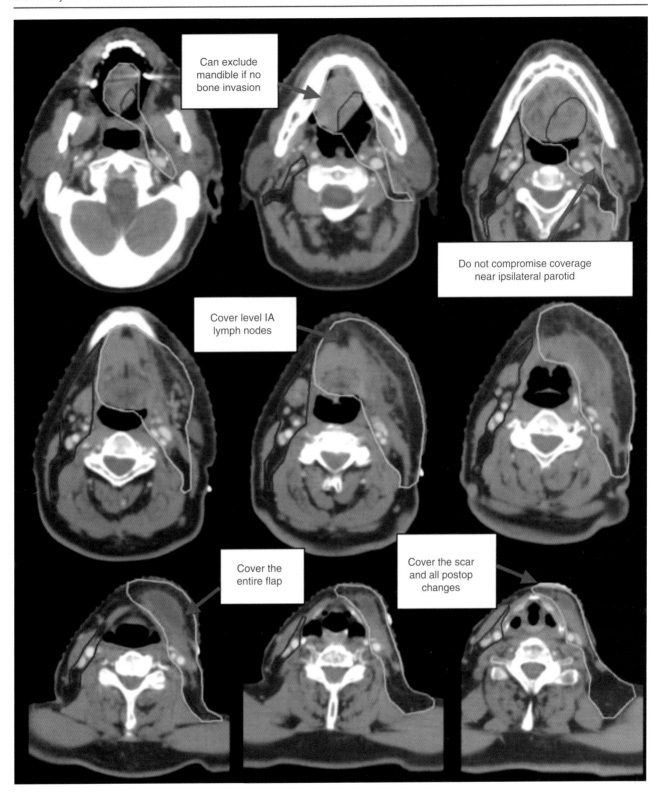

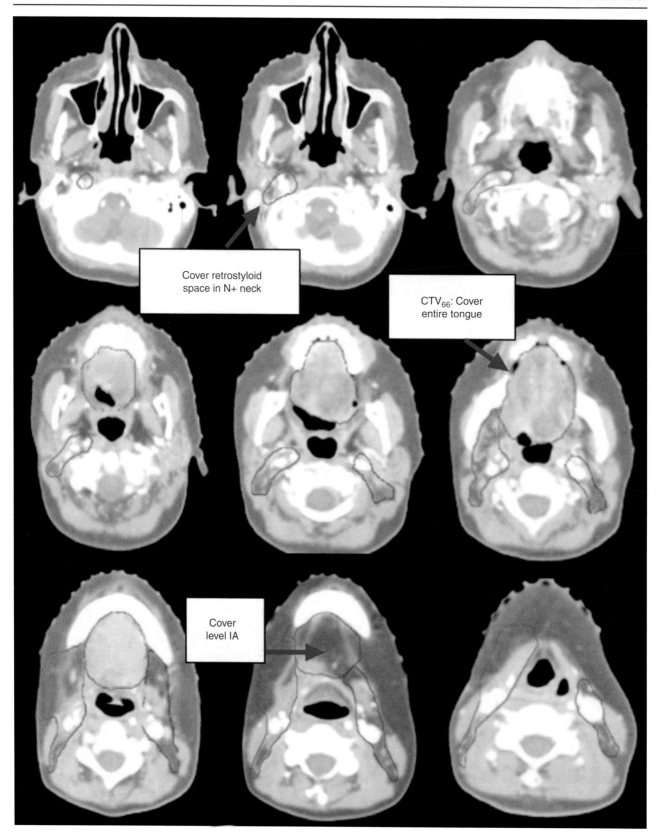

**Fig. 10** A patient with squamous cell carcinoma of the oral tongue, pathologic stage T3N2b, status post partial glossectomy with microscopically positive surgical margins. The high-risk $CTV_{66}$ is shown in *red* and covers the positive margin. The high-risk $CTV_{60}$ is shown in *green* and the low-risk $CTV_{54}$ is shown in *blue*. Neck nodal levels I–V are included on the ipsilateral side, and levels I–IV are included on the contralateral uninvolved side. Level IA should be covered, as should the ipsilateral level V lymph nodes, especially after surgical manipulation of the neck. We put bolus and flash anteriorly to adequately dose level IA. The ipsilateral retrostyloid space is at risk for nodal metastasis, especially with level II nodal involvement. Retropharyngeal nodes are at low risk and are not included

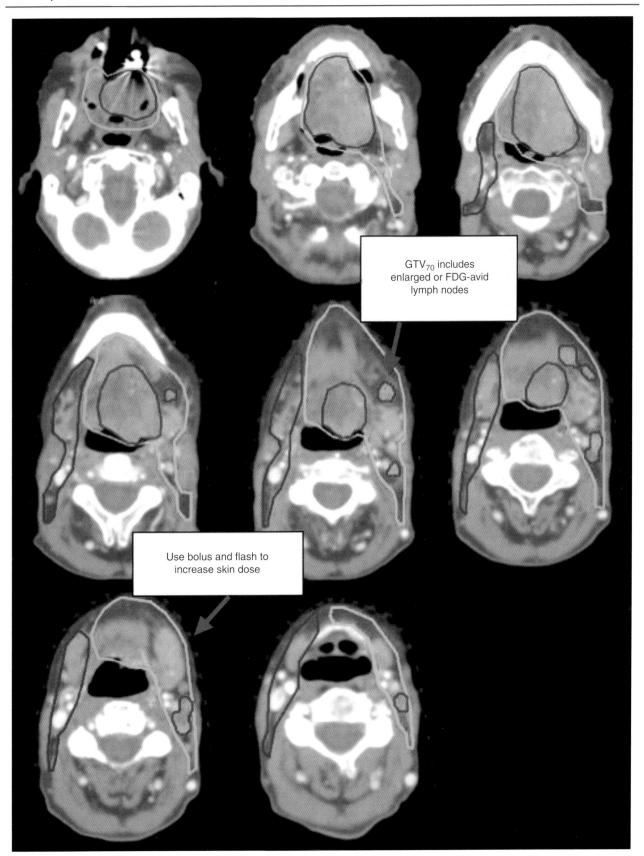

GTV$_{70}$ includes enlarged or FDG-avid lymph nodes

Use bolus and flash to increase skin dose

**Fig. 11** A patient with locally advanced squamous cell carcinoma of the oral tongue, clinical stage T4aN2b, with extension to the floor of the mouth and involvement of extrinsic muscles of the tongue. Given the extensive nature of the resection required, the patient decided to proceed with definitive cisplatin-based concurrent chemoradiation. The GTV$_{70}$ is shown in *red* and encompasses all gross disease visible on CT and PET. The CTV$_{70}$ is equal to the GTV$_{70}$, although a margin could be added if uncertainty exists regarding the extent of gross tumor extension. The high-risk CTV$_{59.4}$ is shown in *green* and includes the ipsilateral levels I–V. The low-risk CTV$_{54}$ encompasses the contralateral neck and is shown in *blue*. Volumes should be generous when treating carcinomas of the oral tongue, and bolus and flash should be used anteriorly to increase dose to the skin and underlying soft tissue

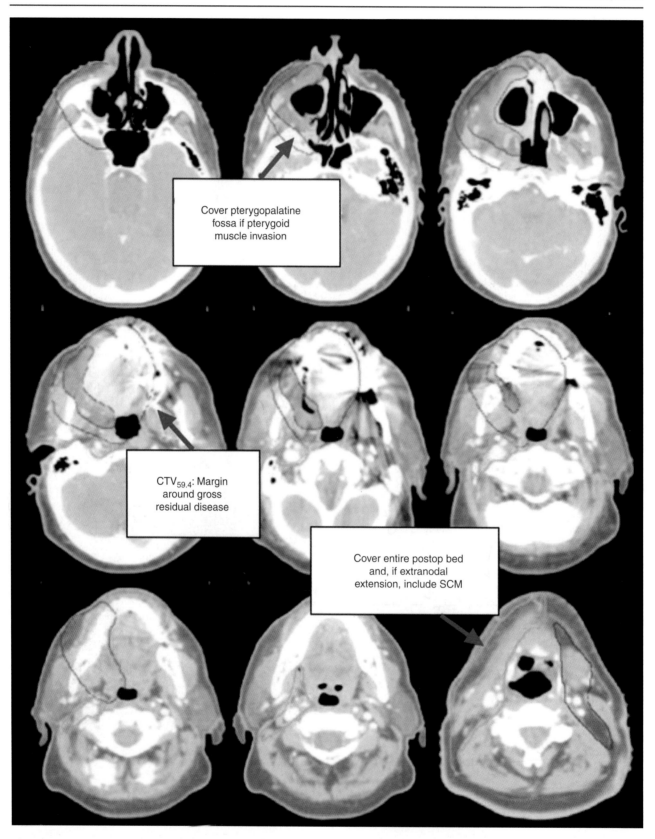

**Fig. 12** A patient with squamous cell carcinoma of the retromolar trigone, pathologic stage T4aN2b, with medial pterygoid involvement. The patient is status post resection and right neck dissection, with gross residual disease within the tumor bed. The gross disease (GTV$_{70}$) is shaded in *red* and delineated based on operative findings, as well as pre- and postoperative imaging. The high-risk CTV (CTV$_{59.4}$) is shown in *red* in the region of the tumor bed and in *green* in the ipsilateral neck. This includes pterygopalatine fossa, given the pterygoid muscle invasion, and ipsilateral levels I–V. If extracapsular extension is identified, the sternocleidomastoid muscle should be well covered. The low-risk CTV (CTV$_{54}$) is in *blue* and includes contralateral levels IB–IV

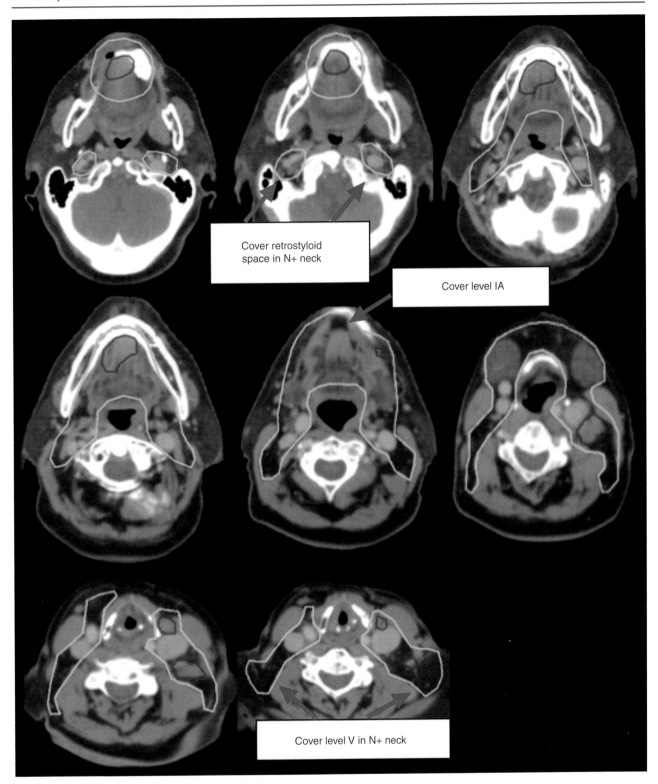

**Fig. 13** A patient with locally advanced squamous cell carcinoma of the floor of the mouth, clinical stage T2N2c, who is not a surgical candidate. The $GTV_{70}$, shown in red, includes all gross disease within the primary site and all positive neck nodes. Given the high reliability of available imaging, the $CTV_{70}$ was equal to the $GTV_{70}$. Bolus should be placed anteriorly to provide adequate dose to anterior floor of the mouth tumors. Given that lymph nodes are involved bilaterally, both the ipsilateral and contralateral neck are included in the high-risk $CTV_{59.4}$ highlighted in *green*. This should include the retrostyloid space and levels I–V

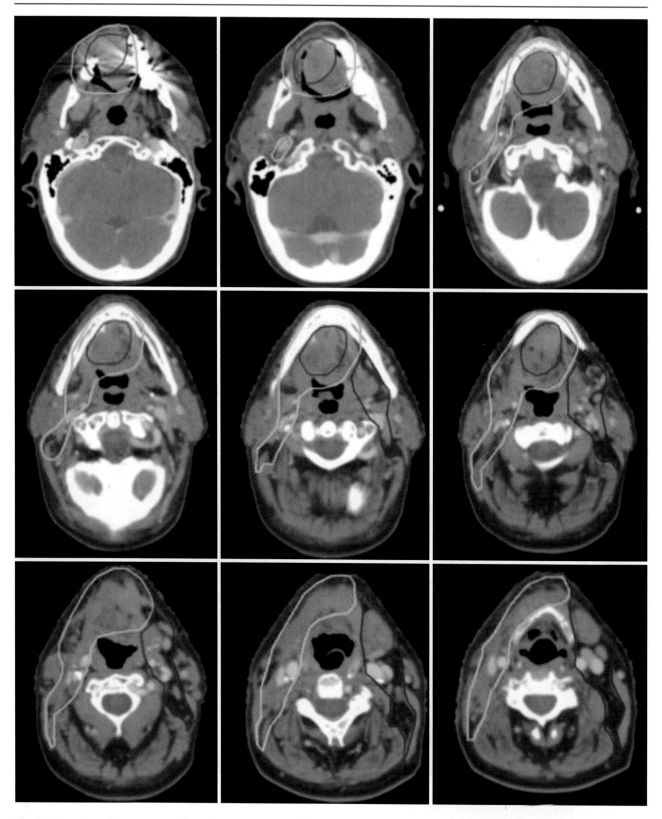

**Fig. 14** A patient with squamous cell carcinoma of the floor of the mouth, pathologic stage T2N2b, status post resection and right modified radical neck dissection. The CTV$_{66}$, shown in red, denotes the highest risk region based on pathologic findings, while the CTV$_{60}$, shown in green, includes the entire postoperative bed and levels I–V within the ipsilateral neck. The CTV$_{54}$, shown in blue, encompasses the CTV$_{60}$ in the region of the primary tumor and extends an additional 0.5–1 cm superiorly. The CTV$_{54}$ also includes levels IB to IV within the clinically N0 contralateral neck

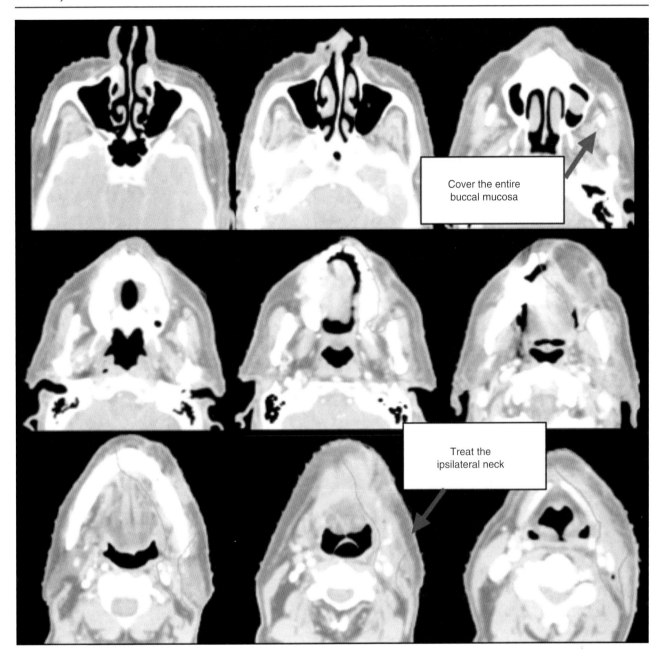

**Fig. 15** A patient with squamous cell carcinoma of the buccal mucosa, pathologic stage T4aN0 with minimal cortical bone invasion. The patient is status post tumor resection, marginal mandibulectomy and left neck dissection. Surgical margins were widely clear. The high-risk CTV (CTV$_{60}$) is shown in *green*. Neck nodal levels I–IV are included on the ipsilateral side. The CTV extends cranially to the buccal-gingival sulcus and infratemporal fossa, caudally to the buccal-gingival sulcus and submandibular gland, anteriorly to the lip commissure, and posteriorly to the retromolar trigone. The high-risk CTV should extend superiorly to the inferior orbital rim (not shown). Wide margins should be used, even in the case of small T1 tumors. Bolus is placed on the skin to provide adequate coverage of the high-risk CTV

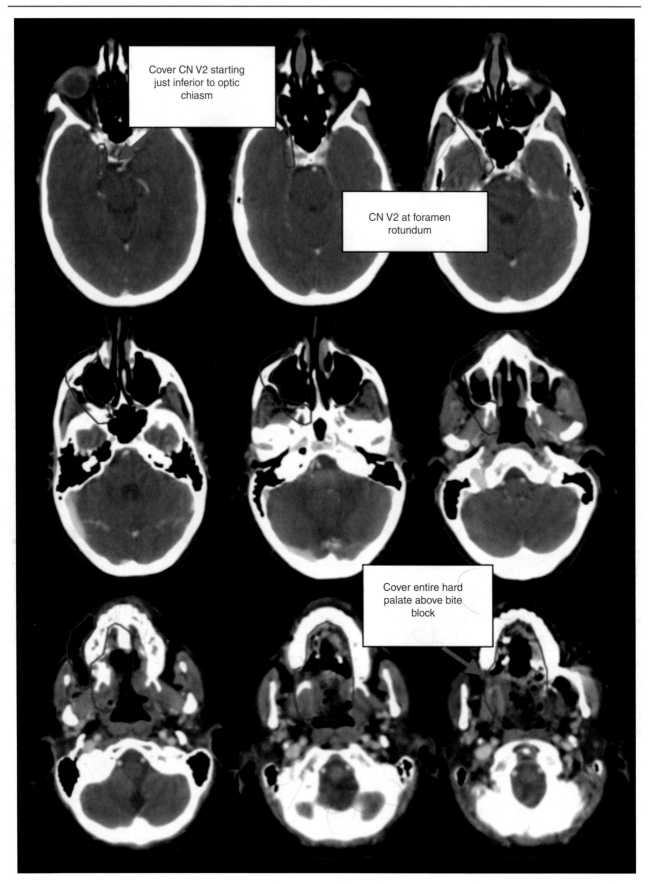

**Fig. 16** A patient with adenoid cystic carcinoma of the right hard palate, pathologic stage T2N0. The patient is status post bilateral partial maxillectomy, with extensive perineural invasion and positive margins. The patient was randomized to treatment with cisplatin-based chemoradiation on protocol RTOG 1008. A bite block was used at the time of simulation. The high-risk $CTV_{60}$ is shown in *red*. It encompasses the entire postoperative bed and extends at least 1.5–2 cm beyond the preoperative GTV. Given the presence of extensive perineural invasion, the low-risk $CTV_{50}$, shown in *blue*, includes the path of cranial nerve $V_2$ through the pterygopalatine fossa and foramen rotundum to the cavernous sinus and Meckel's cave

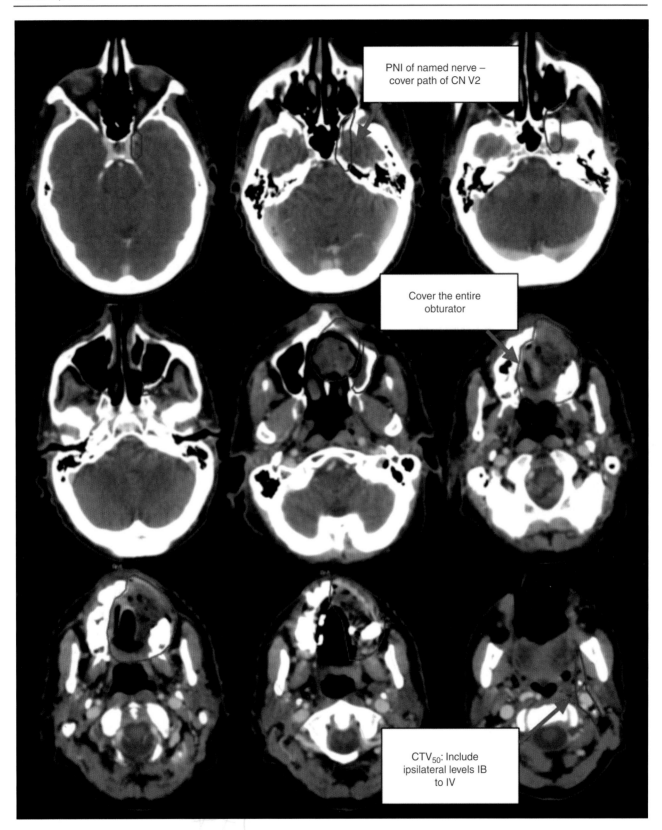

**Fig. 17** A patient with squamous cell carcinoma of the left maxillary alveolar ridge, pathologic stage T4N0 with bone invasion and perineural invasion, status post left inferior maxillectomy with obturator reconstruction. The high-risk $CTV_{66}$, shown in *red*, covers the obturator and postoperative changes in the region of the primary tumor bed. This is treated to 66 Gy due to the presence of bone invasion. The $CTV_{50}$, shown in *blue*, includes the ipsilateral levels IB to IV. When extensive perineural invasion or named nerve invasion is present, the $CTV_{50}$ can include adjacent nerves to the skull base. In this case, the greater palatine nerve is included, extending to cranial nerve $V_2$ and the base of skull (Fig. 3)

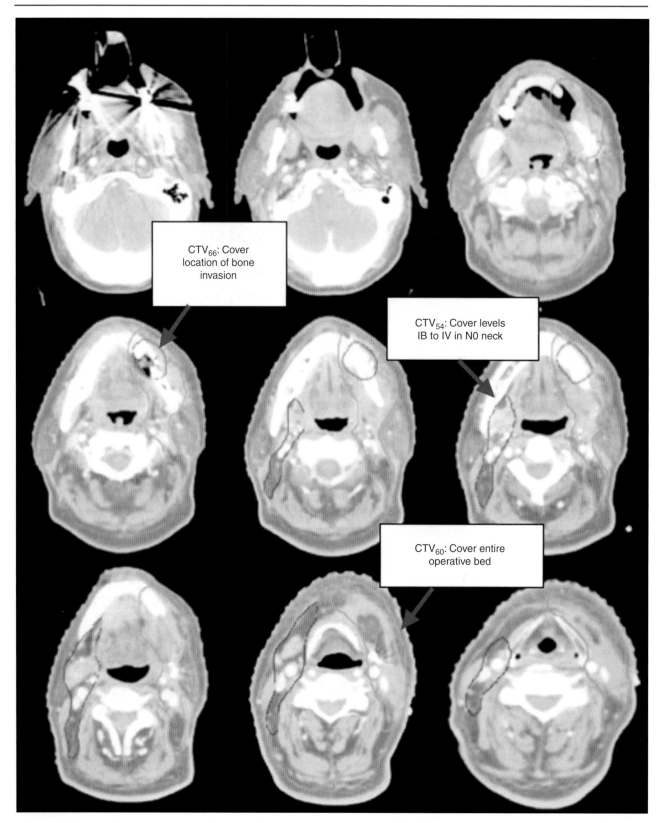

**Fig. 18** A patient with squamous cell carcinoma of the left mandibular alveolar ridge, pathologic stage T4aN1, with bone invasion. The patient is status post tumor resection with marginal mandibulectomy and left neck dissection. The high-risk $CTV_{66}$ is shown in *red* and encompasses the region of bone invasion by tumor. The high-risk $CTV_{60}$ is shown in *green* and includes the operative bed and ipsilateral levels I–IV. The low-risk $CTV_{54}$ is shown in *blue* and covers the contralateral levels I–IV

## 5 Plan Assessment

- If contralateral lymph nodes are uninvolved, efforts should be made to spare the contralateral parotid gland to help preserve salivary function. The dose to the ipsilateral parotid gland and the submandibular glands can be compromised for maximal coverage of the PTV.
- Ideally, at least 95 % of the PTV for each dose level should receive the prescription dose. For advanced tumors, coverage can be compromised to meet normal tissue constraints if necessary.
- Critical normal structures surrounding the oral cavity include the brainstem, spinal cord, optic nerves, optic chiasm, lenses, cochlea, parotid glands, submandibular glands, mandible, skin, brachial plexus, and glottic larynx. Each of these should be outlined. Suggested normal tissue constraints are listed in Table 4.

**Table 4** Intensity-modulated radiation therapy: normal tissue dose constraints[a]

| Critical structures | Constraints |
| --- | --- |
| Brainstem | Max < 50 Gy |
| Optic nerves | Max < 54 Gy |
| Optic chiasm | Max < 54 Gy |
| Spinal cord | Max < 45 Gy or 1 cc of the PTV cannot exceed 50 Gy |
| Mandible | Max < 70 Gy outside high dose PTV, avoid hot spots |
| Brachial plexus | Max < 65 Gy outside high dose PTV |
| Other normal structures | Constraints |
| Parotid gland | (a) Mean ≤26 Gy in one gland |
| | (b) Or at least 20 cc of the combined volume of both parotid glands will receive <20 Gy |
| | (c) Or at least 50 % of one gland will receive <30 Gy |
| Submandibular gland | Mean dose <39 Gy |
| Cochlea | Max < 50 Gy or $D_{05}$ < 55 Gy |
| Lens | Max < 5 Gy |
| Glottic larynx | Mean < 45 Gy |

## References

Ginsberg LE, DeMonte F (1998) Imaging of perineural tumor spread from palatal carcinoma. AJNR Am J Neuroradiol 19:1417–1422

Hermans R (2012) Head and neck cancer imaging, 2nd edn. Springer, Berlin/New York

Ng SH, Yen TC, Chang JTC et al (2006) Propsective study of [18F]fluorodeoxyglucose positron emission tomography and computed tomography and magnetic resonance imaging in oral cavity squamous cell carcinoma with palpably negative neck. Journal of Clinical Onconolgy, 24:4371–4376

Shah JP (1990) Patterns of cervical lymph node metastasis from squamous carcinomas of the upper aerodigestive tract. Am J Surg 160:405–409

Yao M, Chang K, Funk GF et al (2007) The failure patterns of oral cavity squamous cell carcinoma after intensity-modulated radiotherapy – the University of Iowa experience. Int J Radiat Oncol Biol Phys 67:1332–1341

# Early Stage Larynx Cancer

Zachary S. Zumsteg, Nadeem Riaz, and Nancy Lee

## Contents

Z.S. Zumsteg • N. Riaz • N. Lee (✉)
Department of Radiation Oncology, Memorial Sloan Kettering
Cancer Center, New York, NY, USA
e-mail: leen2@mskcc.org

## 1 Introduction

Laryngeal cancer affects approximately 12,000 people in the United States each year, and nearly half of tumors present as an early-stage tumor (T1–2 N0) arising from the true vocal cords. The major risk factor for laryngeal carcinoma is tobacco use, and greater the 95 % of patients with laryngeal cancer have a history of smoking (Wydner et al. 1956). Other risk factors, like alcohol and gastroesophageal reflux disease, also may play a role in the in development of laryngeal cancers, although they rarely lead to this malignancy without a concomitant smoking history. The role of HPV in the etiology of laryngeal cancer is not clear, although HPV-positive laryngeal cancers have been reported.

The larynx is divided into the supraglottis, glottis, and subglottis. The supraglottic larynx includes the false vocal cords, arytenoids, aryepiglottic folds, and the epiglottis. The glottic larynx is defined as the region including the true vocal cords and extending 0.5 cm inferiorly from the free margin of the true vocal cords. The subglottis extends from the inferior border of the glottis to the superior border of the trachea. The probability of cancer in these regions is markedly different. The glottis is by far the most common origin for cancers of the larynx, and the management of early-stage glottic carcinoma will be the focus of this chapter.

The management of early-stage glottic carcinoma is controversial, and radiotherapy, laser excision, and partial laryngectomy are therapeutic options. These approaches have not been compared in a prospective randomized fashion. Nevertheless, definitive radiation not only provides excellent rates of disease eradication, with long-term local control in about 90 % of T1N0 and 75 % of T2N0 patients, but also allows larynx preservation and excellent posttreatment voice quality in most cases (Frata et al. 2005; Cellai et al. 2005). The necessity for laryngectomy due to late toxicity, such as

N.Y. Lee et al. (eds.), *Target Volume Delineation for Conformal and Intensity-Modulated Radiation Therapy*,
Medical Radiology. Radiation Oncology, DOI: 10.1007/174_2014_1012, © Springer International Publishing Switzerland 2014
Published Online: 22 October 2014

radiation-induced necrosis, is very rare and occurs in less than 1 % of patients.

Early-stage glottic carcinoma is unique among cancers of the head and neck in that metastatic spread to the cervical lymph nodes is extremely rare, given that the true vocal cords lack a rich lymphatic drainage network. Because of this, it is one of the only head and neck cancers where elective cervical nodal irradiation is not recommended. Therefore, a much smaller radiation field is employed to treat early-stage glottic carcinoma than other cancers of the head and neck, and acute and late toxicity is much lower.

## 2    Diagnostic Workup

Given the marked difference in the management of early and advanced-stage glottic carcinoma, a careful workup is critical. A thorough physical exam, including indirect of flexible fiberoptic laryngoscopy with biopsy of all suspicious lesions and confirmation of vocal cord mobility, is imperative. In addition, exam under anesthesia by an experienced head and neck surgeon is helpful to evaluate the mucosal extent of disease, especially for subglottic extension, which can be difficult to appreciate on imaging and office laryngoscopy. High-quality imaging is essential for accurate staging and treatment of laryngeal cancer. Although imaging of the cervical lymph nodes in early-stage glottic carcinoma has a low likelihood of changing management, a high-resolution CT scan with thin cuts through the larynx can be useful for determining extralaryngeal spread of disease, including thyroid cartilage invasion. Because of motion artifact from swallowing, CT scan is often preferable to MRI. PET scan is generally not employed for early-stage disease.

## 3    Simulation and Daily Localization

CT simulation should be used for all patients, typically with a 3 mm slice thickness. IV contrast, although not required, may be helpful in delineating the carotid arteries. The patient should be set up in the supine position with the head extended. Immobilization of the head, neck, and shoulders should be achieved utilizing a customized aquaplast mask. The isocenter may be placed at the top of the arytenoids or in the center of the true vocal cords.

For IMRT treatment, daily 2D kV imaging pretreatment is recommended. Additionally, at our institution, we perform weekly CBCT and a posttreatment 2D kV imaging to ensure accurate patient setup. For disease affecting the anterior third of the vocal cord or anterior commissure, anterior bolus should be used if any part of the PTV in this region is receiving less than the prescription dose.

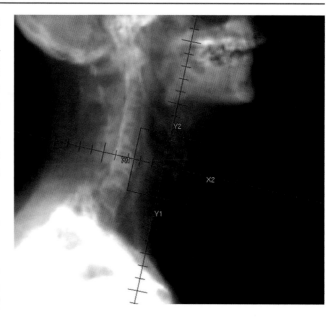

**Fig. 1** A typical 5×5 cm field used for conventional radiotherapy with opposed laterals for T1N0 glottic carcinoma

## 4    Radiation Techniques and Target Delineation

Two main techniques may be employed for definitive radiotherapy of early-stage glottic carcinoma. Conventional radiation with CT-based planning can be delivered with opposed lateral beams collimated to align parallel to the axis of the larynx. In this case, for T1N0 tumors, the opposed lateral fields should consist of a 5×5 cm square extending to the bottom of the hyoid bone or the top of the thyroid notch superiorly, the bottom of the cricoid inferiorly, the anterior edge of the vertebral bodies posteriorly, and 1 cm flash anteriorly (Figs. 1 and 2). For T2N0 tumors, the field may be expanded to a 6×6 cm box to extend inferiorly to include the first tracheal ring. Occasionally, it may be necessary to angle the beams approximately 5°–10° inferiorly in order to avoid treating through the shoulders, especially in patients with relatively short necks or who have difficulty positioning their shoulders inferiorly (Fig. 3). Fifteen or 30° wedges are often used to ensure a more homogeneous dose distribution throughout the larynx. For unilateral lesions, some advocate more heavily weighting the beam entering from the side of the tumor, for example, using a 3:2 ratio.

An alternative to conventional radiotherapy is carotid-sparing IMRT (Gomez et al. 2010; Rosenthal et al. 2010; Chera et al. 2010). For IMRT, a GTV should be delineated to encompass all suspicious lesions identified from laryngoscopy and imaging studies. The CTV should encompass the entire larynx, including the both the anterior and posterior commissures and the arytenoids. Although the inferior piriform sinuses are not part of the target volume, they are often

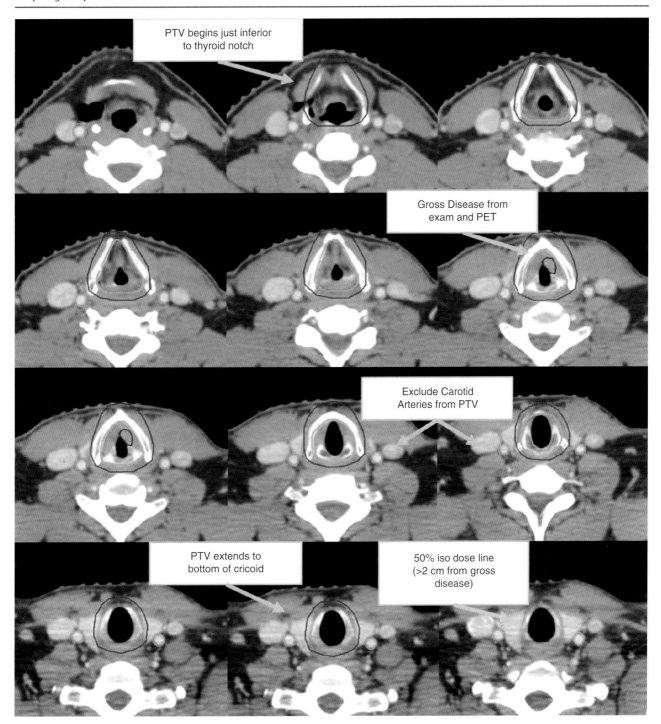

**Fig. 2** A patient with T1N0 squamous cell carcinoma of the left vocal cord. Because of the low rate (<5 %) of nodal metastases for early-stage glottis cancer, there is no elective nodal irradiation. Please note that these are representative slices and not all slices are included. *Blue* = GTV, *Green* = CTV, *Red* = PTV. GTV is delineated by laryngoscopy findings only. For T1 larynx tumors, there are typically no CT abnormalities.

The entire larynx is delineated as CTV to include both false and true vocal cords, anterior and posterior commissures, arytenoids and aryepiglottic folds, as well as the subglottic region. The PTV extends from thyroid notch to the bottom of the cricoid cartilage. A 5 mm margin is added in all directions except posterolaterally where it is limited to 3 mm to spare the carotid artery

included in the CTV at our institution given the relatively small increase in total volume. The PTV is typically a 0.5–1 cm three-dimensional expansion on the CTV, although the margin may be reduced to as little as 0.3 cm near the

carotid arteries. The superior and inferior borders should be similar to the respective borders used in conventional radiotherapy. The superior extent of the PTV should extend to the thyroid notch. The inferior extent of the PTV varies

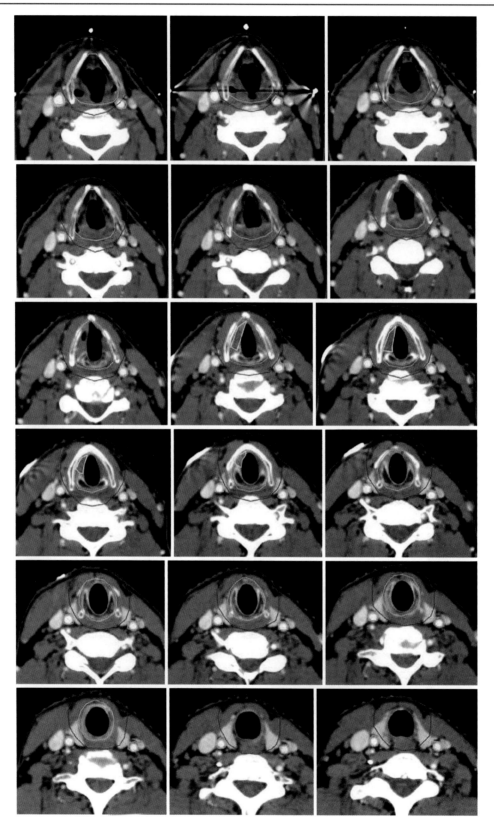

**Fig. 3** A patient with T2N0 squamous cell carcinoma of the right vocal cord with subglottic extension. *Yellow* = GTV, *Orange* = CTV, *Red* = PTV. GTV is delineated by laryngoscopy findings only. The entire larynx is delineated as CTV to include both false and true vocal cords, anterior and posterior commissures, arytenoids and aryepiglottic folds, as well as the subglottic region. Note in these images, the piriform sinuses are included in the CTV, as has been the historical practice at our institution. However, given that the piriform sinuses are not part of the true larynx, they may be excluded from the CTV to enhance carotid sparing. The PTV extends from thyroid notch to the bottom of the first tracheal ring inferiorly. A 1 cm margin is added in all directions except posterolaterally, where it is reduced to as little as 3 mm to exclude the carotid artery

**Table 1** Suggest target volumes for carotid-sparing IMRT in early-stage glottic carcinoma

| Target volumes | Definition and description |
| --- | --- |
| GTV | All gross disease on laryngoscopy and imaging |
| CTV | The entire larynx, including the both the anterior and posterior commissures and the arytenoids. The superior and inferior extents of the CTV are defined based on the PTV borders below |
| PTV | A 0.5–1 cm three-dimensional expansion of the CTV, with allowable reduction of the margin to as little as 3 cm near the carotid arteries. In general, the superior extent of the PTV should be at the thyroid notch. For T1N0 tumors, the inferior border of the PTV should extend to the bottom of the cricoid cartilage. For T2N0 tumors, the field should extend 1 cm more inferiorly to include the first tracheal ring. Additionally, the PTV should be modified to extend at least 2 cm above and below the GTV if it does not do so using traditional borders |

depending on the tumor stage. For T1N0 tumors, generally the inferior border of the PTV is the bottom of the cricoid. For T2N0 tumors, especially if there is subglottic extension, the inferior border of the PTV should be extended an additional 1 cm to include the first tracheal ring. In general, the PTV should also extend a minimum of 2 cm above and below the GTV (Table 1).

In terms of radiation dose and fractionation, there is prospective randomized evidence to suggest that using 2.25 Gy fractions improves local control compared to 2 Gy fractions (Yamazaki et al. 2006). Therefore, we recommend treating patients to 63 Gy in 28 fractions or 65.25 Gy in 29 fractions for T1N0 and T2N0 tumors, respectively.

Hyperfractionation has also been investigated for T2N0 tumors. A randomized phase III trial by the RTOG compared 70 Gy in 35 daily fractions to 79.2Gy delivered in 66 twice daily fractions in 250 patients with T2N0 tumors. Although the authors reported a trend toward improved 5-year local control (79 % vs. 70 %, $P=0.11$) and disease-free survival (51 % vs. 37 %, $P=0.07$) with hyperfractionation, this did not reach statistical significance (Trotti et al. 2006). Nevertheless, 79.2 Gy in 66 twice daily fractions is an alternative acceptable regimen for patients with T2N0 tumors.

Concurrent chemotherapy is not recommended for early-stage glottic carcinoma.

- For T1N0 glottic tumors, a dose of 63 Gy in 2.25 Gy/fraction is typically used.
- For T2 N0 glottic tumors, a dose of 65.25 Gy in 2.25 Gy/fraction is typically used.
- For T2 N0 glottic tumors, a dose of 79.2 Gy in 1.2 Gy/fraction bid is also used.

# References

Cellai E, Frata P, Magrini SM et al (2005) Radical radiotherapy for early glottic cancer: results in a series of 1087 patients from two Italian radiation oncology centers. I. The case of T1N0 disease. Int J Radiat Oncol Biol Phys 63(5):1378–1386

Chera BS, Amdur RJ, Morris CG, Mendenhall WM (2010) Carotid-sparing intensity-modulated radiotherapy for early-stage squamous cell carcinoma of the true vocal cord. Int J Radiat Oncol Biol Phys 77(5):1380–1385

Frata P, Cellai E, Magrini SM et al (2005) Radical radiotherapy for early glottic cancer: results in a series of 1087 patients from two Italian radiation oncology centers. II. The case of T2N0 disease. Int J Radiat Oncol Biol Phys 63(5):1387–1394

Gomez D, Cahlon O, Mechalakos J, Lee N (2010) An investigation of intensity-modulated radiation therapy versus conventional two-dimensional and 3D-conformal radiation therapy for early stage larynx cancer. Radiat Oncol 5:74

Rosenthal DI, Fuller CD, Barker JL Jr et al (2010) Simple carotid-sparing intensity-modulated radiotherapy technique and preliminary experience for T1-2 glottic cancer. Int J Radiat Oncol Biol Phys 77(2):455–461

Trotti A, Pajak T, Emami B et al (2006) A randomized trial of hyperfractionation versus standard fractionation in T2 squamous cell carcinoma of the vocal cord. Int J Radiat Oncol Biol Phys 66(Suppl):S15

Wydner EL, Bross IJ, Day E (1956) Epidemiological approach to the etiology of cancer of the larynx. JAMA 160:1384

Yamazaki H, Nishiyama K, Tanaka E et al (2006) Radiotherapy for early glottic carcinoma (T1N0M0): results of prospective randomized study of radiation fraction size and overall treatment time. Int J Radiat Oncol Biol Phys 64:77–82

# Advanced Laryngeal Carcinoma

Daniel Higginson, Oren Cahlon, and Bhisham Chera

## Contents

D. Higginson (✉) • O. Cahlon
Department of Radiation Oncology, Memorial Sloan Kettering,
New York, NY, USA
e-mail: higginsd@mskcc.org

B. Chera
Department of Radiation Oncology, University of North Carolina,
Chapel Hill, NC, USA

## 1 Anatomy and Patterns of Spread

- Advanced laryngeal cases are defined here as T stages ≥3 and/or N+disease, i.e., cases for which limited larynx-only fields are not appropriate.
- The larynx is divided into three sites: supraglottis, glottis, and subglottis.
- The subglottic space extends from the first tracheal ring to 5 mm inferior to the free edge true vocal cords (TVCs).
- The glottic larynx contains the true vocal folds, anterior commissure, posterior commissure, and the infraglottic space (5 mm inferior to the free edge of the TVCs).
- The supraglottic larynx contains the following subsites of the larynx: ventricles, false vocal folds (FVCs), aryepiglottic folds, and epiglottis (infrahyoid, suprahyoid, laryngeal surface, lingual surface).
- For cases involving the TVC and the ventricle, there can be uncertainty about whether the primary is a T2N0 glottic cancer (for which the limited fields are appropriate) or a T2N0 supraglottic cancer (for which elective nodal coverage is appropriate). In these cases, the physician should make a best possible determination of the epicenter of the tumor in order to decide the appropriate approach.
- Similarly, a glottic tumor can have subglottic extension (more than 5 mm of involvement inferiorly from the TVC) and remain a T2 glottic case as long as the epicenter of the tumor is glottic. True subglottic cases are rare (1 % of laryngeal cases) and have a significantly worse prognosis, and elective nodes should be treated.
- TVC mobility must be assessed on laryngoscopy to document mobility (normal, hypomobility, fixation). A medialized fixed cord is caused by recurrent laryngeal nerve injury, whereas a lateralized fixed or hypomobile is caused by injury of intrinsic laryngeal muscles. Lateralized fixed/hypomobile TVCs are often seen with laryngeal cancer.

N.Y. Lee et al. (eds.), *Target Volume Delineation for Conformal and Intensity-Modulated Radiation Therapy*,
Medical Radiology. Radiation Oncology, DOI: 10.1007/174_2014_1001, © Springer International Publishing Switzerland 2014
Published Online: 22 October 2014

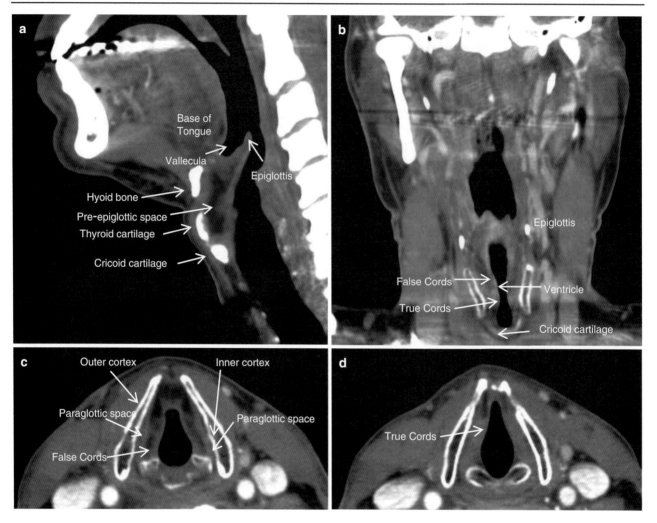

**Fig. 1** CT anatomy of the larynx. (**a**) Sagittal CT of the larynx. The pre-epiglottic space is anterior to the epiglottis and superior to the vocal folds. It is contiguous with the paraglottic space and base of tongue. The hyoid bone divides the epiglottis into infra- and suprahyoid portions. (**b**)   Coronal CT  demonstrates the false cord, the true cord, and the ventricle in between. (**c**) The paraglottic space is a small fat plane adjacent to the thryoid cartilage. (**c, d**) FVCs can be distinguished from the TVCs because the FVCs have a band of fatty tissue and the TVCs do not

- The paraglottic and pre-epiglottic spaces are connected fat planes. The paraglottic space is bounded by the thyroid cartilage laterally and the TVCs, FVCs medially. The pre-epiglottic fat space is bounded by the mucosal surface of the vallecula superiorly, hyoid/thyroid strap muscles anteriorly, and root of the epiglottis posteriorly and inferiorly communicates with the paraglottic spaces.
- Laryngeal cancer often invades the paraglottic and pre-epiglottic spaces. There are no barriers to spread to the adjacent space if one is involved.
- The AJCC 6th edition added paraglottic space invasion to the staging system, denoting laryngeal tumors with this clinical feature as T3. Some practitioners continue to treat a T3N0 glottic SCC (T3 due only to paraglottic invasion) with limited fields (Dagan et al. 2007).
- The thyroid cartilage has an inner and outer cortex. Invasion of the inner cortex only signifies T3 disease and invasion through the outer cortex signifies T4 disease. The degree of invasion can only be assessed through CT imaging with appropriate windowing and must be carefully reviewed by the treating radiation oncologist.
- Surgeries relevant to advanced laryngeal cancer include total laryngectomy, supraglottic laryngectomy (also called horizontal partial laryngectomy), and vertical hemilaryngectomy transoral laser microsurgery (TLM). Supraglottic laryngectomy is appropriate only for cases without vocal fold fixation, involvement of the arytenoids, and/or thyroid cartilage invasion. Patient must also have good respiratory function in case of aspiration postsurgery. Historically, the inferior extent of the tumor must not exceed the level of the FVCs for this surgery, as the inferior surgical margin is the ventricles.
- In general TLM is contraindicated for T3 or T4 disease.

**Table 1** Regional nodal involvement

| | Overall involvement at presentation (pre-CT era) (Lindberg 1972; Candela et al. 1990) (%) | Overall involvement at presentation (CT era) (Buckley and MacLennan 2000) (%) | Occult involvement at neck dissection for a N0 neck (Zhang et al. 2006) (%) |
|---|---|---|---|
| IB | 1–3 | 0 | |
| II | 33–37 | 24 | 18–20 |
| III | 26–34 | 19 | |
| IV | 8 | 14 | |
| V | 5 | 2 | |

## 2 Diagnostic Workup Relevant for Target Volume Delineation

- Critical parts of the history include an assessment of voice, swallowing (i.e., modified barium swallow), respiratory, and constitutional status. A history of an emergent tracheostomy for respiratory dysfunction is a recurrence risk factor for T3 cases using organ preserving radiation, and thus total laryngectomy is a reasonable recommendation. Smoking cessation interventions should be instituted.
- On examination, the larynx should be palpated and gently moved. Very advanced disease may exhibit absence of laryngeal crepitus because of invasion of the post-cricoid area. The nodal basins should be carefully palpated. In postoperative cases, the surroundings of the stoma should be carefully palpated and viewed. Cranial nerves are rarely involved but should be assessed. The examiner should ask the patient to extrude the tongue and check for trismus, in case of very advanced disease. The tongue and tongue base should be palpated.
- Fiberoptic nasopharyngolaryngoscopy should be performed to define the location of the disease. An assessment should start by identifying the bulk and boundaries of disease and determining the origin: supraglottic, glottic, or subglottic and subsites involved. Then vocal fold mobility should be assessed carefully and repeated. Careful attention should be paid to hypopharynx, vallecula, and base of tongue involvement.
- Outpatient nasopharyngolaryngoscopy may be inadequate for truly visualizing the ventricle, the post-cricoid, and subglottic regions. For this reason, a dedicated examination under anesthesia by an otolaryngologist is needed.
- Imaging should include a dedicated, thin slice (1–2 mm cuts) CT of the head and neck with IV contrast. Preepiglottic and paraglottic space invasion as well as thyroid cartilage invasion can only be assessed by CT accurately. Examine if there is more than 1 cm of base of tongue invasion, which was an exclusion criterion for larynx preservation trials.

- A PET/CT is not required to treat this disease but may be informative in some cases, particularly when borderline nodes are identified on CT.

## 3 Organ Preservation Versus Total Laryngectomy

- Fifty-six percent of T4 patients required a salvage laryngectomy in the VA larynx trial, which led to the general recommendations for total laryngectomy for T4 cases and organ preservation for T1–T3. However, the decision is often more nuanced.
- In our practice there have been successes with organ preservation for some carefully selected T4 candidates such as those with small T4 disease with a good functional larynx (normal swallowing study, no airway compromise).
- In addition, some T3 cases may not be appropriate for organ preservation. We offer the following considerations:
  - RTOG 91-11 excluded cases with more than 1 cm invasion of the base of tongue.
  - It has been suggested that one possible reason survival statistics for laryngeal cancer have worsened is inappropriate usage of chemoradiation for advanced cases (Olsen 2010).
  - Retrospective evidence suggests that if an emergent tracheostomy was required for respiratory compromise, these patients may exhibit worse locoregional control after chemoradiation and may be better served by total laryngectomy.
  - Retrospective evidence also suggests that tumor bulk predicts outcome following chemoradiation (Mendenhall et al. 2003). Volume >6 cm$^3$ is considered bulky for supraglottic disease and >3.5 cm$^3$ is bulky for glottic cancers. One system in use is to offer chemoradiation for all true glottic and supraglottic cases <6 cm$^3$ and for supraglottic cases up to 6–12 cm$^3$ if there is no vocal fold fixation.

## 4 Simulation and Daily Localization

- Patient is supine with neck extended. The arms are at the sides and shoulders are immobilized and extended down toward the feet. An arm strap can be used to keep the arms and shoulders in position, or an immobilization device can secure both the head and the shoulders. The head and neck should be immobilized with the head comfortably and securely opposed to a head cushion.
- The CT simulation should use ≤3 mm slices with IV contrast. The CT should include the entire vertex of the head through the carina. Historically with 2D and 3DCRT techniques, the isocenter should be placed at the bottom of the cricoid if there is no subglottic or hypopharyngeal extension. If either is present, then the isocenter is placed 1 cm below the cricoid.
- For postoperative cases, it may be helpful to place a radiopaque marker on the scar if there is a positive margin or extra-nodal extension.
- A variety of IGRT approaches are used in laryngeal cancer. The most common approaches are daily kV or MV cone beam CTs or daily cone beam CT for the first 5 days of treatment and if stable, biweekly thereafter.

## 5 Target Volume Delineation and Treatment Planning

### 5.1 Intact Larynx

- Typically 3 CTVs are drawn: CTV70, CTV60 (actually 59.4–63 Gy), and CTV54 (actually 46–54 Gy). Depending on the clinical situation, the CTV60 may be omitted. All 3 (or 2) CTVs can be treated in one dose-painting IMRT plan. However, if one is concerned with the low-dose per fraction (i.e., <1.8 Gy) for the CTV low risk, 2 sequential IMRT plans may be created: one that includes the CTV60 and CTV54 and one for the CTV70.
- In Table 2, common target volumes and fractionation schemes are presented. Many other variations exist, however. Out of concern for higher long-term toxicity (i.e. laryngeal necrosis), we do not use the 70 Gy/33 fraction regimen involving 2.12 Gy doses.
- The terms high, intermediate, and low risk are used differently by practitioners to describe the IMRT volumes that roughly correspond to the 70, 60, and 50 Gy volumes used with non-IMRT conventional planning. In this chapter, we use terms such as CTV70, CTV60, and CTV54 to avoid confusion.
- The two-volume approach can be used for all cases and is especially attractive for node-negative cases. The three-volume approach is attractive for when there are nodes of indeterminate significance or when a tracheostomy/stoma

**Table 2** Variations in treatment approaches for the intact larynx

| Two-volume approach | Three-volume approach |
|---|---|
| *CTV70*: whole larynx, primary, involved nodes | *CTV70*: primary, involved nodes |
| *CTV54*: elective nodal areas | *CTV60*: remaining larynx, involved and adjacent nodal levels, indeterminate nodes, stoma, tracheostomy site. |
| | *CTV54:* elective nodal areas |
| *Sequential:* 46–54 Gy in 2 Gy daily fractions, followed by a sequential IMRT plan to the CTV70 in 2 Gy daily fractions to 70 Gy | *Sequential:* two consecutive IMRT plans: (1) 60 Gy/30 fractions to CTV60 and 54 Gy/30 fractions to CTV54 and (2) 10 Gy/5 fractions to CTV70 |
| *Dose painting:* 54–63 Gy in 35 daily fractions and 70 Gy in 35 daily fractions of 2 Gy to the CTV70 | *One IMRT plan*: 70, 63, and 54 Gy in 35 daily fractions to the CTV70, CTV63, and CTV54, respectively. Another scheme is 33 daily fractions of 2.12, 1.8, and 1.64 Gy fractions to these volumes |

site needs to be boosted to ~60 Gy. Another consideration is the practicality of developing sequential IMRT plans (dose painting abrogates this challenge). Furthermore the dose conformality and the ability to spare normal tissues are better when dose painting is used.

- Indications for boosting a tracheostomy site include (1) cases when an emergent tracheostomy was required, (2) soft tissue extension into level VI, and (3) subglottic extension (especially when the tracheostomy had to be inserted in close proximity to the primary tumor).
- The typical treatment plan at MSKCC is the three-volume approach above, whereas at the University of North Carolina, a two-volume approach is more typical.
- If the patient is not a candidate for either concurrent cisplatin chemotherapy or cetuximab, then altered fractionation is indicated. Options include:
  - Six fractions per week (DAHANCA trials). Two fractions, 6 h apart, can be given once per week. Any of the planning and dose fractionation strategies above can be used.
  - Concomitant boost (RTOG 90-03). A second afternoon boost treatment is given in the afternoons (>6 h after the AM fractions). Thus the two-volume, sequential approach described above is the only feasible method. The low risk is treated with 54 Gy in 30 fractions of 1.8 Gy and during the last 12 days of treatment, the high risk is boosted in 1.5 Gy fractions in the afternoons to 72 Gy.
  - Hyperfractionation (RTOG 90-03). Daily BID 1.2 Gy fractions are applied. Thus only the sequential plan strategy can be used rather than dose painting. The low-risk volume can be treated to 57.6 Gy in 48 fractions of 1.2 Gy BID. The high-risk volume can be then be boosted to 76.8–79.2 Gy in 16–18 additional

fractions of 1.2 Gy BID. If an intermediate-risk volume is used, then 64.8 Gy may be an appropriate dose. Note the high-risk dose used now is typically lower than that used in RTOG 90-03 (81.6 Gy).

- Of these three options, we recommend the hyperfraction-ation regimen. The MARCH meta-analysis suggests that hyperfractionation produces the best locoregional control (Baujat et al. 2010). The concomitant boost technique led to more late toxicity in RTOG 90-03.

- The gross tumor volume (GTV) is defined as all known gross disease determined from CT, MRI, clinical information, and endoscopic findings.

- Positive nodes in the neck should be defined as those with central necrosis, extracapsular extension, and/or a short axis diameter of >1 cm. For borderline cases, those with FDG avidity should be considered disease. Small nodes that are bean-shaped or exhibit a fatty hilum are more likely benign. Enlarged RP nodes, although unusual in laryngeal cancer, should be considered positive even if small.

- For ≥T3, the bilateral necks must be electively treated (at least levels II–IV). Unilateral treatment is never appropriate.

- Before the IMRT era, levels I–VII were covered at least in the 50 Gy volume even though nodal involvement is most common in II–IV. The low anterior neck covered levels V, VI, and VII, and level IB was unavoidable in the lateral fields. Surgeons have traditionally resected only levels II–IV for the node-negative neck in larynx cancer, then and now. In the IMRT era, level V can clearly be omitted in the node-negative neck. Elective coverage of levels IB, VI, and VII is more varied among practitioners.

- Level IB is in close proximity to the larynx and the sub-mandibular gland cannot easily be spared with IMRT without sacrificing laryngeal coverage. Thus part or most of it is generally included.

- Level VI is a small nodal region without critical structures apart from part of the thyroid gland, which is unavoidably treated to a high dose in any case. We generally include it for all cases, but others reserve coverage only for subglottic extension/subglottic primary tumors, hypopharyngeal extension, gross level IV adenopathy, emergent tracheostomy, or soft tissue extension from the primary into the neck. The tracheoesophageal nodes (part of level VI) must be covered in these cases.

- Level VII (upper mediastinum) is recommended for node-positive cases, subglottic extension, or hypopharyngeal involvement. Prior to IMRT, this region was always included in the low anterior neck AP field, which extended to 1 cm below the inferior clavicular head.

- Regional involvement is very common for supraglottic cases and thus elective treatment (surgery or radiation) to both necks is always required, regardless of T stage. Level VI should also be treated including the tracheoesophageal

nodes. Some practitioners cover only levels II and III for T1 and T2N0 supraglottic cases.

- In an electively treated neck, the superior border of level II can be where the posterior belly of the digastric muscle crosses the internal jugular vein. This represents the superior most region that is dissected in elective neck dissections and is often at the same level as the caudal edge of the lateral process of C1. This allows for sparing of the ipsilateral parotid.

- When there are positive nodes in a hemi-neck, then the ipsilateral V is included. The entire level II to the base of skull and the ipsilateral retropharyngeal nodes are included because of the possibility of "backed up" lymphatics in the involved neck. Some would neither treat the retropharyngeal nodes nor treat level II all the way to the jugular foramen.

**Table 3** Suggested target volumes for 70 Gy

| Target volumes | Definition and description |
|---|---|
| GTV | Primary: all gross disease on physical examination and imaging |
| | Neck nodes: all nodes ≥1 cm or PET positive should be included as GTV – include borderline lymph nodes in doubt as GTV to avoid undertreatment |
| CTV70 | Primary: 5–10 mm expansion of the GTV. If a 2-volume approach is taken, the entire larynx should be in the 70 Gy volume |
| | Nodes: 6–8 mm expansion on involved nodes |
| PTV70 | CTV70+3–5 mm, depending on immobilization, localization, etc. We use 3 mm with on-board CT imaging |

**Table 4** Suggested targeted regions for 59.4–63 Gy

| Target volumes | Definition and description |
|---|---|
| CTV59.4–63 | CTV should encompass the entire CTV70 |
| | Includes the entire larynx, from the top of the thyroid notch to the bottom of the cricoid cartilage |
| | High-risk nodal regions, such as levels II–IV on the involved N+neck |
| PTV59.4–63 | CTV59.4–63+3–5 mm |

**Table 5** Suggested target volumes for low-risk subclinical regions

| Target volumes | Definition and description |
|---|---|
| CTV54 | CTV 54 should encompass the entire CTV59.4–63 |
| | At least levels II–IV of the uninvolved neck. At least I–V for the involved neck. See discussion above and Table 6 for recommendations on levels I, VI, VII and RP nodes |
| PTV54 | CTV54+3–5 mm |

## 5.2  Postoperative RT for Laryngeal Cancer

- Postoperative radiation is indicated for any of these pathological features: pT3–4 disease, pN2–3, extra-nodal extension, and close/positive margin. PNI/LVSI is a minor indication and radiation is often still recommended. Concurrent chemotherapy should be added for + margin and extracapsular extension. The addition of chemotherapy is debatable for the weaker pathological indications of ≥2 nodes, PNI, or LVSI.

- The stoma is always included in the low-risk volume. The stoma is boosted to ~60–70 Gy for subglottic extension and positive level IV nodes and if an emergent tracheostomy was performed. Anatomically a stomal recurrence is a tracheoesophageal node.

- Historically, placement of bolus over the scar was done for positive margins and extracapsular extension. In IMRT treatment planning, the target volumes are purposefully pulled away from the skin to prevent severe dermatitis. The practice of placing bolus over the scar when IMRT is used is variable. If concerned, one may place 5 mm to 1 mm bolus over the scar. The bolus should be accounted for in the treatment planning by either simulating the patient with applied bolus or mocking up a "ghost" bolus in the treatment planning system.

**Table 6**  Management of the neck in advanced laryngeal carcinoma

| Target volumes | Notes about coverage |
|---|---|
| IA | Not included |
| IB | Hard to avoid while preserving coverage of the larynx. Generally included, definitely included in node-positive hemi-neck |
| II | Always covered. If neck is negative, superior border is where the posterior belly of the digastric crosses the IJ (or transverse process of C1). If neck is positive, level II is covered to skull base |
| III | Always covered |
| IV | Always covered |
| V | Covered if ipsilateral neck is involved |
| VI (including tracheoesophageal nodes) | Covered for subglottic extension/subglottic primary tumors, hypopharyngeal involvement, gross level IV adenopathy, emergent tracheostomy, or soft tissue extension from the primary into the neck. Some practitioners always cover level VI, some do not |
| RP nodes | Covered only if ipsilateral bulky neck nodes, which can cause "backed" lymphatics to RP nodes |
| VII (upper mediastinum) | Recommend covering for node-positive cases and for subglottic extension or hypopharyngeal involvement |

- If there is a positive margin or extracapsular extension, the at-risk operative bed/nodal region is treated to 66 Gy rather than 60 Gy.

**Table 7**  Fractionation/dose regimens for postoperative larynx cases

| Negative margins, no ECE | Positive margins and/or ECE |
|---|---|
| *CTV60:* 60 Gy in 30 fractions (2.0 Gy per fraction) | *Option 1:* three volumes, all dose painting. 66, 60, and 54 Gy in 33 fractions |
| *CTV54:* 54 Gy in 30 fractions (1.8 Gy per fraction) | *Option 2:* three volumes, sequential. 60 and 54 Gy in 30 fractions (dose painting) followed by a separate sequential 6 Gy/3fx |
| | *Option 3:* two volumes, dose painting. 66 Gy/33fx and 54–60 Gy/33fx |

**Table 8**  Suggested target volumes at the high-risk subclinical region

| Target volumes | Definition and description |
|---|---|
| CTV66 (if needed) | Operative bed if positive margins |
| | Operative bed + areas of ECE if there is ECE |
| | Stoma boost if indicated |
| CTV60 | Entire operative bed, including scar |
| | Stoma boost if indicated |
| | Lymph node stations where nodes positive |
| CTV54 | CTV60–66 volume |
| | Elective nodal areas, at least levels II–IV |
| | Stoma |
| | Same nodal coverage rules apply as in intact larynx. Note that the stoma is created within level VI and thus is always covered |
| PTV | CTVs + 3–5 mm |

# 6  Plan Assessment

**Table 9**  Constraints used at the University of North Carolina

| *PTVs* |
|---|
| ≥95 % of the PTV should receive 100 % of the prescription dose |
| ≥99 % of the PTV receives ≥93 % of the prescription dose (i.e., cold spot) |
| ≤20 % of the PTV >110 % of the prescription dose (i.e., hot spot) |
| *Normal tissues* |
| Nonspecified tissue outside PTV: ≤1 % receives >110 % of the prescription dose |
| Brain stem: max dose (voxel or 0.1 cc) 54 Gy |
| Spinal cord: max dose (voxel or 0.1 cc) 50 Gy |
| Parotid: mean dose <26 Gy and/or 50 % receives <30 Gy |
| Cochlea: mean dose <45 Gy |
| Oral cavity: mean dose <39 Gy |

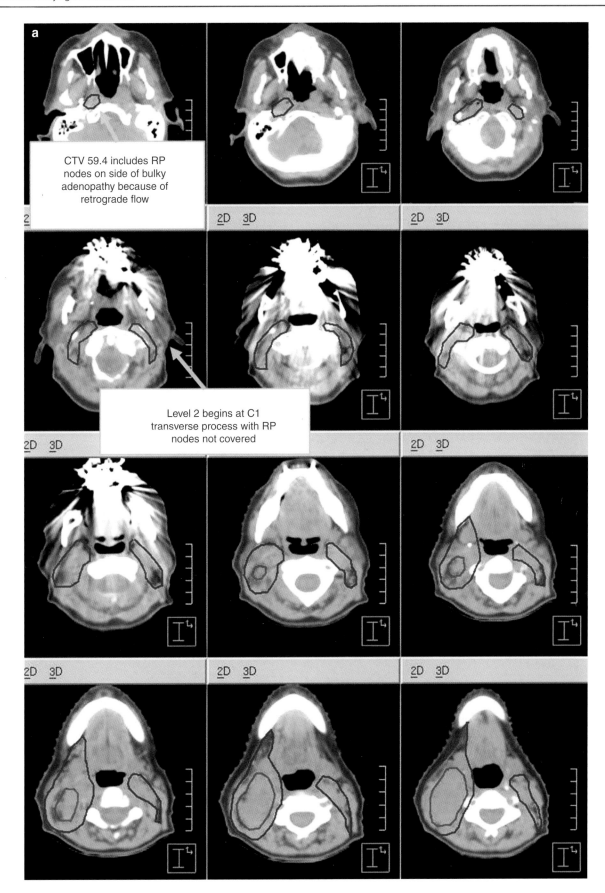

**Fig. 2** T2N2cM0 squamous cell carcinoma of the epiglottis involving right AE fold and bilateral cervical lymph nodes. Please note that these are representative slices and not all slices are included. For this case, a three-volume approach was employed. (**a**) *Magenta* GTV LN, *purple* GTV primary, *blue* CTV 59.4, *orange* CTV 54. (**b**) Additional axial slices. (**c**) Additional axial slices. PET/CT imaging in lower panels. *Green* GTV designed with assistance from PET imaging

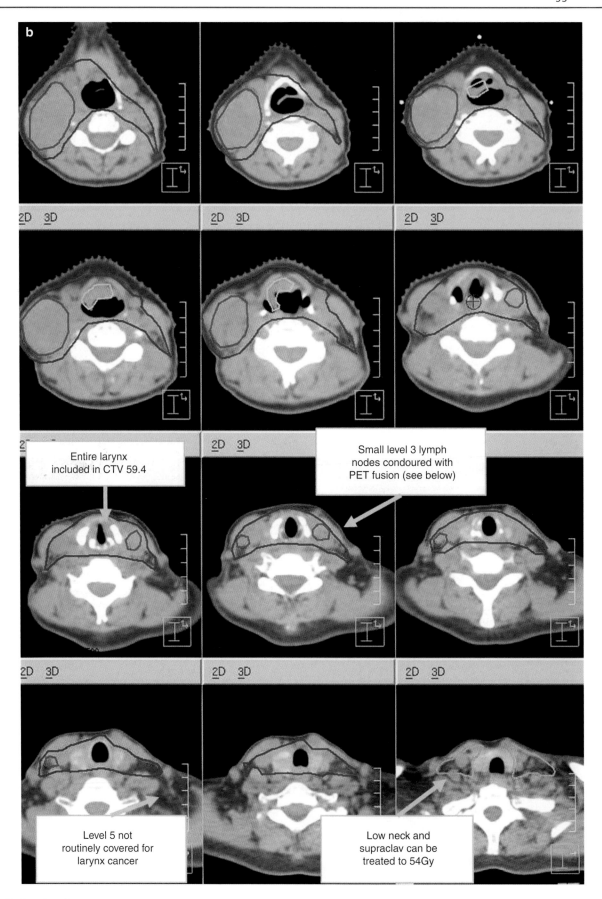

**Fig. 2** (continued)

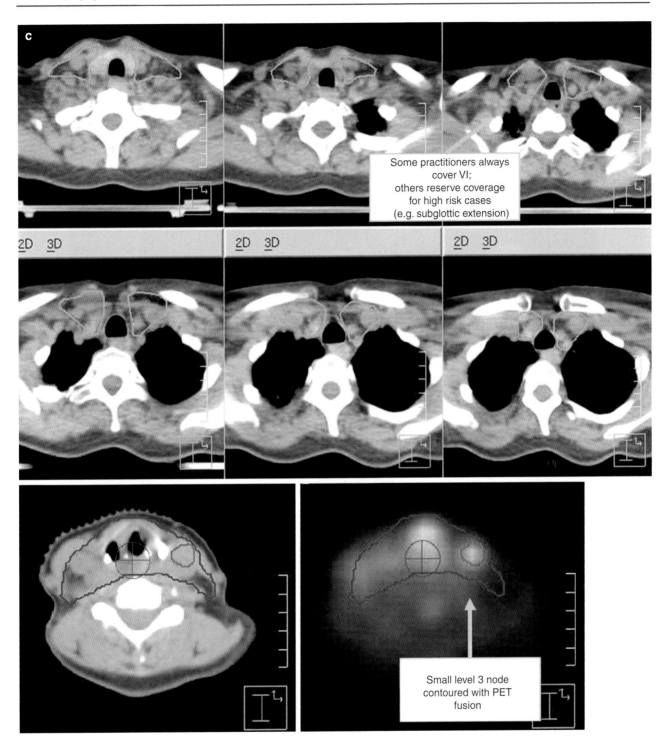

**Fig. 2** (continued)

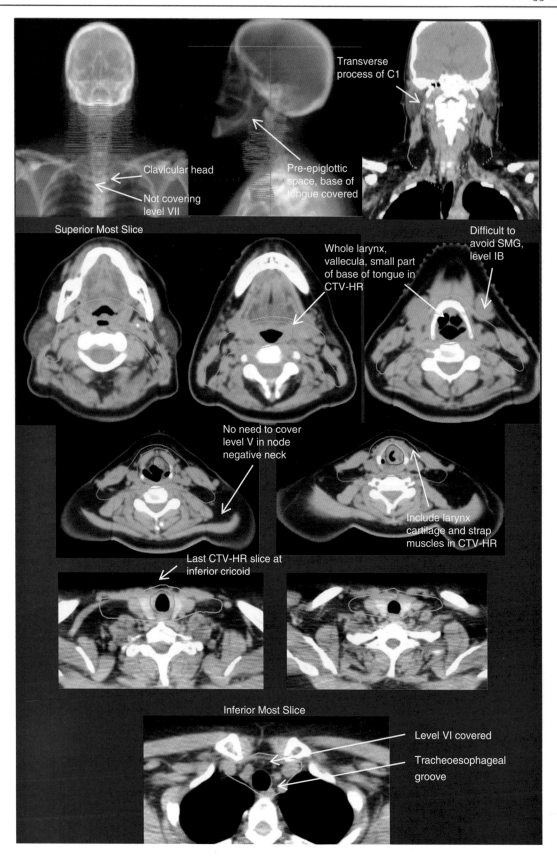

**Fig. 3** T3N0M0 supraglottic squamous cell carcinoma of the larynx. IMRT was required because target straddles the shoulders. Case illustrates bilateral parotid sparing. A two-volume approach was taken. Levels II–IV are covered as well as level VI and part of level IB. GTV is in *red*. CTV70 is in *green*. PTV54 is in *blue*

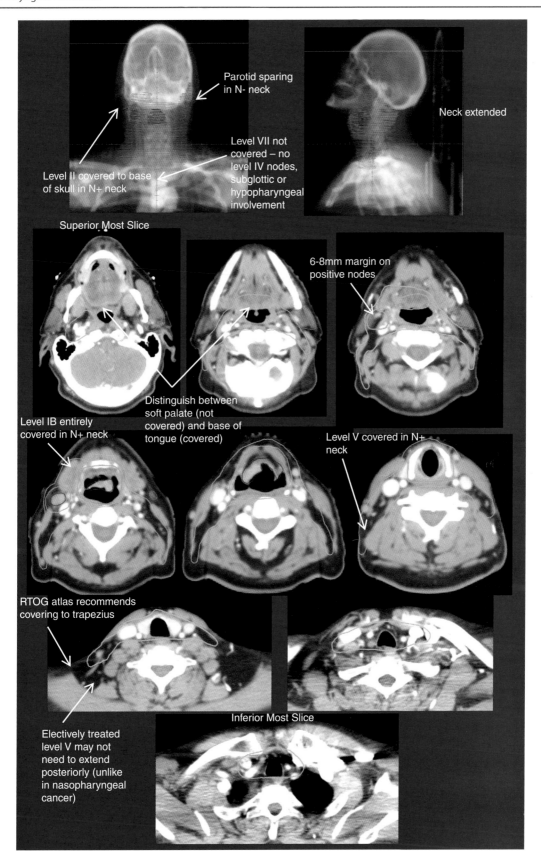

**Fig. 4** T3N1M0 supraglottic squamous cell carcinoma of the larynx. A two-volume approach was taken. Levels II–IV are covered as well as ipsilateral level V and IB on the involved side. Level VI is covered. Though this patient is node positive, level VII is not covered because there was no subglottic extension, hypopharyngeal involvement, or level IV nodes. GTV is in *red*. CTV70 is in *green*. PTV54 is in *blue*. L parotid gland is in *orange*

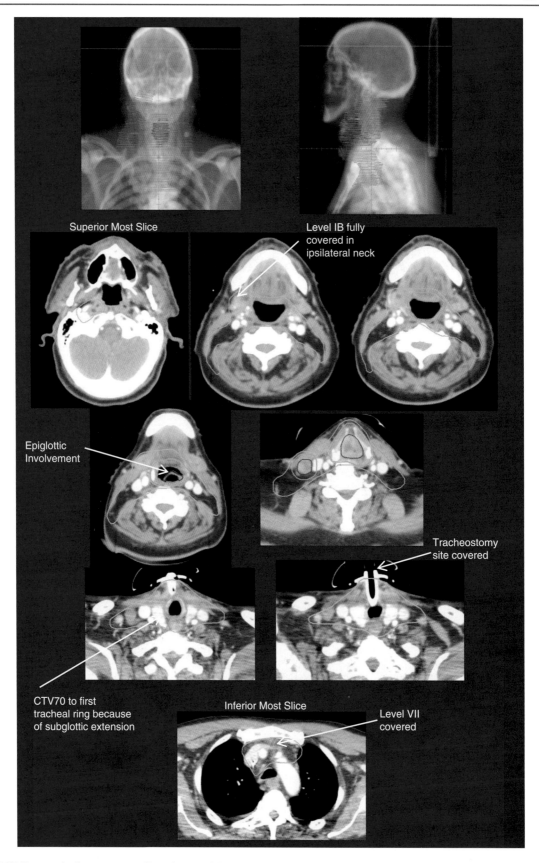

**Fig. 5** T3N1M0 supraglottic squamous cell carcinoma of the larynx with subglottic extension. A two-volume approach is taken. Due to the history of a need for an emergent tracheostomy and because of large tumor bulk, this patient should have ideally undergone a total laryngectomy. However, due to hypercarbic respiratory failure, the patient was not a candidate for surgery. Case illustrates coverage of the tracheostomy site. Levels II–IV, ipsilateral V and IB, and level VI are covered. In contrast to Fig. 4, level VII is covered because of the subglottic extension. GTV is in *red*. CTV70 is in *green*. PTV54 is in *blue*

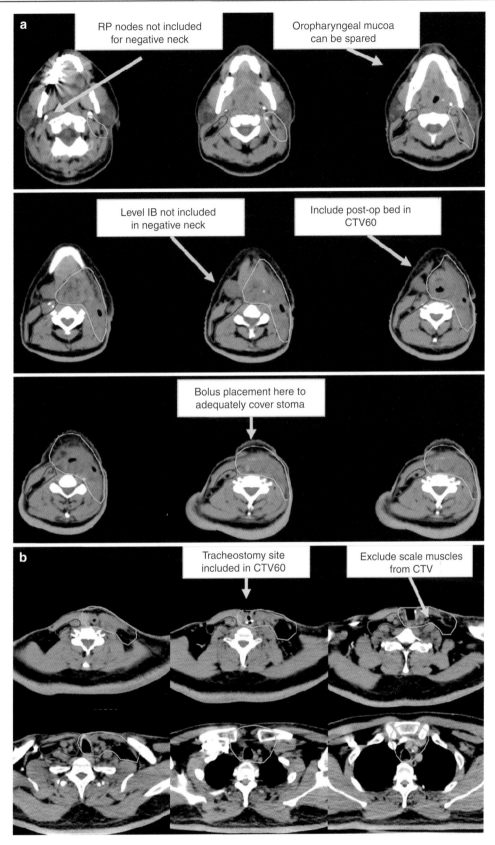

**Fig. 6** (**a**, **b**) Axial slices with contours drawn. pT4N0M0 squamous cell carcinoma of the left glottis status total laryngectomy and left neck dissection. In the postoperative setting, the high-risk CTV (operative bed) receives 60 Gy in 2 Gy/fraction and the low-risk CTV receives 54 Gy in 2 Gy/fraction. *Blue* CTV 54, *green* CTV 60

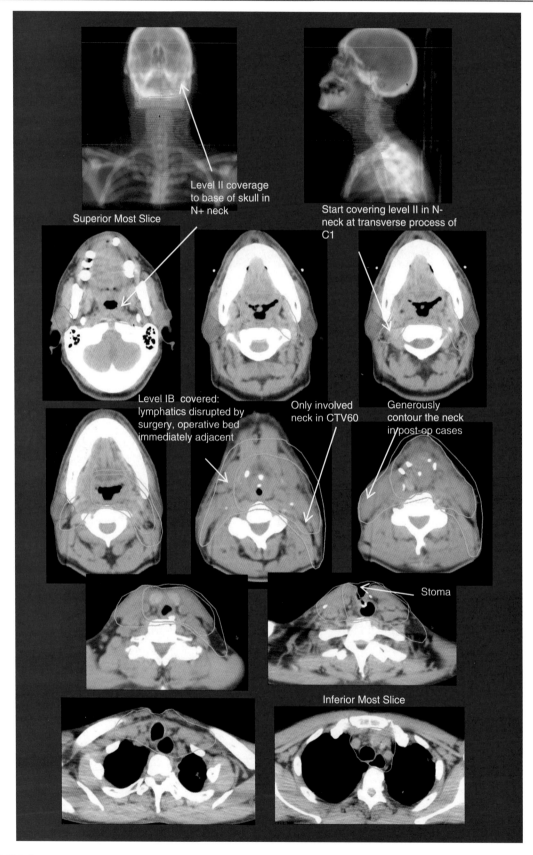

**Fig. 7** T3N2bM0 squamous cell carcinoma of the supraglottis larynx. Pathology indicates close margins (4 mm), +LVSI, 2 positive left level II nodes with no ECE. CTV60 includes the operative bed, the involved level II nodal region, and the stoma. Level II is covered ipsilaterally to base of skull. CTV60 is in *green*. CTV54 is in *blue*. The R parotid gland is contoured in *orange*

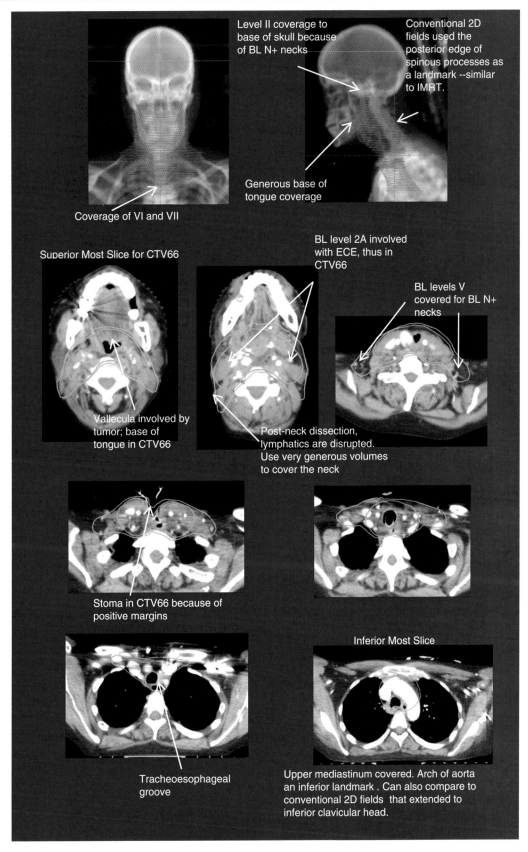

**Fig. 8** pT4aN2cM0 squamous cell carcinoma of the supraglottic larynx that involved the vallecula/base of tongue and hypopharynx. Close margins; bilateral level 2A nodes with extracapsular extension. CTV66 is in *green*. CTV60 in *blue*. 66 Gy was used because of the ECE and close margins. Bilateral level II treated to the base of skull. Lower level II included in 66 Gy volume because of ECE

## Suggested Reading

VA Larynx Trial. Foundational trial for organ preserving radiation in advanced laryngeal cancer (The Department of Veterans Affairs Laryngeal Cancer Study Group 1991)

RTOG 91-11. Chemoradiation for laryngeal cancer and other subsites of head and neck (Forastiere et al. 2013)

RTOG contouring atlas (Gregoire et al. 2003)

RTOG 1216 protocol. Current RTOG trial for post-operative radiation in head and neck cancer

Debate about organ preservation versus total laryngectomy (Olsen 2010)

## References

Baujat B, Bourhis J, Blanchard P, et al (2010) Hyperfractionated or accelerated radiotherapy for head and neck cancer. The Cochrane Database Syst Rev 12:CD002026. doi: 10.1002/14651858.CD002026

Buckley JG, MacLennan K (2000) Cervical node metastases in laryngeal and hypopharyngeal cancer: a prospective analysis of prevalence and distribution. Head Neck 22:380–385

Candela FC, Shah J, Jaques DP, Shah JP (1990) Patterns of cervical node metastases from squamous carcinoma of the larynx. Arch Otolaryngol Head Neck Surg 116:432–435

Dagan R, Morris CG, Bennett JA et al (2007) Prognostic significance of paraglottic space invasion in T2N0 glottic carcinoma. Am J Clin Oncol 30:186–190

Forastiere AA, Zhang Q, Weber RS et al (2013) Long-term results of RTOG 91-11: a comparison of three nonsurgical treatment strategies to preserve the larynx in patients with locally advanced larynx cancer. J Clin Oncol 31:845–852

Gregoire V, Levendag P, Ang KK et al (2003) CT-based delineation of lymph node levels and related CTVs in the node-negative neck: DAHANCA, EORTC, GORTEC, NCIC, RTOG consensus guidelines. Radiother Oncol 69:227–236

Induction chemotherapy plus radiation compared with surgery plus radiation in patients with advanced laryngeal cancer. The Department of Veterans Affairs Laryngeal Cancer Study Group (1991) N Engl J Med 324:1685–1690

Lindberg R (1972) Distribution of cervical lymph node metastases from squamous cell carcinoma of the upper respiratory and digestive tracts. Cancer 29:1446–1449

Mendenhall WM, Morris CG, Amdur RJ, Hinerman RW, Mancuso AA (2003) Parameters that predict local control after definitive radiotherapy for squamous cell carcinoma of the head and neck. Head Neck 25:535–542

Olsen KD (2010) Reexamining the treatment of advanced laryngeal cancer. Head Neck 32:1–7

Zhang B, Xu ZG, Tang PZ (2006) Elective lateral neck dissection for laryngeal cancer in the clinically negative neck. J Surg Oncol 93: 464–467

# Hypopharyngeal Carcinoma

Benjamin H. Lok, Gaorav P. Gupta, Nadeem Riaz,
Sean McBride, and Nancy Y. Lee

## Contents

B.H. Lok (✉) • G.P. Gupta • N. Riaz • S. McBride • N.Y. Lee
Department of Radiation Oncology,
Memorial Sloan Kettering Cancer Center,
New York, NY, USA
e-mail: mcbrides@mskcc.org; leen2@mskcc.org

## 1 Anatomy and Patterns of Spread

- The hypopharynx extends from the level of the hyoid bone to the inferiormost level of the cricoid cartilage. Anteriorly, the border is formed by the connection of the two pyriform sinuses at the postcricoid region and with the posterior extent defined by the posterior pharyngeal wall.
- The three subdivisions and their distribution of tumor involvement according to the SEER database, from 2000 to 2008, are the pyriform sinuses (83 %), posterior pharyngeal wall (9 %), and postcricoid region (4 %).
  - Pyriform sinus
    - "Pear-shaped" structure that begins superiorly at the glossoepiglottic fold with its apex extending inferiorly to the level of the cricopharyngeus. It is laterally bound by the thyroid cartilage and medially defined by the cricoid cartilages, arytenoids, and the lateral surface of the aryepiglottic fold.
      - Superiorly, cancers can invade the arytenoids and aryepiglottic folds as well as the paraglottic and preepiglottic space.
        - Involvement of thyrohyoid membrane, which surrounds the pyriform sinuses superiorly and where internal branch of superior laryngeal nerve passes through cause referred otalgia.
      - Laterally, tumors can invade into the segments of the thyroid cartilage and then further into the lateral neck compartments.
      - Medially, intrinsic laryngeal muscles can be involved causing vocal cord fixation.
      - Inferiorly, extension past the apex can involve the thyroid gland.
  - Posterior pharyngeal wall
    - Formed by the constrictor muscles and directly contacts the paravertebral fascia. Extends from hyoid bone to the inferior aspect of the cricoid.

N.Y. Lee et al. (eds.), *Target Volume Delineation for Conformal and Intensity-Modulated Radiation Therapy*,
Medical Radiology. Radiation Oncology, DOI: 10.1007/174_2014_987, © Springer International Publishing Switzerland 2014
Published Online: 22 October 2014

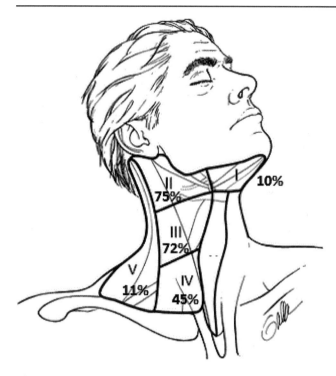

**Fig. 1** Distribution of nodal metastases by neck level based on radical neck dissections in 104 patients (Candela et al. 1990)

- Tumors can extend to involve the oropharynx superiorly, the prevertebral fascia and retropharyngeal space posteriorly, and the cervical esophagus inferiorly.
  - Postcricoid region
    - Extends from the posterior surface of the aryepiglottic fold and arytenoids to the cricoid cartilage.
      - Anteriorly, tumors can invade the larynx causing vocal cord fixation.
      - Radially, the cricoid cartilage can be involved.
      - Other areas at risk from advanced local extension are the esophagus, trachea, and pyriform sinuses.
- Dosimetric coverage of the primary site can be a challenge because hypopharyngeal cancers have a propensity for submucosal spread. Approximately 60 % microscopic spread of about 10 mm (superiorly), 20 mm (laterally and inferiorly), and 25 mm (medially) (Ho et al. 1993).
- The rich lymphatic network of the hypopharynx drains primarily into the jugulodigastric lymph nodes and middle jugular chains (see Fig. 1).
  - Pyriform sinuses drain primarily to the upper and middle jugular nodes, posterior cervical nodes, and retropharyngeal lymph nodes.
  - Posterior pharyngeal wall empties into the jugular nodes and retropharyngeal nodes (Allen et al. 2007).
  - Postcricoid region drains to the middle and lower jugular nodes and to the paratracheal nodes.

## 2 Diagnostic Workup Relevant for Target Volume Delineation

- Clinical examination with a thorough laryngoscopic evaluation is critical in defining the mucosal extent of hypopharyngeal cancers, particularly for those arising in the pyriform sinus.
- MRI may better delineate primary tumor borders, inform regarding potential cartilage or esophageal invasion, and may also facilitate identification of abnormally enhancing lymph nodes (Castelijns et al. 1988; Roychowdhury et al. 2000; Rumboldt et al. 2006; Wenig et al. 1995).
- The sensitivity and specificity of PET are superior to CT alone (Di Martino et al. 2000). FDG-PET provides metabolic information and may identify hypermetabolic cancer cells within morphologically normal-appearing lymph nodes (Adams et al. 1998; Schwartz et al. 2005), which should be included within the high-dose PTV.

## 3 Simulation and Daily Localization

- CT simulation using 3-mm slice thickness with IV contrast is used (unless medically contraindicated) to delineate the primary tumor, gross lymphadenopathy, and additional regions at risk. The simulation scan should extend from the top of the skull to the carina with the isocenter generally placed immediately above the arytenoids.
- The patient should be immobilized with a 5-point thermoplastic head and neck mask or with a 3-point thermoplastic head and neck mask and a shoulder pull board. The neck should be maximally hyperextended to pull as much of the oral cavity and mandible out of the field as possible, and the shoulders should be pulled inferiorly to minimize the risk of beam interference.

## 4 Target Volume Delineation and Treatment Planning

- Due to concerns regarding treatment-related late toxicities, hypofractionation and/or simultaneous integrated boost with IMRT is not recommended for this disease site.
- We utilize dose-painting IMRT (Lee et al. 2007) and prescribe to 70 Gy in 2 Gy fractions to sites of gross disease, 59.5 Gy in 1.7 Gy fractions to high-risk subclinical regions, and 56 Gy in 1.6 Gy fractions to lower-risk subclinical regions. Additional fractionation regimens as well as cone-down IMRT approaches are also appropriate.
- We routinely use all-in-one IMRT for hypopharynx cancers, as a match line to a low anterior neck field would

**Table 1** Suggested target volumes at the gross disease region

| Target volumes | Definition and description |
|---|---|
| $GTV_{70}$[a] (the subscript denotes the total radiation dose prescribed, in Gy) | Primary: all gross disease on physical examination and imaging<br>Neck nodes: all nodes $\geq 1$ cm in short axis; grossly abnormal as well as suspicious lymph nodes should be contoured as GTV |
| $CTV_{70}$[a] | Usually the same as $GTV_{70}$ (no need to add margin); if a margin is needed due to uncertainty of macroscopic disease, add 5 mm so that $GTV_{70} + 5$ mm $= CTV_{70}$<br>For suspicious nodes that are small (i.e., $\leq 1$ cm), a lower dose of 66 Gy may be considered |
| $PTV_{70}$[a] | $CTV_{70} + 10$ mm for the primary tumor, depending on comfort level of daily patient positioning. Hypopharynx structures are highly mobile, so we do not recommend smaller PTV margins. An exception might be posterior pharyngeal wall disease, where posterior expansion margins are minimized due to decreased motion in that direction and to maintain adequate separation from the spinal cord<br>$CTV_{70} + 3$–$5$ mm for lymph nodes, depending on precision of daily positioning |

[a]Suggested dose to gross disease is 2 Gy/fraction to 70 Gy

**Table 2** Suggested target volumes at the high-risk subclinical region: primary tumor expansion and N+neck

| Target volumes | Definition and description |
|---|---|
| $CTV_{59.5}$[a] | Primary: the $CTV_{59.5}$ should encompass the entire $CTV_{70}$ with at least 1-cm margin and should include the entire subsite of the involved hypopharynx as well as adjacent superior and inferior structures. Potential directions of microscopic mucosal and submucosal spread should be considered and targeted. The larynx (from hyoid to cricoid) is at high risk for subclinical disease and should be included in the $CTV_{59.5}$. Adjacent fat spaces, such as the preepiglottic fat and prevertebral fascia, should be included in this high-risk region<br>Neck nodes: CTV59.5 should encompass at least 3-mm margin on $CTV_{70}$ lymph node regions. Include ipsilateral cervical LN levels Ib–IV as well as the lateral retropharyngeal lymph nodes. If there is gross adenopathy in levels II–IV, coverage of ipsilateral level V should be considered. For postcricoid and posterior pharyngeal wall tumors that are close to midline, the same RT dose may be prescribed to both sides of the neck. For an N+neck, retropharyngeal lymph node coverage should extend superiorly to the entrance of the carotid canal at the skull base. Similarly, upper level II lymph nodes in the retrostyloid space should also be included in the target volume, superior to the level where the posterior belly of the digastric muscle crosses over the internal jugular vein. Inferior hypopharyngeal cancers that involve the postcricoid region mandate coverage of the paratracheal lymph nodes in the superior mediastinum as well<br>Any tissue that lies between the primary tumor and level III–IV lymphadenopathy should be contoured in the $CTV_{59.5}$, as it is at high risk for submucosal microscopic invasion |
| $PTV_{59.5}$[a] | $CTV_{59.5} + 3$–$5$ mm, depending on comfort level of daily patient positioning |

[a]Example high-risk subclinical dose: 1.7 Gy/fraction to 59.5 Gy

**Table 3** Suggested target volumes at the lower-risk subclinical region

| Target volumes | Definition and description |
|---|---|
| $CTV_{56}$[a] | The $CTV_{56}$ should include lymph node levels II–IV and retropharyngeal LNs in the N0 neck. The only exception is for midline tumors, where an N0 neck might also be considered high risk if there is contralateral nodal disease. For the contralateral N0 neck considered lower risk, the superior extent of level II coverage need not extend beyond where the posterior belly of the digastric muscle crosses over the internal jugular vein. Similarly, coverage of the superior retropharyngeal nodes in the contralateral N0 neck can terminate at the level of the C1 vertebral body |
| $PTV_{56}$[a] | $CTV_{56} + 3$–$5$ mm, depending on comfort level of daily patient positioning |

[a]Example lower-risk subclinical dose: 1.6 Gy/fraction to 56 Gy

frequently fall in the region of the primary tumor or involved lymph nodes.

- Suggested treatment target volumes for gross disease (Table 1), high-risk subclinical (Table 2), and lower-risk subclinical regions (Table 3) are described in the following tables. The principles of target delineation are similar for early and advanced stages (Figs. 2 vs 3, 4, and 5). Shown here are examples of each subsite: pyriform sinus (Figs. 2 and 3), posterior pharyngeal wall (Fig. 4), and postcricoid region (Fig. 5).

## 5 Plan Assessment

- Coverage should attempt to achieve at least 95 % of the volume of the $PTV_{70}$ receiving prescription dose. The minimum dose to 99 % of the $CTV_{70}$ should be >65.1 Gy. The maximum dose received by 0.03 cc of the $PTV_{70}$ should be <80.5 Gy.
- We typically prioritize normal structure constraints, particularly critical structures. Below are suggested dose constraints utilized at our center (Table 4).

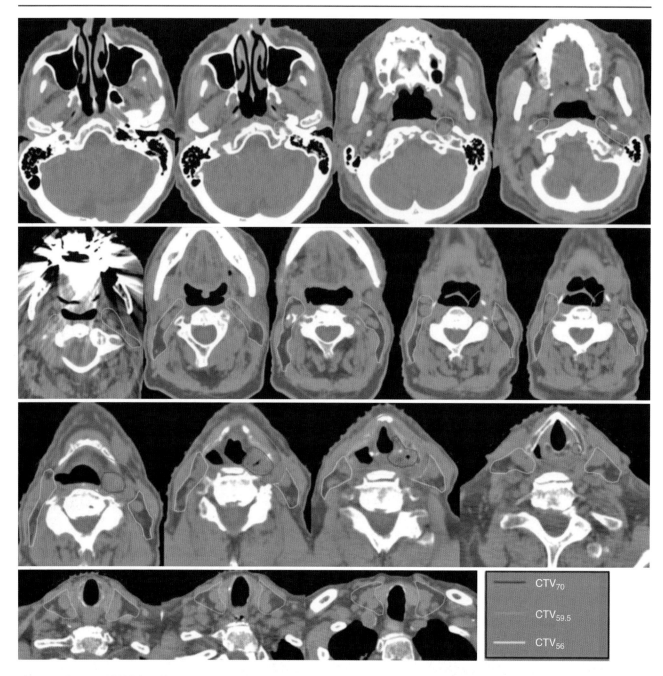

**Fig. 2** Early-stage T2N0 left pyriform sinus HNSCC. The principles of targeting early-stage hypopharyngeal cancers are shared among all subsites. It is critical to perform multiple imaging studies including CT with IV contrast, MRI, and/or PET to confirm with highest certainty that there is no detectable nodal disease. For high confidence cN0 disease, the bilateral neck may receive the lower-risk RT dose, e.g., 56 Gy

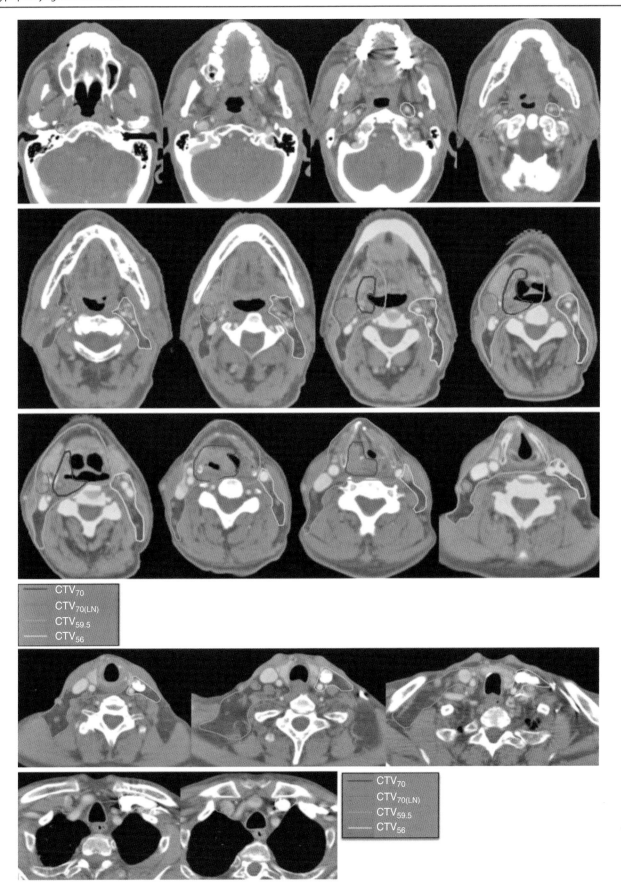

**Fig. 3** Advanced-stage T2N2b pyriform sinus HNSCC. Similar principles are used to delineate IMRT targeting for all subsites of advanced-stage hypopharyngeal cancer. Inferior tumors involving the postcricoid region must include the paratracheal LNs of the superior mediastinum as well as consideration of the central compartment of the neck in the high-risk subclinical treatment volume. It is important that targeting of the N+neck extends superiorly to the base of skull

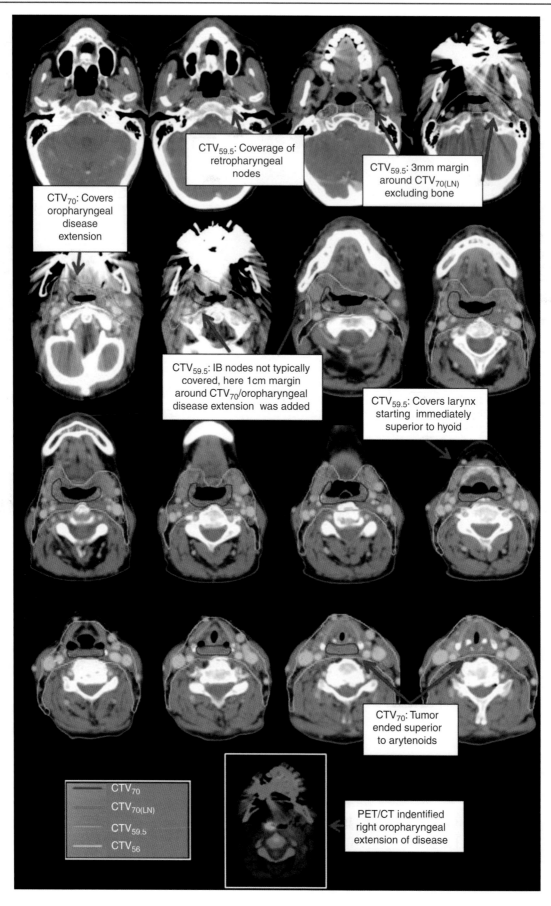

**Fig. 4** Advanced-stage T3N2a posterior pharyngeal wall HNSCC. PET/CT identified right oropharyngeal extension with additional FDG-avid disease in a left retropharyngeal node; left level II, III, and IV cervical nodes; and a right level II cervical node. Though contoured here, level V nodes are not routinely treated at our center, but at the discretion of the prescribing physician

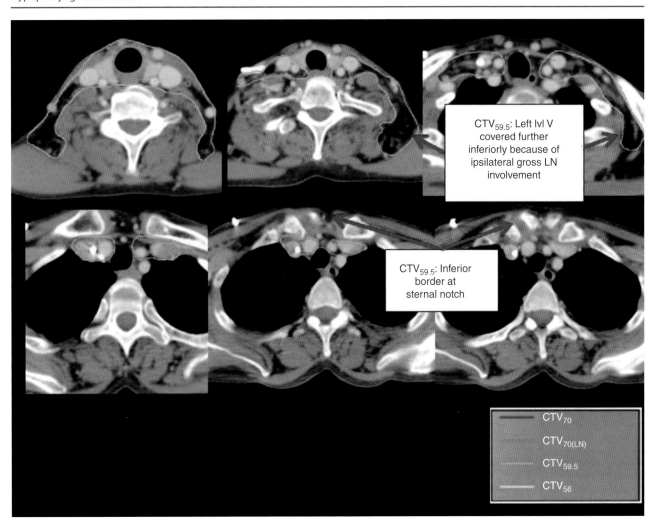

CTV$_{59.5}$: Left lvl V covered further inferiorly because of ipsilateral gross LN involvement

CTV$_{59.5}$: Inferior border at sternal notch

CTV$_{70}$
CTV$_{70(LN)}$
CTV$_{59.5}$
CTV$_{56}$

**Fig. 4** (continued)

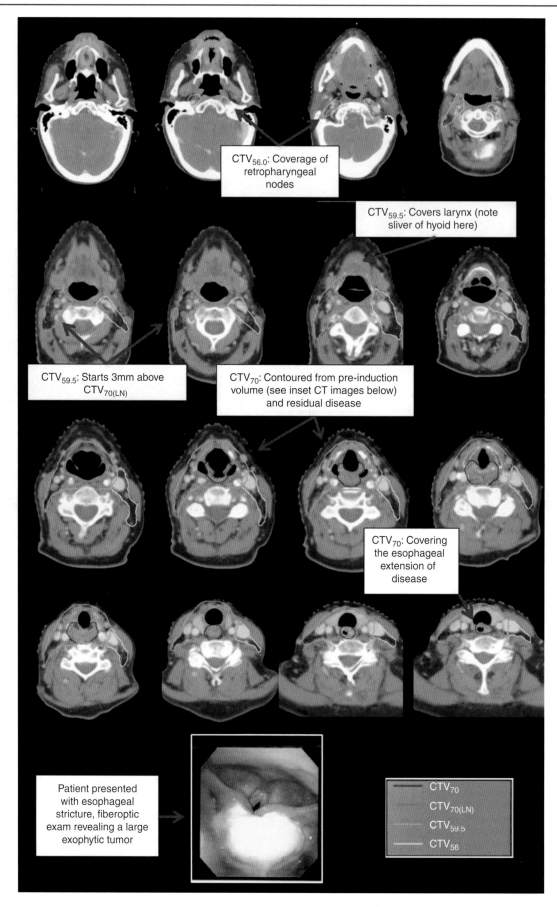

**Fig. 5** Advanced-stage T3N1 postcricoid HNSCC who underwent induction chemotherapy. A large exophytic tumor was appreciated on fiber-optic examination. CTV was contoured from the preinduction CT and PET imaging. PET demonstrated esophageal extension, which was included in the CTV

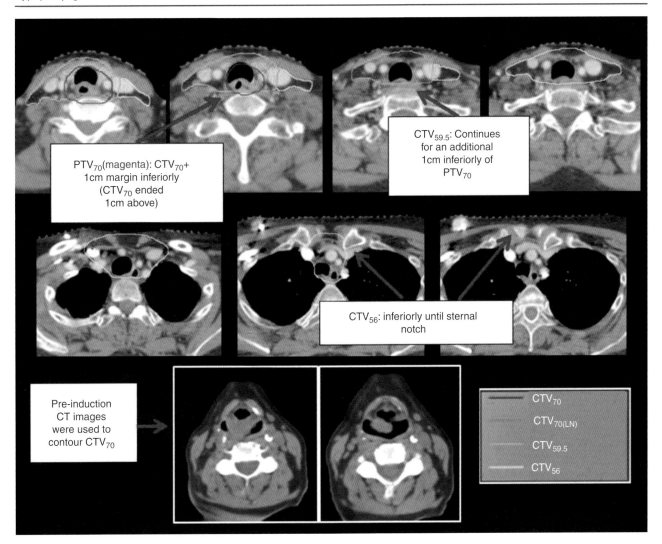

**Fig. 5** (continued)

**Table 4** Intensity-modulated radiation therapy: normal tissue dose constraints

| Critical structures | Constraints |
|---|---|
| Brainstem | Max < 54 Gy or 1 % of PTV cannot exceed 60 Gy |
| Optic nerves | Max < 54 Gy or 1 % of PTV cannot exceed 60 Gy |
| Optic chiasm | Max < 54 Gy or 1 % of PTV cannot exceed 60 Gy |
| Spinal cord | Max < 45 Gy or 1 cc of the PTV cannot exceed 50 Gy |
| Mandible and TMJ | Max < 70 Gy or 1 cc of the PTV cannot exceed 75 Gy |
| Brachial plexus | Max < 65 Gy |
| Temporal lobes | Max < 60 Gy or 1 % of PTV cannot exceed 65 Gy |
| Other normal structures | Constraints |
| Oral cavity | Mean ≤ 40 Gy |
| Parotid gland | (a) Mean ≤ 26 Gy in one gland |
| | (b) Or at least 20 cc of the combined volume of both parotid glands will receive < 20 Gy |
| | (c) Or at least 50 % of one gland will receive < 30 Gy |
| Submandibular gland | Mean ≤ 39 Gy |
| Cochlea | (a) Max ≤ 50 Gy |
| | (b) V55 < 5 %, if max dose constraint not possible |
| Eyes | Mean < 35 Gy, max < 50 Gy |
| Lens | Max < 5 Gy |

*PTV* planning target volume
Based on guidelines presently used at Memorial Sloan Kettering Cancer Center

## Suggested Reading

EORTC 24891 (Lefebvre et al. 1996): Demonstrated laryngeal preservation and equivalent overall survival with induction chemotherapy followed by radiotherapy when compared to surgery followed by radiotherapy for pyriform sinus and aryepiglottic fold cancers

Lee et al. (2007): Concurrent chemotherapy with IMRT experience at MSKCC for laryngeal and hypopharyngeal carcinoma

Prades et al. (2010): Phase III trial demonstrating increased survival in concurrent chemoradiotherapy for pyriform sinus carcinoma when compared to induction chemotherapy

RTOG neck contouring atlas (Gregoire et al. 2003)

## References

Adams S, Baum RP, Stuckensen T et al (1998) Prospective comparison of 18 F-FDG PET with conventional imaging modalities (CT, MRI, US) in lymph node staging of head and neck cancer. Eur J Nucl Med 25(9):1255–1260

Allen AM, Haddad RI, Tishler RB (2007) Retropharyngeal nodes in hypopharynx cancer on positron emission tomography. J Clin Oncol 25(5):599–601

Candela FC, Kothari K, Shah JP (1990) Patterns of cervical node metastases from squamous carcinoma of the oropharynx and hypopharynx. Head Neck 12(3):197–203

Castelijns JA, Gerritsen GJ, Kaiser MC et al (1988) Invasion of laryngeal cartilage by cancer: comparison of CT and MR imaging. Radiology 167(1):199–206

Di Martino E, Nowak B, Hassan HA et al (2000) Diagnosis and staging of head and neck cancer: a comparison of modern imaging modalities (positron emission tomography, computed tomography, color-coded duplex sonography) with panendoscopic and histopathologic findings. Arch Otolaryngol Head Neck Surg 126(12):1457–1461

Gregoire V, Levendag P, Ang KK et al (2003) CT-based delineation of lymph node levels and related CTVs in the node-negative neck: DAHANCA, EORTC, GORTEC, NCIC, RTOG consensus guidelines. Radiother Oncol 69(3):227–236

Ho CM, Lam KH, Wei WI et al (1993) Squamous cell carcinoma of the hypopharynx–analysis of treatment results. Head Neck 15(5):405–412

Lee NY, O'Meara W, Chan K et al (2007) Concurrent chemotherapy and intensity-modulated radiotherapy for locoregionally advanced laryngeal and hypopharyngeal cancers. Int J Radiat Oncol Biol Phys 69(2):459–468

Lefebvre JL, Chevalier D, Luboinski B et al (1996) Larynx preservation in pyriform sinus cancer: preliminary results of a European Organization for Research and Treatment of Cancer phase III trial. EORTC Head and Neck Cancer Cooperative Group. J Natl Cancer Inst 88(13):890–899

Prades JM, Lallemant B, Garrel R et al (2010) Randomized phase III trial comparing induction chemotherapy followed by radiotherapy to concomitant chemoradiotherapy for laryngeal preservation in T3M0 pyriform sinus carcinoma. Acta Otolaryngol 130(1):150–155

Roychowdhury S, Loevner LA, Yousem DM et al (2000) MR imaging for predicting neoplastic invasion of the cervical esophagus. AJNR Am J Neuroradiol 21(9):1681–1687

Rumboldt Z, Gordon L, Gordon L et al (2006) Imaging in head and neck cancer. Curr Treat Options Oncol 7(1):23–34

Schwartz DL, Ford E, Rajendran J et al (2005) FDG-PET/CT imaging for preradiotherapy staging of head-and-neck squamous cell carcinoma. Int J Radiat Oncol Biol Phys 61(1):129–136

Wenig BL, Ziffra KL, Mafee MF et al (1995) MR imaging of squamous cell carcinoma of the larynx and hypopharynx. Otolaryngol Clin North Am 28(3):609–619

# Carcinoma of the Paranasal Sinuses

Daniel E. Spratt and Nancy Y. Lee

## Contents

D.E. Spratt, MD (✉) • N.Y. Lee, MD
Memorial Sloan Kettering Cancer Center,
New York, 10065, NY
e-mail: leen2@mskcc.org

## 1   Anatomy

- The paranasal sinuses are composed of seven bones (ethmoid, maxilla, palatine, lacrimal, pterygoid plate of sphenoid, nasal, and inferior turbinate), four paired sinuses (frontal, ethmoid, maxillary, and sphenoid), and complex networks of nervous, vascular, and lymphatic structures.

## 2   Patterns of Spread

- Paranasal sinus cancers often spread via local extension into adjacent sinuses and bony structures. The paranasal sinuses (and nasal cavity) are all interconnected via multiple ostia and are separated by thin septi allowing for invasion into adjacent air cavities.
  - Maxillary Sinus (as a representative example):
    - Medial infrastructure lesions invade the nasal cavity early via the porous medial wall.
    - Lateral infrastructure lesions erode the lateral wall of the antrum and may present as a submucosal mass in the maxillary gingiva.
    - Posterior infrastructure lesions may invade the infratemporal fossa or extend into the pterygopalatine fossa and pterygoid plates. These lesions may invade the orbit by direct superior extension or via extension into the ethmoids.
    - Suprastructure lesions spread either laterally, invading the malar process of the maxilla and the zygoma, or medially, invading the nasal cavity and ethmoid sinuses.
- Involvement of nerve branches (see Table 1) by tumor often leads to numbness and paresthesias in the skin and mucous membranes of this region. It is of critical importance if cranial nerve involvement is present to cover the involved nerve(s) back to the skull base.

N.Y. Lee et al. (eds.), *Target Volume Delineation for Conformal and Intensity-Modulated Radiation Therapy*,
Medical Radiology. Radiation Oncology, DOI: 10.1007/174_2014_1006, © Springer International Publishing Switzerland 2014
Published Online: 22 October 2014

**Table 1** Anatomy of paranasal sinuses

| Sinus | Overview and boundaries | Blood supply and innervation |
|---|---|---|
| Frontal | Located in the frontal bone superior to the orbits in the forehead | Supraorbital and supratrochlear arteries of the ophthalmic artery |
| | Funnel-shaped structure | Supraorbital and supratrochlear nerves of the first division of the trigeminal nerve |
| | An upward extension of anterior ethmoid cells | |
| | The posterior wall separates the sinus from the anterior cranial fossa. The floor is formed from the upper part of the orbit | |
| Sphenoid | Located in the sphenoid bone at the center of the head | Sphenopalatine artery (and branches), except for the planum sphenoidale, which is supplied by the posterior ethmoidal artery |
| | Closely related to many critical structures: pituitary gland, superiorly; optic nerve and carotid artery, laterally; and nerve(s) of the pterygoid canal at the floor | Branches of the first and second divisions of the trigeminal nerve |
| | May extend as far as the foramen magnum | |
| Maxillary | Pyramidal shaped (the base is along the nasal wall and the apex points laterally toward the zygoma) | Branches of the internal maxillary artery (infraorbital, alveolar, greater palatine, and sphenopalatine arteries) |
| | The roof is the floor of the orbit. The floor is made from the alveolar process of the maxilla and hard palate | Branches of the second division of the trigeminal nerve, the infraorbital nerve, and the greater palatine nerves |
| | Behind the posteromedial wall of this sinus lays the pterygopalatine fossa (houses important neurovascular structures and communicates with skull base foramina) | |
| | The infratemporal fossa lies behind the posterolateral wall of the maxillary sinus | |
| Ethmoid | Located in the ethmoid bone, forming multiple air cells (~6–15) between the eyes | Anterior and posterior ethmoidal arteries from the ophthalmic artery (internal carotid system), as well as by the sphenopalatine artery from the terminal branches of the internal maxillary artery (external carotid system) |
| | The ethmoid cells are shaped like pyramids and are divided by thin septa | V1 supplies the more superior aspect with V2 innervating the inferior regions. Parasympathetic innervation is via the Vidian nerve |
| | Bordered by the middle turbinate medially and the medial orbital wall laterally. The roof is formed from frontal bones anteriorly, and the sphenoid and orbital process of palatine bones posteriorly | |

- Lymphatic drainage of the paranasal sinuses is thought to have limited capillary lymphatic supply. Hence, the frequency of lymph node involvement is low, unless the tumor involves adjacent areas with extensive lymphatic supply (the nasal cavity, nasopharynx, or skin).
  - Ten percent of patients present with cervical lymph node involvement, and an additional 10–15 % develop cervical neck lymph node metastases.

## 3 Diagnostic Workup Relevant for Target Volume Delineation

- Physical examination: bimanual palpation of the orbit, oral and nasal cavities, and nasopharynx and direct fiberoptic endoscopy. Neurologic examination should emphasize cranial nerve function, because nasal cavity and paranasal sinus tumors can be associated with cranial nerve palsies, especially of the trigeminal branches. Cervical lymph nodes should be palpated for adenopathy.
- Imaging has essentially replaced surgical exploration for staging and tumor mapping in this region. The most useful studies are computed tomography (CT) and magnetic resonance imaging (MRI). CT defines early cortical bone erosion more clearly, whereas MRI better delineates soft tissue. CT performs better than MRI in evaluating thin bony structures, such as paranasal sinuses and orbita. MRI may demonstrate subtle perineural spread and involvement of the cranial nerve foramen and canals.
- Paranasal sinus tumors are best approached using endoscopic sinus surgery instruments or by an open transcutaneous or transoral procedure. Caldwell-Luc procedures have been used to gain access to the maxillary antrum.

## 4 Simulation and Daily Localization

- Set up the patient in supine position with head extended. The immobilization device should include at least the head and neck. If possible, shoulders should also be immobilized to ensure accurate patient setup on a daily basis especially when an extended-field IMRT plan is used. A bite block can be placed during simulation and throughout radiation to push the tongue away from the high-dose nasopharynx region.

- CT simulation using 3 mm thickness with IV contrast should be performed to help guide the GTV target, particularly for the lymph nodes. We typically recommend a simulation scan from the top of the head including the brain to the carina. 5 mm thickness can be reconstructed below the clavicle to the level of the carina. The isocenter is typically placed just above the arytenoids.

- Image registration and fusion applications with MRI and PET scans should be used to help in the delineation of target volumes, especially for regions of interest encompassing the GTV, skull base, brain stem, and optic chiasm. The GTV and CTV and normal tissues should be outlined on all CT slices in which the structures exist.

## 5 General Principles of Target Delineation

- The surgical approach (midfacial degloving, lateral rhinotomy, craniofacial, or endoscopic) can complicate the radiation field. If a craniofacial resection has been performed, the frontal graft should be included in the target volume. Fiducial markers implanted during surgery can help to delineate the tumor bed.

- Preoperative CT and MRI should be evaluated to ensure that the initial tumor volume is covered in the high-risk

CTV. Detailed description of the surgical procedure and pathology report is mandatory to properly define the CTV that should encompass all initial sites of disease and the subclinical tumor spread. MRI should be used in all cases to help delineation of the tumor unless medically contraindicated.

- Adenoid cystic carcinomas are highly neurotrophic so radiotherapy volumes must encompass the afferent and efferent local nerves to the skull base. Esthesioneuroblastomas arise in the superior nasal cavity and in their early stages tend to invade the cribriform plate and anterior cranial fossa, and therefore, these regions should be encompassed in the target volume.

- Lymph node metastases are unusual, so elective treatment of the neck is not mandatory but can be done at the discretion of the treating physician. However, elective neck irradiation should be considered for esthesioneuroblastoma; high-grade, high-stage squamous cell carcinoma, especially if originating from the maxillary sinus or there is invasion of the mucosa of the palate or of the nasopharynx; when there is involvement of the skin of the cheek or of the anterior nose; and invasion of the maxillary gingiva or the alveolus. Depending on the clinical situation, cover either ipsilateral or bilateral levels Ib–IV. The need to include level V is determined by the location of the primary (i.e., level V should be encompassed in ethmoid carcinomas invading the nasopharynx).

- Suggested target volumes at the gross disease, high- and low-risk regions are detailed in Tables 2 and 3.

**Table 2** Suggested target volumes for gross disease

| Target volumes | Definition and description |
| --- | --- |
| GTV$_{70}$ | All gross disease on physical examination and imaging (CT and MRI). PET can help further define the tumor extent |
| CTV$_{70}$ | Usually same as GTV$_{70}$. If a margin is needed due to uncertainness during gross disease delineation, add 3–5 mm so that GTV$_{70}$+3–5 mm=CTV$_{70}$ |
| PTV$_{70}$ | CTV$_{70}$+3–5 mm depending on comfort level and can be as small as 1 mm when near critical normal structures |

**Table 3** Suggested target volumes at the high- and low-risk subclinical regions

|  | Definition and description | |
|---|---|---|
| Target volumes | Ethmoid | Maxillary |
| $CTV_{66}$ | Tumor implantation area or microscopically affected margins | |
| $CTV_{60}$ | The $CTV_{60}$ should encompass the areas at high risk of microscopic tumor spread from initial macroscopic tumor. Although the $CTV_{60}$ has to be defined in a case-by-case evaluation, the general proposed limits are: | |
|  | *Superior*: if the cribriform plate has not been resected, it should be included for ethmoid sinus tumors; if it has been resected, the $CTV_{60}$ should encompass the dura or the dural graft, extending at least 10 mm superior to the cribriform plate, or encompass the initial gross tumor volume | |
|  | *Inferior*: the inferior turbinate; if the inferior border of the tumor allows a 10 mm margin around the original disease, then the entire hard palate does not need to be included | *Inferior*: the inferior border of the maxilla and the hard palate but should encompass a 10 mm margin around the initial gross disease |
|  | *Lateral*: the nasal cavity, ethmoid sinuses, and the ipsilateral maxillary sinus and when indicated the volume should extend to the rectus muscle | *Lateral*: medial aspect should be the nasal septum, unless violation of midline structures occurs |
|  | *Posterior*: include the sphenoid sinus. The retropharyngeal lymph nodes should be encompassed if the tumor extended close to the nasopharynx or if there are metastatic neck nodes from an ethmoidal carcinoma | *Posterior*: the pterygopalatine and the infratemporal fossa should be included, paying special attention to encompass the masticator space and the infraorbital fissure |
| $PTV_{66}$[a] | CTV66 + 3–5 mm, depending on comfort level of daily patient positioning. Image guidance is recommended to reduce random and systematic setup errors. The PTV can be further modified to produce expansions as small as 1 mm in areas adjacent to critical normal structures | |
| $PTV_{60}$[a] | CTV60 + 3–5 mm, depending on comfort level of patient positioning but can be as small as 1 mm in areas adjacent to critical normal tissues | |

[a]High-risk subclinical dose: postoperatively, 2Gy/fraction to 60 Gy or 66 Gy (any region that has been surgically violated should be kept at least to 2Gy per fraction); for the nonsurgically violated neck or prophylactic cranial nerves coverage, can consider 1.8Gy/fraction to 54 Gy ($PTV_{54}$). In the radical setting when a simultaneous integrated boost is used with chemotherapy, the suggested doses are 1.8 Gy/fraction to 59.4 Gy and 1.64 Gy/fraction to 54 Gy. $PTV_{70}$ can be treated either in 2Gy or 2.12Gy/fraction

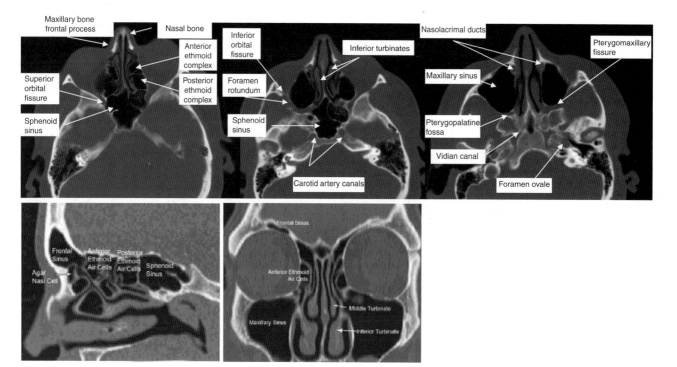

**Fig. 1** Representative normal anatomy from axial CT slices

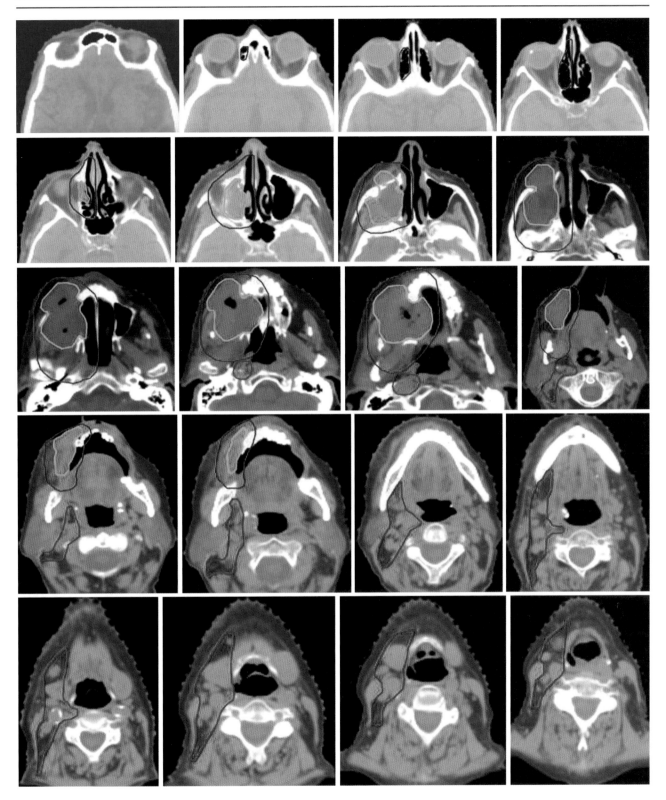

**Fig. 2** An example of a 91-year-old patient with a T4aN0 squamous cell carcinoma of the maxillary sinus. Patient refused surgery and was treated with definitive chemoradiation. The GTV is noted in *green color*, while the high-risk subclinical CTV is noted in *red color*. Only the ipsilateral neck was treated given the tumor involved only the right maxillary sinus and hard palate and his elderly age. The *pink color* shows the ipsilateral CTV nodal coverage

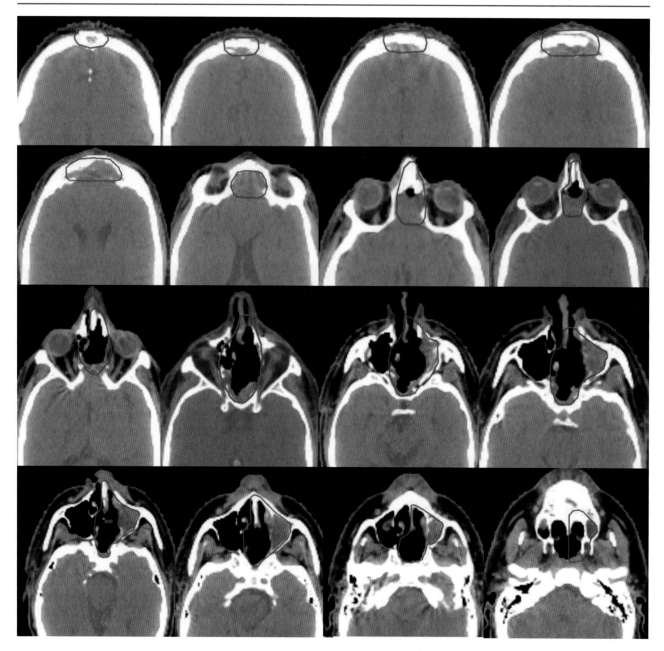

**Fig. 3** An example of a 43-year-old patient with a pT4aN0 squamous cell carcinoma of the ethmoid sinus. Patient is s/p ethmoidectomy, sphenoidectomy, nasal exenteration, and anterior craniotomy. Patient then received adjuvant chemoradiation. The CTV is noted in *pink color*. As this was a low-grade tumor with no neck involvement, no LN regions were treated

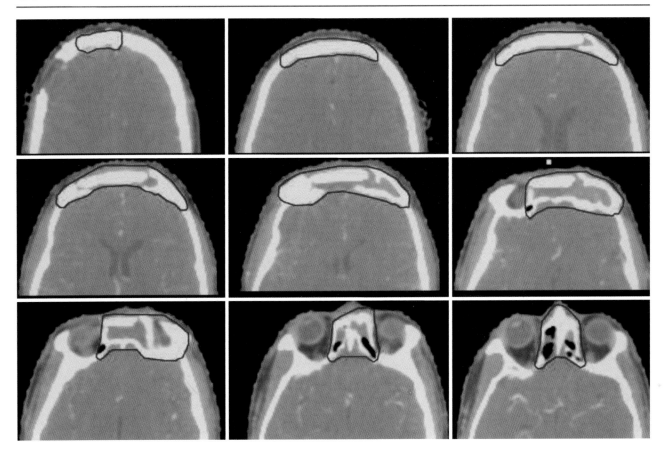

**Fig. 4** An example of a 36-year-old patient with a squamous cell carcinoma of the frontal sinus. Patient is s/p en bloc resection of frontal sinus with autologous calvarial graft with positive margins. Patient then received adjuvant radiation. The CTV is noted in *pink color*. As this was a well-differentiated tumor with no perineural invasion or neck involvement, no adjuvant chemotherapy or LN regions were treated

## References

Bristol IJ, Ahamad A, Garden AS et al (2007) Postoperative radiotherapy for maxillary sinus cancer: long-term outcomes and toxicities of treatment. Int J Radiat Oncol Biol Phys 68:719–730

Chen AM, Daly ME, Bucci MK et al (2007) Carcinomas of the paranasal sinuses and nasal cavity treated with radiotherapy at a single institution over five decades: are we making improvement? Int J Radiat Oncol Biol Phys 69:141–147

Le QT, Fu KK, Kaplan MJ et al (2000) Lymph node metastasis in maxillary sinus carcinoma. Int J Radiat Oncol Biol Phys 46:541–549

# Major Salivary Glands

Yiat Horng Leong, Eli Scher, Nancy Lee,
and Ivan WK Tham

## Contents

Y.H. Leong • I.W. Tham (✉)
National University Health System, Singapore, Singapore
e-mail: ivan_wk_tham@nuhs.edu.sg

E. Scher • N. Lee
Department of Radiation Oncology, MSKCC, New York, NY, USA
e-mail: leen2@mskcc.org

# 1    Anatomy and Patterns of Spread

## 1.1    Parotid Gland

- The parotid gland is a paired, irregular wedge-shaped uni-lobular organ in the preauricular region deep to the skin and subcutaneous tissues.
- The parotid compartment contains the parotid gland and associated vessels, nerves, and lymphatics and is bounded by the following landmarks:
    - Superior – zygomatic arch
    - Inferior – styloid process, styloid muscles, and internal carotid and jugular vessels
    - Anterior – anterior border of masseter
    - Posterior – mastoid process and external auditory canal
- Stensen's duct is the parotid duct which lies anterior and exits the buccal mucosa at the level of the second upper molar.
- The facial nerve exits the skull base through the stylomastoid foramen, which lies medial to the mastoid tip and lateral to the styloid process. After giving off 3 motor branches to the stylohyoid, postauricular, and posterior belly of the digastric muscles, it turns laterally to enter the parotid gland posteriorly, dividing the gland into a larger supraneural and smaller infraneural component. Within the parotid gland, the nerve divides at the pes anserinus (goose's foot) or parotid plexus into the upper temporofacial and lower cervicofacial divisions, which then form the 5 major branches: temporal, zygomatic, buccal, mandibular, (marginal) and cervical.
- Lymphatic drainage is via two layers of lymph nodes. The superficial layer consists of 3 to 20 nodes and drains the gland, external auditory canal, pinna, scalp, eyelids, and lacrimal glands. The deep layer lies deep in parotid tissue and drains the gland, external auditory canal,

N.Y. Lee et al. (eds.), *Target Volume Delineation for Conformal and Intensity-Modulated Radiation Therapy*,
Medical Radiology. Radiation Oncology, DOI: 10.1007/174_2014_1013, © Springer International Publishing Switzerland 2014
Published Online: 11 October 2014

middle ear, nasopharynx, and soft palate. Both systems empty into the superficial and deep cervical lymphatic systems.

- The main pattern of spread is local invasion of surrounding tissues adjacent to the parotid gland, following the anatomical borders of the parotid gland. Perineural invasion can occur along the facial nerve to the stylomastoid foramen.

## 1.2    Submandibular Gland

- The paired submandibular gland lies within the submandibular triangle, formed by the anterior and posterior bellies of the digastric muscle and the inferior margin of the mandible. It is medial and inferior to the mandibular ramus and wraps around the mylohyoid muscle, forming a smaller superficial and a larger deep lobe.
- The Wharton duct exits the medial surface of the gland and travels between the mylohyoid and hyoglossus muscles to the genioglossus muscle, opening intraorally lateral to the lingual frenulum at the floor of the mouth.
- The hypoglossal nerve lies inferiorly, and the lingual nerve superiorly, as the duct exits the gland. The mandibular and cervical branches of the facial nerve lie laterally. These nerves provide a potential pathway for perineural spread to the base of the skull. Hence, a named nerve with perineural invasion is tracked to the base of the skull and encompassed in the CTV.

## 2    Diagnostic Imaging for Target Volume Delineation

- Contrast-enhanced computed tomography (CT) or magnetic resonance imaging (MRI) of the head and neck region, from the base of skull to the clavicles, should be performed for salivary gland cancers. As far as possible, the head and neck imaging should be performed in the radiation therapy treatment position.
- The MRI signal intensity of the parotid gland is hyperintense (bright), intermediate between fat and muscle, on T1-weighted sequences and closer to the signal intensity of fat on T2-weighted sequences. The submandibular gland has less fat and appears closer to the signal intensity of muscle on both T1- and T2-weighted sequences.
- Neoplastic lesions are better visualized and delineated with MRI compared to CT, given the superior soft tissue contrast in the gland. The T1-weighted images can give an excellent assessment of the margin of the tumor, its deep extent, and its pattern of infiltration. With the addition of fat-saturated, contrast-enhanced T1-weighted imaging, perineural spread, bone invasion, or meningeal

infiltration can be better visualized. CT is more useful than MRI in imaging calcifications.

- Systemic staging can be completed with CT thorax and liver. Hybrid positron emission tomography (PET)/CT imaging is more sensitive for distant metastases than conventional modalities and has an increasing important role in staging. However, PET/CT should not replace MRI head and neck because it has inferior spatial and soft tissue resolution, especially close to the skull base, compared to MRI.

## 3    Simulation and Daily Localization

- The patient is typically set up in a supine position with head extended. The immobilization shell would encompass the head and neck down to the shoulders. Surgical scars are wired if present.
- CT simulation is performed from the vertex to the carina using 3 mm slices at the region of interest and 5 mm elsewhere.
- IV contrast should be performed to help guide the gross target volume (GTV) delineation, particularly for lymph nodes. Fusion with diagnostic MRI is recommended, typically with the sagittal gadolinium-enhanced T1 sequence.
- Image-guided radiation therapy should be considered in all cases treated with radical intent. Typically, cone-beam CT images will be acquired on the first 4 fractions, then on a weekly basis. Matching is at the PTV, except in locally advanced cases where the high-dose PTV abuts critical structures, e.g., brain stem, whereby matching to the critical structure may take precedence over PTV.
- Change in contour over the treatment course is to be expected, due to weight loss or tumor/surgical bed changes. Repeat shell and CT simulation should be individualized. Currently, there is no evidence that adaptive radiation therapy (e.g., reducing dose or volume as tumor shrinks) provides an improved therapeutic index and is discouraged.

## 4    Target Volume Delineation and Treatment Planning

Doses for curative treatment are outlined in tables 1 and 2. Doses for treatment with palliative intent vary according to the clinical circumstances and must be individualized. Typical hypofractionated doses include:

- 20 Gy in 5 fractions over 1 week
- 30 Gy in 10 fractions over 2 weeks
- 14 Gy in 4 fractions over 2 or 4 days, repeated monthly to a total of 28 Gy in 8 fractions (2 cycles, within cord

tolerance), or 42 Gy in 12 fractions (3 cycles, off-cord)

- 40 Gy in 16 fractions over 3½ weeks
- 50–55 Gy in 20 fractions over 4 weeks

**Table 1** Suggested target volumes at the gross disease region

| Target volumes | Definition and description |
|---|---|
| $GTV_{70}$[a] (the subscript 70 denotes radiation dose delivered) | Parotid or submandibular primary: all gross disease on physical examination and imaging |
| | Neck nodes: all nodes ≥ 1 cm in short axis diameter or nodes with necrotic center |
| $CTV_{70}$ | Add 5 mm so that $GTV_{70}+5$ mm $=CTV_{70}$ |
| | For nodes that are small but suspicious for disease (i.e., <1 cm), can consider a lower dose of 63–66 Gy |
| $PTV_{70}$ | Margin specific to treatment center and less if image guidance available |
| | Typically $CTV_{70}+3$ to 5 mm $=PTV_{70}$ |

[a]Suggested dose to gross disease is 2 Gy/fraction to 70 Gy.

**Table 2** Suggested target volumes at the high-risk subclinical region

| Target volumes | Definition and description |
|---|---|
| $CTV_{60}$ | Parotid or submandibular $CTV_{60}$ should encompass the entire GTV or the surgical bed for postoperative patients |
| | Landmarks for the parotid surgical bed |
| | Superior: zygomatic arch |
| | Anterior: masseter muscle |
| | Lateral: soft tissue of neck |
| | Medial and inferior: styloid process at depth |
| | Posterior: mastoid bone |
| | Landmarks for the submandibular surgical bed: include the entire surgical bed, all postoperative changes, and use the contralateral submandibular gland as a guide |
| | Highly consider a boost of 6–10 Gy to residual disease or positive margins. The surgeon should be encouraged to leave clips where possible for localization |
| $CTV_{50}$ | *Clinically node-positive tumors* |
| | Electively irradiate rest of the ipsilateral neck (levels Ib–V) to 50 Gy |
| | *Clinically node-negative tumors* |
| | *Ipsilateral neck*: include at least levels Ib–III for high-grade or large (T3–T4) tumors. Adenoid cystic or acinic cell cancers typically do not require elective nodal irradiation because of the low risk of lymphatic spread |
| | *Contralateral neck* |
| | *Parotid tumors*: consider treating when clinically concerned, e.g., multiple nodes <1 cm |
| | *Submandibular tumors*: treat contralateral levels I–III for tumors close to midline |
| $PTV_{60}$ | Margin specific to treatment center and less if image guidance available |
| | Typically $CTV_{60}+3$ to 5 mm $=PTV_{60}$ |

## 5 Plan Assessment

- For superficial tumors or tumors with skin infiltration, a bolus of 0.5 to 1 cm should be applied to ensure adequate surface coverage.
- Suggested target volumes at the gross disease and high-risk regions are detailed in Tables 1 and 2.
- Intensity-modulated radiation therapy (IMRT) planning parameters follow the standard head and neck radiation therapy norms. Normal tissue constraints follow the Quantitative Analyses of Normal Tissue Effects in the Clinic (QUANTEC) recommendations. Of note, for unilateral radiation, we recommend a stricter dose constraint for the contralateral parotid gland (<20 Gy mean dose) compared to <25 Gy mean dose if there is bilateral irradiation (Figs. 1, 2, 3, 4, 5, 6, 7, 8, 9, 10, 11, and 12).

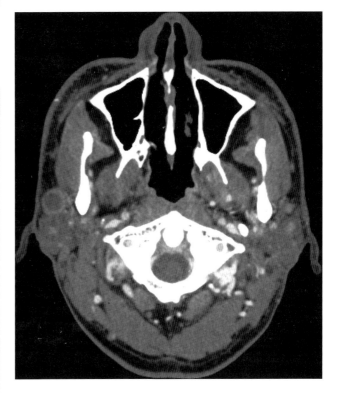

**Fig. 1** Axial contrast-enhanced CT image of a patient with a history of excision of a cutaneous squamous cell carcinoma (*SCC*) in the right temporal region, who now presents with an ipsilateral parotid mass, confirmed on biopsy to be metastatic SCC

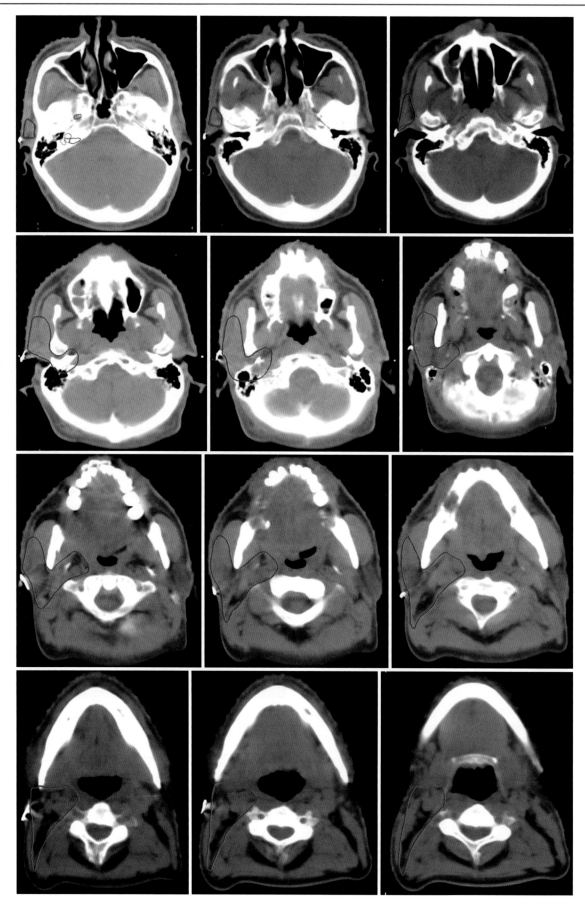

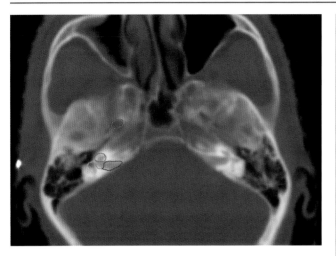

**Fig. 3** Base of the skull. Delineation of structures in the base of skull should be done using bone windows. Structures as follows: *Red*, foramen ovale; *blue*, cochlea; *orange*, vestibule; *violet*, internal auditory canal; *green*, semicircular canals

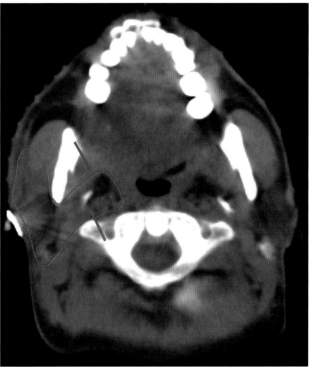

**Fig. 4** The parapharyngeal space (*red arrow*) is a predominantly fat-filled space extending from the base of the skull to the hyoid and should be included for large or deep parotid tumors. The retrostyloid space (*green arrow*) is posterolateral to the styloid process, may contain lymph nodes, and should be included in the $CTV_{60}$

**Fig. 2** CT simulation with 3 mm slices in a head shell was performed in the same patient following superficial parotidectomy with clear margins. These are representative slices and not all slices are included. Of note, the temporal region where the skin cancer was should also be included using either electrons matching to IMRT or 3D CRT, or all inclusive IMRT or 3D CRT plan, especially if primary site treatment was less than a year prior

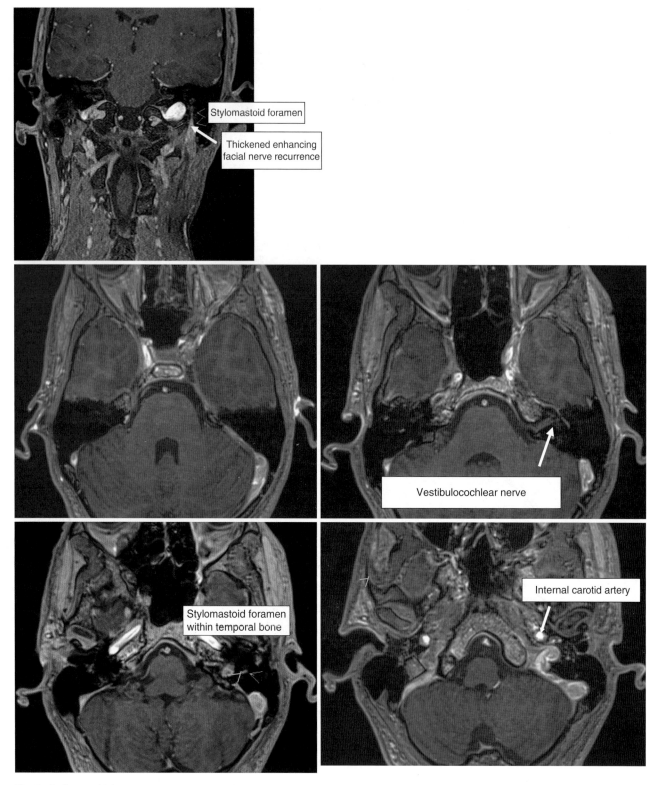

**Fig. 5** Stylomastoid foramen. Note pattern of perineural recurrence in these T1-weighted contrast-enhanced MRI images, which show recurrent mucoepidermoid carcinoma of the left parotid gland infiltrating the left facial nerve through the stylomastoid foramen (*green arrowheads*). For parotid tumors, include facial nerve when involved, or if histology is adenoid cystic carcinoma. Include intra-temporal course of the nerve, via the facial canal, which extends from the internal auditory canal to the stylomastoid foramen

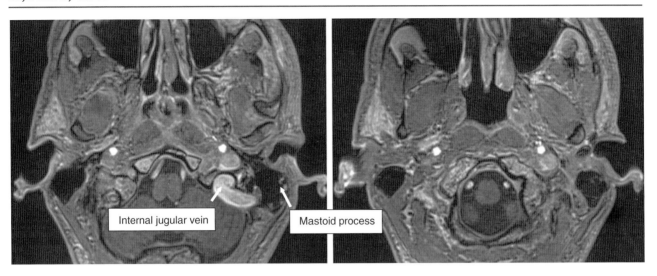

Internal jugular vein    Mastoid process

**Fig. 5** (continued)

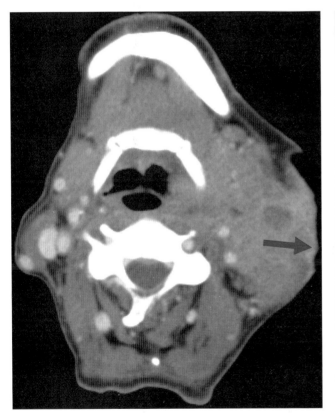

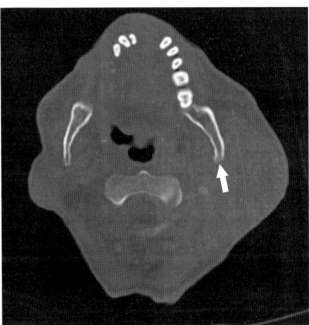

**Fig. 7** Mandible. Assess bone involvement with bone windows on CT scans and include in CTV if required. *White arrow* indicates periosteal reaction at posterior aspect of left ramus of mandible, suggesting involvement

**Fig. 6** Skin. Include involved skin as a target structure by utilizing a bolus if there is clinical or radiological (*red arrow*) evidence of dermal infiltration. Include the scar in cases with perioperative tumor spillage

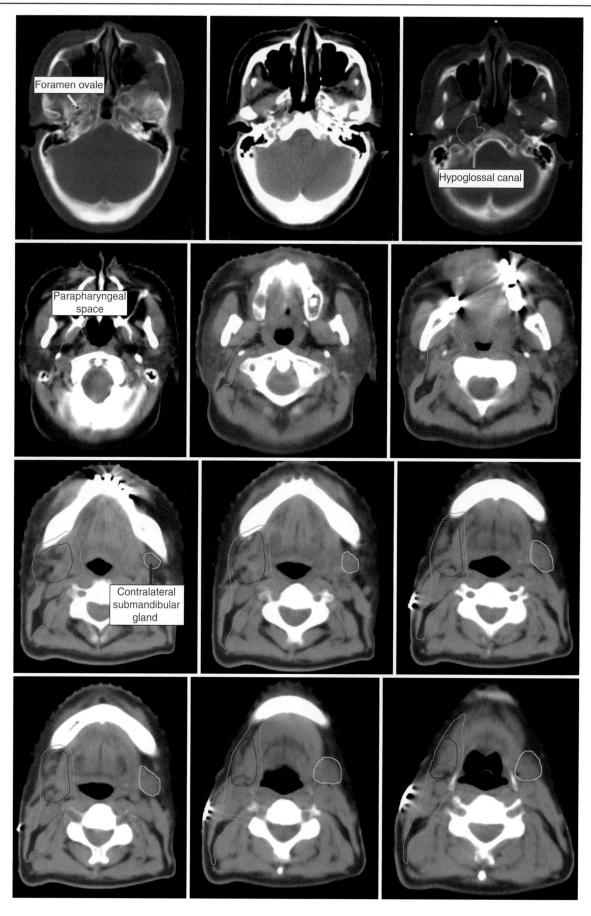

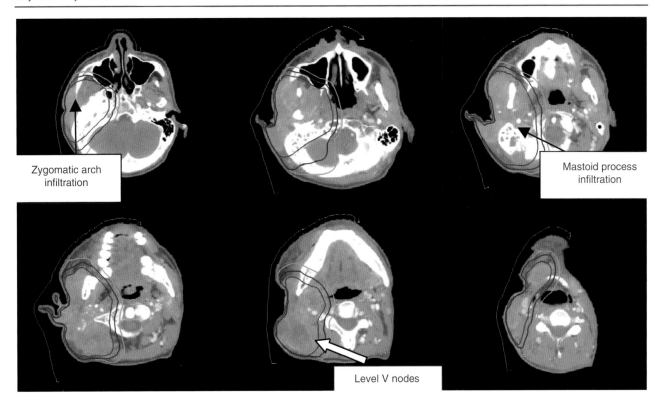

**Fig. 9** Inoperable parotid gland porocarcinoma. Representative slices of a CT simulation in a patient with a history of right temporal porocarcinoma and who now has an inoperable ipsilateral parotid recurrence and distant metastases. There is extensive bony infiltration and disease in the right level I, II, III, and IV cervical lymph nodes which are included in the high-dose CTV (55 Gy in 20 fractions over 4 weeks). The rest of the ipsilateral neck is irradiated to 50Gy. Structures as follows: *red* GTV, *green* phase 1 CTV$_{54}$, *blue* phase 2 boost CTV. A 0.5 cm bolus is applied to ensure adequate coverage at the skin

**Fig. 8** Submandibular gland. Selected CT simulation images of a patient who underwent complete excision of a cT1N1M0 high-grade mucoepidermoid carcinoma of the right submandibular gland with clear margins. Structures as follows: *Red* – CTV$_{60-66}$ (surgical bed), *green* – CTV$_{50-54}$ (ipsilateral nodal stations and parapharyngeal space to base of skull). Lingual or hypoglossal nerves should be treated to the base of the skull especially when these named nerves are involved. The lingual nerve originates from the mandibular (V3) branch of the trigeminal nerve at the foramen ovale and courses via the parapharyngeal space to the medial aspect of the submandibular gland before terminating in the tongue

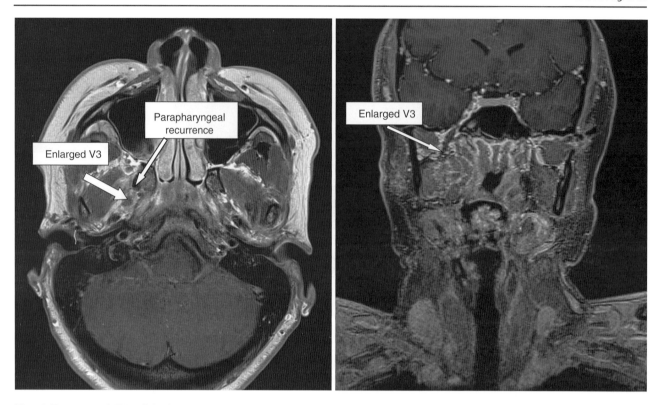

**Fig. 10** Foramen ovale T1-weighted contrast-enhanced MRI images in a patient with a history of right parotid acinic cell carcinoma and who now has a parapharyngeal recurrence. Note the disease involvement of the right mandibular branch (V3) of the trigeminal nerve which is abnormally enlarged

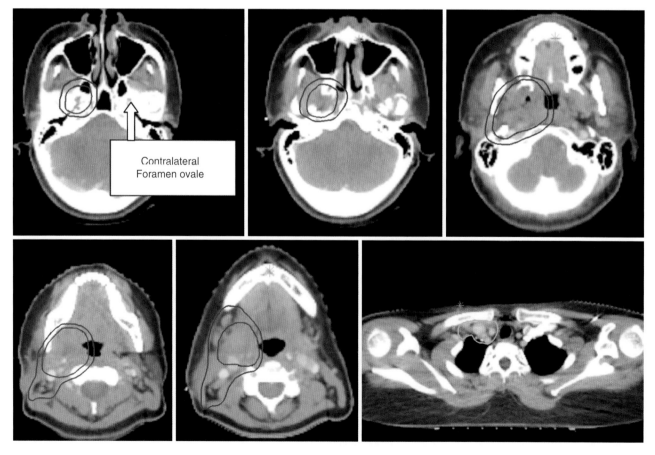

**Fig. 11** CT simulation images of the same patient. The V3 nerve is tracked to the foramen ovale and covered in the high-dose PTV due to the risk of perineural recurrence. The ipsilateral neck was electively irradiated in view of tumor recurrence. Structures as follows: *red* PTV$_{70}$, *blue* PTV$_{60}$, *green* PTV$_{50}$. See chapter on cranial nerves for additional details

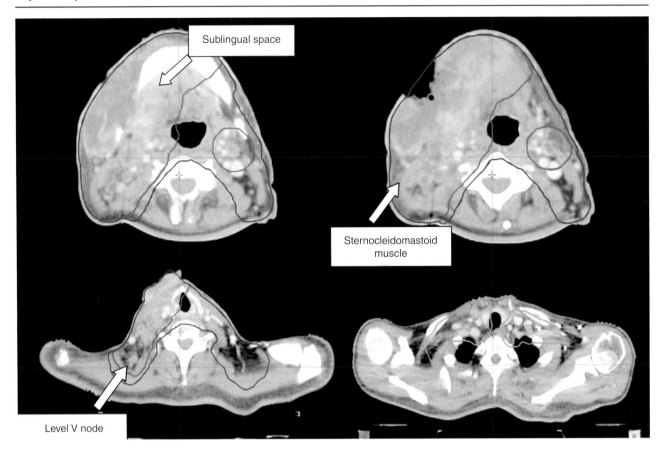

**Fig. 12** Inoperable submandibular carcinoma. Representative slices of a CT simulation in a patient who presented with a fungating right submandibular mass that was biopsy proven to be a poorly differentiated carcinoma. There is extensive locoregional infiltration, rendering it inoperable. The right sternocleidomastoid muscle, right sublingual space, right hyoglossus muscle, and right masseter muscle were all involved with disease. There is bony destruction of the right hemimandible as well. Right level II to V and left level II cervical nodes were enlarged. Structures as follows: *magenta* PTV$_{70}$, *blue* PTV$_{60}$, *green* PTV$_{50}$. A 0.5 cm bolus was applied (not shown)

## Suggested Reading

Adelstein DJ, Koyfman SA, El-Naggar AK, Hanna EY (2012) Biology and management of salivary gland cancers. Semin Radiat Oncol 22(3):245–53

Andry G, Hamoir M, Locati LD, Licitra L, Langendijk JA (2012) Management of salivary gland tumors. Expert Rev Anticancer Ther 12(9):1161–8

Grégoire V, Ang K, Budach W, Grau C, Hamoir M, Langendijk JA, Lee A, Le QT, Maingon P, Nutting C, O'Sullivan B, Porceddu SV, Lengele B (2013) Delineation of the neck node levels for head and neck tumors: a 2013 update. DAHANCA, EORTC, HKNPCSG, NCIC CTG, NCRI, RTOG, TROG consensus guidelines. Radiother Oncol. pii: S0167-8140(13)00514-8.

Marks LB, Yorke ED, Jackson A et al (2010) Use of normal tissue complication probability models in the clinic. Int J Radiat Oncol Biol Phys 76(3 Suppl):S10–9

# Thyroid Carcinoma

Paul B. Romesser and Nancy Y. Lee

## Contents

## 1 Anatomy and Patterns of Spread

- The thyroid gland is a highly vascular endocrine organ in the anterior low neck that spans from the fifth cervical vertebrae to the first thoracic vertebrae (Strandring 2005; Harnsberger et al. 2011).
- The gland consists of a right lobe and a left lobe connected by a narrow, median isthmus. A pyramidal lobe, ascending from the isthmus toward the hyoid, is present in approximately 40 % of patients (Harnsberger et al. 2011).
- The lobes are conical with ascending apices diverging laterally to the level of the oblique lines on the lamina of the thyroid cartilage (Strandring 2005).
- Small detached masses of thyroid tissue may occur above the lobes or isthmus as accessory thyroid glands.
- Importantly, the medial surface of the gland abuts the larynx and trachea. The posterolateral surface of the gland is close to the carotid sheath and overlaps with the common carotid artery.
- The thyroid has a thin capsule of connective tissue, which extends into the glandular parenchyma and divides each lobe into irregularly shaped lobules. The follicles contain a colloid core, which comprises mostly iodo-thyroglobulin, an inactive storage form of thyroid hormone T4 produced by follicular epithelial cells (follicular cells).
- The thyroid parenchyma also contains C-cells, which produce the peptide hormone calcitonin.
- An enlarged thyroid from malignancy or benign conditions can result in pressure on the trachea, recurrent laryngeal nerve, or venous engorgement (Strandring 2005).
- The thyroid is usually supplied by the superior and inferior thyroid arteries.
  - The superior thyroid artery usually arises from the first branch of the external carotid artery (a common anatomical variant occurs where it arises more inferiorly

P.B. Romesser • N.Y. Lee, MD (✉)
Department of Radiation Oncology, Memorial Sloan Kettering
Cancer Center, New York, NY, USA
e-mail: leen2@mskcc.org

N.Y. Lee et al. (eds.), *Target Volume Delineation for Conformal and Intensity-Modulated Radiation Therapy*,
Medical Radiology. Radiation Oncology, DOI: 10.1007/174_2014_1014, © Springer International Publishing Switzerland 2014
Published Online: 1 November 2014

from the common carotid artery) and divides into anterior and posterior branches. The anterior branch will form an anastomosis with the contralateral anterior branch of the superior thyroid artery (Oertli and Udelsman 2012). Conversely, the posterior branch will form an anastomosis with the superior branch of the inferior thyroid artery (Oertli and Udelsman 2012).

- The inferior thyroid artery divides into an inferior and superior branch. The superior branch forms an anastomosis with the posterior branch of the superior thyroid artery. The inferior branch supplies the inferior part of the gland.

• Approximately 3 % of the population has a thyroid ima artery, which arises from the aortic arch or brachiocephalic artery (Harnsberger et al. 2011).

• Venous drainage is usually via three pairs of veins: the superior, middle, and inferior thyroid veins (Strandring 2005; Harrison et al. 2014).

- The superior thyroid vein emerges from the upper aspect of the gland and runs with the superior thyroid artery toward the carotid sheath to drain into the internal jugular vein.

- The middle vein drains the inferior aspect of the gland, emerges laterally, and drains into the internal jugular vein.

- The tracheal plexus, formed from the inferior thyroid veins, is located below the thyroid gland in front of the trachea.

• The thyroid lymphatic drainage consists of a rich intraglandular network, which has been implicated in the high rates of multifocal disease, and an extraglandular component (Harrison et al. 2014).

• Thyroid lymphatic vessels communicate with the tracheal plexus and pass to the prelaryngeal nodes (neck lymph node level VI) just above the thyroid isthmus and to the pretracheal and paratracheal nodes (thoracic lymph node levels II, III, and IV) (Strandring 2005).

• Laterally the gland is drained by vessels lying along the superior thyroid veins to the deep cervical nodes.

• In addition, thyroid lymphatics may drain directly to the thoracic duct.

• Many important nerves lie in close proximity to the thyroid gland.

- The external laryngeal nerve is a division of the superior laryngeal nerve and a branch of the vagus nerve and supplies the cricothyroid muscle (Oertli and Udelsman 2012). Damage to the external laryngeal nerve will impair phonation (Oertli and Udelsman 2012).

- The recurrent laryngeal nerve, a branch of the vagus nerve, supplies the remainder of the laryngeal musculature as well as sensation on and inferior to the vocal folds (Oertli and Udelsman 2012). Its path differs on the

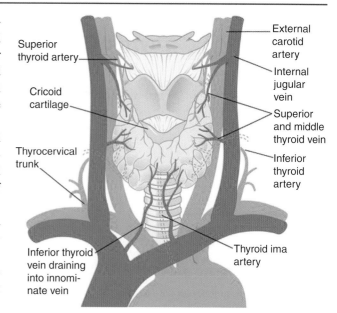

**Fig. 1** Arterial supply and venous drainage of the thyroid gland. The superior and inferior thyroid arteries (STA and ITA) arise from the external carotid arteries and the thyrocervical trunks, respectively. Rarely, the thyroid ima artery, a branch of the brachiocephalic artery, may enter the inferior margin of the thyroid isthmus. The STA is usually the first branch of the external carotid artery, and it has an intimate relationship with the superior laryngeal nerve, making this nerve and its motor branch, the external laryngeal nerve, susceptible to injury during thyroidectomy or from direct compression in patients with locally advanced thyroid cancers. The venous drainage of the thyroid gland is variable as in other organs. Generally, the superior and middle thyroid veins drain into the internal jugular vein, and the inferior thyroid veins drain into the brachiocephalic vein (From Springer reference https://www.springerimages.com/Images/MedicineAndPublicHealth/2-ACE0101-14-001A)

right and left side. On the right side, the recurrent laryngeal nerve loops posterior to the subclavian artery to ascend obliquely until it reaches the tracheoesophageal groove near the inferior extent of the thyroid (Oertli and Udelsman 2012). On the left side, the nerve loops posterior to the aortic arch and ascends to the larynx in the tracheoesophageal groove. The recurrent laryngeal nerve has a close but variable relationship with the inferior thyroid artery and is closely related to or within the ligament of Berry (fascia attachment between the thyroid and the cricoid cartilage) (Figs. 1, 2, and 3).

## 2 Diagnostic Workup Relevant for Target Volume Delineation

• In addition to a focused head and neck examination, radiographic imaging should be obtained for diagnosis, staging, and treatment planning.

• All patients should undergo a CT of the neck, preferably with contrast, though this will ultimately delay radioactive

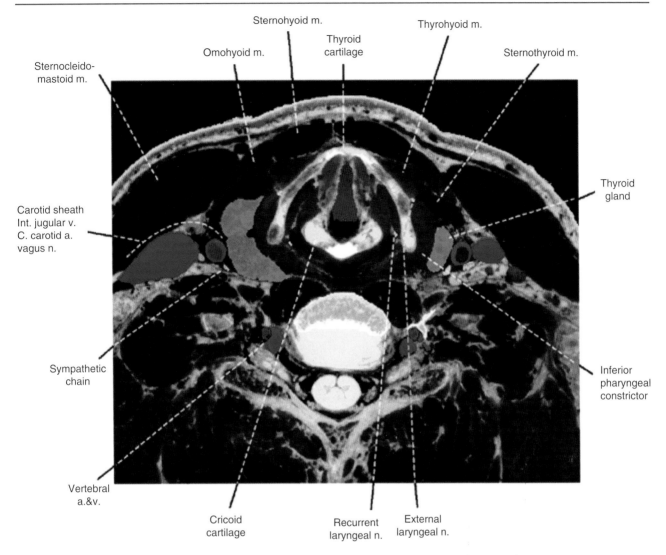

**Fig. 2** Thyroid gland and its relations at the level of the thyroid cartilage. Color enhancement demonstrates major arteries (*red*), veins (*blue*), and nerves (*yellow*). The thyroid gland is enhanced with *pink*. It is important to note the close relationship of the superior pole of the thyroid gland, with the carotid sheath and sympathetic chain (From Springer reference: Oertli and Udelsman 2012. http://link.springer.com/chapter/10.1007%2F978-3-642-23459-0_2/fulltext.html)

iodine therapy if applicable. It is important to include the superior mediastinum in the scan to assess for the presence of superior mediastinal lymphadenopathy.
- If there is concern for cervical esophagus involvement, a MR neck with gadolinium may aid in the diagnosis.
- Laboratory workup should include complete blood count (CBC), comprehensive metabolic panel (CMP), thyroid-stimulating hormone (TSH), T3, free T4, and thyroglobulin level.
- As the definitive treatment for non-anaplastic thyroid carcinomas is surgical resection, all patients should be evaluated by an experienced head and neck surgeon to assess resectability.

## 3 General Treatment Considerations

- Thyroid malignancies constitute the widest range of clinically aggressive tumors. Patients with well-differentiated carcinoma carry an extremely favorable prognosis, whereas anaplastic thyroid carcinoma is among the deadliest of all human cancers.
- The role of external beam radiation therapy (EBRT) in the treatment of differentiated thyroid cancer remains controversial but is better established for medullary carcinoma and anaplastic carcinoma.
- There is a lack of prospective trials evaluating the efficacy of EBRT in patients with well-differentiated thyroid carcinoma.

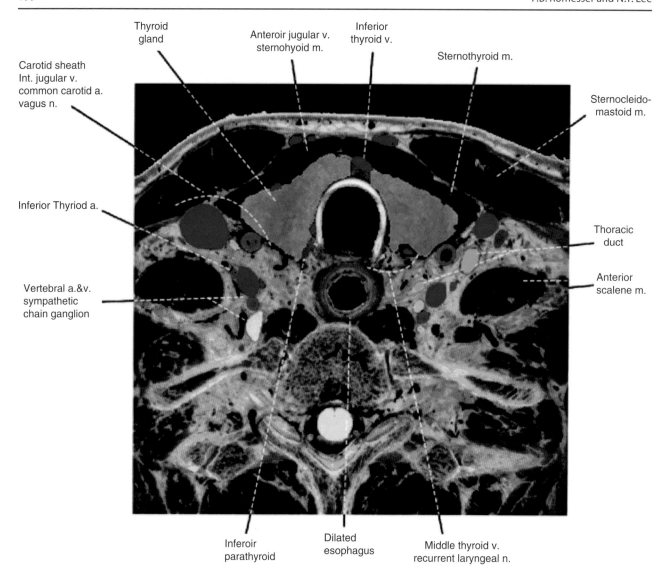

**Fig. 3** Thyroid gland and its relations at the level of the third tracheal ring. Note the posteromedial relationships of the thyroid gland with the recurrent laryngeal nerve and the middle thyroid veins. The thoracic duct (*green*) is atypically dilated close to where it joins the left internal jugular and subclavian veins. The inferior thyroid artery follows a looping course. An inferior right parathyroid gland (*purple*) is evident near the recurrent laryngeal nerve and middle thyroid veins. Major nerves (*yellow*), arteries (*red*), veins (*blue*), and thyroid (*pink*) are indicated (From Springer reference: Oertli and Udelsman 2012. http://link.springer.com/chapter/10.1007%2F978-3-642-23459-0_2/fulltext.html)

- – Multiple single-institution experiences have demonstrated that EBRT improves locoregional control in patients with microscopic/gross residual disease after surgical resection and those with unresectable disease.
- Postoperative radiation therapy for patients with extrathyroid extension or even extranodal extension with well-differentiated histology remains controversial, as alternative adjuvant therapies, such as radioactive iodine (RAI), are often preferred.
- Postoperative radiation therapy should be considered for any patient with well-differentiated RAI-refractory disease or medullary carcinoma with concern for microscopic or gross residual disease.
- Patients with anaplastic carcinoma require immediate referral to a tertiary cancer center and mandate multidisciplinary care given their poor prognosis.

- Intensity-modulated radiation therapy (IMRT) is the recommended technique for definitive or postoperative radiation therapy for thyroid cancer to decrease treatment-related morbidity (Schwartz et al. 2009).

## 4    Principles of Simulation and Target Delineation

- Given the accuracy of IMRT treatment, efficacy is largely dependent on tumor localization.
- Imaging may be difficult to interpret as many of these patients have undergone multiple head and neck surgeries.
- Fludeoxyglucose positron emission tomography (FDG-PET) can be useful for the delineation of tumor in patients with anaplastic and RAI-refractory-differentiated carcinomas.

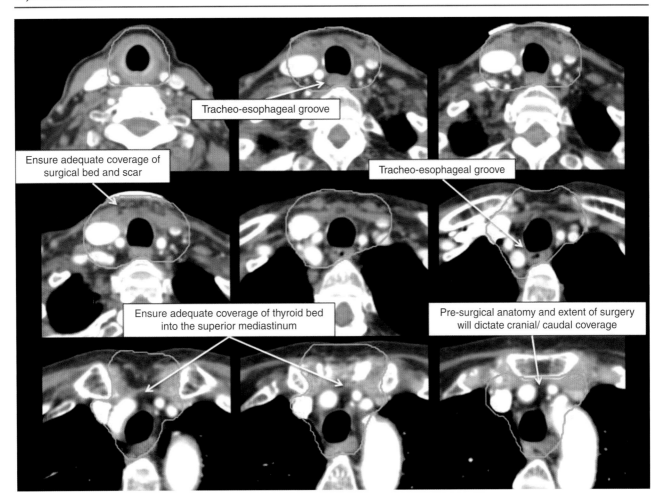

**Fig. 4** A 75-year-old woman with a 1.5 cm medullary carcinoma status post total thyroidectomy with a microscopic positive surgical margin who refused re-excision. Postoperative radiation therapy was recommended to decrease the risk of local recurrence. The $CTV_{60Gy}$ is in green. As she had early-stage disease with no evidence of lymph node involvement, a neck dissection and hence neck irradiation were deferred. These are representative slices, and not all slices are included

- FDG uptake has been inversely correlated with RAI uptake and thus is of particular benefit in patients with RAI-refractory, well-differentiated thyroid carcinoma (Wang et al. 2001; Grunwald et al. 1999).
- We generally recommend PET-CT simulation. The use of iodinated contrast is preferable, though it needs to be justified clinically as stated above.
- We generally recommend 3 mm or less slice thickness.
- A thermoplastic mask is used for immobilization (Orfit Industries, Wijnegem, Belgium).
  - Immobilization of the head, neck, and shoulders is preferable to immobilizing only the head and neck region.
- The head should be slightly extended to allow sparing of the oral cavity.
- Gross disease, as documented by clinical or radiographic examination, should be treated to 7,000 cGy (Lee and Lu 2012).

- Microscopic residual disease should be treated to 6,600 cGy (Lee and Lu 2012).
- High-risk areas, including the operative or tumor bed, operative thyroid gland volume, tracheoesophageal grooves, and central nodal compartment (covered superiorly to the caudal edge of hyoid bone), should be treated to 6,000 cGy.
- Low-risk areas including the upper and lower paratracheal lymph node levels and uninvolved cervical lymph node levels should be treated to 5,400 cGy. In some patients the lateral neck can be omitted if after thorough discussions with the surgeon, it is deemed to be low risk and surgical salvage remains available.
- Patients may be treated in 30–35 fractions with an all-in-one dose-painting IMRT plan or alternatively an initial IMRT course followed by a boost.
- Suggested target volumes for gross disease and at-risk regions are detailed in Tables 1 and 2.
- Suggested normal tissue dose constraints are detailed in Table 3.

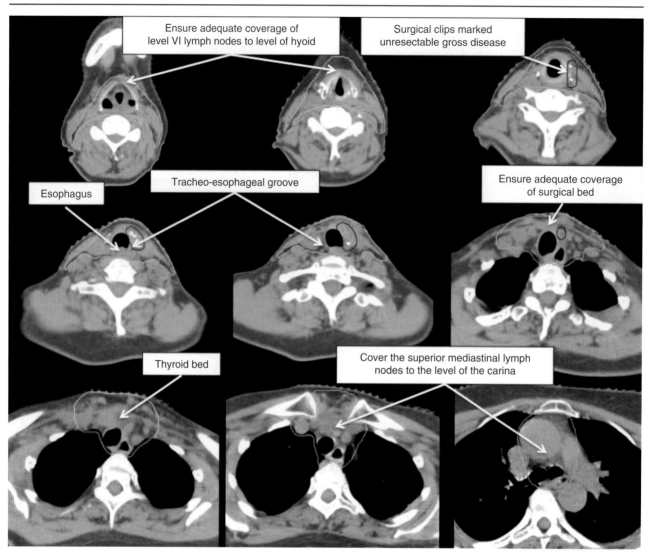

**Fig. 5** A 59-year-old woman with multiply recurrent papillary carcinoma, tall-cell variant, with gross residual disease involving the recurrent laryngeal nerve and left subglottic larynx after a repeat total thyroidectomy and left neck dissection. Definitive radiation therapy to the thyroid bed, central compartment, and cervical neck levels II–IV was recommended. The clinical target volume $(CTV)_{70Gy}$ is in *red*, and the $CTV_{60Gy}$ is in *green*. Please note the omission of IV contrast given the plan for postradiation radioactive iodine (RAI) therapy to assess and treat micrometastatic disease

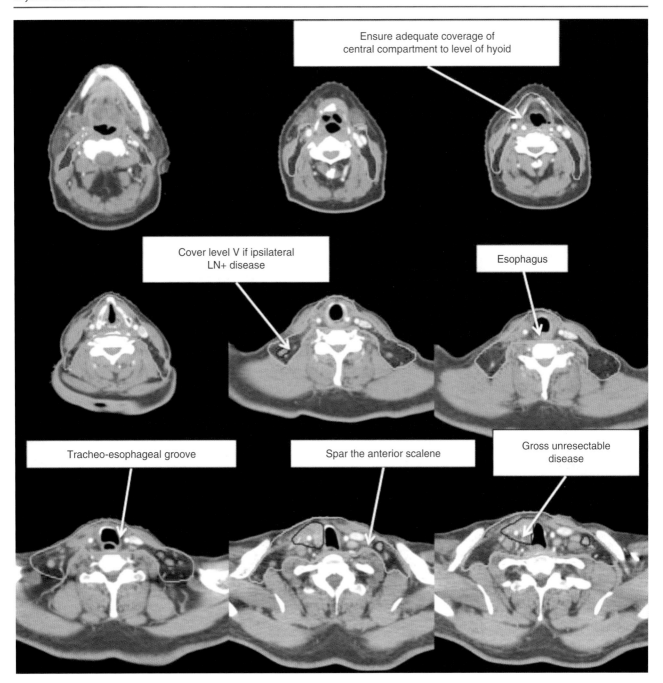

**Fig. 6** A 58-year-old man with multiply recurrent metastatic papillary thyroid carcinoma status post multiple surgical resections now with an unresectable local recurrence and multiple involved mediastinal lymph nodes. Chemoradiation with concurrent doxorubicin was recommended to prevent local progression. The $CTV_{70Gy}$ is in *red* and the $CTV_{60Gy}$ is in *green*. These are representative slices and not all slices are included

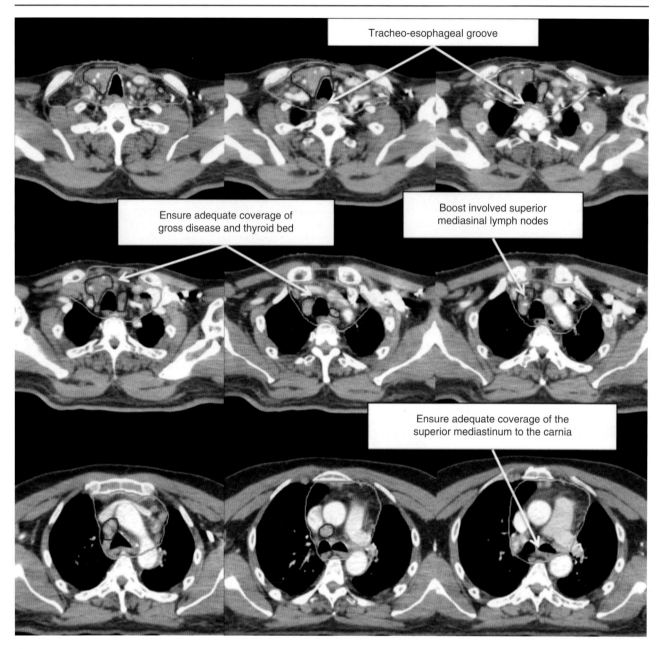

**Fig. 6** (continued)

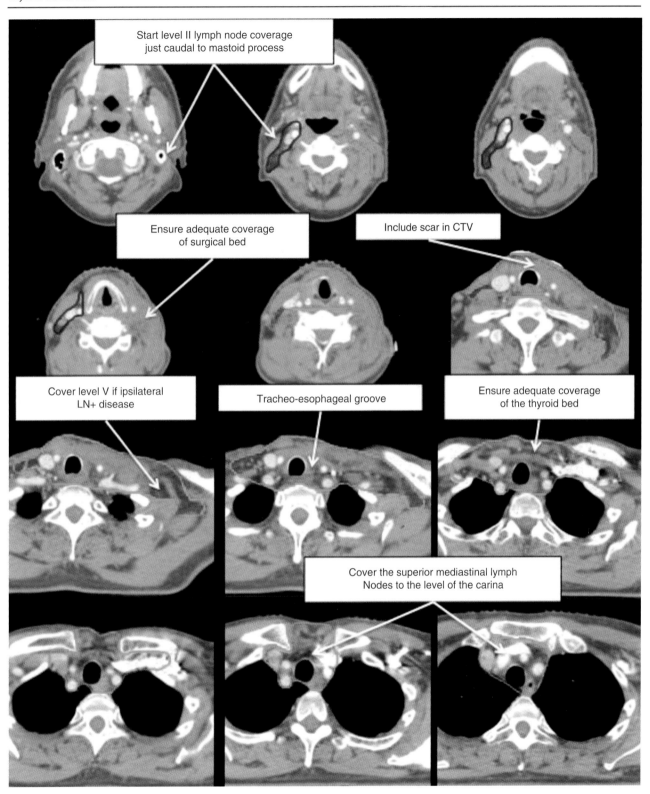

**Fig. 7** A 69-year-old man presented with left neck adenopathy. A fine-needle aspiration was consistent with papillary thyroid carcinoma. He subsequently underwent a total thyroidectomy and left neck dissection. Pathology noted papillary carcinoma, tall-cell variant, with associated anaplastic carcinoma involving 6 of 122 lymph nodes with extranodal extension in the left neck. No disease was identified within the thyroid gland itself. Postoperative chemoradiation with concurrent doxorubicin was recommended. The clinical target volume (CTV)$_{60Gy}$ is in *green* and the CTV$_{54Gy}$ is in *blue*. These are representative slices and not all slices are included

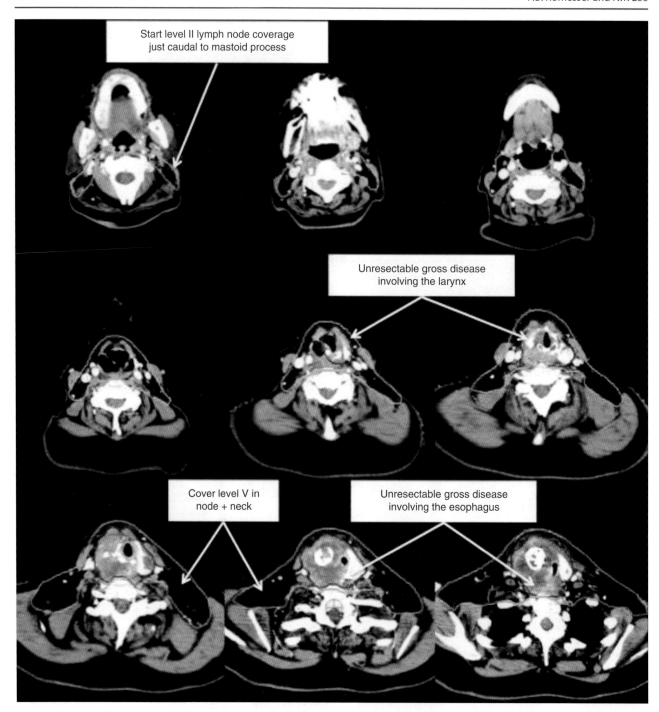

**Fig. 8** A 73-year-old woman with unresectable anaplastic thyroid carcinoma invading the trachea and esophagus. Definitive chemoradiation with concurrent doxorubicin was recommended after multidisciplinary evaluation and discussion to prevent further local progression. Clinical target volume $(CTV)_{70Gy}$ is in *red* and the $CTV_{60Gy}$ is in *green*. Although the manubrium is not routinely encompassed in the at-risk volume, it was included for this patient with aggressive bulky anterior neck disease. These are representative slices and not all slices are included

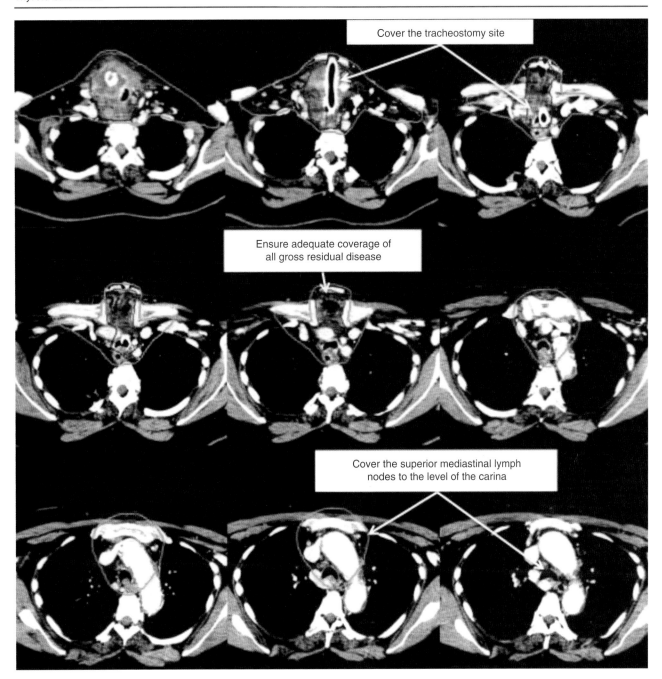

**Fig. 8** (continued)

**Table 1** Suggested target volumes for gross disease

| Target volumes | Definition and description |
|---|---|
| GTV$_{70-66}$[a] | Primary: All gross disease on physical examination and imaging<br><br>Neck nodes: All nodes $\geq 1$ cm or with necrotic center |
| CTV$_{70-66}$[a] | Usually same as GTV$_{70-66}$. If a margin is needed due to uncertainty of the gross disease, add 3–5 mm so that GTV$_{70-66}$ + 3–5 mm = CTV$_{70-66}$<br><br>If the GTV is adjacent to the spinal cord, a 1 mm margin is acceptable, as protection of the spinal cord is required<br><br>For suspicious nodes that are small (i.e., ~1 cm), a lower dose of 66 Gy (CTV$_{66}$) can be considered |
| PTV$_{70-66}$[a] | CTV$_{70-66}$ + 3–5 mm, depending on variability in daily patient positioning. If the CTV is adjacent to the spinal cord, a 1 mm margin is acceptable |

[a]Suggested dose for gross disease is 70 Gy. In cases where there is concern for brachial plexus, laryngeal, spinal cord, lung, or esophageal toxicity, 66 Gy may be considered. In postoperative cases with gross resection but significant concern for residual disease based on positive margin(s), the tumor bed or region of concern can be treated to 66 Gy

**Table 2** Suggested target volumes for at-risk subclinical region

| Target volumes | Definition and description |
|---|---|
| CTV$_{60-54}$[a] | Primary: Should include tracheoesophageal groove and >5 mm margin around any CTV$_{70-66}$<br><br>In the postoperative setting, should encompass tumor bed, surgical bed, and tracheoesophageal groove on the involved side(s). If tracheostomy performed, should also encompass tracheostomy stoma to the skin surface<br><br>Optimally, the upper larynx (vocal cords/arytenoid cartilage and above) and posterior esophagus should be excluded, if not adjacent to tumor/tumor bed (See Table 9–1, regarding positive margins.)<br><br>Neck regions: In locally advanced or node-positive disease generally include nodal levels II–VII. The upper mediastinum (thoracic lymph node levels II, III, and IV) should be covered to the level of the carina. Level V should be covered in the node-positive neck but can be spared in the node-negative neck if clinical suspicion is low. Omission of the lateral cervical neck can be considered in a node-negative neck if after thorough discussions with the surgeon it is deemed to be low risk and surgical salvage remains available<br><br>Level I and retropharyngeal nodes may be covered if there is bulky neck disease |
| PTV$_{60-54}$[a] | CTV$_{60-54}$ + 3–5 mm, depending on variability in daily patient positioning. If the CTV is adjacent to the spinal cord, a 1 mm margin is acceptable |

[a]Suggested at-risk subclinical dose: 60 Gy. Uninvolved nodal regions may be deemed as low-risk subclinical regions and treated to 54 Gy at the discretion of the treating physician

**Table 3** Normal tissue dose constraints

| Organ at risk (OAR) | Constraints |
|---|---|
| Parotid | Mean <26 Gy |
| Larynx | Mean <45 Gy |
| Esophagus | Mean <34 Gy |
| Brachial plexus | Max point dose <65 Gy |
| Spinal cord | Max point dose <45 Gy |
| Lung | Mean dose <21 Gy, V20<37 %, NTCP <25 % |

Based on guidelines presently used at Memorial Sloan-Kettering Cancer Center
*PTV* planning target volume

# References

Grunwald F, Kalicke T, Feine U et al (1999) Fluorine-18 fluorodeoxyglucose positron emission tomography in thyroid cancer: results of a multicentre study. Eur J Nucl Med 26:1547–1552

Harnsberger HR, Osborn AG, Ross JS et al (eds) (2011) Diagnostic and surgical imaging anatomy. Amirsys, Salt Lake City

Harrison LB, Sessions SB, Kies MS (eds) (2014) Head and Neck Cancer: A Multidisciplinary Approach, 4th edn. Lippincott Williams & Wilkins, New York

Lee NY, Lu JJ (eds) (2012) Target volume delineation and field setup: a practical guide for conformal and intensity-modulated radiation therapy. Springer, New York

Oertli D, Udelsman R (eds) (2012) Surgery of the thyroid and parathyroid glands. Springer, New York

Schwartz DL, Lobo MJ, Ang KK et al (2009) Postoperative external beam radiotherapy for differentiated thyroid cancer: outcomes and morbidity with conformal treatment. Int J Radiat Oncol Biol Phys 74:1083–1091

Strandring S (ed) (2005) Gray's anatomy: the anatomical basis of clinical practice, 39th edn. Elsevier Churchill Livingstone, New York

Wang W, Larson SM, Tuttle RM et al (2001) Resistance of [18f]-fluorodeoxyglucose-avid metastatic thyroid cancer lesions to treatment with high-dose radioactive iodine. Thyroid 11:1169–1175

# Squamous Cell Carcinoma of Unknown Primary in the Head and Neck

John Cuaron, Nadeem Riaz, and Nancy Lee

## Contents

J. Cuaron, MD • N. Riaz, MD • N. Lee, MD (✉)
Department of Radiation Oncology, Memorial Sloan Kettering,
New York, NY, USA
e-mail: leen2@mskcc.org

## 1 Anatomy and Patterns of Spread

- Squamous cell carcinoma of unknown primary (SQCUP) in the head and neck is defined by malignancy in the cervical lymph nodes without identification of the primary tumor after extensive workup.

- Potential sites of the occult primary tumor include the nasopharynx, oropharynx, larynx, and hypopharynx (Fig. 1).

- The most common primary sites that are eventually identified upon workup for patients with SQCUP are the tonsils and base of the tongue (~90 %) (Cianchetti et al. 2009).

- The distribution of lymph node metastases from a SQCUP of the head and neck is shown in Fig. 2. The most common sites of involvement are levels II and III.

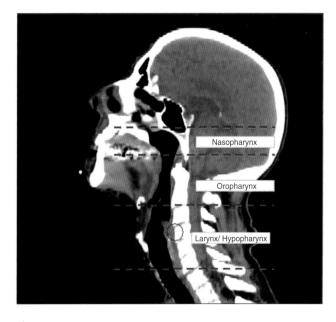

**Fig. 1** Potential sites of occult primary tumor in SQCUP. The *red circle* represents the level of the isocenter for an intensity modulated radiation therapy plan for squamous cell carcinoma of unknown primary. The *red dotted* lines delineate the anatomical divisions between the nasopharynx, oropharynx and larynx and hypopharynx, respectively

N.Y. Lee et al. (eds.), *Target Volume Delineation for Conformal and Intensity-Modulated Radiation Therapy*,
Medical Radiology. Radiation Oncology, DOI: 10.1007/174_2014_1002, © Springer International Publishing Switzerland 2014
Published Online: 22 October 2014

**All patients**
**(n=352)**

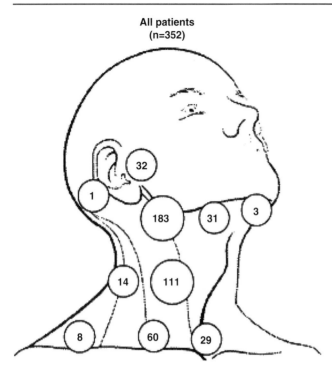

**Fig. 2** Distribution of involved lymph nodes in SQCUP (Grau et al. 2000)

## 2 Diagnostic Workup Relevant for Target Volume Delineation

- A thorough workup is necessary to rule out a site of origin before proceeding with a diagnosis of an unknown primary. At a minimum, this should consist of a careful physical examination including testing of the cranial nerves; fiberoptic examination visualizing the nasopharynx, oropharynx, larynx, and hypopharynx; and cross-sectional imaging with at least a high-resolution CT scan with contrast. Obtaining a careful patient history, including a smoking history, is also critical to determine risk factors for cancer and to consider possible infraclavicular primary sources (e.g., thoracic, gynecologic, or gastrointestinal). Panendoscopy may also be useful.
- HPV and EBV testing should be performed to help determine possible primary locations.
- Directed biopsies of all suspicious lesions in the pharyngeal axis are mandatory; blind biopsies of normal-appearing mucosa have tradiationally been recommended but are only occasionally helpful in identifying the primary tumor.
- PET/CT is able to identify the primary site in 25 % of tumors that are undetected by other modalities, with a sensitivity, specificity, and accuracy of 88.3, 74.9, and 78.8 %, respectively (Rusthoven et al. 2004).

- PET/CT should be performed before biopsy when possible to decrease the incidence of false-positive findings.
- The chapter on lymph node contouring in the head and neck contains further details of diagnostic imaging to assess lymphatic involvement.

## 3 Simulation and Daily Localization

- Set up the patient in supine position with head extended. The immobilization device should include at least the head and neck. If possible, shoulders should also be immobilized to ensure accurate patient setup on a daily basis especially when an extended-field IMRT plan is used.
- CT simulation using 3 mm thickness with IV contrast should be performed to help guide the GTV and CTV targets, particularly for the lymph nodes. We typically recommend a simulation scan from the top of the head including the brain to the carina. Five millimeter thickness can be reconstructed below the clavicle to the level of the carina.
- Image registration and fusion applications with MRI and PET scans should be used to help in the delineation of target volumes, especially for regions of interest encompassing the GTV, skull base, brainstem, and optic chiasm. The GTV and CTV and normal tissues should be outlined on all CT slices in which the structures exist.

## 4 Target Volume Delineation and Treatment Planning

- Treatment to the bilateral neck and areas of pharynx at risk for harboring a primary is typically recommended.
- Generally, cervical lymph nodes (levels IB-V) and retropharyngeal nodes should be included for the node-positive neck. For the contralateral neck, nodal levels II–IV and the retropharyngeal nodes should be targetted to a prophylactic dose (50–54 Gy). Inclusion of level IB and V can be considered on a case-by-case basis.
- Irradiation of the ipsilateral neck alone is controversial. Several single institutional reports have shown a low risk of contralateral neck failure and no difference in disease-free or overall survival when an ipsilateral approach is used (Grau et al. 2000; Ligey et al. 2009; Lu et al. 2009; Perkins et al. 2012; Weir et al. 1995), whereas other studies have demonstrated improved outcomes with more extensive treatment volumes (Reddy and Marks 1997).
- The extent of the pharynx to irradiate must be determined on a case-by-case basis and remains an area of active investigation. The pattern of lymph node spread can further help guide decisions on how much of the pharynx to treat.

**Table 1** Suggested target volumes

| Target volumes | Definition and description |
|---|---|
| $GTV_{70}$[a] (The subscript 70 denotes the radiation dose delivered) | All lymph nodes $\geq 1$ cm in short axis, significantly FDG avid, or positive on biopsy. Contour any lymph nodes in doubt as GTV |
| $PTV_{70}$[a] | $GTV_{70}$ + 3–5 mm depending on institutional accuracy of daily patient positioning |
| $CTV_{nasopharynx}$[b] | Extends from the base of skull superiorly to the soft palate inferiorly. Anteriorly extends from the posterior choana to the posterior pharyngeal wall. Laterally ensure adequate coverage on the fossa of Rosenmüller |
| $CTV_{oropharynx}$[b] | Extends superiorly from the surface of the soft palate to the floor of the vallecula inferiorly (or hyoid bone). Anteriorly, the base of tongue should be covered; however, an additional margin covering the oral tongue is not necessary. Laterally, the tonsils should be covered adequately. Posteriorly, the entire pharyngeal wall should be covered |
| $CTV_{larynx}\&_{hypopharynx}$[b] | Extends superiorly from the hyoid bone to the bottom of cricoid cartilage |
| $PTV_{mucosa}$[b] | A 3–5 mm expansion on the mucosal surface CTVs depending on institutional accuracy of daily patient positioning |
| $CTV_{neck\ nodes}$[c] | RPN, levels IB-V in the node-positive neck. RPN, levels II–IV on the node-negative neck |
| $PTV_{neck\ nodes}$[c] | A 3–5 mm expansion on the neck node CTVs depending on institutional accuracy of daily patient positioning |

*Note*: If the patient underwent surgery, the postoperative dissected neck should be treated anywhere from 60 to 66 Gy in 2 Gy per fractions
[a]Suggested dose to gross disease is 2.12 Gy/fraction to 69.96 Gy
[b]Suggested dose to mucosal surfaces at risk for harboring a primary is 54–60 Gy in 1.64 and 1.8 Gy fraction sizes, respectively
[c]High-risk subclinical dose, 1.8 Gy/fraction to 59.4 Gy. Lower risk subclinical regions can consider 1.64 Gy/fraction to 54 Gy

- – Some authors have advocated sparing the larynx when there are no low lymph nodes involved (Barker et al. 2005) (see Fig. 7).
- – Irradiating the oropharynx alone may be sufficient for an HPV + patient; however, the nasopharynx should be included if there is any suspicion of a nasopharyngeal primary, as recent data demonstrated poor outcomes for patients with HPV + nasopharyngeal carcinoma (Stenmark et al. 2013).
- – EBV + patients may only need treatment to the nasopharynx.
- When in doubt, the entire pharynx should be treated.
- In the postoperative setting, concurrent chemotherapy should be considered when extracapsular extension is present (ECE). In the definitive setting, advanced nodal disease is a consideration for concurrent chemotherapy.

## 5 Plan Assessment

- Ideally, 95 % of the volume of each PTV should receive the prescription dose (D95% $\geq$ Rx).
- The dose to the 5 % of the PTV receiving the highest dose should not exceed 108 % of the presecription (D05 $\leq$108 % Rx).
- Many critical normal structures surround the pharyngeal axis and neck and therefore need to be outlined for dose constraints (Table 2). These structures including the brain stem, spinal cord, optic nerves, chiasm, parotid glands, pituitary, temporomandibular (T-M) joints and middle and inner ears, skin (in the region of the target volumes), oral cavity, mandible, eyes, lens, temporal lobe, brachial plexus, esophagus (including postcricoid pharynx), and glottic larynx should be outlined.

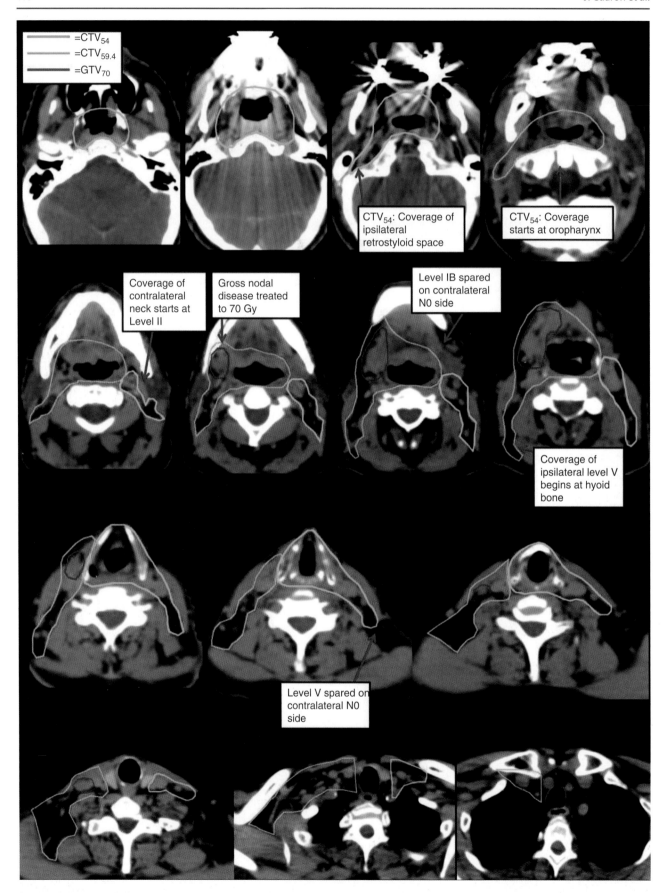

**Fig. 3** 52M with TxN2bM0 SQCUP. He underwent an excisional biopsy of a right submandibular lymph node that demonstrated metastatic SCC. A PET/CT showed multiple hypermetabolic lymph nodes in right level IB, level II, and level IV. There was also asymmetric uptake in the right base of the tongue, but biopsy of this area failed to demonstrate tumor. He was treated with concurrent chemoradiation therapy to a total dose of 54 Gy to the nasopharynx, larynx, and uninvolved left neck (CTV$_{54}$ = *green* contour). Given the high suspicion of an oropharyngeal primary, the oropharynx was treated to 59.4 Gy along with the right neck (CTV$_{59.4}$ = *orange* contour). The gross nodal disease was treated to 70 Gy using concomitant boost technique (GTV$_{70}$ = *red* contour). Please note that these are representative slices and not all slices are included

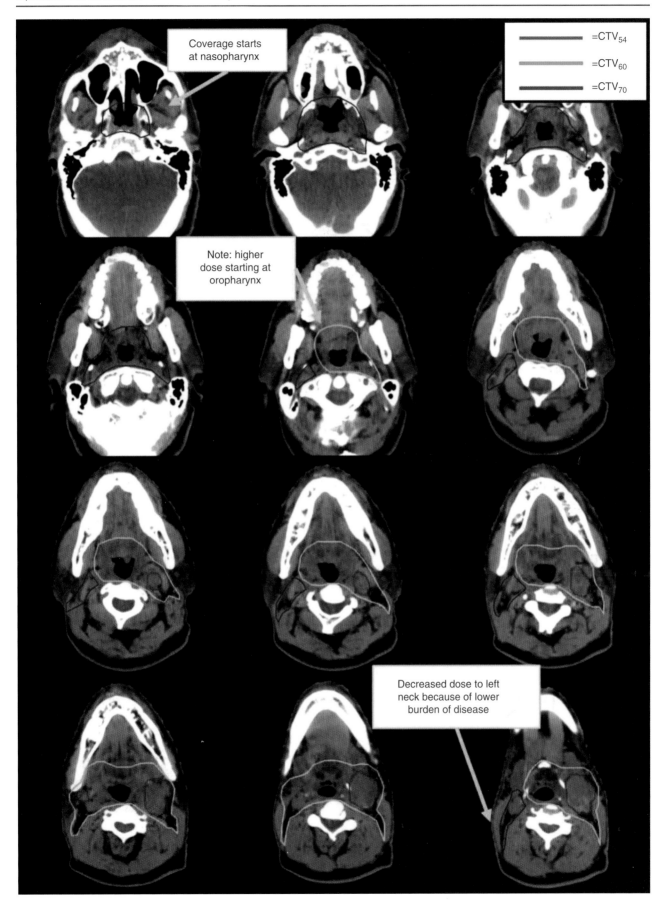

**Fig. 4** A 50-year-old gentleman with a TxN2c squamous cell carcinoma referred for definitive treatment. An open biopsy of a left lymph node demonstrated extra-nodal extension. HPV ISH and p16 testing were negative. He received definitive chemoradiotherapy. The CTV$_{70Gy}$ is in *red*, the CTV$_{60Gy}$ is in *green*, and the CTV$_{54Gy}$ is in *blue*. Please note that these are representative slices and not all slices are included

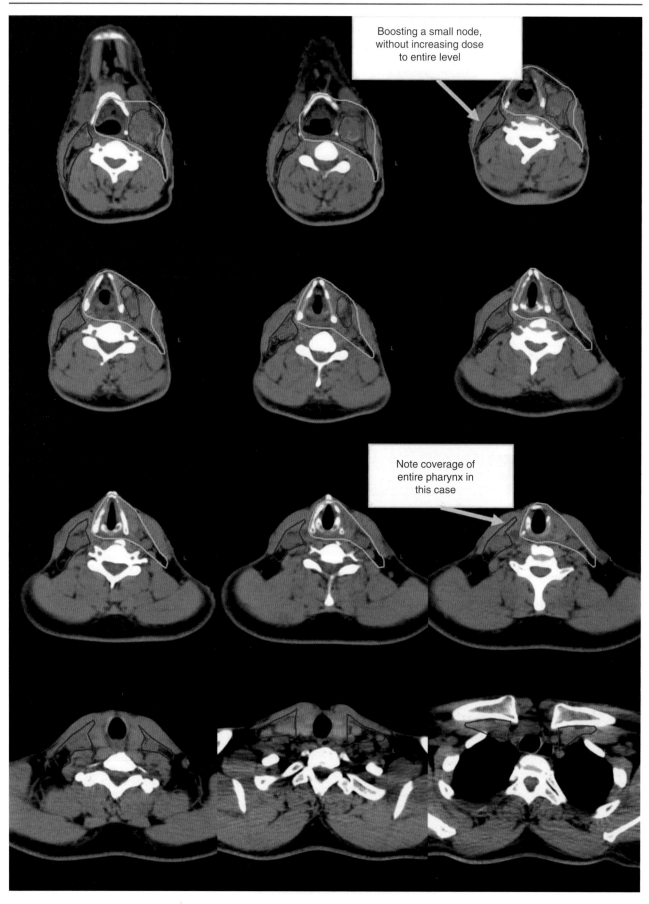

**Fig. 4** (continued)

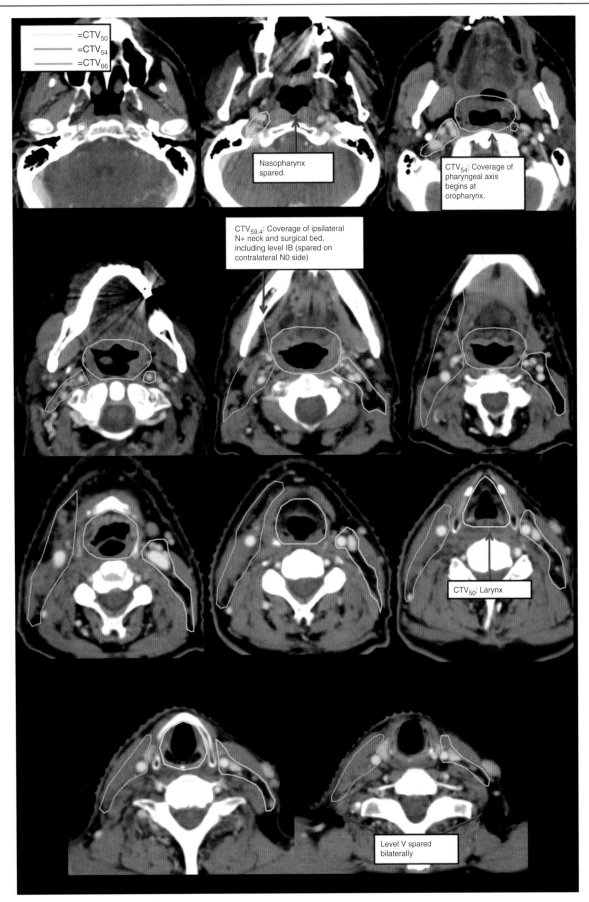

**Fig. 5** 64M with TxN2bM0 SCC. He underwent a tonsillectomy and right-sided neck dissection that showed 2/21 lymph nodes positive with extracapsular extension. Immunostaining for p16 and HPV in situ hybridization was positive. Given the HPV positivity of the tumor and the high suspicion of an oropharyngeal primary, the nasopharynx and bilateral level V were spared and the larynx was treated to a reduced dose of 50 Gy (CTV$_{50}$ = *yellow* contour). The oropharynx and left neck were treated to 54 Gy (CTV$_{54}$ = *green* contour) and the right neck was treated to 66 Gy (CTV$_{66}$ = *orange* contour). Please note that these are representative slices and not all slices are included

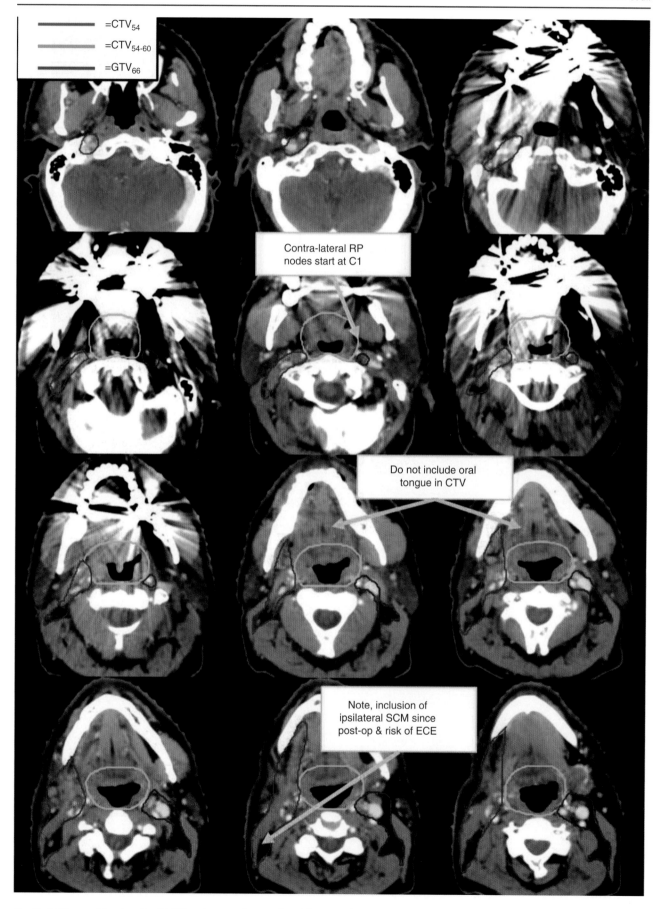

**Fig. 6** A 62-year-old male with a TxN2a unknown primary referred for postoperative treatment. He underwent bilateral tonsillectomy and a right neck dissection which revealed a single 4.6 cm level II lymph node. Notice the difference in the target delineation in the involved neck versus the contralateral neck. The $CTV_{66Gy}$ is in *red*, the $CTV_{54-60Gy}$ is in *green*, and the $CTV_{54Gy}$ is in *blue*. Please note that these are representative slices and not all slices are included

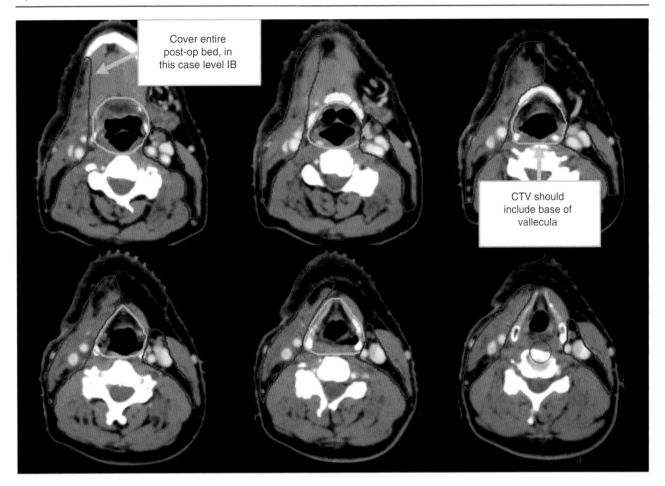

**Fig. 6** (continued)

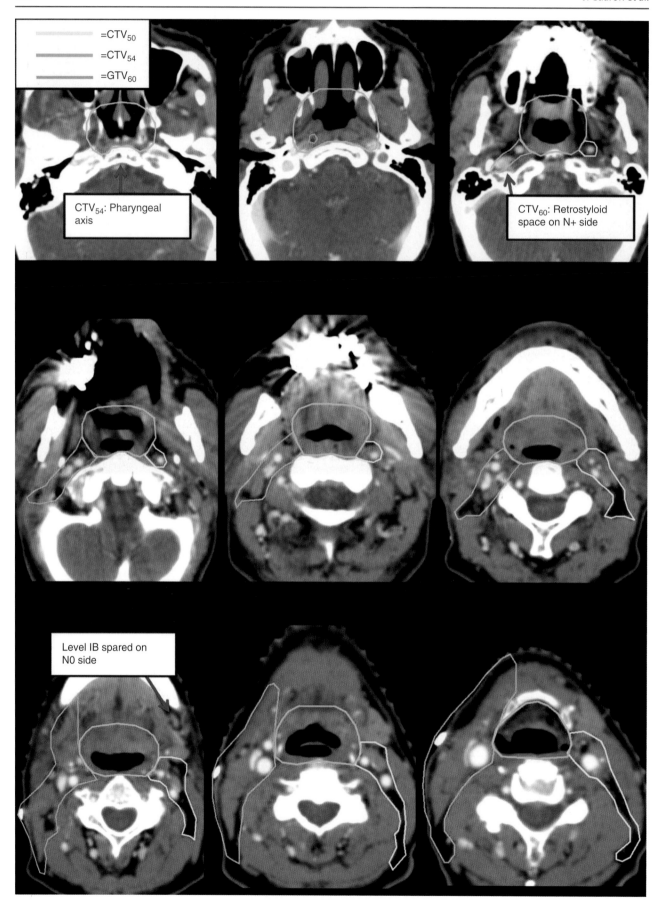

**Fig. 7** 76M Hx of TxN1M0 SQCUP. He underwent a right neck dissection that showed 1/26 lymph nodes positive at level III of the right neck, without ECE. On examination, there was fullness in the nasopharynx, but imaging, biopsy, and EBV staining failed to identify a nasopharyngeal primary tumor. The suspicion for a nasopharyngeal primary remained high. He was treated with comprehensive pharyngeal irradiation to a total dose of 54 Gy (CTV$_{54}$ = *green* contour). The larynx and left neck were treated to 50 Gy (CTV$_{50}$ = *yellow* contour) and the surgical bed and right neck were treated to 60 Gy (CTV$_{60}$ = *orange* contour). Please note that these are representative slices and not all slices are included

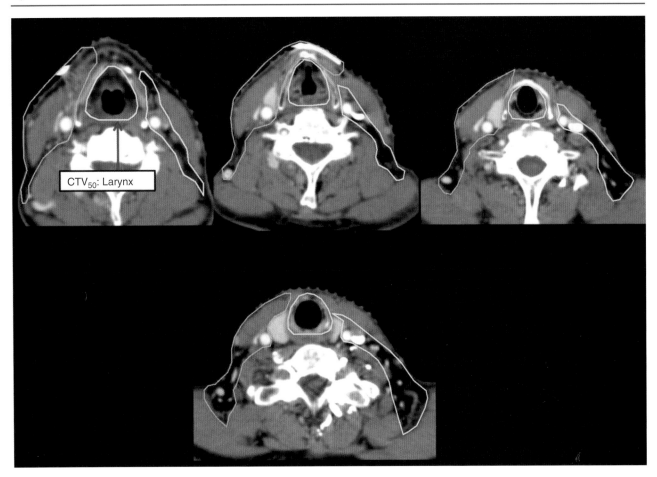

**Fig. 7** (continued)

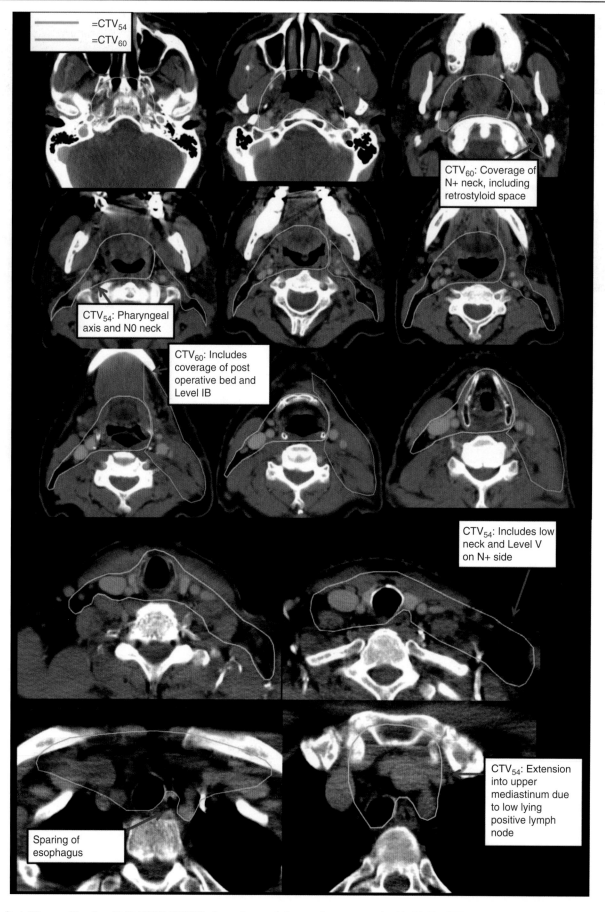

**Fig. 8** A 57-year-old male with TxN1M0 SQCUP who underwent left modified radical neck dissection showing 2/44 positive lymph nodes with extracapsular extension in the left posterior triangle. He was treated with concurrent chemoradiation therapy. The pharyngeal axis and right neck were treated with 54 Gy (CTV$_{54}$ = *green* contour), the upper left neck and postoperative bed were treated to 60 Gy (CTV$_{60}$ = *orange* contour), and the left low neck was treated to 54 Gy. Please note that these are representative slices and not all slices are included

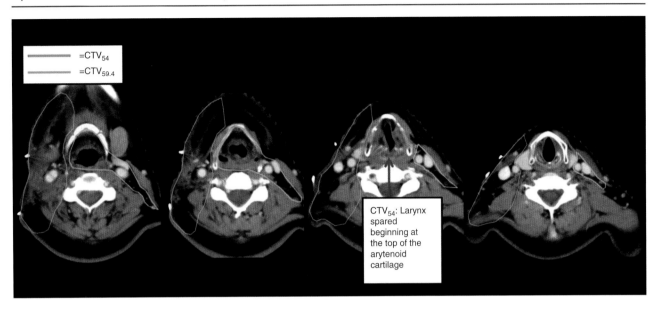

**Fig. 9** 56M TxN3M0 SQCUP. He underwent resection and was treated with postoperative chemoradiation therapy. The postoperative bed and ipsilateral neck were treated to a dose of 66 Gy (CTV$_{66}$ = *orange* contour). The pharyngeal axis was treated to 54 Gy (CTV$_{54}$ = *green* contour) with sparing of the larynx. Please note that these are representative slices and not all slices are included

**Table 2** Intensity-modulated radiation therapy: normal tissue dose constraints

| Critical structures | Constraints |
|---|---|
| Brain stem | Max <50 Gy or 1 % of PTV cannot exceed 60 Gy |
| Optic nerves | Max <54 Gy or 1 % of PTV cannot exceed 60 Gy |
| Optic chiasm | Max <54 Gy or 1 % of PTV cannot exceed 60 Gy |
| Spinal cord | Max <45 Gy or 1 cc of the PTV cannot exceed 50 Gy |
| Mandible and TMJ | Max <70 Gy or 1 cc of the PTV cannot exceed 75 Gy |
| Brachial plexus | Max <65 Gy |
| Temporal lobes | Max <60 Gy or 1 % of PTV cannot exceed 65 Gy |
| Other normal structures | Constraints |
| Oral cavity | Mean <40 Gy |
| Parotid gland | (a) Mean ≤26 Gy in one gland |
| | (b) Or at least 20 cc of the combined volume of both parotid glands will receive <20 Gy |
| | (c) Or at least 50 % of one gland will receive <30 Gy |
| Cochlea | (a) Max <50 Gy |
| | (b) Or V55 <5 % |
| Eyes | Mean <35 Gy, max <50 Gy |
| Lens | Max <5 Gy |
| Esophagus, postcricoid pharynx | Mean <45 Gy |

*PTV* planning target volume

Based on guidelines presently used at Memorial Sloan Kettering Cancer Center

## Suggested Reading

Gillison ML, D'Souza G, Westra W et al (2008) Distinct risk factor profiles for human papillomavirus type 16-positive and human papillomavirus type 16-negative head and neck cancers. J Natl Cancer Inst 100:407–420

Mendenhall WM, Mancuso AA, Werning JW (2012) Unknown head and neck primary site. In: Gunderson LL, Tepper JE, Bogart JA (eds) Clinical radiation oncology, 3rd edn. Saunders/Elsevier, Philadelphia, pp 723–729

Nieder C, Gregoirc V, Ang KK (2001) Cervical lymph node metastases from occult squamous cell carcinoma: cut down a tree to get an apple? Int J Radiat Oncol Biol Phys 50:727–733

Strojan P, Ferlito A, Medina JE et al (2011a) Contemporary management of lymph node metastases from an unknown primary to the neck: I. A review of diagnostic approaches. Head Neck

Strojan P, Ferlito A, Langendijk JA et al (2011b) Contemporary management of lymph node metastases from an unknown primary to the neck: II. A review of therapeutic options. Head Neck

## References

Barker CA, Morris CG, Mendenhall WM (2005) Larynx-sparing radiotherapy for squamous cell carcinoma from an unknown head and neck primary site. Am J Clin Oncol 28:445–448

Cianchetti M et al (2009) Diagnostic evaluation of squamous cell carcinoma metastatic to cervical lymph nodes from an unknown head and neck primary site. Laryngoscope 119:2348–2354. doi:10.1002/lary.20638

Grau C et al (2000) Cervical lymph node metastases from unknown primary tumours. Results from a national survey by the Danish Society for Head and Neck Oncology. Radiother Oncol 55:121–129

Ligey A et al (2009) Impact of target volumes and radiation technique on loco-regional control and survival for patients with unilateral cervical lymph node metastases from an unknown primary. Radiother Oncol 93:483–487. doi:10.1016/j.radonc.2009.08.027

Lu X, Hu C, Ji Q, Shen C, Feng Y (2009) Squamous cell carcinoma metastatic to cervical lymph nodes from an unknown primary site: the impact of radiotherapy. Tumori 95:185–190

Perkins SM et al (2012) Radiotherapeutic management of cervical lymph node metastases from an unknown primary site. Arch Otolaryngol Head Neck Surg 138:656–661. doi:10.1001/archoto.2012.1110

Reddy SP, Marks JE (1997) Metastatic carcinoma in the cervical lymph nodes from an unknown primary site: results of bilateral neck plus mucosal irradiation vs. ipsilateral neck irradiation. Int J Radiat Oncol Biol Phys 37:797–802

Rusthoven KE, Koshy M, Paulino AC (2004) The role of fluorodeoxyglucose positron emission tomography in cervical lymph node metastases from an unknown primary tumor. Cancer 101:2641–2649. doi:10.1002/cncr.20687

Stenmark MH et al (2013) High frequency of HPV-Associated Nasopharyngeal Carcinoma (NPC) in North American Patients: association with poor prognosis [abstract]. In: Proceedings of the annual meeting of the American Society for Radiation Oncology, Atlanta. 22–25 Sept 2013, Abstract No. 194

Weir L et al (1995) Radiation treatment of cervical lymph node metastases from an unknown primary: an analysis of outcome by treatment volume and other prognostic factors. Radiother Oncol 35:206–211

# Locally Advanced and High-Risk Cutaneous Malignancies

Christopher A. Barker

## Contents

C.A. Barker
Department of Radiation Oncology,
Memorial Sloan Kettering Cancer Center,
New York, New York 10065 USA
e-mail: barkerc@mskcc.org

## 1 Anatomy and Patterns of Spread

The skin is composed of two layers: the more superficial and thinner epidermis and the deeper and thicker dermis.

The epidermis (average thickness 0.05 mm) contains keratinocytes (basal cells and squamous epithelial cells), melanocytes, and Langerhans cells among others. Structures such as hair and glandular ducts project through the epidermis.

The dermis (average thickness 2 mm) contains Merkel cells, lymphatic and vascular channels, nerves, mast cells, fibroblasts, macrophages, and dendritic cells among others. Structures such as hair follicles, sweat glands, and small muscles are present in the dermis.

The division between the epidermis and the dermis is the basement membrane.

The hypodermis (subcutis or subcutaneous tissue) is deep to the dermis and also contains lymphatic and vascular channels, nerves, adipose, and other tissues that connect the skin to underlying muscles, bones, and cartilage (Fig. 1).

The thickness of the skin (epidermis and dermis) varies between 0.5 and 4 mm in locations such as the eyelids and palms/soles, respectively.

The skin covers almost all external surfaces of the body, for an average surface area of $1.79 \ m^2$ (men $1.91 \ m^2$, women $1.71 \ m^2$) (Sacco et al. 2010). Body surface area can be approximated by height and mass using the Dubois and Dubois method:

$$\text{Body surface area}\left(\text{in} \ m^2\right) = \text{mass}\left(\text{in kg}\right)^{0.425} \times \text{height}\left(\text{in cm}\right)^{0.725} \times 0.007184$$

The palm of a patient's hand is estimated to be approximately 0.5 % of the total body surface area (Rhodes et al. 2013).

N.Y. Lee et al. (eds.), *Target Volume Delineation for Conformal and Intensity-Modulated Radiation Therapy*, Medical Radiology. Radiation Oncology, DOI: 10.1007/174_2014_975, © Springer International Publishing Switzerland 2014
Published Online: 22 October 2014

**Fig. 1** Composition of the skin.
(*sq*) squamous cells, (*b*) basal
cell, (*m*) melanocytes,
(*f*) fibroblast, (*dc*) dendritic cell,
(*lc*) Langerhans cell, (*mc*) mast
cell, (*Mc*) Merkel cell, (*h*) hair,
(*n*) nerve, (*P*) Pacinian corpuscle,
(*v*) vessels, (*s*) sebaceous gland,
(*mu*) muscle, erector pili,
(*ec*) eccrine gland,
(*Me*) Meissner's corpuscle.
(Credited to MSKCC)

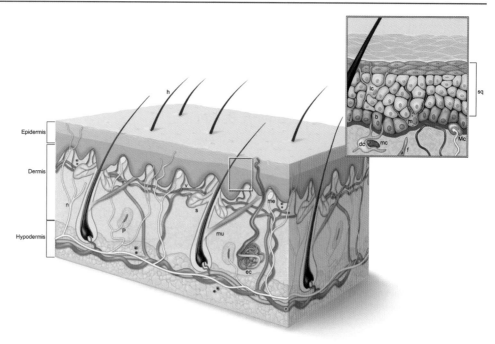

The lymphatic channels of the skin are within the dermis and drain to lymphatic channels of the hypodermis and eventually to the regional lymph node basins. Note that some skin regions will drain to multiple lymph node basins.

An interactive tool is available to aid in the prediction of the draining lymph node basin for primary skin cancers of the head and neck (http://sites.bioeng.auckland.ac.nz/hrey004/head/) and trunk and extremities (http://sites.bioeng.auckland.ac.nz/hrey004/) (Figs. 2, 3, 4, 5, and 6).

Different types of skin cancer have different proclivities for spread.

Local spread can occur superficially along planes of the skin and hypodermis (SCC, especially sclerosing or desmoplastic subtypes; BCC, especially infiltrative or morpheaform subtypes; angiosarcoma), along cutaneous nerves (SCC, BCC, and melanoma, especially desmoplastic and/or neurotropic subtypes), and through direct invasion of subcutaneous and deeper tissues (SCC, BCC, especially deeply invasive subtypes).

Regional spread can develop via "in-transit" dermal lymphatics to lymph node basins (Merkel cell carcinoma, melanoma, angiosarcoma, SCC, especially deeply invasive subtypes).

Distant spread can occur hematogenously (Merkel cell carcinoma, melanoma, SCC, especially those that have spread regionally).

# 2 Diagnostic Workup for Relevant Target Volume Delineation

## 2.1 Clinical Evaluation

Symptom assessment is critical to help determine if a skin cancer harbors high-risk features.

Local neurologic symptoms such as pain, paresthesias, anesthesia, dysesthesia, pruritus, and formications can herald neurotropic cancer and should be routinely queried and investigated further if present.

Physical examination for abnormal local neurologic signs in the case of potentially neurotropic skin cancers is essential. Strength, sensory, or reflex impairments should prompt further evaluation when abnormalities are present.

Examination of regional lymph node basins at risk for disease is also vital. Primary skin cancers at or approaching midline require examination of the lymph node basins bilaterally.

Direct visualization of the skin under bright light (projected at different angles) and magnification is the best means of determining the extent of superficial disease. Carefully observing the color, texture, creases, follicles, and hair growth pattern of the skin harboring cancer and comparing this to normal skin can be helpful.

Palpation of the skin can also help delineate the extent of superficial disease. For skin cancers on surfaces that can be palpated between gloved fingers from opposing surfaces (lip, ear, cheek), this practice is encouraged. Assess fixation to underlying structures by moving the lesion along the plane of the skin surface. Fixation of the skin cancer to the structures beneath subcutaneous tissues can suggest local invasion and requires further evaluation when present.

## 2.2 Imaging

Calibrated clinical digital photography is encouraged to characterize and record the appearance of skin cancer. Appropriate lighting, positioning, focus, exposure, and zoom are encouraged (Bhatia 2006).

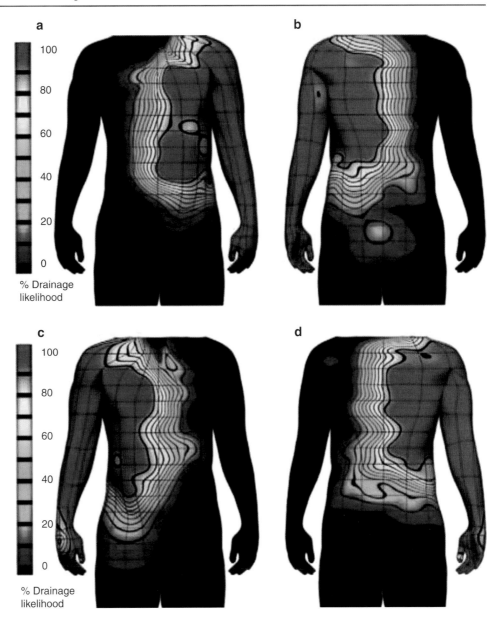

**Fig. 2** Likelihood of lymphatic drainage to axillary lymph nodes from different sites of primary skin cancer (Reynolds et al. 2007). Drainage to left axillary lymphatics (**a**, **b**); and right axillary lymphatics (**c**, **d**). Regions of skin with no lymphatic drainage to axilla are colored black. (**a**, **c**) are anterior projections and (**b**, **d**) are posterior projections

Wood's lamp (ultraviolet light at ~365 nm) can help delineate the extent of pigmented skin cancers (Paraskevas et al. 2005).

Investigational modalities for determining the superficial extent of skin cancer include, but are not limited to, reflectance confocal microscopy, high-frequency ultrasonography, optical coherence microscopy, and in vivo fluorescence microscopy.

Gadolinium-enhanced MRI can help assess the extent of perineural invasion (PNI) in cases of neurotropic skin cancer. Typically, patients with radiographic evidence of perineural spread will also have symptoms or signs of PNI (clinical PNI or cPNI) and pathologic evidence of PNI (pPNI). The absence of radiographic evidence of perineural spread does not exclude the possibility of neurotropic skin cancer.

CT provides a superior assessment of cortical bone and is the preferred modality for determining the extent of local bone invasion. MRI can identify marrow involvement.

MRI and CT with or without PET can all be valuable in the assessment of regional lymphadenopathy. Nodes are considered involved with cancer when they exhibit abnormal morphology (metabolically active, centrally necrotic, irregular capsule, rounded shape without fatty hilum) or size (>10 mm in short axis) (Schwartz et al. 2009).

## 2.3 Tissue Sampling

Punch, rather than shave, biopsy to the superficial reticular dermis through the tumor is the preferred method of diagnosis of skin cancer. Shave biopsy may be preferable

**Fig. 3** Likelihood of lymphatic drainage to the groin lymphatics from different sites of primary skin cancer (Reynolds et al. 2007). Drainage to left groin lymphatics (**a**, **b**); and right groin lymphatics (**c**, **d**). (**a**, **c**) are anterior projections and (**b**, **d**) are posterior projections

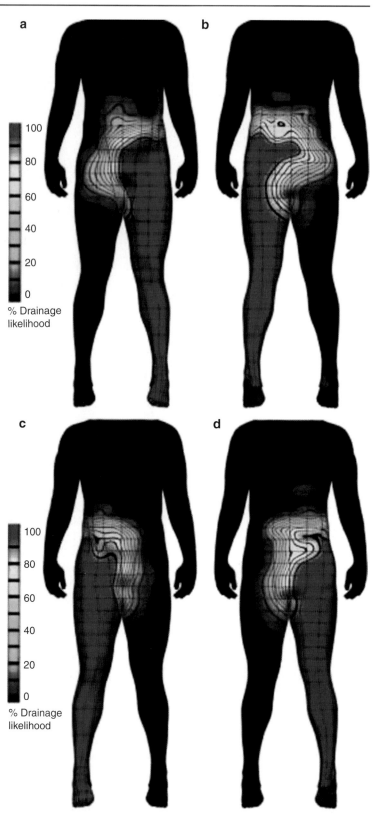

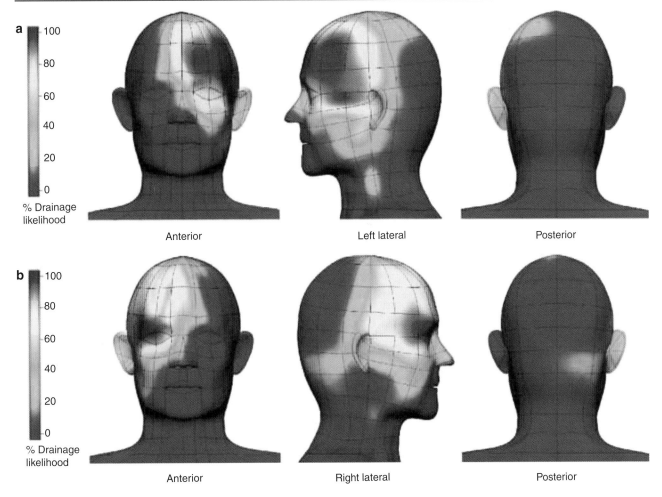

**Fig. 4** Likelihood of lymphatic drainage to the left (**a**) and right (**b**) preauricular lymphatics from different sites of primary skin cancer (Reynolds et al. 2009)

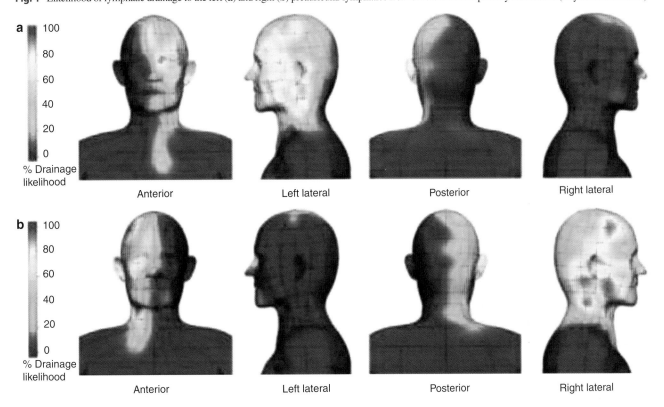

**Fig. 5** Likelihood of lymphatic drainage to the left (**a**) and right (**b**) upper cervical (level II) lymphatics from different sites of primary skin cancer (Reynolds et al. 2009)

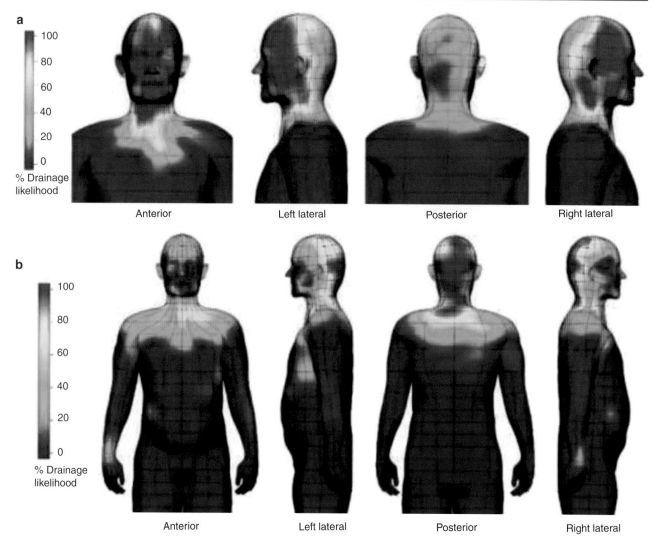

**Fig. 6** Likelihood of lymphatic drainage to anterior (preauricular, submental, cervical I–IV, **a**) or posterior (postauricular, suboccipital, cervical V, supraclavicular, **b**) neck lymphatics from different sites of primary skin cancer (Reynolds et al. 2009)

in cosmetically sensitive areas or in certain patient populations; however, the depth of invasion and high-risk histopathologic features are often difficult to ascertain on shave biopsy.

Some "infiltrative" types of skin cancers are superficially occult. Mapping biopsies at the periphery of a poorly defined skin cancer can help determine the extent of disease not apparent on visual inspection.

Sentinel lymph node biopsy should be considered for several forms of skin cancer when there is no clinical evidence of regional lymph node metastasis: cutaneous melanoma >0.75 mm thick, all Merkel cell carcinoma (regardless of size or thickness), cutaneous SCC >2 mm thick.

## 3 Simulation and Daily Localization

### 3.1 General Guidelines

Patient positioning for the treatment of skin cancer is highly dependent on the location of the target volume and radiotherapy technique.

CT (with or without PET, with or without MRI) is performed for simulation. Intravenous contrast media is recommended for all sites, when not medically contraindicated. Oral contrast is recommended for patients with a target volume near the gastrointestinal tract. Slice thickness of 2 mm is preferred for target volumes incorporating cranial nerves or the skull base. Otherwise, a slice thickness of 3 mm is preferred. Head and neck scans should include the entire head and neck through the carina. Upper trunk and extremity scans should include the mastoid processes through the entire volume of the lungs. Lower trunk and extremity scans should include the iliac crests through the popliteal fossa. Isocenter is placed in the center of the target volume.

Image registration and fusion of MR and PET with CT should be performed to help guide target delineation or relevant targets (nerves, ganglia, hypermetabolic tumors).

## 3.2 Skin Surface Targets

Prior to simulation, patients should be reexamined and the superficial extent of the skin cancer marked on the skin surface with a single use sterile marker. Fiducial markers (radiopaque wires with adhesive) should be placed on these marks to aid in target volume delineation in CT datasets. Of note, patients with clinical or pathologic evidence of extranodal extension of carcinoma are at risk for dermal disease in proximity to any surgical scars. A 2 cm perimeter is marked around surgical scars, and this along with the surgical scars themselves (incision and drain sites) should be marked with fiducial markers. Prior radiotherapy sites should also be delineated on the skin surface using fiducial markers.

Patients with skin, in-transit lymphatics, or regional node basins at risk for dermal disease should have appropriate tissue equivalent bolus fabricated prior to fabrication of the immobilization equipment. Bolus thickness will depend on radiotherapy technique (generally, we use 0.5 cm for conformal plans incorporating beams oblique to the skin surface and 1.0–1.5 cm for single-field and parallel-opposed beam arrangements when beams are normally incident to the skin surface). Tissue equivalent bolus should be positioned between the skin surface at risk and the immobilization equipment. When possible, the tissue equivalent bolus should be fixed to the immobilization equipment to aid in setup reproducibility.

When the skin surface is at risk, in vivo dosimetry is encouraged to confirm adequate dose at the skin surface. This is particularly important with heavily modulated planning techniques (e.g., IMRT) (Price et al. 2006).

## 3.3 Head and Neck Targets

Patients with skin cancers of the head and neck are usually immobilized supine with a thermoplastic mask. In some cases, the prone position may be preferable for posterior targets. For the treatment of the neck lymphatics only, the neck is extended. For the treatment of cranial nerves V1 and V2 or the skull base, the neck is kept in a neutral position, with the hard palate normal to the table top. Gaze fixation and intraoral stent may also be valuable in this situation.

## 3.4 Upper Trunk or Extremity Targets

Patients with skin cancers of the upper trunk or extremities are immobilized supine in an alpha cradle. In some cases, the prone position may be preferable for posterior targets. For patients with a target volume in the axilla, the ipsilateral arm is placed akimbo. This position is preferred to arm maximally abducted as patients are often elderly and have very recently undergone axillary surgery, which limits the ability to abduct the arm. Absent these conditions, maximal arm abduction is an acceptable alternative position. CT bore and linear accelerator gantry permitting, the arm should be abducted enough so that no skin folds are present in the axilla. This helps reduce dermatitis in the axilla. Rotation of the arm and immobilization at the hand may be necessary for patients with target volumes along the length of the extremity or in the epitrochlear fossa.

## 3.5 Lower Trunk or Extremity Targets

Patients with skin cancers of the lower trunk or extremities are immobilized supine in an alpha cradle. In some cases, the prone position may be preferable for posterior targets. For patients with a target volume in the groin, the ipsilateral hip is abducted ("frog-leg"). CT bore and linear accelerator gantry permitting, the leg should be abducted enough so that no skin folds are present in the groin. This helps prevent dermatitis in the groin. Rotation of the leg and immobilization of the foot may be necessary for patients with target volumes along the length of the leg or in the popliteal fossa.

## 3.6 Daily Localization

Localization is dependent on the anatomic region being treated. Generally, for skin cancers of the head and neck, daily orthogonal kV images are used for localization. This is particularly important when targeting cranial nerves and the skull base. For skin cancers of the extremity and trunk, weekly MV images are used for localization.

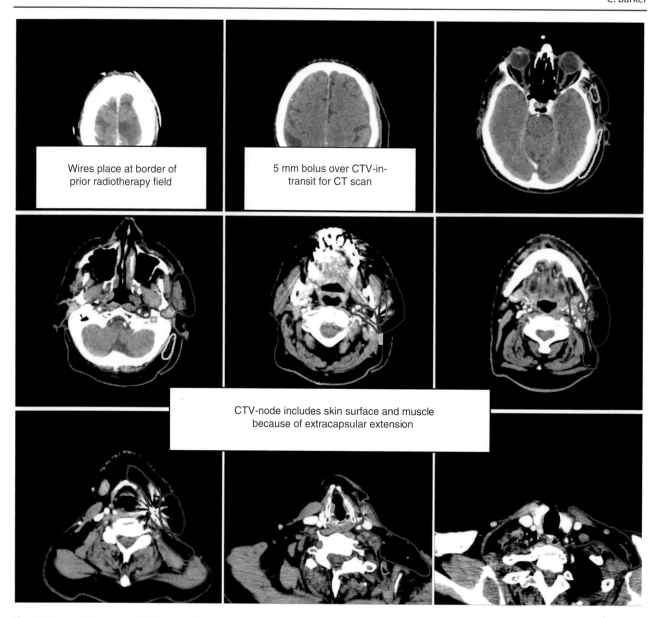

**Fig. 7** Target delineation of CTVs in a 75-year-old man with rpT0N-2bM0R0 cutaneous squamous cell carcinoma of the vertex of the scalp in axial CT displayed from cranial to caudal direction. He underwent wide excision of the primary tumor, adjuvant radiotherapy to the scalp vertex, and recurrence in left temporal in-transit and preauricular lymphatics. He underwent excision of the left temporal in-transit metastasis and left superficial parotidectomy. Pathology revealed squamous cell carcinoma within the left temporal dermis and parotid gland, not within a lymph node. Adjuvant radiotherapy was recommended to the left temporal in-transit lymphatics (*orange*, intact; *dark blue*, free flap), left preauricular (*light blue*), postauricular (*yellow*) and cervical (IB-VB, *pink*) lymphatics, and the facial nerve (*green*) to a dose of 60 Gy in 30 fractions, with a cone-down boost to the sites of resected carcinoma (*turquoise* and *light blue*) to a total dose of 70 Gy in 35 fractions over 7 weeks. Please note that these are representative images and not all images are included

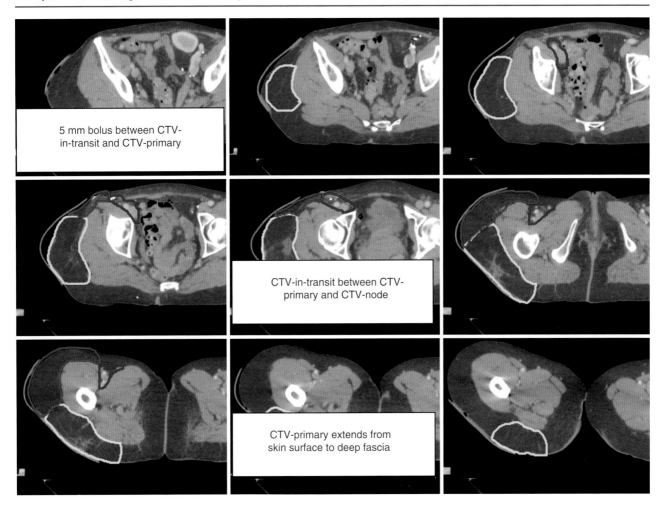

**Fig. 8** Target delineation of CTVs in a 54-year-old woman with pT2N1aM0R0 Merkel cell carcinoma of the left posterior thigh in axial CT displayed from cranial to caudal direction. She has a history of renal allograft (note left pelvic kidney) and underwent wide excision of the primary tumor and sentinel lymph node biopsy of a left inguinofemoral lymph node. Pathology revealed a 4.5 cm Merkel cell carcinoma, with microscopic involvement of the sentinel lymph node. Adjuvant radio-therapy was recommended to the left posterior thigh primary tumor site (*yellow*), in-transit lymphatics (*pink*), and left inguinofemoral lymphatics (*blue*) to a dose of 50 Gy in 25 fractions, with a cone-down boost to the site of resected carcinoma to a total dose of 60 Gy in 30 fractions over 6 weeks. Please note that these are representative images and not all images are included

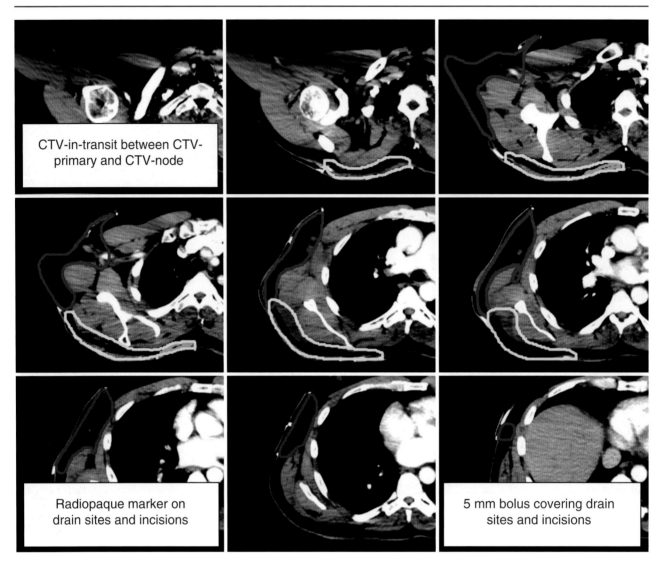

**Fig. 9** Target delineation of CTVs in a 54-year-old man with rpT0N-2bM0R0 basal cell carcinoma of the right posterior trunk in axial CT displayed from cranial to caudal direction. He has a history of acquired immunodeficiency syndrome and underwent excision and subsequent re-excision of the primary tumor for recurrence. He subsequently recurred in the in-transit lymphatics of the posterior trunk between the primary tumor and the draining lymph node basin in the right axilla. Excision of the in-transit metastasis and axillary lymphadenectomy revealed carcinoma, not within a node. Adjuvant radiotherapy was recommended to the left posterior trunk primary tumor site (*green*), in-transit lymphatics (*yellow*), and axilla (*blue*) to a dose of 60 Gy in 30 fractions, with an integrated boost to the site of resected carcinoma to a total dose of 66 Gy in 30 fractions over 6 weeks. Please note that these are representative images and not all images are included

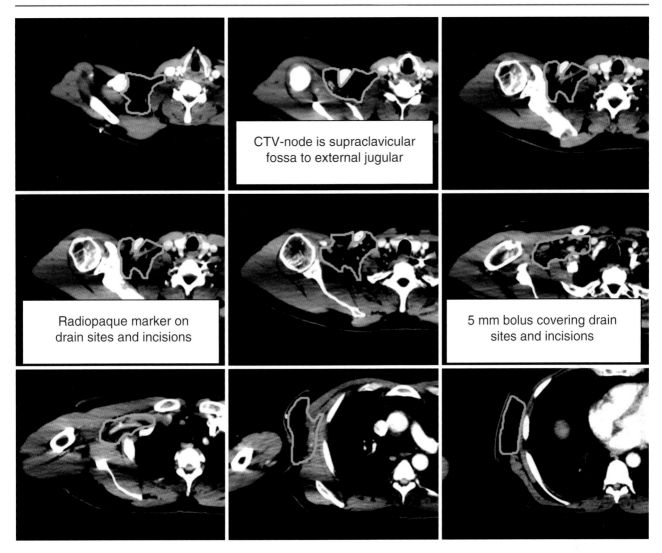

**Fig. 10** Target delineation of CTVs in a 55-year-old man with pT4bN-2bM0R0 cutaneous melanoma of the right shoulder in axial CT displayed from cranial to caudal direction. He underwent wide local excision of the primary tumor and axillary lymphadenectomy revealing 3 nodes involved with melanoma, measuring up to 5.3 cm in size, with extranodal extension. Adjuvant radiotherapy was recommended to the right axilla and supraclavicular fossa (*green*). The patient requested an abbreviated course of therapy and was therefore given a dose of 30 Gy in 5 fractions over 2.5 weeks. Please note that these are representative images and not all images are included

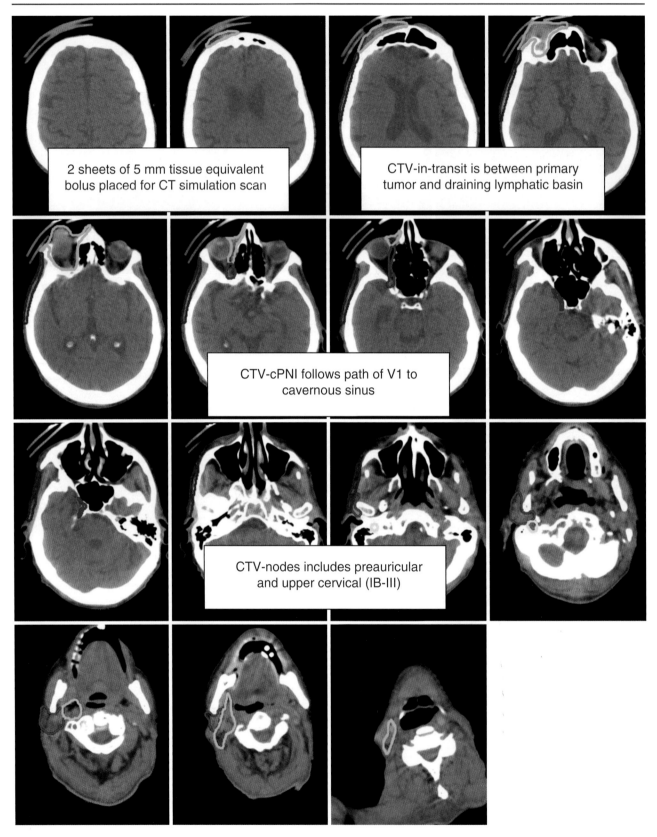

**Fig. 11** Target delineation CTVs in a 79-year-old man with cT3N0M0 cutaneous squamous cell carcinoma of the right brow in axial CT displayed from cranial to caudal direction. Imaging revealed perineural invasion along the distal right ophthalmic branch of the trigeminal nerve (V1) at the supraorbital notch. Definitive radiotherapy was recommended to the primary tumor (*green*), the V1 nerve (*blue*), and the in-transit (*purple*), preauricular (*pink*), and upper cervical (IB-III, *turquoise*) lymphatics and facial nerve (*yellow*) to a dose of 56 Gy using in 23 fractions, with an cone-down boost (using electrons and an internal eye shield) to the primary tumor to a total dose of 86 Gy in 43 fractions over 8.6 weeks. Please note that these are representative images and not all images are included

## 4 Target Volume Delineation and Treatment Planning
(Figs. 7, 8, 9, 10, and 11)

GTV-T – tumor (clinically apparent tumor on physical exam or imaging)

GTV-N – nodes (clinically apparent nodes on physical exam or imaging)

CTV-T – peritumor (subclinical disease on skin surface adjacent to primary tumor [radial distance along skin surface from primary tumor according to Table 1], and deep to this including the dermis, and hypodermis to deep fascia); tumors with clinical evidence of deep invasion may require more extensive CTV-T (i.e., when primary tumor invading paranasal sinus, adjacent paranasal sinuses may need to be included as CTV-T)

CTV-IT – in-transit (subclinical disease in dermal lymphatics between primary tumor and draining node basin for distances <20 cm)

CTV-N – node (subclinical disease in draining node basin; see Figs. 2, 3, 4, 5, 6, 12, 13, and 14 and Table 2)[1]

CTV-lpPNI – limited pathologic perineural invasion (subclinical disease surrounding primary tumor, 2 cm surrounding primary tumor)

---

[1] For patients with node basin recurrence <1 year after treatment of primary skin cancer, generally the primary tumor and in-transit lymphatics are irradiated, if feasible and not previously treated.

**Table 1** CTV skin surface margin on GTV (respecting natural anatomic barriers to spread)

| Skin cancer | GTV to CTV margin (mm) |
|---|---|
| Low-risk SCC/BCC | 4 |
| High-risk SCC/BCC | 20 |
| Melanoma in situ | 5 |
| Desmoplastic neurotropic melanoma | 20 |
| Merkel cell carcinoma | 40 |

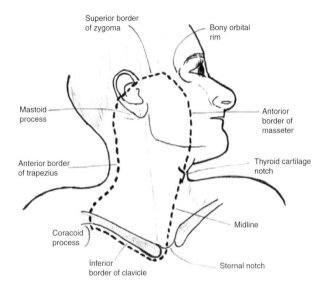

**Fig. 12** Skin surface borders for adjuvant electron beam radiotherapy after lymphadenectomy for cutaneous melanoma metastatic to the pre-auricular or cervical lymphatics (Burmeister et al. 2006)

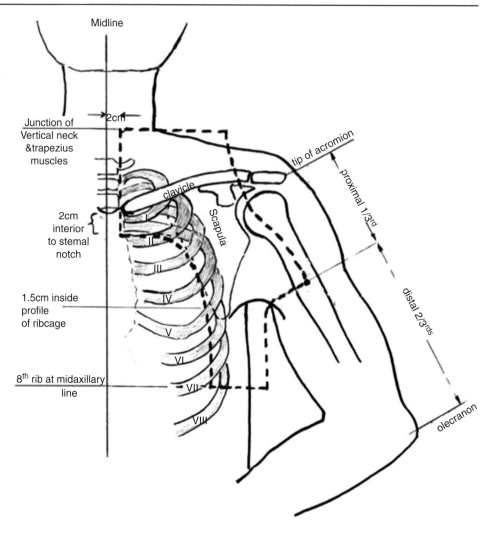

**Fig. 13** Field borders for adjuvant high-energy photon radiotherapy after lymphadenectomy for cutaneous melanoma metastatic to the axillary lymphatics (Burmeister et al. 2006)

Midline

Junction of
Vertical neck
&trapezius
muscles

2cm
interior
to stemal
notch

1.5cm inside
profile
of ribcage

8th rib at midaxillary
line

2cm

clavicle

Scapula

tip of acromion

proximal 1/3rd

distal 2/3rds

olecranon

I

II

III

IV

V

VI

VII

VIII

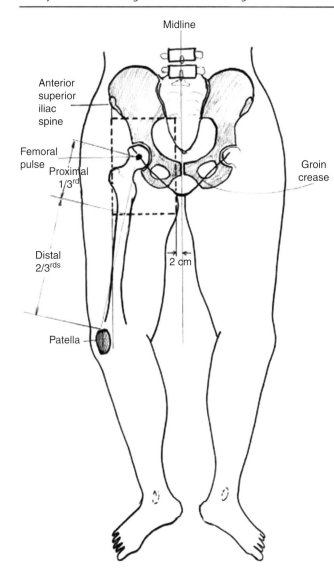

**Fig. 14** Field borders for adjuvant high-energy photon radiotherapy after lymphadenectomy for cutaneous melanoma metastatic to the inguinofemoral lymphatics (Burmeister et al. 2006)

**Table 2** Expert consensus of cervical lymphatics at risk in cutaneous SCC metastatic to the preauricular/parotid region based on primary tumor location (O'Hara et al. 2011)

| Location of primary tumor | Cervical lymphatics at risk |
|---|---|
| Face | I–III and external jugular node |
| Anterior scalp and external ear | II–III and external jugular node |
| Posterior scalp and neck | II–IV and external jugular node |

CTV-epPNI – extensive pathologic perineural invasion (CTV – limited PNI+sensory dermatome+motor myotome (when feasible) to distal bony foraminal origin)

CTV-cPNI – clinical perineural invasion (CTV – extensive PNI+nerve pathway to origin at brainstem or spinal cord)

PTV – depends on immobilization and daily localization, but generally 2–10 mm. Smaller for HN and larger for trunk and extremities (Table 3)

## 5    Plan Assessment

Standard planning goals for conventional fractionation set forth in other chapters of this textbook are generally used for skin cancers. Prospective studies of hypofractionated radiotherapy for skin cancer have used specific dose constraints detailed below:

*TROG constraints.* The TROG 96.06 and 02.01 studies using standardized fields (Figs. 12–14, depicted above) also limited doses to several organs and tissues when delivering a dose of 48 Gy in 20 fractions of 2.4 Gy.

Brain and spinal cord $\leq$40 Gy

Bowel (small volume), brachial plexus, mandible, and larynx $\leq$45 Gy

Femoral neck, bowel (V1000 cm$^3$) $\leq$35 Gy

**Table 3** Dose and fractionation schema for selected locally advanced and high-risk cutaneous malignancies

| Disease | Source | Site | Condition | Total dose (Gy) | Fractions (number) | Margins |
|---------|--------|------|-----------|-----------------|--------------------|---------|
| MCC | NCCN (2014a) | Primary tumor | R0 resection | 50–56 | 25–28 | 5 cm if possible |
| | NCCN (2014a) | Primary tumor | R1 resection | 56–60 | 28–30 | 5 cm if possible |
| | NCCN (2014a) | Primary tumor | R2 resection or unresectable | 60–66 | 30–33 | 5 cm if possible |
| | Jouary et al. (2012) | Primary tumor | Local excision with ≥1.5 cm radial margin deep to perimuscular aponeurosis | 60 | 30 | 3 cm around excision if possible |
| | NCCN (2014a) | Lymph node basin | cN0, not sampled or dissected | 46–50 | 23–25 | |
| | NCCN (2014a) | Lymph node basin | cN0, sampled and negative (axilla or groin) | Radiation not indicated | | |
| | NCCN (2014a) | Lymph node basin | cN0, sampled and negative (head and neck) | 46–50 | 23–25 | |
| | NCCN (2014a) | Lymph node basin | cN0, sampled and positive (axilla or groin) | 50 | 25 | |
| | NCCN (2014a) | Lymph node basin | cN0, sampled and positive (head and neck) | 50–56 | 25–28 | |
| | NCCN (2014a) | Lymph node basin | cN+, not dissected | 60–66 | 30–33 | |
| | NCCN (2014a) | Lymph node basin | cN+, dissected (axilla or groin) | 50–54 | 25–27 | |
| | NCCN (2014a) | Lymph node basin | cN+, dissected (head and neck) | 50–60 | 25–30 | |
| | Jouary et al. (2012) | Lymph node basin | cN0, not sampled or dissected | 50 | 25 | |
| Melanoma | TROG | Lymph node basin | cN+, dissected | 48 | 20 | |
| | MDACC | Lymph node basin | cN+, dissected | 30 | 5 | |
| BCC/SCC | NCCN (2014b) | Primary tumor | Intact, <2 cm tumor | 64 | 32 | 1–1.5 cm |
| | NCCN (2014b) | Primary tumor | Intact, <2 cm tumor | 55 | 20 | 1–1.5 cm |
| | NCCN (2014b) | Primary tumor | Intact, <2 cm tumor | 50 | 15 | 1–1.5 cm |
| | NCCN (2014b) | Primary tumor | Intact, <2 cm tumor | 35 | 5 | 1–1.5 cm |
| | NCCN (2014b) | Primary tumor | Intact, ≥2 cm tumor | 66 | 33 | 1.5–2 cm |
| | NCCN (2014b) | Primary tumor | Intact, ≥2 cm tumor | 55 | 20 | 1.5–2 cm |
| | NCCN (2014b) | Primary tumor | Excised | 60 | 30 | 1.5–2 cm |
| | NCCN (2014b) | Primary tumor | Excised | 50 | 20 | 1.5–2 cm |
| | Mendenhall et al. (2009) | Primary tumor | Large, untreated with bone/cartilage invasion or recurrent | 71.5 | 35 | |
| | Mendenhall et al. (2009) | Primary tumor | Large, untreated with minimal or suspected bone/cartilage invasion | 66 | 35 | |
| | Mendenhall et al. (2009) | Primary tumor | Moderate to large inner canthus, eyelid, nasal, or pinna | 60.5 | 30 | |
| | Mendenhall et al. (2009) | Primary tumor | Small, thin lesion around the eye, nose, or ear | 55 | 20 | |
| | Mendenhall et al. (2009) | Primary tumor | Moderate-sized lesion on free skin | 50.5 | 15 | |
| | Mendenhall et al. (2009) | Primary tumor | Small lesion on free skin | 44 | 10 | |
| | Mendenhall et al. (2009) | Primary tumor | Small lesion on free skin | 33 | 5 | |
| | Mendenhall et al. (2009) | Primary tumor | Excised with positive margins | 50.5 | 15 | |

**Table 3** (continued)

| Disease | Source | Site | Condition | Total dose (Gy) | Fractions (number) | Margins |
|---|---|---|---|---|---|---|
| SCC | NCCN (2014b) | Lymph node basin | cN0, not sampled or dissected | 50 | 25 | |
| | NCCN (2014b) | Lymph node basin | cN+, not dissected (axilla or groin) | 66 | 33 | |
| | NCCN (2014b) | Lymph node basin | cN+, not dissected (head and neck) | 66–70 | 33–35 | |
| | NCCN (2014b) | Lymph node basin | Dissected, ECE not noted (axilla and groin) | 54 | 27 | |
| | NCCN (2014b) | Lymph node basin | Dissected, ECE noted (axilla and groin) | 60 | 30 | |
| | NCCN (2014b) | Lymph node basin | Dissected, ECE not noted (head and neck) | 56 | 28 | |
| | NCCN (2014b) | Lymph node basin | Dissected, ECE noted (head and neck) | 60–66 | 30–33 | |
| | Mendenhall et al. (2009) | Lymph node basin | Dissected, negative margins | 60 | 30 | |
| | Mendenhall et al. (2009) | Lymph node basin | Dissected, positive margins | 66–70 | 33–35 | |
| | Mendenhall et al. (2009) | Lymph node basin | Dissected, positive margins | 74.4 | 62 (bid) | |

*MDACC constraints.* The MDACC phase II study of adjuvant radiotherapy for cutaneous melanoma of the head and neck limited doses to several organs and tissues. Subsequent application of this regimen (30 Gy in 5 fractions of 6 Gy) has been described in other non-head and neck sites.

Brain, spinal cord, and bowel ≤24 Gy.

## Suggested Reading

Melanoma (Burmeister et al. 2006, 2012; Ang et al. 1990, 1994)

Basal cell and squamous cell carcinoma (O'Hara et al. 2011; Mendenhall et al. 2009; Brantsch et al. 2008)

Merkel cell carcinoma (Jouary et al. 2012)

Perineural invasion (Balamucki et al. 2013; Barnett et al. 2013; Gluck et al. 2009)

## References

Ang KK, Byers RM, Peters LJ et al (1990) Regional radiotherapy as adjuvant treatment for head and neck malignant melanoma. Preliminary results. Arch Otolaryngol Head Neck Surg 116:169–172

Ang KK, Peters LJ, Weber RS et al (1994) Postoperative radiotherapy for cutaneous melanoma of the head and neck region. Int J Radiat Oncol Biol Phys 30:795–798

Balamucki CJ, Dejesus R, Galloway TJ et al (2013) Impact of radiographic findings on for prognosis skin cancer with perineural invasion. Am J Clin Oncol, [Epub ahead of print]

Barnett CM, Foote MC, Panizza B (2013) Cutaneous head and neck malignancies with perineural spread to contralateral cranial nerves: an argument for extending postoperative radiotherapy volume. J Clin Oncol 31:e291–e293

Bhatia AC (2006) The clinical image: archiving clinical processes and an entire specialty. Arch Dermatol 142:96–98

Brantsch KD, Meisner C, Schonfisch B et al (2008) Analysis of risk factors determining prognosis of cutaneous squamous-cell carcinoma: a prospective study. Lancet Oncol 9:713–720

Burmeister BH, Mark Smithers B, Burmeister E et al (2006) A prospective phase II study of adjuvant postoperative radiation therapy following nodal surgery in malignant melanoma-Trans Tasman Radiation Oncology Group (TROG) Study 96.06. Radiother Oncol 81:136–142

Burmeister BH, Henderson MA, Ainslie J et al (2012) Adjuvant radiotherapy versus observation alone for patients at risk of lymph-node field relapse after therapeutic lymphadenectomy for melanoma: a randomised trial. Lancet Oncol 13:589–597

Ellis F (1942) Tolerance dosage in radiotherapy with 200 kV X rays. Br J Radiol 15:348–350

Gluck I, Ibrahim M, Popovtzer A et al (2009) Skin cancer of the head and neck with perineural invasion: defining the clinical target volumes based on the pattern of failure. Int J Radiat Oncol Biol Phys 74:38–46

Jouary T, Leyral C, Dreno B et al (2012) Adjuvant prophylactic regional radiotherapy versus observation in stage I Merkel cell carcinoma: a multicentric prospective randomized study. Ann Oncol 23:1074–1080

Mendenhall WM, Amdur RJ, Hinerman RW, Cognetta AB, Mendenhall NP (2009) Radiotherapy for cutaneous squamous and basal cell carcinomas of the head and neck. Laryngoscope 119:1994–1999

National Comprehensive Cancer Network. Merkel Cell Carcinoma (Version 1.2014). http://www.nccn.org/professionals/physician_gls/pdf/mcc.pdf. Accessed May 28, 2014

National Comprehensive Cancer Network. Basal Cell and Squamous Cell Skin Cancers (Version 2.2014). http://www.nccn.org/professionals/physician_gls/pdf/nmsc.pdf. Accessed May 28, 2014

O'Hara J, Ferlito A, Takes RP et al (2011) Cutaneous squamous cell carcinoma of the head and neck metastasizing to the parotid gland–a review of current recommendations. Head Neck 33:1789–1795

Paraskevas LR, Halpern AC, Marghoob AA (2005) Utility of the Wood's light: five cases from a pigmented lesion clinic. Br J Dermatol 152: 1039–1044

Price S, Williams M, Butson M, Metcalfe P (2006) Comparison of skin dose between conventional radiotherapy and IMRT. Australas Phys Eng Sci Med 29:272–277

Reynolds HM, Dunbar PR, Uren RF, Blackett SA, Thompson JF, Smith NP (2007) Three-dimensional visualisation of lymphatic drainage patterns in patients with cutaneous melanoma. Lancet Oncol 8: 806–812

Reynolds HM, Smith NP, Uren RF, Thompson JF, Dunbar PR (2009) Three-dimensional visualization of skin lymphatic drainage patterns of the head and neck. Head Neck 31:1316–1325

Rhodes J, Clay C, Phillips M (2013) The surface area of the hand and the palm for estimating percentage of total body surface area: results of a meta-analysis. Br J Dermatol 169: 76–84

Sacco JJ, Botten J, Macbeth F, Bagust A, Clark P (2010) The average body surface area of adult cancer patients in the UK: a multicentre retrospective study. PloS One 5:e8933

Schwartz LH, Bogaerts J, Ford R et al (2009) Evaluation of lymph nodes with RECIST 1.1. Eur J Cancer 45:261–267

# Target Delineation of the Neck in Head and Neck Carcinomas

Joanne Zhung, Eli Scher, Nancy Lee,
and Ruben Cabanillas

## Contents

J. Zhung (✉)
Department of Radiation Oncology, Tufts Medical Center,
New York, NY, USA
e-mail: jzhung@gmail.com

E. Scher • N. Lee
Department of Radiation Oncology, Memorial Sloan-Kettering,
New York, NY, USA

R. Cabanillas
Department of Radiation Oncology, Institute of Molecular and
Oncological Medicine of Asturias (IMOMA), Oviedo, Spain

## 1 Anatomy and Patterns of Spread

IMRT is utilized for treatment in head and neck sites to maximize target coverage and decrease normal tissue toxicity, such as xerostomia and dysphagia. The most common at-risk nodal levels for head and neck cancers typically include levels I to VII and the lateral retropharyngeal lymph nodes (RPLN).

Ipsilateral neck treatment is reasonable for the clinically N0 neck in small T1–2 oropharyngeal carcinomas that are well lateralized (>1 cm between midline and medial extent of tumor), without significant soft palate or base of tongue involvement, as well as small carcinomas of the parotid gland, buccal mucosa, retromolar trigone, gingiva, or lateral border of the oral tongue (O'Sullivan et al. 2001). Early stage, small glottic larynx carcinomas (T1–2) do not require additional prophylactic neck treatment.

Typically, one ipsilateral nodal region beyond the pathologically involved level must be covered. Often, the N + neck requires coverage of levels IB to V, as well as coverage of the RPLN.

Lateral RPLN should be electively covered in clinically N0 pharyngeal tumors (naso-, oro-, and hypopharynx), supraglottic carcinomas, and high-risk paranasal carcinomas. The medial RPLN are not contoured in this chapter given low locoregional rates of relapse and the ability to spare pharyngeal constrictors (Feng et al. 2010). However, with posterior pharyngeal wall or gross RPLN involvement, it is recommended to include the medial and lateral RPLN. In the N0 neck, it is possible to start the superior extent of the RPLN at the inferior level of C1 and stop caudally at the superior edge of the hyoid bone. In the N + neck, especially in the presence of high level II adenopathy, RPLN should be treated up to the skull base. Routine inclusion of uninvolved RPLN will increase the dose to the pharyngeal constrictors and therefore should be carefully considered.

High level II and the retrostyloid (RS) lymph nodes (a cranial continuation of level II up to the skull base) can be spared in the N0 neck in order to reduce parotid gland dose. The N0 level II contours may begin where the posterior belly of the digastric muscle crosses the internal jugular vein (usually at the level of C1). In the N + neck, level II and the RS nodes should be treated up to the skull base (Figs. 2 and 3). The primary sites at highest risk of RS involvement include the nasopharynx and bulky involvement of upper level II due to retrograde flow.

Level I is at high risk for nodal involvement in oral cavity tumors. Specifically, IA drains the anterior oral cavity including the lip, the anterior mandibular alveolar ridge, the anterior oral tongue, and the floor of the mouth. Level IB is at highest risk in oral cavity tumors, the anterior nasal cavity, and cheek.

Levels II, III, and IV will be the most commonly treated nodal levels in the vast majority of mucosal head and neck cancers, given drainage patterns following the internal carotid artery and internal jugular vein. Levels II and III are at risk in nasopharynx, oropharynx, hypopharynx, and laryngeal tumors. Level IV is at risk of involvement in hypopharynx, larynx, and thyroid tumors.

Level V is infrequently involved in oral cavity, oropharyngeal, hypopharyngeal, and laryngeal tumors in the N0 neck. Posterior level V (Vb) has to be carefully included in thyroid, nasopharyngeal, parotid gland, and cutaneous carcinomas.

Level VI should be treated in laryngeal carcinomas with subglottic extension and in thyroid tumors.

Level VII should be treated in thyroid tumors, extending inferiorly for node-positive disease from the brachiocephalic vein to the carina.

Supraclavicular (SCV) nodes include part of the historically referenced "triangle of Ho." Nasopharyngeal tumors are highest risk of metastases to the SCV region, bilaterally.

Surgical dissection of the neck may be performed prior to radiation treatment, depending on the location and treatment of the primary tumor (Table 1). All surgical clips should be covered in the clinical target volume, and microscopically positive mar-gins or ECE should be included in the high-risk tumor vol-ume.

Well-lateralized N + tumors after unilateral neck dissection strongly warrant bilateral postoperative radiation therapy, due to altered lymphatic drainage.

Factors strongly recommended for postoperative chemoradiation, per EORTC 22931 and RTOG 9501, are extracapsular extension and positive margins.

**Table 1** Types of neck dissection

| Surgical neck management | Definition |
|---|---|
| Radical neck dissection | En bloc removal of neck levels I–V, sternocleidomastoid, internal jugular vein, spinal accessory nerve (CN XI) |
| Modified radical neck dissection | Removal of neck levels I–V but sparing of at least one uninvolved non-lymphatic structure (sternocleidomastoid, internal jugular vein, and/or accessory nerve) |
| Selective neck dissection | Removal of neck levels I–V, with preservation of at least one nodal level |
| Types | |
| Supraomohyoid | Typically performed in oral cavity carcinomas, levels I–III, or in occasional skip metastases, to level IV (referred to as extended supraomohyoid neck dissection) |
| Lateral | Typically performed in oropharyngeal, hypopharyngeal, and laryngeal carcinomas: levels II–IV |
| Anterior compartment | Thyroid carcinomas at highest risk: level VI |

Selected procedures from 2001 American Head and Neck Society

## 2 Diagnostic Workup Relevant for Target Volume Delineation

Clinical examination, CT with IV contrast, and PET scan are the best modalities for the majority of cases. PET scan is helpful for small FDG-avid nodes that fall under size criteria on CT scan. Note the PET fusion may be misleading due to patient movement and should be evaluated closely for any inconsistencies without CT correlate. Ultrasound can be helpful when combined with fine-needle aspiration for staging the neck when other radiographic modalities are nondiagnostic.

MRI with contrast may be helpful in those who cannot receive CT with IV contrast and in cases where nodal adenopathy is obscured or is not easily delineated with contrast CT.

## 3 Simulation and Daily Localization

CT simulation with 3 mm slice thickness and IV contrast is preferred to ease delineation of vascular structures from lymph nodes. Supine patient positioning with rigid head cradle with the neck extended to reduce oral cavity exit dose is recommended. A custom thermoplastic mask to immobilize the nose, chin, and forehead is utilized. Shoulder pulls or other reproducible devices are used to reduce beam interference and allow adequate neck exposure. The CT simulation scan should encompass adequate superior extent of coverage of the primary disease and inferiorly to the level of the carina.

Image fusion depending upon the primary disease may include MRI and/or PET to aid in delineating involved gross disease in the neck. Attention should be paid to image fusion between primary disease and fusion to nodal disease, as patients will not have PET images in the CT simulation position (neck extended, shoulders pulled down).

Mediastinal windows should be used for contouring the neck nodal contents.

IGRT is recommended to aid in decreasing the PTV margins, depending upon patient positioning reproducibility and treatment machine considerations.

Uninvolved glottic larynx may be spared to limit RT-related speech disorders. Two possible techniques to treat the entire neck include an extended field IMRT or split field using an upper IMRT field matched to a lower anterior neck field (Fig. 1). Advantages of a split field include significantly reduced mean dose to the uninvolved larynx and inferior pharyngeal constrictors (Caudell et al. 2010). This technique is not recommended in laryngeal,

hypopharyngeal, or unknown primary head and neck cases or when gross primary or nodal disease is present at the matchline or inferior to the larynx. In these cases, extended field IMRT will provide excellent coverage, whereas a split field may contribute to matchline failures or underdosage (Lee et al. 2007).

# 4 Target Volume Delineation and Treatment Planning

Fractionation schemes may vary between dose-painting IMRT and conventional IMRT (Table 2.) Suggested target volumes for nodal GTV and CTVs are detailed in Tables 3, 4, and 5.

# 5 Plan Assessment

The spinal cord is the only structure within the neck that carries the highest priority over tumor coverage. The brachial plexus (Hall et al. 2008), parotids and submandibular glands, mandible, temporomandibular joint, and constrictors are important normal tissue structures that need to be weighed appropriately when evaluating target coverage.

Occasionally, treatment of involved cranial nerves will warrant coverage to the base of the skull. In this case, the brainstem will therefore carry higher priority over tumor coverage.

Ideally, at least 95 % of the PTV should receive the prescription dose. The minimum dose to 99 % of the CTV should be >93 % of the dose. The maximum dose to the PTV should not exceed 115 %.

Several critical normal structures at risk in the neck should be carefully outlined to calculate dose. The spinal

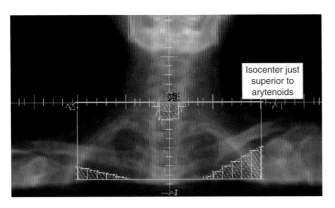

Isocenter just superior to arytenoids

**Fig. 1** Beam's eye view of low anterior neck field

**Table 2** Selected IMRT dose fractionation schemes for the neck

| | Concomitant dose-painting IMRT | Postoperative dose-painting IMRT | Definitive dose-painting IMRT |
|---|---|---|---|
| | Total dose/dose per fraction (Gy) | | |
| GTV | 69.96/2.12, 66/2.0[a] 70/2.0[b] | 70/2.0[c] | 69.96/2.12 |
| CTV_high risk | 59.4/1.8 59.5/1.7[b] | 66-60/2.2-2.0 | 59.4/1.8 |
| CTV_low risk | 54/1.64 56/1.70[b] | 54/1.8 not surgically manipulated | 56/1.7 |
| *Optional CTV* | | | |
| CTV_low neck | 50.4/1.8 | | |

[a]Small, suspicious involved nodal disease
[b]Suggested dose levels without simultaneous integrated boost
[c]If gross disease is present postoperatively

**Table 3** Suggested target volumes for involved nodal disease

| Target volumes | Definition and description |
| --- | --- |
| *Concomitant or definitive dose-painting IMRT* | |
| GTV$_{70}$ | Neck nodes: clinically involved, nodes ≥ 1 cm, central necrosis, FDG-avid on PET, or biopsy proven. Include any suspicious or questionable nodes |
| GTV$_{66}$ | Small, involved nodal disease can be treated to 66 Gy |
| CTV$_{70\ or\ 66}$ | No margin from GTV. Consider GTV$_{70\ or\ 66}$+5–10 mm margin if unclear or imaging quality is reduced |
| PTV$_{70\ or\ 66}$ | CTV$_{70}$+3–5 mm, variable |
| *Postoperative IMRT* | |
| CTV$_{postop66}$ | Extracapsular involvement. 70 Gy may be needed for residual gross disease |
| PTV$_{postop66}$ | CTV$_{postop66}$+3–5 mm, variable |

**Table 4** Suggested target volumes for high-risk nodes

| Target volumes | Definition and description |
| --- | --- |
| *Concomitant or definitive dose-painting IMRT* | |
| CTV$_{59.4}$ | Typically, one level above and below grossly involved nodal disease. May involve entire involved muscle or at least one level above and below the muscle if ECE is present |
| PTV$_{59.4}$ | CTV$_{59.4}$+3–5 mm, variable |
| *Postoperative IMRT* | |
| CTV$_{postop60}$ | Preoperative gross nodal disease with negative margins, entire operative bed without ECE. Include entire muscle (at least one level above and below the level of involvement) if involved. May include bilateral necks, depending on primary site |
| PTV$_{postop60}$ | CTV$_{postop60}$+3–5 mm, variable |

**Table 5** Suggested volumes for low-risk nodes

| Target volumes | Definition and description |
| --- | --- |
| *Concomitant or definitive dose-painting IMRT* | |
| CTV$_{54–56}$ | Low-risk ipsilateral and/or contralateral neck |
| PTV$_{54–56}$ | CTV$_{54–56}$+3–5 mm, variable |
| *Postoperative IMRT* | |
| CTV$_{postop54}$ | Contralateral neck and occasionally the uninvolved, low-risk, nonsurgically violated ipsilateral neck |
| PTV$_{postop54}$ | CTV$_{postop54}$+3–5 mm, variable |

**Table 6** Intensity-modulated radiation therapy: normal tissue dose constraints

| Target coverage | Constraints |
| --- | --- |
| PTV$_{GTV}$ | D95 ≥ prescription dose (70 Gy) |
| | D05 ≤ 108 % of prescription dose |
| PTV$_{CTV\ high\ risk}$ | D95 ≥ prescription dose (59.4 Gy) |
| | D05 ≤ GTV prescription dose |
| PTV$_{CTV\ low\ risk}$ | D95 ≥ prescription dose (54 Gy) |
| | D05 ≤ CTV$_{high\ risk}$ prescription dose |
| Critical structures | Constraints |
| Spinal cord | Max <45 Gy or 1 cc of the PRV cannot exceed 50 Gy |
| Brainstem | Max <54 Gy or 1 % of PRV cannot exceed 60 Gy |
| Pharyngeal constrictors | V50 <33 %, V60 <15 % and mean <45 Gy |
| Brachial plexus | Max <66 Gy, D05 <60 Gy |
| Mandible and TMJ | Max <70–66 Gy or 1 cc of the organ cannot exceed 75 Gy |
| Oral cavity | Mean <40 Gy, mean <30 Gy if uninvolved |
| Parotid gland | (a) Mean ≤ 26 Gy in one gland |
| | (b) Or at least 20 cc of the combined volume of both parotid glands will receive <20 Gy |
| | (c) Or at least 50 % of one gland will receive <30 Gy |
| Submandibular gland | Mean <39 Gy |
| Glottic larynx | Mean <45 Gy or 20 Gy if uninvolved |
| Esophagus/postcricoid pharynx | Mean <45–30 Gy |

Based on guidelines used at Memorial Sloan Kettering Cancer Center and RTOG 1016. Dmax =0.03 cc or 3 mm×3 mm×3 mm cube

cord should be contoured at the top of vertebral body C1 down to T4 or 2 cm beyond the lowest extent of the target volume. The uninvolved pharyngeal constrictors should be contoured as suggested by Levendag et al. (2007). The glottic larynx should be contoured superiorly from the hyoid to the cricoid cartilage and including the arytenoids. Critical structures that traverse the length of the treated organ should be contoured 2 cm above and below the superior and inferior most extent of the combined target volumes. The structures at risk are detailed in Table 6.

A PRV or planning risk volume may be created for at-risk organs, such as the spinal cord (+5 mm) or brainstem (+3 mm).

## 6    Target Volumes for the Node-Negative and Node-Positive Neck

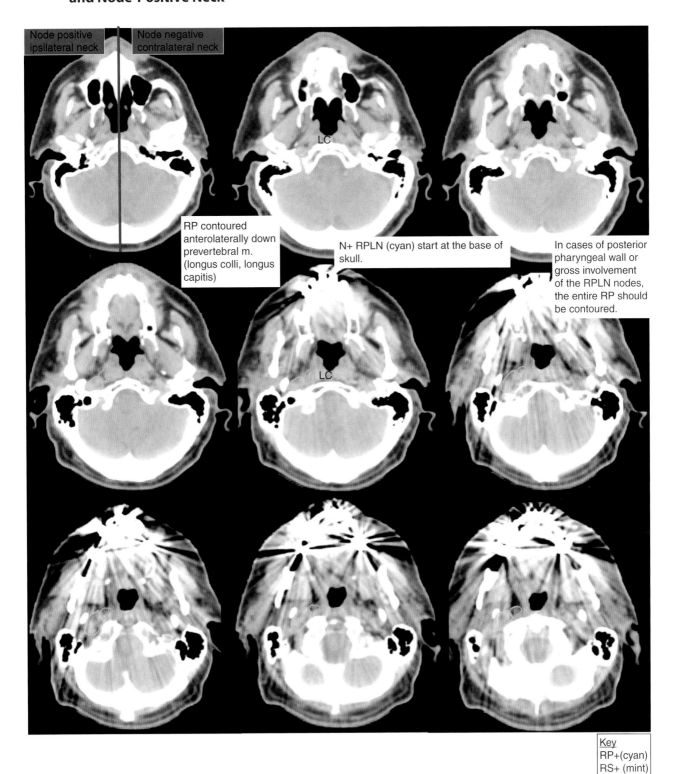

Fig. 2 Intact neck target delineation volumes. Patient with multiple level II and III nodal involvement with strongly suggestive extracapsular muscle involvement on CT. Each nodal level contoured with the left side showing examples of node-positive contours (*right neck*) and the right side showing examples of node-negative contours (*left neck*). *LC* longus capitis, *PD* posterior belly of the digastric muscle, *AD* anterior belly of the digastric muscle, *GH* geniohyoid muscle, *ECA* external carotid artery, *ICA* internal carotid artery, *IJV* internal jugular vein, *CA* common carotid artery, *SCM* sternocleidomastoid, *SP* superficial lobe of the parotid gland, *DP* deep lobe of the parotid gland, *SG* submandibular gland, *BH* body of hyoid, *TZ* trapezius muscle, *LS* levator scapulae muscle, *SL* splenius capitis muscle, *CR* cricoid cartilage, *ASC* anterior scalene muscles, *BP* brachial plexus, *MSC* middle scalene muscles, *PSC* posterior scalene muscles, *BT* brachiocephalic trunk, *RBV* right brachiocephalic vein, *RSA* right subclavian artery, *LBV* left brachiocephalic vein, *LCA* left common carotid artery, *LSA* left subclavian artery

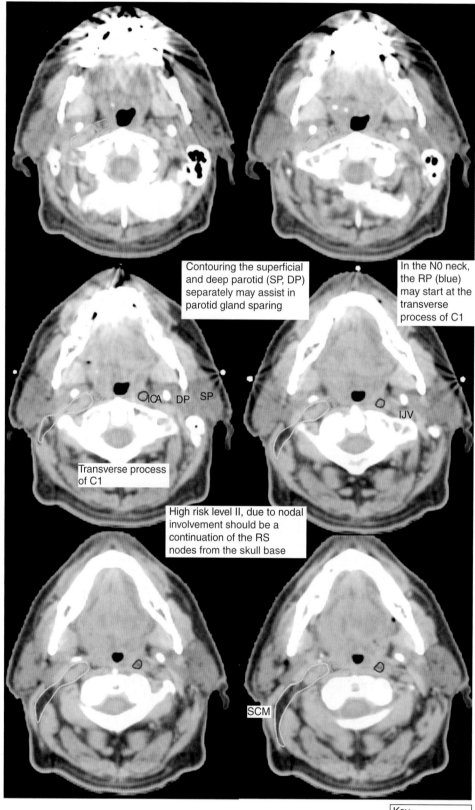

**Fig. 2** (continued)

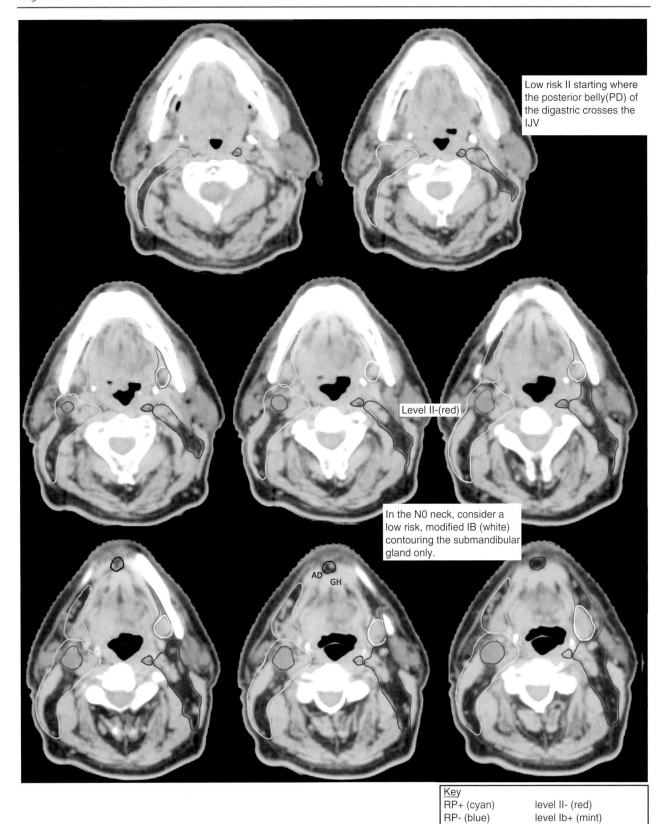

Low risk II starting where the posterior belly(PD) of the digastric crosses the IJV

Level II-(red)

In the N0 neck, consider a low risk, modified IB (white) contouring the submandibular gland only.

AD  GH

Key
RP+ (cyan)            level II- (red)
RP- (blue)            level Ib+ (mint)
Level II+ (yellow)    level Ib- (orange)
Level Ia (black)      involved node (magenta)
Modified level Ib (white)

**Fig. 2** (continued)

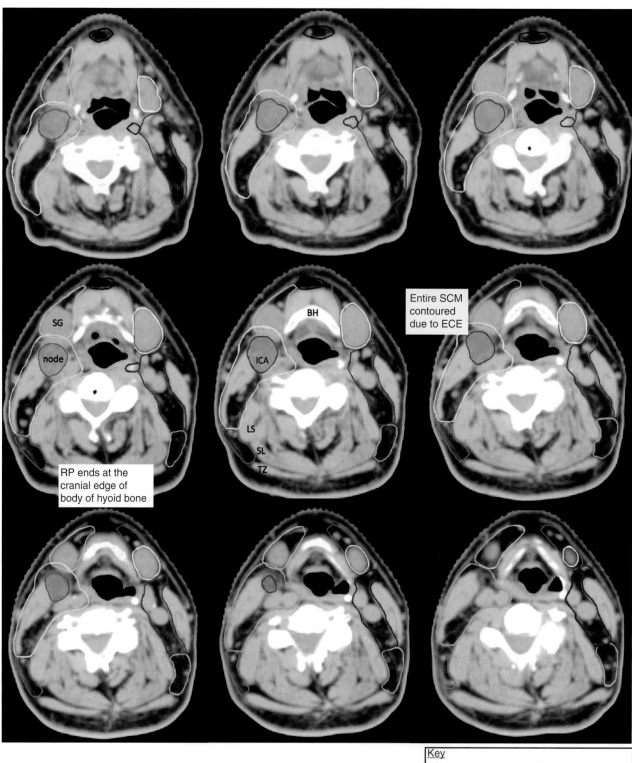

**Fig. 2** (continued)

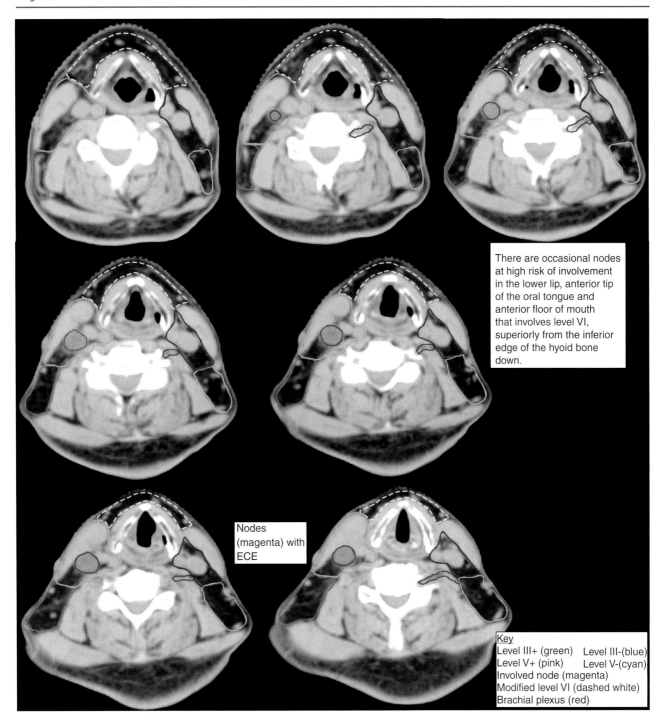

There are occasional nodes at high risk of involvement in the lower lip, anterior tip of the oral tongue and anterior floor of mouth that involves level VI, superiorly from the inferior edge of the hyoid bone down.

Nodes (magenta) with ECE

Key
Level III+ (green)      Level III-(blue)
Level V+ (pink)        Level V-(cyan)
Involved node (magenta)
Modified level VI (dashed white)
Brachial plexus (red)

**Fig. 2** (continued)

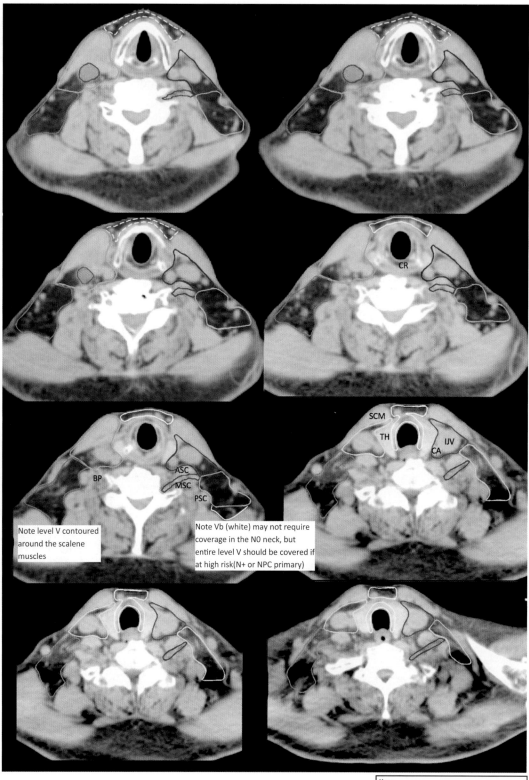

Note level V contoured around the scalene muscles

Note Vb (white) may not require coverage in the N0 neck, but entire level V should be covered if at high risk(N+ or NPC primary)

Key
Level III+ (green)  Level III- (blue)
Level IV+ (yellow)  Level IV-(magenta)
Level V+ (pink)  Level V-(cyan)
SCV+ (green)  SCV- (yellow)
Involved node (magenta)
Modified level VI (dashed white)
Level VI (solid white)
Brachial plexus (red)

**Fig. 2** (continued)

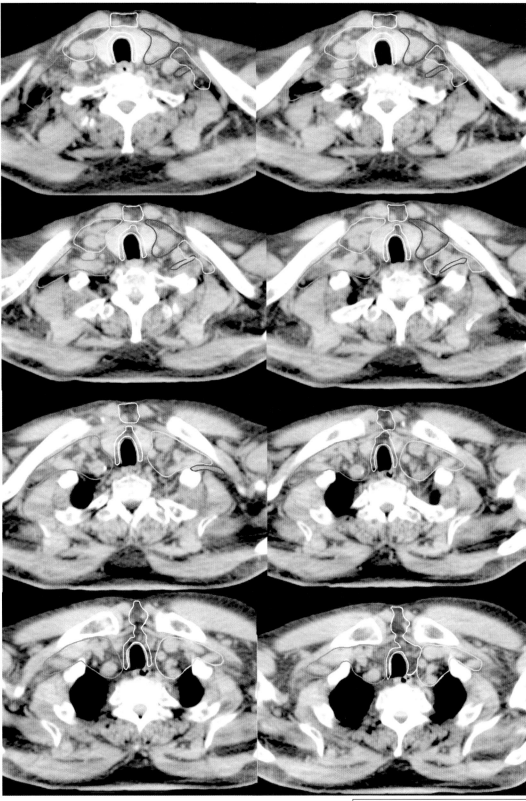

Key
Level IV+ (yellow)  Level IV-(magenta)
Level V+ (pink)     Level V-( cyan)
SCV+ (green)        SCV-(yellow)
Level VI (white)
Brachial plexus (red)

**Fig. 2** (continued)

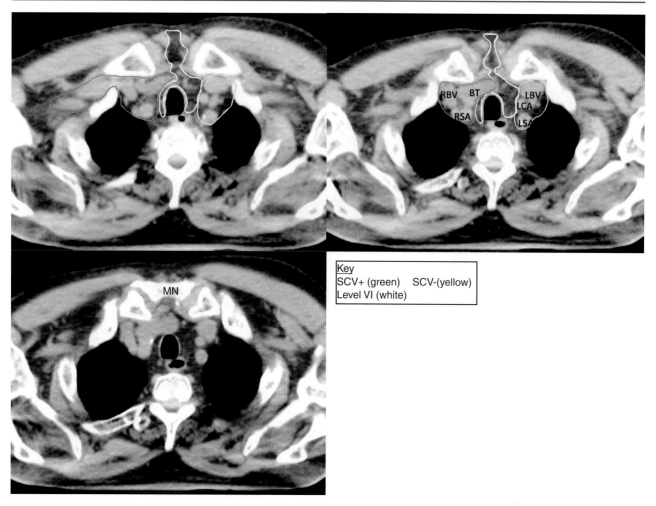

**Fig. 2** (continued)

| Level | Superior/inferior | Medial/lateral | Anterior/posterior |
|---|---|---|---|
| Lateral RPLN | Base of the skull or inferior transverse process of C1 → cranial edge of the hyoid bone | Lateral edge of the longus capitis muscle → medial edge of internal carotid artery | Fascia under pharyngeal mucosa ->prevertebral muscles (longus colli, longus capitis) |
| RS | Jugular foramen → inferior aspect of C1 (top of level II) | Medial edge of internal carotid artery → deep parotid lobe | Parapharyngeal space → skull base and transverse process of C1 |
| IA | Basilar edge of the mandible → body of the hyoid | Space between the anterior bellies of the digastric muscles | Platysma → geniohyoid muscles |
| IB | Superior aspect of the submandibular gland → body of the hyoid | Digastric muscle/ cranially the medial border of the mandible and caudally the platysma | Platysma → posterior submandibular gland |
| II | Inferior border of transverse process of C1 (continuation of the RS nodes) → inferior body of the hyoid bone | Medial internal carotid artery, paraspinal muscles → SCM | Anterior edge of internal carotid artery/ SG → posterior edge of the SCM |
| II (low risk) | Posterior belly of the digastric muscle crosses the internal jugular vein | Same | Same |
| III | Caudal edge of the hyoid bone → inferior cricoid | Medial internal carotid artery and scalenus muscles → SCM | Anterior edge of SCM → posterior edge of SCM |
| IV | Caudal edge of the cricoid cartilage → 2 cm superior to the sternoclavicular joint | Thyroid gland, internal carotid artery and scalenus muscles → SCM | Anterior edge of SCM → posterior edge of SCM |
| Va | Cranial edge of the hyoid bone → CT slice containing the transverse cervical vessels | Paraspinal muscles → platysma and skin | Posterior border of the SCM → anterior edge of the trapezius muscle |
| Vb | Cranial edge of the cricoid → CT slice containing transverse cervical vessels | Same | Anterior edge of the trapezius muscle → posterior border of the trapezius muscle |
| VI | Caudal edge of the thyroid cartilage (hyoid bone in anterior floor of mouth, tip of the tongue or lower lip tumors) → manubrium | Trachea → medial edge of the SCM/ thyroid gland | Platysma → thyroid cartilage/thyro-hyoid membrane/anterior border of the esophagus |
| SCV | Inferior border of IV/V → superior edge of the manubrium | Posterior edge of SCM/medial edge of carotids/medial clavicular edge → trapezius superiorly, medial edge of the clavicle inferiorly | SCM/clavicle → posterior edge of carotids/ anterior surface of scalene muscles |

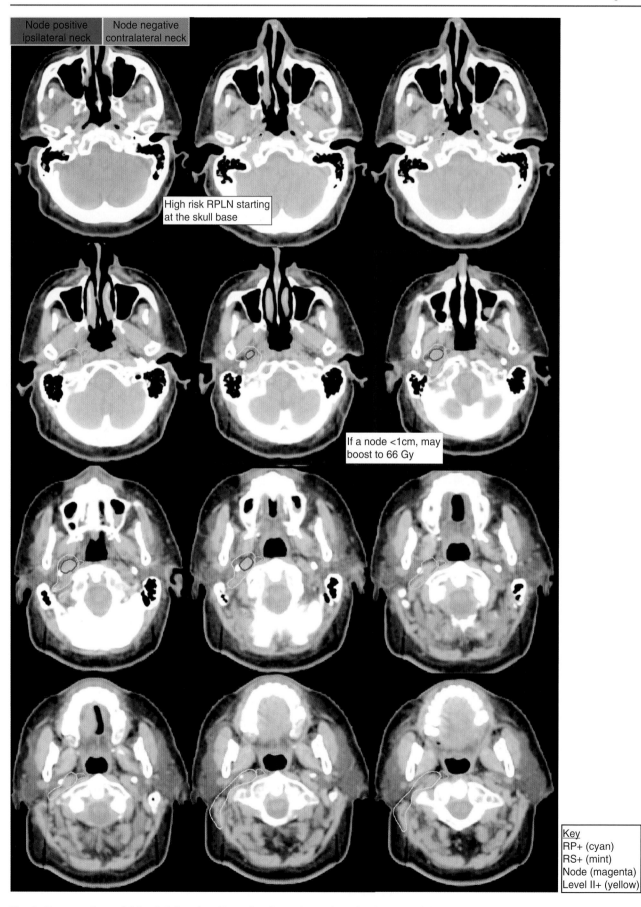

**Fig. 3** Postoperative nodal level delineation. Example of a patient undergoing a modified radical neck dissection, with sacrifice of the sternocleidomastoid, with extracapsular extension in level II and found to have involvement of the ipsilateral retrostyloid. Each nodal contour depicts involved node involved/positive side on the left (patient's right) and uninvolved, node-negative side on the right (patient's left)

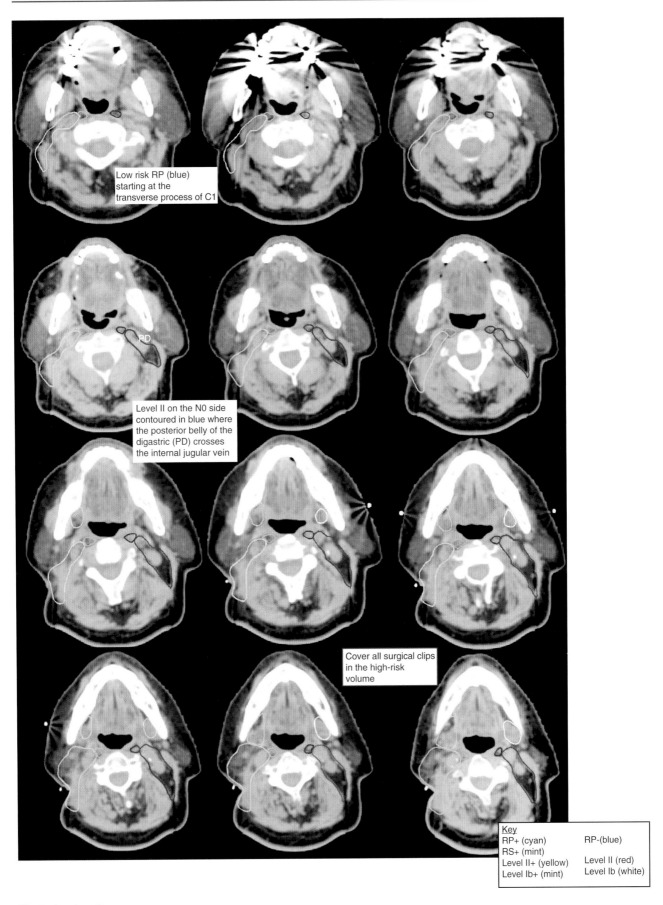

Low risk RP (blue) starting at the transverse process of C1

Level II on the N0 side contoured in blue where the posterior belly of the digastric (PD) crosses the internal jugular vein

Cover all surgical clips in the high-risk volume

Key
RP+ (cyan)          RP-(blue)
RS+ (mint)
Level II+ (yellow)   Level II (red)
Level Ib+ (mint)     Level Ib (white)

**Fig. 3** (continued)

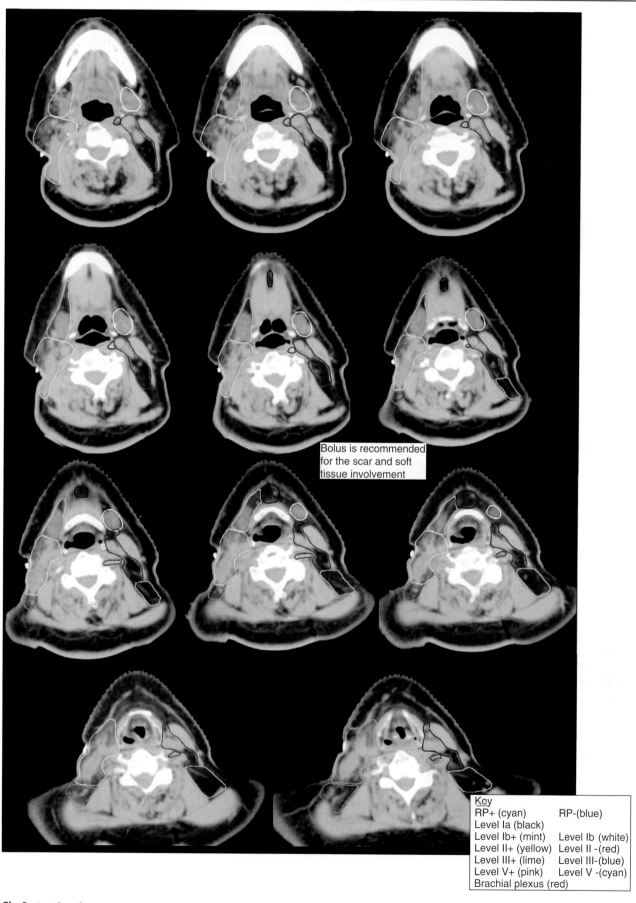

Bolus is recommended
for the scar and soft
tissue involvement

Key
RP+ (cyan)              RP-(blue)
Level Ia (black)
Level Ib+ (mint)       Level Ib (white)
Level II+ (yellow)     Level II -(red)
Level III+ (lime)      Level III-(blue)
Level V+ (pink)        Level V -(cyan)
Brachial plexus (red)

**Fig.3** (continued)

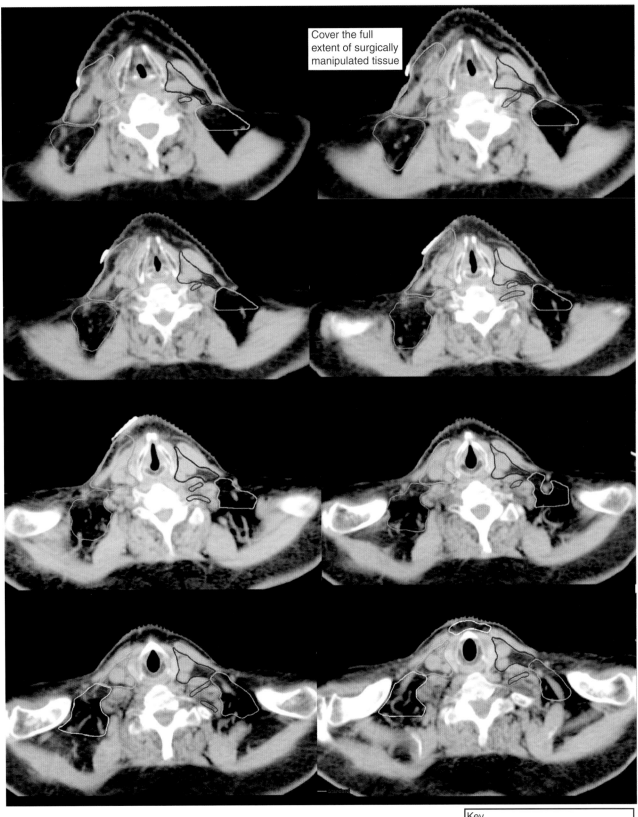

Cover the full extent of surgically manipulated tissue

Key
Level III+ (lime)        Level III- (blue)
Level Ib+ (mint)        Level Ib (white)
Level V+ (pink)         Level V- (cyan)
SCV+ (yellow)          SCV-(green)
Level VI (white)
Brachial plexus (red)

**Fig. 3** (continued)

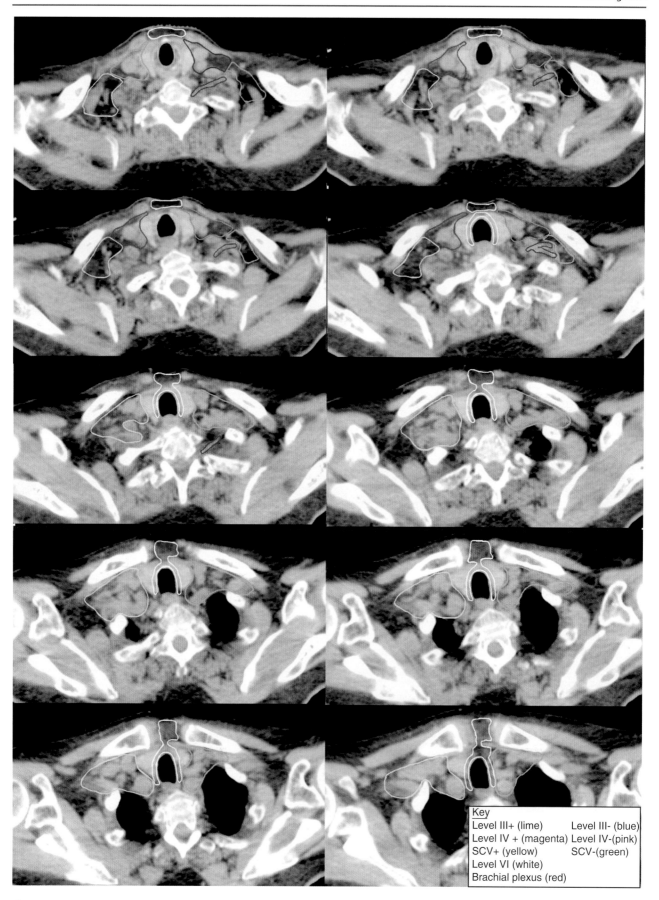

**Key**
Level III+ (lime)          Level III- (blue)
Level IV + (magenta)   Level IV-(pink)
SCV+ (yellow)            SCV-(green)
Level VI (white)
Brachial plexus (red)

**Fig. 3** (continued)

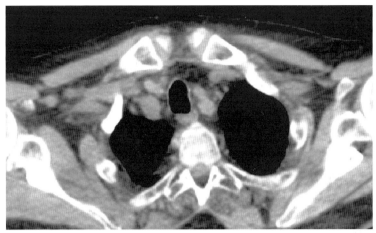

Note for involved cranial nerves :

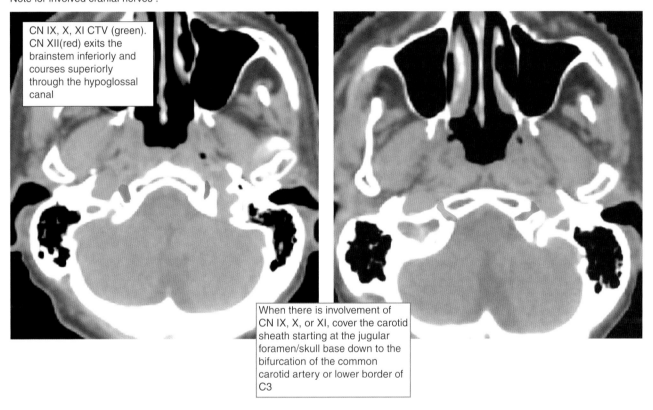

CN IX, X, XI CTV (green). CN XII(red) exits the brainstem inferiorly and courses superiorly through the hypoglossal canal

When there is involvement of CN IX, X, or XI, cover the carotid sheath starting at the jugular foramen/skull base down to the bifurcation of the common carotid artery or lower border of C3

**Fig. 3** (continued)

## Suggested Reading

Gregoire V et al (2003) CT-based delineation of lymph node levels and related CTVs in the node-negative neck: DAHANCA, EORTC, GORTEC, NCIC, RTOG consensus guidelines. Radiother Oncol 69(3):227–36.

Gregoire V et al (2006) Proposal for the delineation of the nodal CTV in the node-positive and the post-operative neck. Radiother Oncol 79(1):15–20.

Gregoire V et al (2013) Delineation of the neck node levels for head and neck tumors: A 2013 update, DAHANCA, EORTC, HKNPCSG, NCIC CTG, NCRI, RTOG, TROG consensus guidelines. Radiother Oncol. Epub ahead of print

Mourad WF et al (2013). Cranial nerves IX-XII contouring atlas for head and neck cancer. *RTOG*.org. Retrieved 5 Oct 2013 from http://www.rtog.org/LinkClick. aspx?fileticket=B7fuSx-B1GU%3D&tabid=229

Young B (2011) Neuroanatomy modules: skull base CT. Retrieved 13 Nov 2013 from http://headneckbrainspine.com/Skull-Base-CT.php

## References

Caudell JJ et al (2010) Comparison of methods to reduce dose to swallow-related structures in head and neck cancer. Int J Radiat Oncol Biol Phys 77(2):462–467

Feng FY et al (2010) Intensity-modulated chemoradiotherapy aiming to reduce dysphagia in patients with oropharyngeal cancer: clinical and functional results. J Clin Oncol 28(16): 2732–2738

Hall WH et al (2008) Development and validation of a standardized method for contouring the brachial plexus: preliminary dosimetric analysis among patients treated with IMRT for head-and-neck cancer. Int J Radiat Oncol Biol Phys 72(5): 1362–1367

Lee NY et al (2007) Choosing an intensity-modulated radiation therapy technique in the treatment of head-and-neck cancer. Int J Radiat Oncol Biol Phys 68(5):1299–1309

Levendag PC et al (2007) Dysphagia disorders in patients with cancer of the oropharynx are significantly affected by the radiation therapy dose to the superior and middle constrictor muscle: a dose-effect relationship. Radiother Oncol 85(1):64–73

O'Sullivan B et al (2001) The benefits and pitfalls of ipsilateral radiotherapy in carcinoma of the tonsillar region. Int J Radiat Oncol Biol Phys 51(2):332–343

# Cranial Nerves

Ryan Lanning, Robert Young, Christopher Barker,
and Nancy Lee

## Contents

## 1   Introduction

For the Radiation Oncologist, knowledge and identification of the cranial nerve pathways in cancers of the head and neck is important for both characterizing extent of disease involvement and determining clinical treatment volumes. There are two processes by which tumors involve nerve pathways. Perineural invasion involves tumor cells directly invading a nerve in close proximity to the primary lesion. Perineural spread is a metastatic process whereby malignant cells travel along a nerve pathway in either retrograde or anterograde directions.

## 2   Anatomy and Contouring

### 2.1   Important Foramina, Fossa, Cavities, and Canals

Understanding relevant anatomic landmarks is critical to defining the pathways of the cranial nerves when contouring clinical cases with possible cranial nerve involvement or to identify them as avoidance structures. Notable are the skull base foramina, osseous canals, and anatomically defined fossa and cavities that contain many of the cranial nerves along their course from the brainstem. Table 1 defines the major foramina, fossa, and cavities with respect to their contents and anatomic boundaries. Figures 1, 2, and 3 identify these structures on a non-contrast planning CT scan.

### 2.2   The Cranial Nerve Pathways

*Cranial Nerve I*: The *cribriform plate* of the ethmoid bone is the primary landmark to identify the location of CN I. It forms the roof of the nasal cavities. Small foramina in the *cribriform plate* allow passage of numerous olfactory nerves

R. Lanning • C. Barker • N. Lee (✉)
Department of Radiation Oncology, Memorial Sloan
Kettering Cancer Center, New York, NY, USA
e-mail: leen2@mskcc.org

R. Young
Department of Radiology, Memorial Sloan Kettering
Cancer Center, New York, NY, USA

N.Y. Lee et al. (eds.), *Target Volume Delineation for Conformal and Intensity-Modulated Radiation Therapy*,
Medical Radiology. Radiation Oncology, DOI: 10.1007/174_2014_1017, © Springer International Publishing Switzerland 2014
Published Online: 11 October 2014

**Table 1** Important foramina, fossa, and canals involving the cranial nerves

| Name | Contents | Anatomic location |
| --- | --- | --- |
| Supraorbital foramen | Supraorbital nerve ($CN\ V_1$) and vessels | Frontal bone – superior to the orbit and inferior to the superciliary arch |
| Superior orbital fissure | $CN\ III$, $CN\ IV$, $CN\ V_1$, $CN\ VI$, ophthalmic vein, and sympathetic fibers from the cavernous plexus | Between lesser and greater wings of the sphenoid bone |
| Optic canal | Optic nerve ($CN\ II$) and ophthalmic artery | Superior aspect of the body and small wing of the sphenoid bone |
| Cavernous sinus | $CN\ III$, $CN\ IV$, $CN\ V_1$, $CN\ V_2$, $CN\ VI$, internal carotid artery, and sympathetic plexus | Lateral to the sella turcica, on superior portion of the body of the sphenoid bone, and anterior to apex of the petrous part of the temporal bone |
| Foramen rotundum | Maxillary nerve ($V_2$) | Within the anteromedial portion of the sphenoid bone and inferolateral to the superior orbital fissure |
| Inferior orbital fissure | Zygomatic branch of $V_2$ and ascending branches of pterygopalatine ganglion | Junction of sphenoid bone and maxilla in the floor of the orbit |
| Internal auditory canal | $CN\ VII$, $CN\ VIII$, and nervous intermedius ($VII$) | Opening in the posterior portion of the petrous temporal bone |
| Meckel's cave[a] | Trigeminal ganglion ($CN\ V$) | Bounded by clivus medially, lateral wall of the cavernous sinus superomedially, cerebellar tentorium superolaterally, and apex of the petrous temporal bone inferolaterally |
| Pterygopalatine fossa (PPF) | Maxillary nerve ($V_2$), Vidian nerve (junction of greater and deep petrosal nerves), terminal portion of the maxillary artery, and pterygopalatine ganglion | Bounded by the infratemporal surface of the maxilla anteriorly, root of the pterygoid process posteriorly, palatine bone medially, pterygomaxillary fissure laterally, and pyramidal process of the palatine bone inferiorly |
| Palatovaginal canal | Pharyngeal branch of $V_2$ | Connects sphenoid and palatine bones connecting nasopharynx to the pterygopalatine fossa |
| Zygomaticofacial foramen | Zygomaticofacial nerve ($V_2$) | Malar/lateral surface of the zygomatic bone |
| Foramen ovale | Mandibular nerve ($V_3$), lesser petrosal nerve (branch of $IX$), accessory meningeal artery, emissary veins from the cavernous sinus, and the otic ganglion | Posterior portion of the greater wing of the sphenoid bone, posterolateral to foramen rotundum, and anteromedial to foramen spinosum |
| Sphenopalatine foramen | Nasopalatine nerve ($V_2$) and sphenopalatine vessels | Processes of the superior border of the palatine bone and superiorly by the body of the sphenoid bone |
| Pterygoid/vidian canal | Nerve (junction of greater and deep petrosal nerves), artery, and vein of the pterygoid canal | Within medial pterygoid plate of the sphenoid bone |
| Foramen spinosum | Meningeal branch of $V_3$ and middle meningeal vessels | Posteromedial to the foramen ovale, medial to the mandibular fossa, and anterior to the Eustachian tube |
| Greater petrosal foramen | Greater petrosal nerve ($VII$) and petrosal branch of middle meningeal artery | An oblique extension of the facial canal emerging from the anterior surface of the petrous temporal bone |
| Tympanic canaliculus | Tympanic nerve or *nerve of Jacobson* ($IX$) | Small canal within the ridge of the temporal bone separating the carotid canal from the jugular foramen |
| Carotid canal | Internal carotid artery and carotid plexus of nerves | Within the temporal bone, anterolateral to the jugular foramen, and mediolateral to the Eustachian tube |
| Jugular foramen | *Pars Nervosa – CN IX*, tympanic nerve or *nerve of Jacobson* ($IX$), and inferior petrosal sinus. *Pars vascularis – CN X*, *CN XI*, auricular branch of $X$ or *Arnold's nerve*, superior bulb of the internal jugular vein, and meningeal branches of ascending pharyngeal and occipital arteries | Posterior to the carotid canal at the intersection of the petrous temporal and occipital bones. *Pars nervosa* is the anteromedial portion, while the *pars vascularis* is the larger posteromedial portion |
| Greater palatine foramen | Greater palatine nerve ($V_2$) and descending palatine vessels | Foramen at the termination of the greater palatine canal which begins in the inferior PPF passing through the sphenoid and palatine bones to the posterior angle of the hard palate |
| Infraorbital foramen | Infraorbital nerve ($V_2$) and vessels | Opening in the maxillary bone inferior to the infraorbital margin of the orbit |
| Hypoglossal canal | $CN\ XII$ | Superior to the foramen magnum and between the basiocciput and jugular process of the occipital bone |
| Lesser palatine foramen | Lesser palatine nerve ($V_2$) | Posterior to the greater palatine foramen and within the pyramidal process of the palatine bone |
| Mandibular foramen | Inferior alveolar nerve ($V_3$) and artery | Foramen on internal surface of the ramus of the mandible |
| Mental foramen | Mental nerve ($V_3$) and vessels | Anterior surface of the mandible |

[a]Meckel's cave has relatively indistinct borders and is not routinely identifiable on a standard CT scan. Given its importance as the junction of all three branches of the trigeminal nerve, it should be identified when CN V perineural spread is suspected. Using either T1-weighted SPGR or T2-weighted MRI sequences, the images produced reveal Meckel's cave as either a hypointense cavity or hyperintense fluid collection, respectively (Fig. 4)

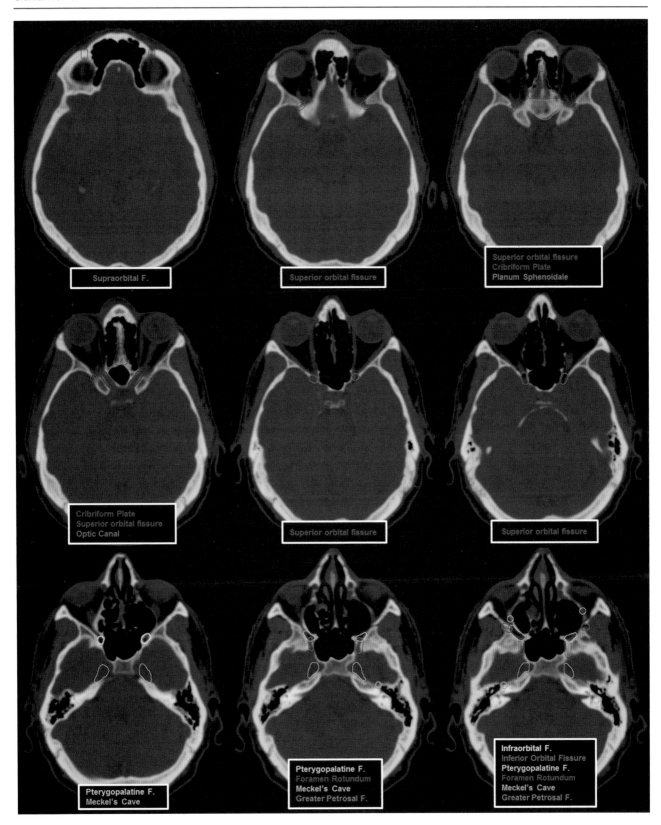

**Fig. 1** Important foramina, fossa, and canals of the cranium and skull base

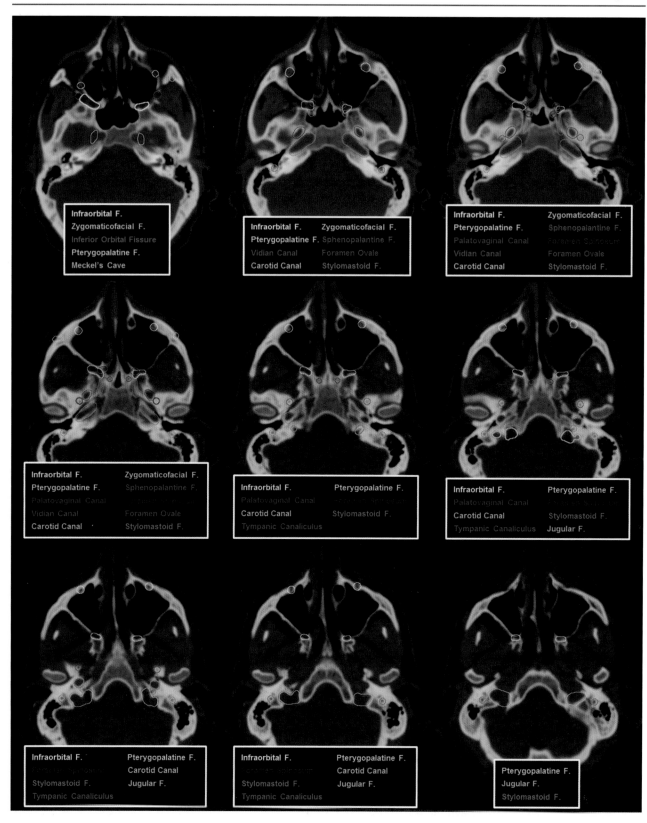

**Fig. 2** Important foramina, fossa, and canals of the cranium and skull base

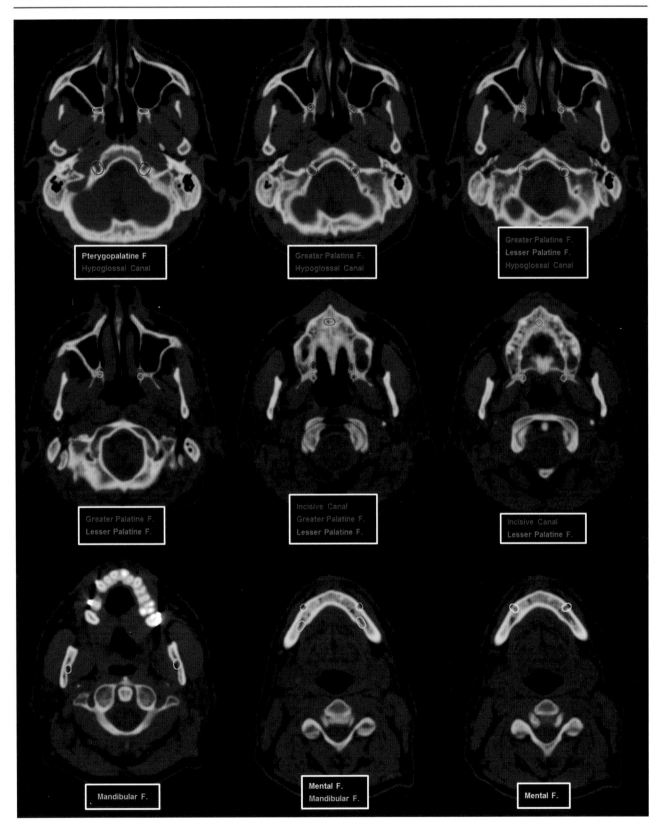

**Fig. 3** Important foramina, fossa, and canals of the cranium and skull base

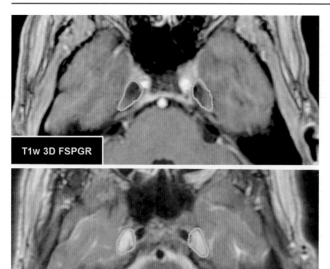

**Fig. 4** Meckel's cave which contains the trigeminal ganglion is easily identifiable on a number of MRI sequences. In this figure, Meckel's cave (in *green*) is seen as a hypointense structure on a T1-weighted FSPGR image and a hyperintense fluid-filled structure on a T2-weighted fast relaxation fast spin echo (*FRFSE*) image

from the roof of the nasal cavity, superior portion of the nasal septum, and superior nasal concha. After passing through the *cribriform plate*, these nerves traverse the dura mater and subarachnoid space before ending in the olfactory bulb, which is situated under the basal surface of the frontal lobe.

Identification of the olfactory nerve is not routinely performed in planning for radiotherapy. It may be important in the treatment of certain skull base tumors such as olfactory groove meningiomas and esthesioneuroblastomas as recently reported by the University of Pittsburgh Medical Center (Gande et al. 2014). The *cribriform plate* is seen in Fig. 1.

*Cranial Nerve II*: The axons of the retinal ganglion cells in the eye are the basis of CN II which originates where they pass through the sclera. The nerve passes posteromedially beneath the *superior rectus muscle* and between the medial and lateral rectus muscles. It exits the orbit through the *optic canal* located in the *sphenoid bone*. Intracranially, the nerve passes superomedially to the *ophthalmic artery* and terminal segments of the *internal carotid artery*. The nerve ends at the *optic chiasm* which lies superior to the *sella turcica*, anterior to the *pituitary stalk*, and inferior to the supra-optic recess of the *third ventricle*. The *central retinal artery and vein* travel with the optic nerve within the meninges until they rejoin the *ophthalmic artery* and *superior ophthalmic vein*, respectively.

The optic nerve is not often a treatment target unless it is grossly involved with disease (see Case 6). More often it is

contoured as an organ at risk (OAR) for treatment planning assessment. Use of a fused T1-weighted MR image is best for delineating the chiasm. Figure 5 illustrates the path of CN II with respect to the structures discussed above.

*Cranial Nerve III*: The oculomotor nerve originates from two nuclei (somatic and visceral motor) located in the *midbrain* at the level of the *superior colliculus* and anterior to the *cerebral aqueduct*. The nerve exits the midbrain into the *interpeduncular fossa* medial to the *basilar artery*. It immediately passes between the *posterior cerebral artery* and *superior cerebellar artery*. The nerve enters the cavernous sinus lateral to the *internal carotid artery* and superior to *CN IV*. It enters the orbit through the *superior orbital fissure* wherein it divides into the superior and inferior divisions to supply motor innervation to its target extraocular muscles. The inferior division carries the parasympathetic fibers to the ciliary and constrictor pupillae muscles.

The oculomotor nerve is typically not contoured independent of other structures. If there is concern for involvement of the cavernous sinus, all structures within are at risk and the whole region is covered by a treatment volume. As shown in Fig. 6, the path of CN III is traceable into the orbit.

*Cranial Nerve IV*: The trochlear nerve motor nucleus is in the periaqueductal gray matter of the *midbrain* at the level of the *inferior colliculus*. The nerve fibers emerge dorsally from the midbrain, travelling anterolaterally between the *posterior cerebral artery* and *superior cerebellar arteries*. It enters the lateral wall of the cavernous sinus inferolateral to *CN III*. To enter the orbit, the nerve passes medially through the *superior orbital fissure* below the *anterior clinoid process* and *CN III*.

Similar to CN III, the trochlear nerve is not contoured independent of other structures. If there is clinical or radiographic involvement of the nerve, the contents of the entire cavernous sinus are often involved and treated. Figure 7 depicts the course approximate of CN IV into the orbit.

*Cranial Nerve V*: The trigeminal nerve originates from 4 nuclei – 1 motor and 3 sensory. The locations and paths of these nuclei are beyond the scope of this chapter and can be reviewed elsewhere (Bathla and Hegde 2013; Moore and Dalley 1999). CN V emerges from the pons as essentially two separate nerves: a small motor and large sensory root. The collection of cranial nerve roots enters *Meckel's cave* (Fig. 8) wherein the sensory branches coalesce into the *trigeminal ganglion*, while the motor root travels medially and rejoins the sensory portion of $V_3$ to create the mandibular nerve. The trigeminal ganglion splits into the 3 branches of CN V: the *ophthalmic nerve* ($V_1$), *maxillary nerve* ($V_2$), and the sensory component of the *mandibular nerve* ($V_3$). Both

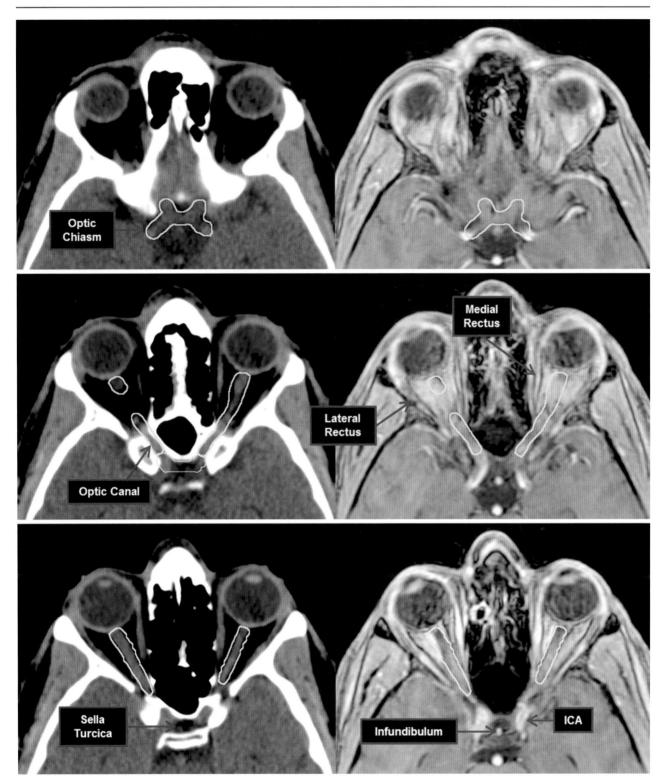

**Fig. 5** Path of the optic nerve (*yellow*) into the optic chiasm. Images on the left are non-contrast CT scans with corresponding images from a T1w 3D FSPGR MRI on the right. *ICA* internal carotid artery

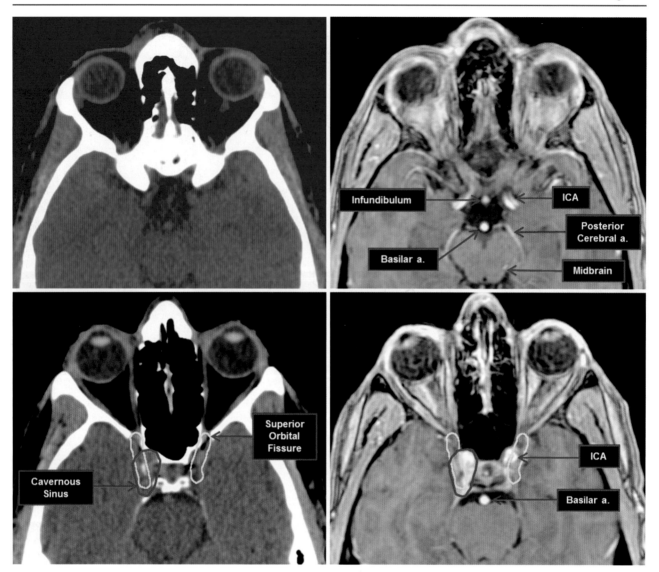

**Fig. 6** Path of cranial nerve III, the oculomotor nerve (*yellow*), from the midbrain through the cavernous sinus and finally into the orbit through the superior orbital fissure. Images on the left are non-contrast CT scans with corresponding images from a T1w 3D FSPGR MRI on the right. *ICA* internal carotid artery

$V_1$ and $V_2$ pass through the lateral wall of the *cavernous sinus* inferolateral to *CN IV* and *III*.

- The *ophthalmic nerve* ($V_1$) enters the orbit through the *superior orbital fissure* where it divides into its terminal branches: the lacrimal, frontal, and nasociliary nerves. The *lacrimal nerve* follows the course of the *lateral rectus* along its superior edge until it reaches the *lacrimal gland*. The *frontal nerve* passes medial to the *lateral rectus muscle* and travels superior to the *superior rectus* finally terminating as the supratrochlear and supraorbital nerves. The *nasociliary nerve* travels medially in the orbit until it divides into its terminal branches that supply sensation to nasal cavity and paranasal sinuses.

If there is perineural spread along $V_1$, the clinical treatment volume (CTV) encompasses nearly the whole of the orbit to Meckel's cave. This covers both retrograde and anterograde spread along the terminal branches. As seen in Fig. 9, the CTV for the *lacrimal nerve* includes the *lateral rectus* and extends superiorly eventually encompassing the *lacrimal gland* on more superior axial slices. A CTV for the *frontal nerve* includes the ophthalmic artery and *superior rectus*. It also encompasses the supraorbital foramen in the most superior aspect. The *nasociliary nerve* spreads out into multiple branches along the medial wall of the orbit of which a CTV would include.

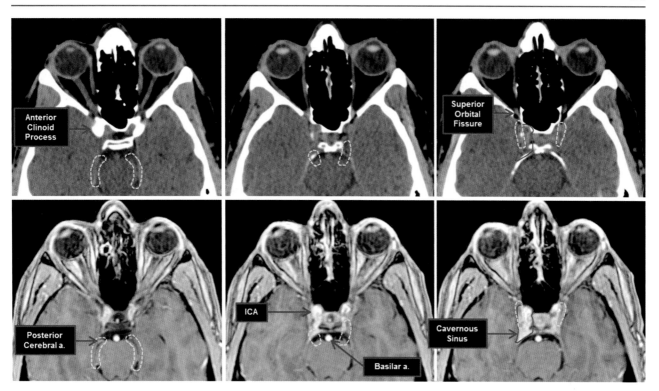

**Fig. 7** Approximate path of cranial nerve IV, the trochlear nerve (*dashed yellow*), from the dorsal midbrain through the cavernous sinus and finally into the orbit through the superior orbital fissure inferior to the anterior clinoid process. Images on *top* are non-contrast CT scans with corresponding images from a T1W 3D FSPGR MRI on the *bottom*. *ICA* internal carotid artery

- After traversing the *cavernous sinus*, the *maxillary nerve* (*V₂*) exits through the *foramen rotundum* and enters the *pterygopalatine fossa*. Prior to entering the *foramen rotundum*, V₂ gives off the *middle meningeal nerve* which enters the *foramen spinosum*. Within the *pterygopalatine fossa*, V₂ divides into its terminal branches: zygomatic, greater palatine, lesser palatine, nasopalatine, posterior-superior alveolar, and infraorbital nerves. The *zygomatic nerve* enters the orbit through the *inferior orbital fissure* and supplies sensation to the skin over the zygomatic and temporal bones. Sphenopalatine branches of V₂ directly supply the pterygopalatine ganglion and continue into the *greater and lesser palatine nerves*. The *greater palatine nerve* moves inferiorly from the *pterygopalatine fossa* and enters the hard palate through the *greater palatine foramen*. The *lesser palatine nerve* follows a similar course and emerges to innervate the soft palate, tonsils, and uvula through the *lesser palatine foramen*. The *posterior-superior alveolar nerve* arises from V2 prior to entering the *infraorbital groove* and descends to supply a portion of the gums and teeth. The *infraorbital nerve* enters the orbit through the *inferior orbital fissure* and enters the *infraorbital canal* exiting to innervate the lower eyelid, upper lip, and part of the nasal vestibule through the *infraorbital foramen*.

- The CTV for CV V₂ is illustrated in Fig. 10. Here the CTV includes all the major branches of V₂ except for the *nasopalatine* and *posterior-superior alveolar nerve*. Inclusion of these branches is important when there is gross tumor involvement of the *pterygopalatine fossa* (see Case 6). A CTV that includes the *nasopalatine nerve* would encompass the nasal septum down to the *incisive foramen* in the anterior hard palate. The osseous structures around the nerves are included in the CTV given variability in nerve position and difficult visualization on MRI unless there is perineural spread.

- The *mandibular nerve* (*V₃*) exits *Meckel's cave* inferiorly through the *foramen ovale*. Upon exiting the *foramen ovale*, the nerve splits into an anterior and posterior branch. The anterior nerve supplies the *masseteric, deep temporal, buccal,* and *medial and lateral pterygoid nerves*. The posterior division divides into the *auriculotemporal, lingual,* and *inferior alveolar nerves* and motor branches to the *mylohyoid* and *anterior belly of the digastric* muscles. The *inferior alveolar nerve* enters the *mandibular foramen* and supplies sensation to the mandibular teeth and finally the lower lip and chin after it exits the mandible through the *mental foramen* as the mental nerve.

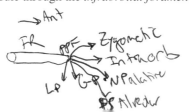

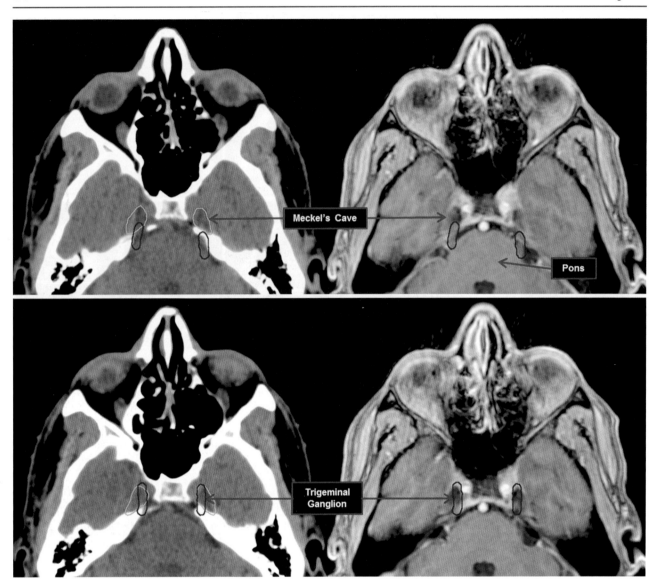

**Fig. 8** The trigeminal trunk is illustrated emerging from the pons (*blue*) and entering Meckel's cave where it forms the trigeminal ganglion. Images on the left are non-contrast CT scans with corresponding images from a T1w 3D FSPGR MRI on the right

The CTV for CN V$_3$ is defined by the parapharyngeal spaces containing the vessels and best highlighted by a T2-weighted MRI (Fig. 11). The CTV begins superiorly at *Meckel's cave* and includes the *foramen ovale* and these parapharyngeal spaces to the mandibular foramen and the sublingual space along the lingual artery. If there is gross perineural spread, the muscles innervated by the V$_3$ should be included in the CTV (Cases 2 and 5).

*Cranial Nerve VI*: The abducens nerve arises in the medial aspect of the pons near the floor of the 4th ventricle and adjacent to the motor nucleus of *CN VII*. It emerges into the pontine cistern at the pontomedullary junction. It travels anteriorly along the basilar artery and enters the *cavernous sinus* through *Dorello's canal* (Fig. 12) after bending over

the petrous portion of the temporal bone. In the cavernous sinus it is immediately posterolateral to the *internal carotid artery* and medial to *CN III and IV*. It enters the orbit through the medial aspect of the *superior orbital fissure* where it innervates *the lateral rectus muscle*. The approximate pathway through the cavernous sinus is seen in Fig. 13.

The abducens nerve is difficult to image except on very dedicated scans as shown in Fig. 12. If it is clinically grossly involved with disease, the entire cavernous sinus is included in the CTV.

*Cranial Nerve VII*: The facial nerve originates from two separate nerves exiting the brainstem at the *cerebellopontine angle*. The motor component arises from the motor nucleus

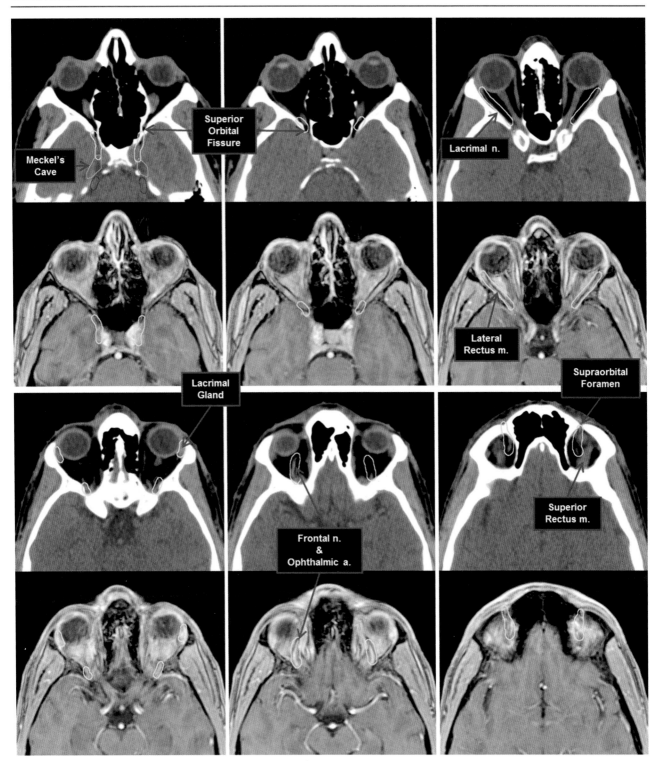

**Fig. 9** The approximate pathway and branches of the ophthalmic branch (CN V₁) of the trigeminal nerve (CN V) are shown here after exiting Meckel's cave. Images on the *top* are non-contrast CT scans with corresponding images from a T1w 3D FSPGR MRI on the *bottom*. *CN V₁* yellow

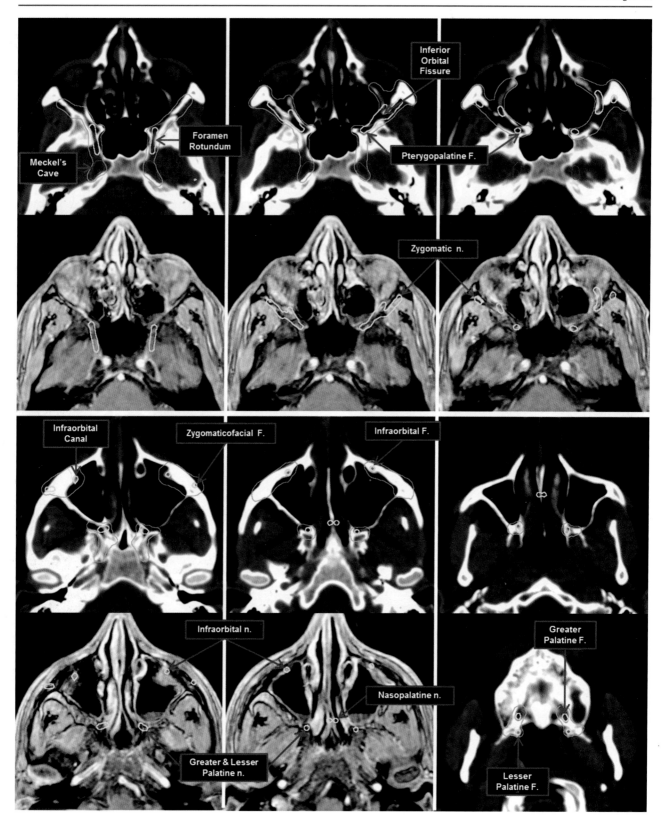

**Fig. 10** The pathway and branches of the maxillary branch (CN V₂) of the trigeminal nerve (CN V) are shown here after exiting Meckel's cave. The CTV is shown in *green*. Images on the *top* are non-contrast CT scans with corresponding images from a T1w 3D FSPGR MRI on the *bottom. CN V₂ yellow*

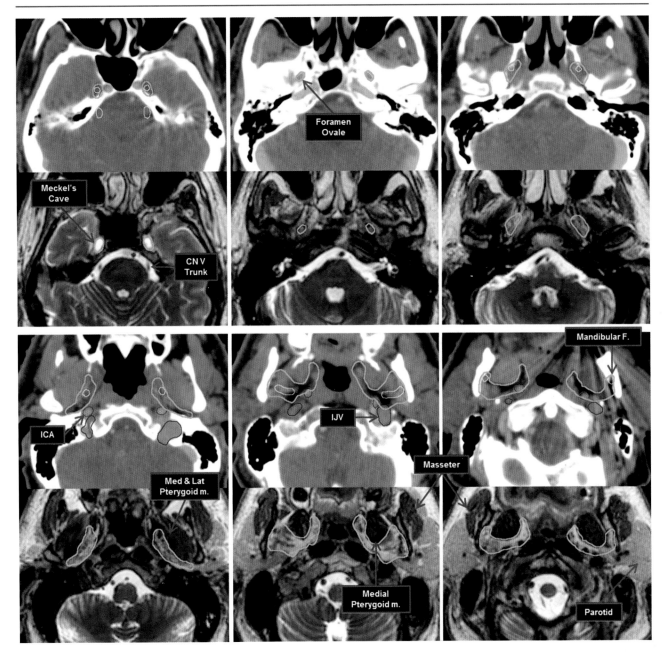

**Fig. 11** The pathway of the mandibular nerve, CN V₃ (*yellow*), of the trigeminal nerve (CN V) is shown here after exiting Meckel's cave and entering the foramen ovale. The CTV is indicated in *green*.

Images on the *top* are contrast CT scans with corresponding images from a T2w 3D MRI on the *bottom*. *ICA* internal carotid artery, *IJV* internal jugular vein

in the dorsal pons. The sensory component, often called the nervus intermedius, arises from a combination of inputs from the spinal nucleus of CN V, the superior salivary nucleus, and the nucleus solitarius. The two nerves cross the *cerebellopontine cistern* and join at the internal acoustic meatus. The facial nerve travels with *CN VIII* until it enters the *facial/fallopian canal* and travels anterolaterally. At the *geniculate ganglion* the nerve abruptly changes direction forming the *first genu*. Here, the *greater petrosal nerve* branches off the facial nerve and travels through the *greater petrosal foramen* into the middle cranial fossa until it reaches

the *vidian canal* where it forms the *vidian nerve* and finally reaches the pterygopalatine ganglion. The facial nerve travels posteriorly along the medial wall of the *tympanic cavity* wherein it gives rise to the *nerve to the stapedius*. At the end of the *tympanic cavity* is the *second genu* where the nerve turns 90° inferiorly and enters the *mastoid bone*. In this segment, the facial nerve gives rise to the *chorda tympani* which eventually joins the *lingual nerve* of CN V₃ to supply taste to the anterior two-thirds of the tongue. The facial nerve then exits the cranium through the *stylomastoid foramen* and enters the substance of the *parotid gland*. The nerve terminates

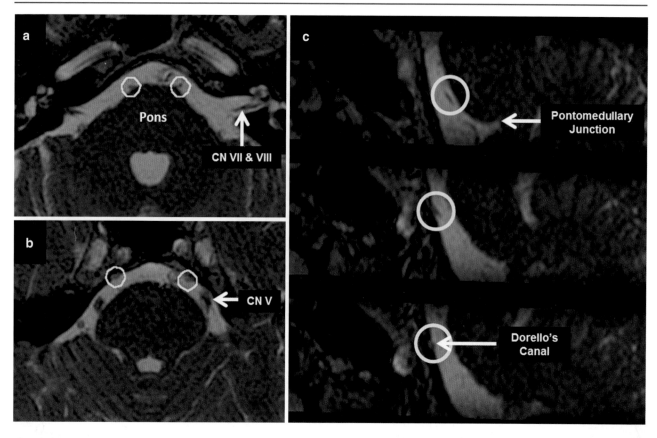

**Fig. 12** The abducens nerve (CN VI) as it exits the pontomedullary junction as seen on a 3D FIESTA MRI (**a**). (**b**, **c**) show CN VI entering Dorello's canal after traveling superiorly in the pontine cistern. Additional cranial nerves are also seen in these images. *Yellow circles* CN VI

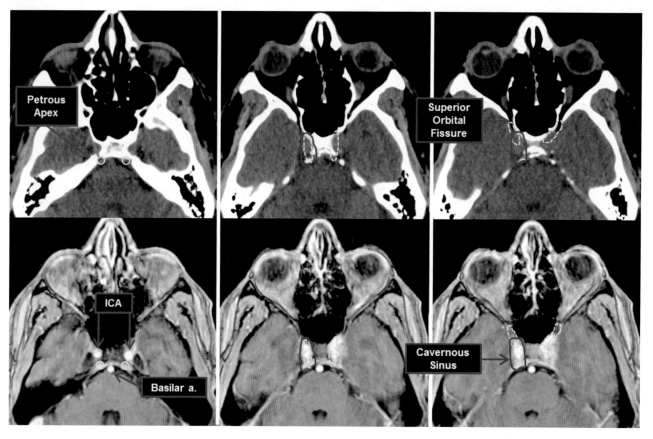

**Fig. 13** The approximate pathway of the abducens nerve, CN VI (*dashed yellow*), is shown here after entering Dorello's canal and crossing the petrous apex. Images on the *top* are non-contrast CT scans with corresponding images from a T1w 3D FSPGR MRI on the *bottom*. *ICA* internal carotid artery

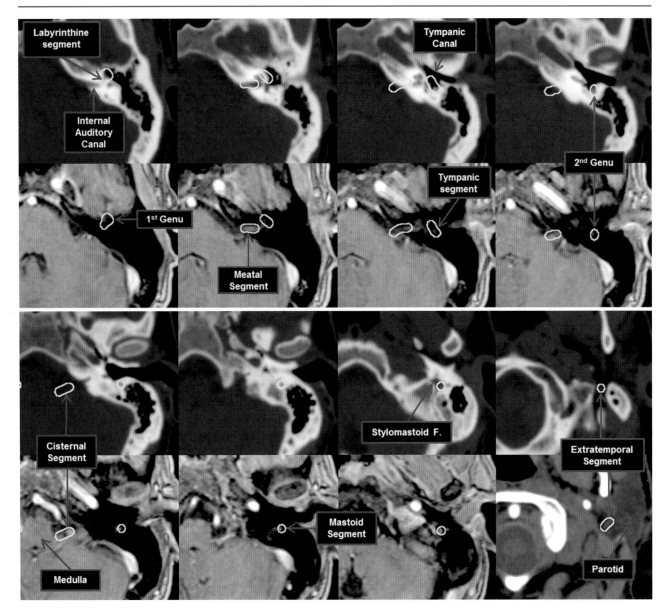

**Fig. 14** Axial slices through the mastoid bone with the pathway of the facial nerve (CN VII) identified. Images on the *top* are non-contrast CT scans with corresponding images from a T1w 3D FSPGR MRI on the *bottom*

in six branches: the posterior auricular, temporal, zygomatic, buccal, mandibular, and cervical nerves. *Additional information on the anatomy and path of the facial nerve can be found elsewhere* (Gilchrist 2009; Veillona et al. 2010).

If there is facial nerve involvement of disease, the CTV typically includes the entire parotid gland as the 6 terminal branches are within its substance. The CTV continues superiorly through the *stylomastoid foramen* in the mastoid bone. Inclusion of the *chorda tympani* in the CTV may also be important based on clinical considerations. Unless there is gross perineural invasion of CN VII into the stylomastoid foramen, the CTV can stop below the 2nd genu given additional toxicity to the cochlea and inner ear. Case 1 demon-

strates a CTV for CN VII involvement. The course of the nerve within the mastoid bone is illustrated in Fig. 14.

*Cranial Nerve VIII* (Fig. 15): The vestibulocochlear nerve comprises a collection of two separate nerve fibers, the vestibular and cochlear. Four vestibular nuclei are found in the lateral aspect of the floor of the fourth ventricle between the pons and medulla. Two cochlear nuclei are located in the rostral medulla adjacent to the inferior cerebellar peduncle. The nerve exits the brainstem at the *pontomedullary junction* and crosses the *cerebellopontine cistern* lateral to *CN VII* and enters the *internal acoustic meatus*. After passing through the *internal acoustic meatus*, CN VIII splits into the *cochlear* and *vestibular* branches which independently form separate ganglia (Fig. 15c).

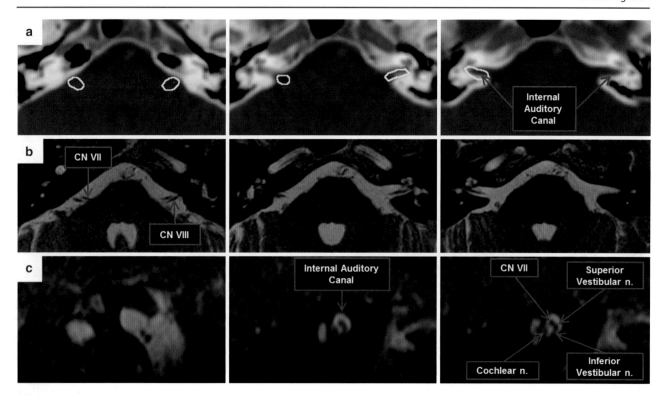

**Fig. 15** The pathway of the vestibulocochlear nerve (CN VIII) depicted on axial slices of a non-contrast CT (**a**) and respective T2-weighted MRI (**b**). Sagittal sections through the internal auditory canal reveal CNVIII splitting into its cochlear and vestibular branches (**c**)

The cochlear ganglion collects afferent fibers from the organ of Corti, while the vestibular ganglion collects afferent fibers from the hair cells in the maculae of the utricle, saccule and ampullae of the semicircular ducts. *A full discussion regarding CN VII can be found elsewhere* (Landau and Barner 2009).

*Cranial Nerve IX*: The glossopharyngeal nerve arises from 4 nuclei in the medulla which it shares with *CN X* and *CN XI*. These are the *nucleus ambiguous* (efferent), *inferior salivary nucleus* (efferent), *nucleus of the solitary tract* (afferent), and *spinal nucleus of the trigeminal nerve* (afferent). The nerve exits the medulla in its posterolateral aspect and traverses the *cerebellopontine cistern* in an anterolateral direction to the *jugular foramen*. It enters the foramen on the medial aspect and travels inferoanteriorly to *CN X* and *CN XI*. In the *jugular foramen*, CN IX forms the *superior* and *inferior (petrous) glossopharyngeal ganglia*. At this point, the *tympanic nerve* (or *nerve of Jacobsen*) branches off the *petrous ganglion* and enters the *tympanic canaliculus* where it supplies innervation to the middle ear, secretory function of the parotid gland via the *lesser petrosal nerve*, and connects with the *auriculotemporal branch* of *CN V₃*. Upon exiting the *jugular foramen*, CN IX passes between the *internal jugular vein* and *internal carotid artery*. Below the *styloid process*, the nerve passes laterally and then anteriorly across the *internal carotid artery* following the trajectory of the *stylopharyngeus muscle*, which it innervates. It passes through the medial aspect of the *parapharyngeal space* where it

eventually reaches its terminal branches supplying sensation (*pharyngeal*, *tonsillar*, and *lingual*) and visceral sensory from the carotid body and carotid sinus. *Further details on the anatomy and course of CN IX can be found elsewhere* (Erman et al. 2009; Roldan-Valadez et al. 2014).

At the level of the skull base and *first cervical vertebrate*, cranial nerves IX, X, and XI travel together and a single CTV encompasses all of them (Fig. 16). The suggested guidelines for contouring these lower cranial nerves are found in the RTOG atlas (http://www.rtog.org/CoreLab/ContouringAtlases/HNAtlases.aspx) and is published in detail elsewhere (Mourad et al. 2013). Briefly, starting at the *jugular foramen*, the CTV encompasses the *internal carotid artery* and the *internal jugular vein*. CN IX traverses the *jugular foramen* medially in the *pars nervosa* compartment. Traveling inferiorly, the CTV encloses the *internal carotid artery* with a 3 mm margin to ensure the *carotid sheath* is covered given it contains the lower cranial nerves. A portion of the anterior aspect of the *internal jugular vein* is also covered. At the level of the end of the styloid process, the CTV for CN IX includes both the carotid sheath and the *stylopharyngeus muscle* (Fig. 17). The CTV includes the medial parapharyngeal space at this level. The contours continue until the fibers of the *stylopharyngeus muscle* are lost in the medial parapharyngeal space near the pharyngeal wall.

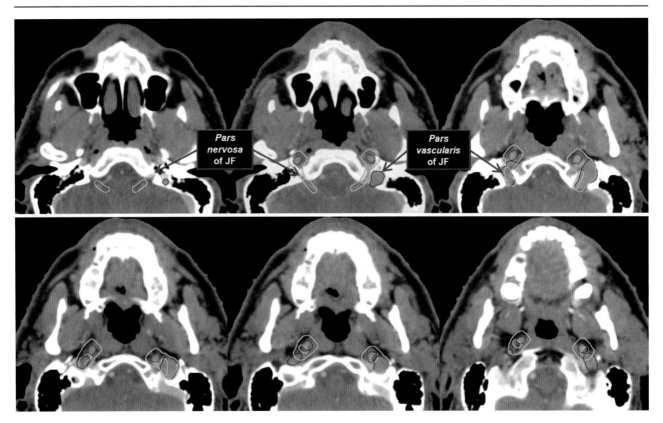

**Fig. 16** Cranial nerves IX, X, and IX all pass extracranially through the jugular foramen (JF). The CTV of the shared portion of their path is shown in *green*. The ICA (*red*) and IJV (*blue*) are also indicated with respect to the CTV. CNIX is shown in *yellow*

**Fig. 17** The clinical treatment volume (*green*) for the glossopharyngeal nerve (CN IX) is depicted on axial slices of a contrast CT (*right*) and respective T2-weighted MRI (*left*). The internal carotid artery (*red*) and internal jugular vein (*blue*) are also identified in relation to the CN IX pathway (*yellow*). *SPM* stylopharyngeus muscle

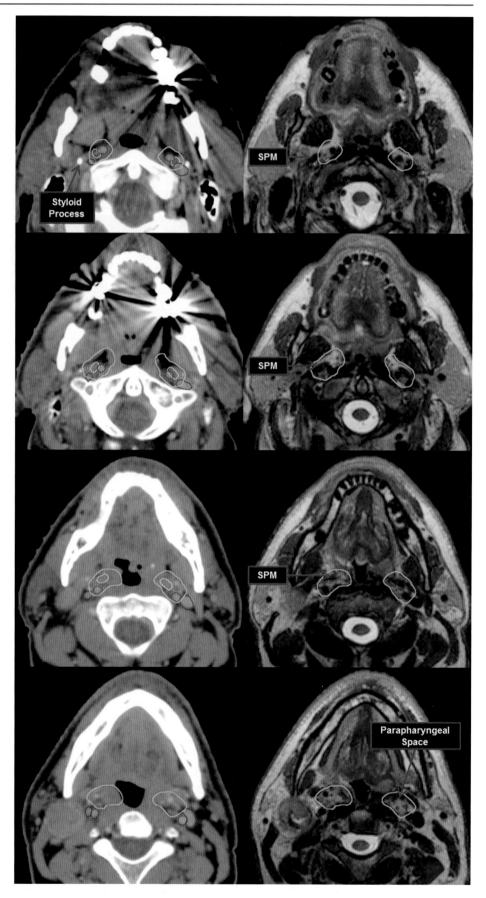

*Cranial Nerve X*: The vagus nerve originates from the brainstem as a series of rootlets emerging from the medulla inferior to *CN IX*. As discussed, the vagus nerve shares the same nuclei with *CN IX* and *CN XI*. The vagus nerve follows *CN IX* into the *jugular foramen* and travels inferiorly along the posteromedial wall of the *internal jugular vein*. Within the *jugular foramen*, the vagus nerve forms the *superior ganglion of the vagus nerve* (or *jugular ganglion*) from which arises the *auricular branch*, also known as *Arnold's nerve* supplying sensation to the skin of the external acoustic meatus. Upon exiting the *jugular foramen*, the vagus nerve forms the *inferior ganglion of the vagus nerve* (or *nodose ganglion*) at the level of the transverse process of *C1*. This carries much of the visceral afferent sensation. Extracranially, the vagus nerve travels lateral to *CN XII* between the *internal carotid artery* and *internal jugular vein* within the *carotid sheath*. Arising from the *nodose ganglion* are the nerve fibers for the *pharyngeal branch* and *superior laryngeal nerves* which both cross the *internal carotid artery* and innervate intrinsic skeletal muscles of the pharynx and larynx. The vagus nerve then passes posterolaterally to the *common carotid artery* as it enters the thorax. Of import to the head and neck, the *right recurrent laryngeal nerve* branches off the right vagus at the level of the *aortic arch* and wraps around the *right subclavian artery* ascending to innervate the larynx via the tracheoesophageal groove. The *left recurrent laryngeal nerve* is longer as it wraps around the *aortic arch* prior to ascending to the larynx. *Descriptions of the innervation of the vagus nerve to the visceral organs can be found elsewhere* (Moore and Dalley 1999).

The CTV for the superior portion of the vagus nerve follows the description above for *CN IX*. After *CN IX* exits the *carotid sheath* at the level of the *1st cervical vertebrate* or tip of the *styloid process*, the CTV for CN X continues inferiorly as a 3 mm margin around the *internal carotid artery* including a portion of the *internal jugular vein* (Fig. 18). As per the RTOG lower cranial nerve atlas, the CTV stops below the level of the 3rd cervical vertebrate. Although if there is gross or clinical involvement below that level, the CTV continues as needed.

*Cranial Nerve XI*: The spinal accessory nerve has both cranial and spinal origins. The cranial component arises from the *nucleus ambiguous* in the medulla which it shares with *CN IX* and *CN X*. The spinal portion originates from rootlets in the dorsal horns of the first 4 or 5 cervical levels and coalesces to form the spinal accessory nerve which passes intracranially through the *foramen magnum*. The two parts temporarily join in the *jugular foramen* as CN XI travels inferiorly through the skull base. Once extracranial, the cranial root separates and joins the *vagus nerve* through the *nodose ganglion* to innervate the striated muscles of the soft palate, pharynx, larynx,

and esophagus. The spinal root continues inferiorly and posteriorly, crossing the *internal jugular vein* along its course into the *posterior cervical triangle*. The spinal component terminates in branches innervating the *sternocleidomastoid* and *trapezius* muscles. Sensory fibers from C2 to C4 join the spinal accessory nerve in the *posterior cervical triangle* to supply pain and proprioceptive fibers. *Further details on CN XI can be found elsewhere* (Massey 2009).

*Cranial Nerve XII*: The hypoglossal nerve arises in the medulla from the *hypoglossal nucleus* and exits as a series of rootlets between the olive and pyramid. The rootlets cross the subarachnoid space posterior to the *vertebral artery* and exit the posterior fossa through the *hypoglossal canal* in which they coalesce. Upon emerging from the skull base, the *meningeal branch* separates from CN XII and travels back through the *hypoglossal canal* to innervate the posterior dural space. CN XII is then joined by a branch of the *cervical plexus* containing fibers from the C1 and C2 spinal nerves. These same fibers eventually separate from CN XII to join a branch of the *ansa cervicalis* to innervate the infrahyoid musculature. The nerve travels inferiorly adjacent to *CN X* and *CN XI* and posteromedial to the *internal carotid artery*. It eventually passes between the *internal carotid artery* and *internal jugular vein* travelling lateral to the *external carotid artery* in the *lateral pharyngeal space*. At the *angle of the mandible* it crosses deep to the *posterior belly of the digastric* into the *sublingual space* and inferior to the *lingual artery*. At this level, the hypoglossal nerve terminates in branches that supply the extrinsic and intrinsic muscles of the tongue.

The CTV for the hypoglossal nerve is also described in the RTOG atlas. The superior extent of the CTV begins at the *hypoglossal canal* and encompasses the *internal carotid artery* with a 3 mm margin (Fig. 19). At the level of the *anterior belly of the digastric muscle* and *common carotid artery*, the CTV expands to include the medial *parapharyngeal space* as well as the anterior portion of the *internal carotid artery*. The parapharyngeal space is included in the CTV below the *anterior belly of the digastric* and the *lingual artery* along the hyoglossus muscle until it reaches the substance of the base of tongue. The horns of the *hyoid bone* are not ideal markers as they move with swallowing.

## 2.3   Anastomoses Between Cranial Nerves

While a primary cranial nerve pathway may be involved with disease, interconnections between cranial nerves may serve as conduits for further dissemination of metastatic cancer in an anterograde or retrograde fashion. Knowledge of the major connections between the cranial nerves helps the radiation oncologist identify potential regions at risk if certain

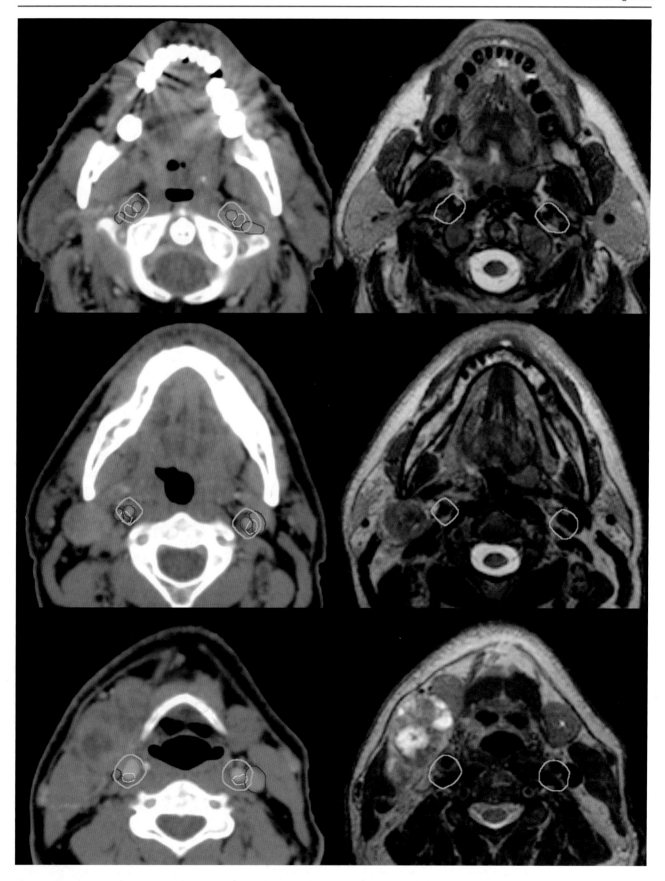

**Fig. 18** The clinical treatment volume (*green*) for the vagus nerve (CN X) is depicted on axial slices of a contrast-enhanced CT (*left*) and respective T2-weighted MRI (*right*) after the glossopharyngeal nerve (CN IX) exits the carotid sheath. The internal carotid artery (*red*), internal jugular vein (*blue*), and common carotid (*pink*) are also identified in relation to the CN X pathway (*yellow*)

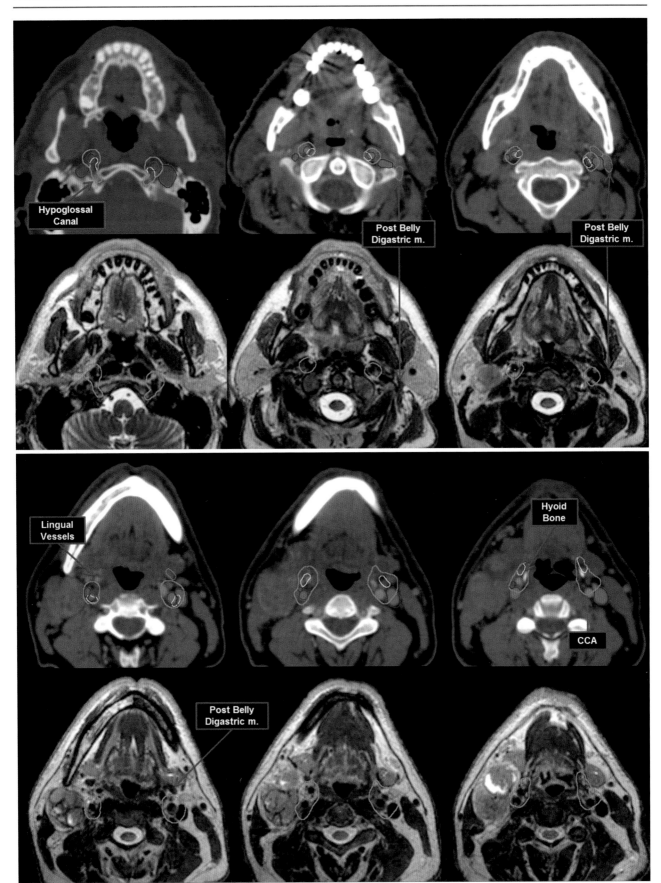

**Fig. 19** The clinical treatment volume (*green*) for the hypoglossal nerve (CN XII) is depicted on axial slices of a contrast-enhanced CT (*top*) and respective T2-weighted MRI (*bottom*) upon exiting the hypoglossal canal. The internal carotid artery (*red*), internal jugular vein (*blue*), and digastric muscle (*orange*) are indicated with respect to the path of CN XII (*yellow*). *CCA* common carotid artery

**Table 2** Important anastomoses between cranial nerves

| Nerve | Interconnection | Innervation | Anatomy | Site of concern |
|---|---|---|---|---|
| Greater petrosal (Fig. 20) | $V_2 \leftrightarrow VII$ | Lacrimal gland, palate (taste), nasal cavity, and pharynx (parasympathetic) | Geniculate ganglion at hiatus → along the temporal bone → Meckel's cave → joins deep petrosal nerve in Vidian canal → PPF → $V_2$ | Tumor in PPF or Meckel's cave |
| Lesser petrosal (Fig. 21) | $IX \leftrightarrow VII$ | Parotid (parasympathetic) | Tympanic plexus → hiatus in temporal bone → floor middle cranial fossa → foramen ovale → otic ganglion → parotid gland | Tumors involving the parotid gland or foramen ovale |
| Auriculotemporal (Fig. 22) | $V_3 \leftrightarrow VII$ (temporofacial n.) $V_3 \leftrightarrow V_2$ (zygomaticotemporal n.) | Parotid gland and sensation to auricle and skin of temporal region | Branch of $V_3$ after exiting the foramen ovale → encircle middle meningeal artery → parotid gland posterior to the mandibular ramus → posterior and superior, deep to superficial temporal artery | Interconnections in parotid gland |
| Chorda tympani (Fig. 23) | $VII \leftrightarrow V_3$ (lingual n.) | Taste to anterior $^2/_3$ of the tongue. Parasympathetic to submandibular and sublingual glands | VII (near exit of the stylomastoid foramen) → petrotympanic fissure → infratemporal fossa → lingual nerve | Tumors of the parotid, tongue, and minor salivary glands |
| Interconnections along extrinsic muscles of tongue | $V_3 \leftrightarrow XII$ (lingual n.) | Sensation to anterior $^2/_3$ of the tongue and motor to tongue | - | Tumors involving the tongue, BOT, and minor salivary glands |

cranial nerves are clinically or radiographically involved. Table 2 highlights some of the most clinically relevant anastomoses between cranial nerves. There are many additional connections that vary between individuals. Further details on these lesser known interconnections are reviewed elsewhere (Shoja et al. 2014a, b).

## 3 Physical Exam

To identify potential cranial nerve involvement in malignancies of the head and neck, it is important for the Radiation Oncologist to perform a thorough clinical exam. Understanding the sensorimotor targets of the individual cranial nerves is essential in identifying both the potential nerves involved with disease and their target tissues which may be at risk for perineural spread. Table 3 lists the cranial nerves and their motor and sensory functions. The reader is directed elsewhere for further details on the cranial nerve exam (Damodaran et al. 2014; Swartz 2002).

## 4 Imaging

- CT Scan: Ideal to image the skull base foramina through which the cranial nerves or their branches pass. To ease identification of the anatomic features, a slice thickness of 2 mm or less should be obtained during treatment planning. CT cisternography, which is routinely used to identify cerebrospinal fluid (CSF) leaks in patients, can also be useful in the identification of the cranial nerve origins from the brainstem (Roldan-Valadez et al. 2014). This technique is not routinely used in treatment planning unless a myelogram is needed for treatment of lesions in close proximity to the spinal cord.
- MRI T1-weighted sequences: Tissues with high adipose content appear bright, while edema and tissues with increased water content appear dark. Gadolinium contrast appears bright on T1-weighted images.

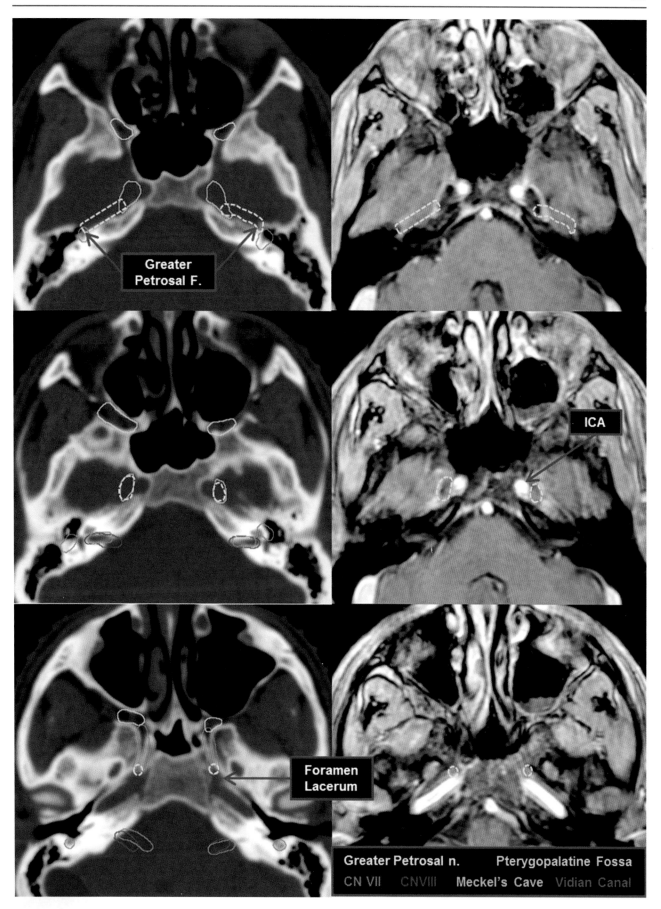

**Fig. 20** Path of the greater petrosal nerve (*GPN*) connecting the facial nerve (VII) to the pterygopalatine fossa (*PPF*) which contains branches of the maxillary branch of the trigeminal nerve (V₃). The GPN passes through both Meckel's cave and the Vidian canal in route to the PPF. Images on the *left* are non-contrast CT scans with corresponding images from a T1w 3D FSPGR MRI on the *right*. *ICA* internal carotid artery

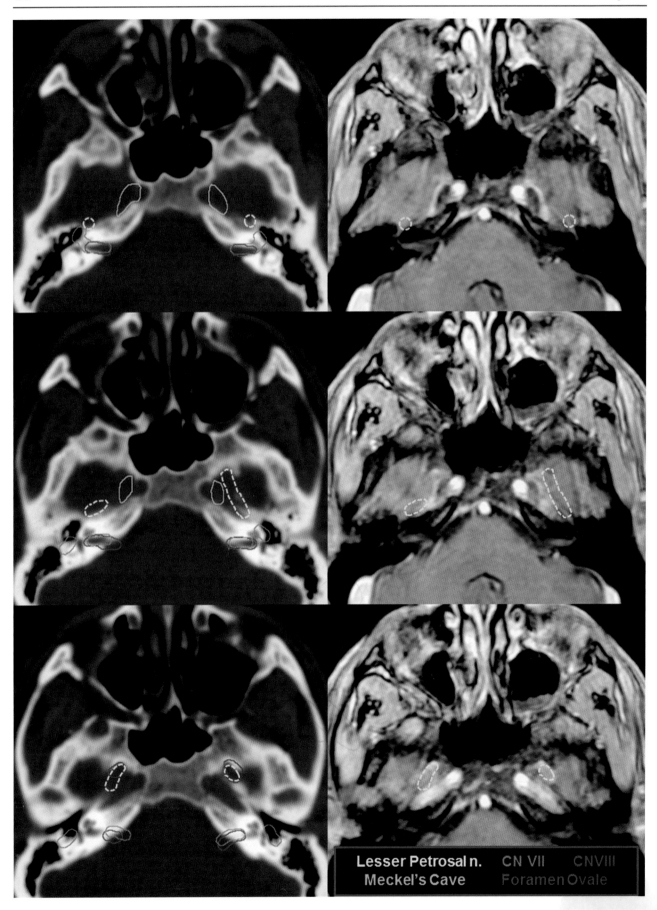

**Fig. 21** Path of the lesser petrosal nerve (*LPN*) connecting the glosso-pharyngeal nerve (IX) to the facial nerve (VII). The LPN enters the floor of the middle cranial fossa through a hiatus in the temporal bone from the tympanic plexus. It courses to the parotid through the foramen ovale and otic ganglion. Images on the *left* are non-contrast CT scans with corresponding images from a T1w 3D FSPGR MRI on the *right*

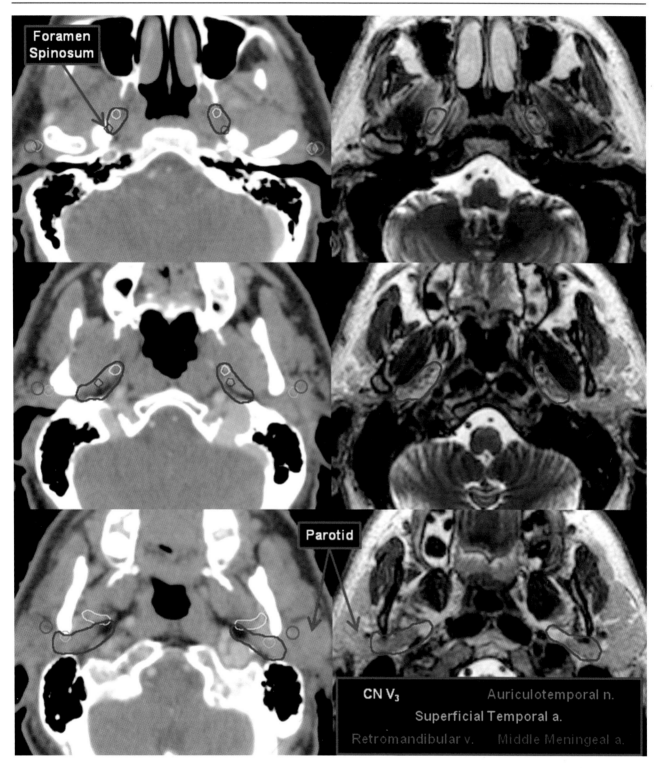

**Fig. 22** CTV of the auriculotemporal nerve (*ATN*) connecting the mandibular branch of the trigeminal nerve (V₃) to both the facial nerve (VII) and maxillary branch of the trigeminal nerve (V₂). The ATN emerges from V3 as two branches shortly after exiting the foramen ovale. It encircles the middle meningeal artery and then enters the substance of the parotid gland along the posterior aspect of the mandibular ramus. If involved by tumor, the remainder of the CTV would include the parotid and pass superiorly with the superficial temporal artery. Images on the *left* are non-contrast CT scans with corresponding images from a T2w 3D post-contrast MRI on the *right*

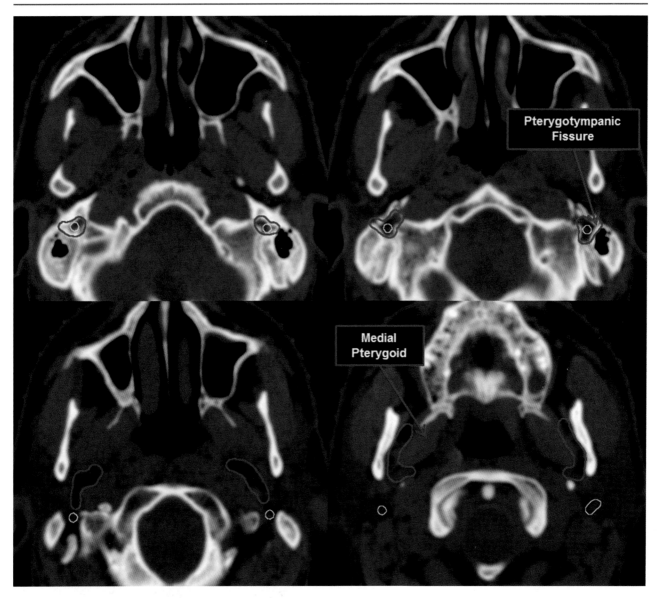

**Fig. 23** CTV for the chorda tympani nerve (*blue*) that connects the facial nerve (VII, *yellow*) with the lingual branch of the mandibular nerve (V₃). The chorda tympani connects to CN VII at the level of the pterygotympanic fissure (*arrow*) near the extracranial portion of the stylomastoid foramen. It then travels through the parapharyngeal space and finally the lateral masticator space adjacent to the medial pterygoid. It is here that it joins the lingual nerve (V₃)

– FSPGR 3D (*Fast Spoiled Gradient Echo*): High-resolution imaging useful for imaging all segments of the cranial nerves (Borges and Casselman 2010).

– Post contrast: Critical for identifying malignant perineural invasion along cranial nerves as well as inflammatory processes. Fat-suppressed T1-weighted post-contrast sequences produce the best images for nerve segments in tissues with high adipose content such as the orbits (Morani et al. 2011).

• MRI T2-weighted sequences: Tissues with increased water content such as edema and tumors are bright on T2-weighted images.

  • FIESTA 3D (*Fast Imaging Employing Steady State Acquisition*): Permits imaging of the *cisternal segments* of the cranial nerves given the hypointensity of the roots surrounded by hyperintense CSF (Morani et al. 2011) and also within other hyperintense structures such as the parotid gland (Li et al. 2012). For optimal imaging, acquisition image thickness should be submillimeter (Alves 2010). Analogous sequences include CISS (constructive interference in steady state) (Borges 2008).

• There are many additional MRI sequence names analogous to those described above that are dependent on the MRI instrument manufacturer.

• *Perineural Spread*: Suggested by obliteration of the fatty tissue within and adjacent to the skull base foramina

**Table 3** Sensorimotor targets of the cranial nerves

| Cranial nerve | | Somatic motor | Sensory | Visceral motor |
|---|---|---|---|---|
| I | Olfactory | – | Smell | – |
| II | Optic | – | Vision | – |
| III | Oculomotor | Superior, medial, and inferior rectus, inferior oblique, and levator palpebrae superioris | – | Sphincter pupillae – *pupillary constriction* Ciliary m. – *accommodation* |
| IV | Trochlear | Superior oblique | – | – |
| V | Ophthalmic (V₁) | – | Cornea; skin of forehead, scalp, eyelids, and nose; mucosa of the nasal cavity and paranasal sinuses | – |
| | Maxillary (V₂) | – | Skin over maxilla and upper lip. Maxillary teeth. Mucosa of nose, maxillary sinus and palate | – |
| | Mandibular (V₃) | M. mastication (temporalis, masseter, and pterygoid), anterior belly digastric, tensor veli palatini, and tensor tympani | Skin over mandible, lower lip and side of head. Mandibular teeth. Temporomandibular joint. Mucosa of mouth. Anterior 2/3 of the tongue | – |
| VI | Abducens | Lateral rectus | – | – |
| VII | Facial | M. facial expression and scalp. Stapedius, stylohyoid, and posterior belly digastric | Skin of external acoustic meatus Taste anterior 2/3. Mucosa of the tongue, floor of the mouth, and palate | Submandibular, sublingual, and lacrimal glands |
| VIII | Vestibular | – | Equilibrium – semicircular ducts, utricle, and saccule | – |
| | Cochlear | – | Hearing | – |
| IX | Glossopharyngeal | Stylopharyngeus | Skin of the external ear Taste posterior 1/3 tongue Parotid, carotid body and sinus, pharynx, and middle ear | Parotid |
| X | Vagus | Pharyngeal constrictor m., intrinsic m. larynx, palatoglossus, m. palate, striated m. in superior 2/3 esophagus | Auricle, external acoustic meatus, and dura mater of the posterior cranial fossa Taste – epiglottis and palate Base of the tongue, pharynx, larynx, trachea, bronchi, heart, esophagus, stomach, and intestine | Smooth m. of the trachea, bronchi, digestive tract, and heart |
| XI | Spinal accessory | Sternocleidomastoid and trapezius Striated m. soft palate, pharynx, and larynx | – | – |
| XII | Hypoglossal | Extrinsic and intrinsic m. tongue (styloglossus, hyoglossus, and geniglossus), thyrohyoid and geniohyoid | Dura of posterior cranial fossa | – |

where cranial nerves pass (Borges 2008; Moonis et al. 2012). On CT this can be seen as alterations in the bony foramina such as widening or destruction. Perineural fat along the nerves and at the foramina is best imaged with a precontrast T1-weighted MRI. Irregularities are suggestive of perineural spread. Tumor spread along the nerves is best appreciated on post-gadolinium T1w images.

# 5 Target Volume Delineation and Treatment Planning

## 5.1 Primary Tumor Site and Cranial Nerves at Risk

The risk of cranial nerve involvement is dependent upon the site of the primary lesion in the head and neck.

**Table 4** Cranial nerves at risk for perineural spread for given primary head and neck sites

| Site | Cranial nerves at risk | Pathways |
|---|---|---|
| Base of tongue | XII | Hypoglossal nerve |
| Cheek | $V_2$, $V_3$, and VII | Zygomaticofacial n. ($V_2$) |
| | | Deep temporal n. ($V_3$) |
| | | Auriculotemporal n. ($V_3$) |
| | | Zygomatic and temporal branches (VII) |
| Ear | $V_3$ and VII | Greater auricular n., auriculotemporal n. |
| Ethmoid sinus | II, III, IV, $V_1$, VI | Nasociliary n. ($V_1$) |
| | | Optic n.(II) |
| | | Nerves of EOM (III, IV, VI) |
| Eyelid | $V_1$ (Upper) | Supraorbital n. ($V_1$) |
| | $V_2$ (Lower) | Infraorbital n. ($V_2$) |
| Forehead | $V_1$ | Supraorbital n. ($V_1$) |
| Frontal sinus | $V_1$ | Supraorbital n. ($V_1$) |
| Lacrimal gland | $V_1$ | Lacrimal n. ($V_1$) |
| Lower lip and chin | $V_3$ and VII | Mental n. ($V_3$) |
| | | Marginal mandibular n. (VII) |
| Mandible | $V_3$ | Inferior alveolar n. ($V_3$) |
| Maxillary sinus | $V_2$ | Superior alveolar n. ($V_2$) |
| Nasal cavity | $V_2$ | Direct extension to PTF |
| Nasopharynx (Chang et al. 2005; Lu et al. 2001) | V and VI (less common II, III, IV, XII) | Direct extension to Meckel's cave, cavernous sinus, and carotid space |
| Nose (Barnett et al. 2013) | $V_1$ (bridge) or $V_2$ (nares) | Supraorbital n. ($V_1$) |
| | | Infraorbital n. ($V_2$) |
| Oral cavity (buccal surface) | $V_3$ and VII | Buccal branches of $V_3$ and VII |
| Oral cavity (floor) | $V_3$ | Lingual n. ($V_3$) |
| Palate | $V_2$ | Greater and lesser palatine n. ($V_2$) |
| Parotid gland | $V_3$, VII, and IX | Auriculotemporal n. ($V_3$) |
| | | Facial nerve branches (VII) |
| | | Lesser petrosal n. (IX) |
| Retromolar trigone | $V_3$, $V_2$, and IX | Lingual nerve and inferior alveolar n. ($V_3$) |
| | | Lesser palatine n. ($V_2$) |
| | | Pharyngeal branches of CN IX |
| Sphenoid sinus | II, III, IV, V, VI (cavernous sinus syndrome) | Direct extension |
| Submandibular and sublingual gland | $V_3$ and XII | Lingual n. ($V_3$) |
| | | Hypoglossal n. (XII) |
| Temple | $V_2$ and VII | Zygomatic n. ($V_2$) |
| | | Temporal branches (VII) |
| Tonsil (palatine) | $V_2$ and IX | Lesser palatine n. ($V_2$) |
| | | Glossopharyngeal n. (IX) |
| Upper lip | $V_2$ and VII | Infraorbital n. ($V_2$) |
| | | Buccal branch of VII |

Adapted from Moonis et al. (2012), Gluck et al. (2009), Ibrahim et al. (2007)

In addition, certain cancer types have an increased predilection for perineural invasion (PNI) and spread. Tropism for PNI is found more commonly in adenoid cystic carcinomas (Gomez et al. 2008), nasopharyngeal carcinoma (Chang et al. 2005), sinonasal carcinoma (undifferentiated) (Gil et al. 2009), squamous cell carcinoma, salivary gland carcinoma, and adenocarcinoma. PNI is fairly uncommon in sarcomas or malignant melanoma. Further reports have suggested that smaller nerves are often more likely invaded by malignant cells (Gil et al. 2009). For cutaneous malignancies, it is important to note that the dermatomal and myotomal distributions of cranial nerves are at risk for perineural invasion and metastatic spread (Gluck et al. 2009). Table 4 identifies primary tumor sites in the head and neck and the associated cranial nerves at risk for perineural spread.

## 5.2   Prescription Doses for Cranial Nerve Target Volumes (Table 5)

**Table 5**  IMRT dose fractionation schemes used at MSKCC for cranial nerve involvement

| Target volumes | Dose/fraction (Gy) | Definition and description |
|---|---|---|
| $GTV_{70}$ | – | Gross perineural spread by imaging (T1-weighted post-contrast MRI) |
| | | Clinical involvement of a cranial nerve on exam |
| $CTV_{70}$ | – | $CTV_{70} = GTV_{70}$ or $GTV_{70} + \geq 5$ mm margin |
| $PTV_{70}$ | 69.96/2.12 | $CTV_{70} + 3$–5 mm, depending upon patient immobilization and positioning |
| $CTV_{60-66}$ | 66.0/2.0 | Extensive perineural invasion noted on surgical pathology |
| | 59.40/1.80 | Nerve sacrificed and excised due to gross involvement of disease |
| | | No gross disease evident on imaging |
| | | Microscopic perineural invasion |
| $CTV_{50-54}$ | 54.12/1.64 | Low risk for perineural spread |
| | 50.0/2.0 | Innervates structures involved with disease that were surgically removed |
| | | No perineural invasion seen on path near CN terminal branches |

PTV = CTV + 3–5 mm depending on comfort level with patient positioning and daily imaging. Treatment volumes typically include the skull base foramina, but not the cranial nerve roots into the brainstem. Margin of target volumes around the foramina can be minimal unless there is evidence of osseous invasion of disease on CT scan in the foramina

## 6   Cases

- Case 1 (Fig. 24): pT2N2b adenoid cystic carcinoma of the left parotid status post a left parotidectomy and left neck dissection. In the OR, cranial nerve VII had gross invasion by carcinoma and the marginal and cervical branches were divided. Surgical pathology was notable for perineural invasion and positive margins. No evidence of PNI along CN VII on imaging.
  - *Cranial nerves at risk: $V_3$, VII, and IX*
  - PTV 66Gy should include the *parotid gland*, *CN VII* to the *stylomastoid foramen,* and the *auriculotemporal nerve*. No gross disease remaining as patient is post-op = no PTV 70 Gy.

- Given connections through the *ATN* and the *lesser petrosal nerve*, both CN $V_3$ and CN IX are at risk for PNS. These are contained within the PTV 54Gy.
  - CTV 54Gy encompasses only the parapharyngeal space and not the innervated targets such as the muscles since there is no clinical or radiographic spread along the nerves.
  - The terminal branches of CN $V_3$ (inferior alveolar nerve and lingual nerve) are not included in any CTV.

- Case 2 (Fig. 25): pT2N0 (stage II) adenoid cystic carcinoma of the right sublingual gland s/p resection, right partial glossectomy including the mylohyoid muscle, lingual nerve, and right submandibular gland en bloc. Surgical pathology was notable for extensive perineural invasion, lymphovascular invasion, close margins, and no metastatic lymph nodes. No MRI evidence of PNI along CN $V_3$ or its terminal branches.
  - *Cranial nerves at risk: $V_2$, $V_3$, chorda tympani (VII), and XII.* CN $V_2$ is at risk due to a close margin to the retromolar trigone.
  - CTV60 includes the post-op bed (inferior slices, not completely shown), but no CN.
  - CTV54 encompasses *Meckel's cave, foramen rotundum, pterygopalatine fossa, foramen ovale,* and *stylomastoid foramen* on the superior slices. This includes CN $V_2$, $V_3$, and VII (*chorda tympani*).
  - At the base of skull, CTV54 includes the *hypoglossal canal* and thus CN XII as well as the *pterygoid plates* (PPF). Further inferiorly it encloses the right *mandible* from the *mandibular* to the *mental foramen*. CN VII is not followed into the substance of the *parotid gland*.
  - There is no specific need to include the muscles of mastication supplied by CN $V_3$, but given the extent of the low dose CTV, the *pterygoid muscles* are partially included.

- Case 3 (Fig. 26): pT2cN0 adenoid cystic carcinoma of the right hard palate s/p bilateral partial maxillectomy. Intraoperative findings were notable for a firm tumor invading the mucosa of the hard palate right of midline and adjacent to the premolar and molar teeth. Surgical pathology revealed extensive perineural and intraneural invasion and invasion of the hard palate. MRI showed no PNI.
  - *Cranial nerves at risk: $V_2$*
  - PTV/CTV66 includes the hard palate and the *greater and lesser palatine, nasopalatine, and posterior-superior alveolar branches* of CN $V_2$ to the level of the PPF. CTV66 extends further on the right inferiorly based on the postoperative volume.
  - PTV/CTV50 includes the *infraorbital* and *zygomaticofacial branches* of CN $V_2$ as these do not directly supply the maxillary teeth and hard palate or pass through the PPF.
  - PTV50 extends superiorly through the *foramen rotundum* and into *Meckel's cave*.

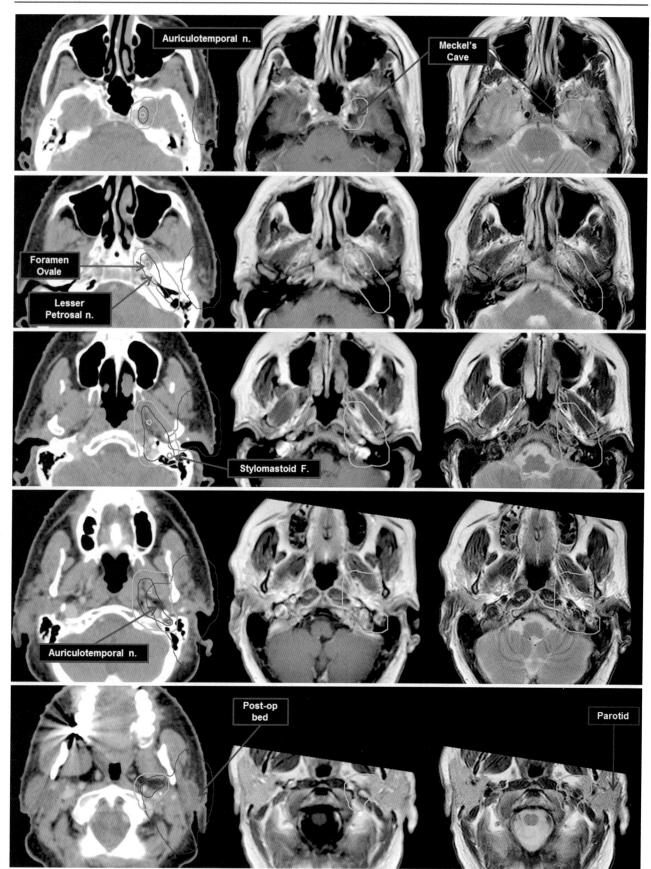

**Fig. 24** *Case 1*: PTV66=*red*. PTV54=*green*. CTV54=*blue*. CN V3=*yellow*. CN VII=*purple*. CN IX=*orange*. MRI sequences are of the brain and obtained prior to surgery. *1st column* contrast-enhanced planning CT scan, *2nd column* T1w post-contrast MRI, *3rd column* T2w fat saturation MRI, *ATN* auriculotemporal nerve, *LPN* lesser petrosal nerve, *SMF* stylomastoid foramen

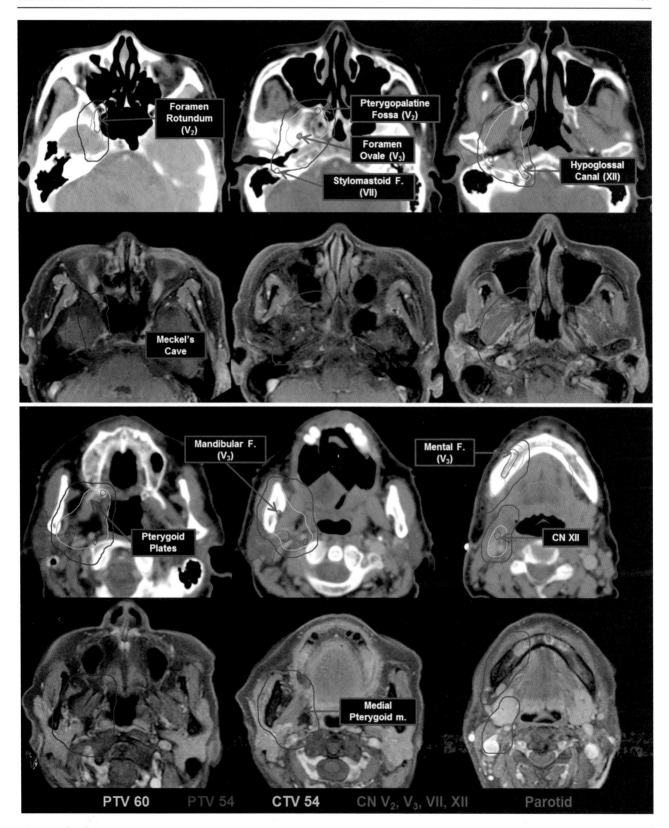

**Fig. 25** *Case 2*: *Top* contrast-enhanced CT, Bottom T1w post-contrast fat saturation MRI oral cavity

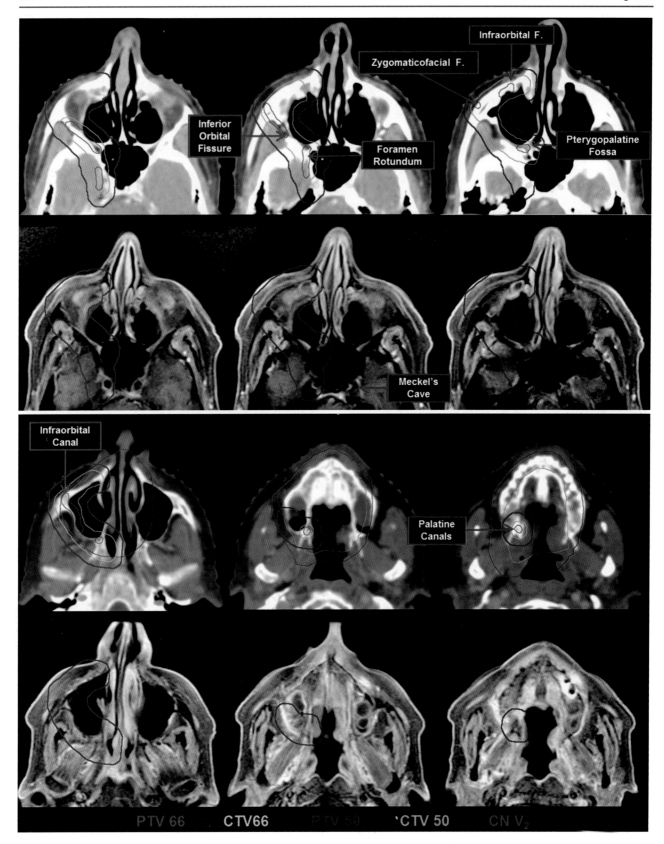

**Fig. 26** *Case 3: Top* contrast-enhanced CT. *Bottom* T1w post-contrast fat saturation MRI oral cavity

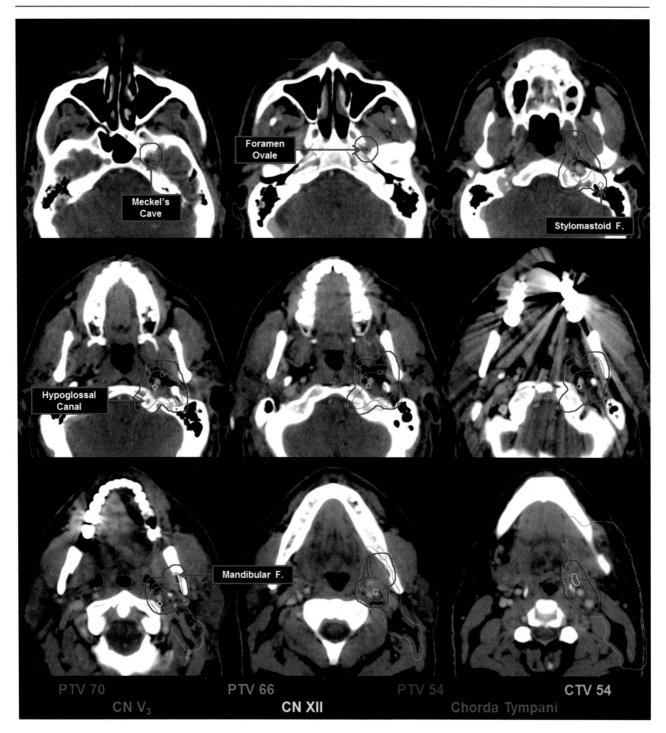

**Fig. 27** *Case 4*: Contrast-enhanced planning CT scan

- Case 4 (Fig. 27): pT2N2b adenoid cystic carcinoma of the left submandibular gland s/p resection. Pathology was notable for scattered soft tissue tumor deposits and perineural invasion.
    - *Cranial nerves at risk*: $V_3$, *XII, and the chorda tympani (VII)*
    - CTV54 begins superiorly at the *foramen ovale*. Slightly inferiorly, it includes the *hypoglossal canal* and the *stylomastoid foramen*.
    - Given tumor deposits, PNI and nodal disease, PTV66 begins just below the level of the hypoglossal canal and encompasses the parapharyngeal space around CN XII and the *chorda tympani*.
    - On inferior slices, PTV66 encompasses much of the level II neck nodes, the *lingual* and *inferior alveolar branches* of $V_3$ and termination of XII at the base of the tongue around the postoperative bed (PTV70) of the submandibular gland where scattered tumor deposits are still present. PTV/CTV54 are shown to illustrate the at risk volume for the cranial nerves. Note that the mandible is included in the treatment volume due to the *inferior alveolar branch* of $V_3$.
- Case 5 (Fig. 28): pT3N0 adenoid cystic carcinoma of the left sublingual gland s/p transoral resection. Pathology demonstrated perineural invasion and a positive surgical margin. MRI revealed perineural tumor spread along CN $V_3$ extending to the inferior aspect of Meckel's cave.
    - *Cranial nerves at risk*: $V_3$, *chorda tympani (VII), and XII*.
    - GTV70 follows the course of $V_3$ from Meckel's cave through the *foramen ovale*, *mandibular foramen*, and finally the *mental foramen*. PTV70 is an expansion of

~1 cm on the GTV. Note that the enhancement indicative of PNI included defines the GTV70 on the superior slices.
- PTV66 includes PTV70 as well as the muscles supplied by $V_3$ (*pterygoid muscles and anterior body of the digastric*) given their high risk of microscopic disease involvement. Inferiorly it includes the base of the tongue and sublingual region on the left side given the primary site.
- PTV54 includes the superior and inferior aspects of CN XII as well as the superior aspect of the *chorda tympani* in the *stylomastoid foramen*.
- Case 6 (Fig. 29): pT2Nx adenoid cystic carcinoma of the upper lip s/p full thickness excision with pathology notable for perineural invasion and a positive margin. MRI of the orbits demonstrated left CN $V_2$ perineural spread involving the left cavernous sinus and extending through the left foramen rotundum and left orbital fissure. Tumor completely surrounds the left orbital nerve.
    - *Cranial nerves at risk*: II, III, IV, $V_2$, and VI
    - GTV70 defines the tumor involving the cavernous sinus, CN II, and proximal portion of $V_2$ in the *foramen rotundum* to the level of the PPF.
    - PTV66 includes Meckel's cave, the PPF, and the *zygomaticofacial, infraorbital, and greater and lesser palatine branches* of $V_2$ on the left. Given the primary site involved, the upper lip on the left, the upper lip, and lower nasal vestibule are included.
    - PTV54 encompasses the minor branches of V2 on the right given concern for spread on the skin surface and retrograde' spread. Given this is a low risk volume; there is no need to cover Meckel's cave.

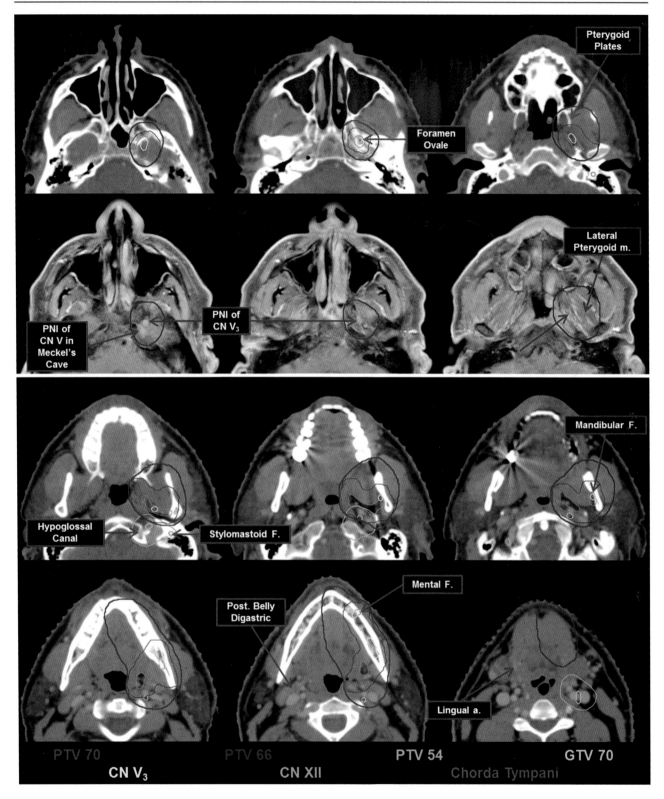

**Fig. 28** *Case 5*: The *2nd row* includes T1w post-contrast MRI oral cavity images

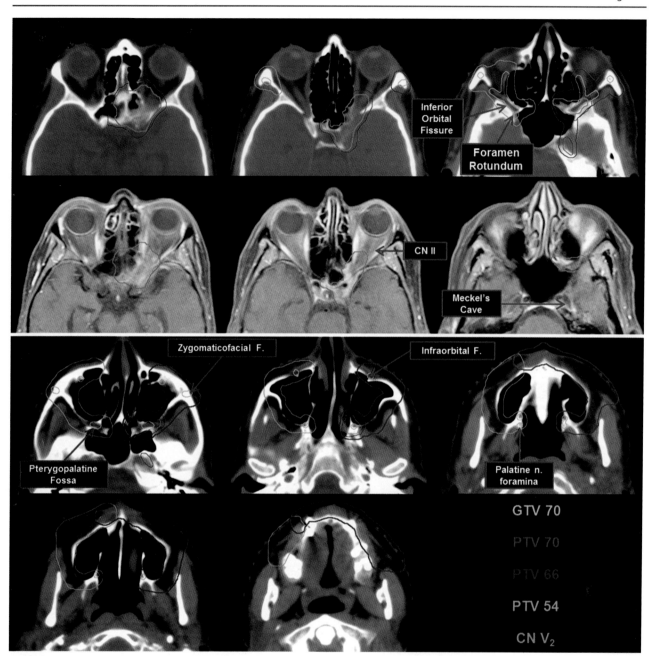

**Fig. 29** *Case 6*: The images in the *2nd row* are T1w post-contrast sequences from an MRI orbit

# References

Alves P (2010) Imaging the hypoglossal nerve. Eur J Radiol 74:368–377

Barnett CM, Foote MC, Panizza B (2013) Cutaneous head and neck malignancies with perineural spread to contralateral cranial nerves: an argument for extending postoperative radiotherapy volume. J Clin Oncol 31:c291 e293

Bathla G, Hegde AN (2013) The trigeminal nerve: an illustrated review of its imaging anatomy and pathology. Clin Radiol 68:203–213

Borges A (2008) Skull base tumours part I: imaging technique, anatomy and anterior skull base tumours. Eur J Radiol 66:338–347

Borges A, Casselman J (2010) Imaging the trigeminal nerve. Eur J Radiol 74:323–340

Chang JT, Lin CY, Chen TM et al (2005) Nasopharyngeal carcinoma with cranial nerve palsy: the importance of MRI for radiotherapy. Int J Radiat Oncol Biol Phys 63:1354–1360

Damodaran O, Rizk E, Rodriguez J et al (2014) Cranial nerve assessment: a concise guide to clinical examination. Clin Anat 27:25–30

Erman AB, Kejner AE, Hogikyan ND et al (2009) Disorders of cranial nerves IX and X. Semin Neurol 29:85–92

Gande A, Kano H, Bowden G et al (2014) Gamma Knife radiosurgery of olfactory groove meningiomas provides a method to preserve subjective olfactory function. J Neurooncol 116:577–583

Gil Z, Carlson DL, Gupta A et al (2009) Patterns and incidence of neural invasion in patients with cancers of the paranasal sinuses. Arch Otolaryngol Head Neck Surg 135:173–179

Gilchrist JM (2009) Seventh cranial neuropathy. Semin Neurol 29:5–13

Gluck I, Ibrahim M, Popovtzer A et al (2009) Skin cancer of the head and neck with perineural invasion: defining the clinical target volumes based on the pattern of failure. Int J Radiat Oncol Biol Phys 74:38–46

Gomez DR, Hoppe BS, Wolden SL et al (2008) Outcomes and prognostic variables in adenoid cystic carcinoma of the head and neck: a recent experience. Int J Radiat Oncol Biol Phys 70:1365–1372

Ibrahim M, Parmar H, Gandhi D et al (2007) Imaging nuances of perineural spread of head and neck malignancies. J Neuroophthalmol 27:129–137

Landau ME, Barner KC (2009) Vestibulocochlear nerve. Semin Neurol 29:66–73

Li C, Li Y, Zhang D et al (2012) 3D-FIESTA MRI at 3 T demonstrating branches of the intraparotid facial nerve, parotid ducts and relation with benign parotid tumours. Clin Radiol 67:1078–1082

Lu TX, Mai WY, Teh BS et al (2001) Important prognostic factors in patients with skull base erosion from nasopharyngeal carcinoma after radiotherapy. Int J Radiat Oncol Biol Phys 51:589–598

Massey EW (2009) Spinal accessory nerve lesions. Semin Neurol 29:82–84

Moonis G, Cunnane MB, Emerick K et al (2012) Patterns of perineural tumor spread in head and neck cancer. Magn Reson Imaging Clin N Am 20:435–446

Moore KL, Dalley AF (1999) Clinically oriented anatomy, 4th edn. Lippincott Williams & Wilkins, Philadelphia

Morani AC, Ramani NS, Wesolowski JR (2011) Skull base, orbits, temporal bone, and cranial nerves: anatomy on MR imaging. Magn Reson Imaging Clin N Am 19:439–456

Mourad WF, Young BM, Young R et al (2013) Clinical validation and applications for CT-based atlas for contouring the lower cranial nerves for head and neck cancer radiation therapy. Oral Oncol 49:956–963

Roldan-Valadez E, Martinez-Anda JJ, Corona-Cedillo R (2014) 3 T MRI and 128-slice dual-source CT cisternography images of the cranial nerves a brief pictorial review for clinicians. Clin Anat 27:31–45

Shoja MM, Oyesiku NM, Griessenauer CJ et al (2014a) Anastomoses between lower cranial and upper cervical nerves: a comprehensive review with potential significance during skull base and neck operations, part I: trigeminal, facial, and vestibulocochlear nerves. Clin Anat 27:118–130

Shoja MM, Oyesiku NM, Shokouhi G et al (2014b) A comprehensive review with potential significance during skull base and neck operations, Part II: glossopharyngeal, vagus, accessory, and hypoglossal nerves and cervical spinal nerves 1–4. Clin Anat 27:131–144

Swartz MH (2002) Textbook of physical diagnosis: history and examination, 4th edn. Saunders, Philadelphia

Veillona F, Ramos-Taboada L, Abu-Eid M et al (2010) Imaging of the facial nerve. Eur J Radiol 74:341–348

# Part II

# Breast

# Early Breast Cancer

Sagar Patel, Brian Napolitano,
and Shannon M. MacDonald

## Contents

S. Patel, MD • B. Napolitano, BS, CMD
S.M. MacDonald, MD (✉)
Harvard Radiation Oncology Program, Department of Radiation
Oncology, Massachusetts General Hospital
e-mail: smacdonald@partners.org

## 1   General Principles of Planning and Target Delineation

Three-dimensional radiation therapy (3D CRT) with appropriate compensation using a field-in-field technique or intensity-modulated radiation therapy (IMRT) to provide homogeneous dose to the breast tissue is the standard modern technique for definitive radiation therapy for early-stage breast cancer. While two-dimensional radiation therapy with planning performed using x-rays has provided excellent outcomes, it does not allow for the use of more advanced compensation for improved homogeneity and does not allow for collection of DVH data or visualization of all structures including the left anterior descending artery (LAD) or chambers of the heart. The highest level of evidence supports whole-breast irradiation followed by a boost to the lumpectomy cavity. At present, this treatment represents the most established optimal radiation course (Fisher et al. 1998, 2002). The use of hypofractionated whole-breast radiation has been studied in the randomized controlled setting and shown to provide similar outcomes for disease control and toxicity (Whelan et al. 2010). This treatment allows for a shorter course of treatment, typically 3–4 weeks, without a change in the treatment volume. Randomized trials included only patients with early-stage invasive breast cancer. While there is less data for patients with preinvasive cancer or those with early-stage cancer that received systemic chemotherapy, retrospective data is available reporting safety, tolerability, and excellent local control for these patients (Ciervide et al. 2012; Hathout et al. 2013). Accelerated partial breast irradiation (APBI), although not yet the standard of care, may be an acceptable alternative for select patients unable to receive several weeks of radiation therapy. Several institutional trials have been published establishing safety and efficacy for early invasive breast cancer. The RTOG/NSABP randomized controlled trial has been completed, but results are not yet available. ASTRO consensus guidelines have been published and may serve as a guide for the use of APBI off protocol (Smith et al. 2009).

## 2 Workup

In addition to thorough history and physical examination, adequate imaging studies and pathological examination should be obtained for diagnosis, staging, and planning. All patients should undergo mammogram at diagnosis. Imaging also often includes ultrasound and magnetic resonance imaging (MRI) of the breast. These imaging studies should be reviewed prior to radiation planning. Image-guided biopsy generally confirms a diagnosis of cancer. Surgery consisting of segmental excision alone for ductal carcinoma in situ (DCIS) and segmental excision and sentinel lymph node biopsy (SLNB) for early invasive disease is standard for breast-conserving therapy. Pathology should be reviewed to ensure adequate margins and confirm an early-stage breast cancer requiring radiation to the breast without inclusion of the regional lymphatics. Surgical clips should be placed at the time of surgery if possible to assist in delineation of the tumor bed and for radiographic localization prior to radiation delivery.

## 3 Anatomy/Imaging

An understanding of breast anatomy and familiarity with breast imaging is critical for the radiation oncologist to facilitate accurate delineation of breast tissue and the regions of the breast at highest risk of recurrence. The female breast is composed of lobules, ducts, fat, and connective tissue, which lies anterior to the pectoralis muscles. A network of ducts connects the lobules together and to the nipple. The lobules and ducts are surrounded by fat, ligaments, and connective tissue. Breast cancer originates from the ducts (ductal carcinoma) or lobules (lobular carcinoma). Mammography is the standard of care for screening. Screening should be performed with two-view mammography including craniocaudal (CC) and mediolateral oblique (MLO) views. The MLO view should include the pectoralis muscle to the level of the nipple. These images should be reviewed prior to radiation planning to determine the highest-risk region of the breast and to assist in contouring the surgical cavity/location of the primary breast tumor. A focal ultrasound of the region showing an abnormality by mammography or a palpable lesion is usually performed and may be useful for treatment planning. Additional alternative imaging that is sometimes acquired includes MRI and tomosynthesis. MRI is used as a screening tool for select high-risk women and sometimes obtained after the diagnosis of a primary breast cancer to better define the known breast cancer and to rule out additional areas of disease in the breast. MRI provides a three-dimensional image in the prone position. MRI can be very helpful in determining the location of primary breast tissue and should be reviewed at the time of radiation planning if available. Digital breast tomosynthesis has recently been introduced into screening mammography. Tomosynthesis images use mammography to provide three-dimensional images through the use of computer software that synthesizes projection images made possible by digital detectors. The resulting images appear as thin slices through the breast. Similar to MRI, these images give a better idea of the location of a breast tumor in 3D images.

## 4 Contours

Target volumes for early-stage breast cancer include the breast tissue and lumpectomy cavity for whole-breast irradiation and lumpectomy cavity, lumpectomy CTV, and lumpectomy PTV for APBI. Organs at risk (OAR) should include the heart, lung, LAD, and left ventricle. Suggested target volumes are described in Table 1.

The breast tissue contour should include all visible glandular tissue as well as tissue encompassed in a wire (if used) or pendulous tissue. For some patients with tissue folds, it may be difficult to determine the lateral or superior edge of the breast tissues. In such cases, bony landmarks may be useful, but one should be careful to ensure all glandular tissue is included in the volume. The lumpectomy cavity should include all visible postsurgical changes and clips (if placed by surgeon). In cases where it is difficult to detect postsurgical changes, mammogram, ultrasound, and MRI should be utilized. Although breast cancers are not well visualized on CT, a preoperative CT may be helpful and should be reviewed if the patient had one completed. The heart should be contoured for all patients with left-sided breast cancer. Most physicians begin the heart OAR just below the pulmonary vessels. The left ventricle and LAD should be contoured if they can be identified (Fig. 1). This may be difficult on a noncontrast CT scan.

## 5 Supine Positioning

For supine positioning, the patient should be positioned on a breast board with arms above the head. We recommend neutral head position, and patient comfort should be ensured. CT images should be obtained to encompass entire breast volume with a generous margin. We recommend scanning from the chin to upper abdomen with a CT slice thickness of

**Table 1** Suggested target volumes for early-stage breast cancer for whole-breast irradiation and APBI

| Target volumes | Definition and description |
|---|---|
| Breast | Clinical reference is required for breast tissue delineation. Breast tissue may be wired or borders may be placed clinically at the time of CT. Contour should include all glandular breast tissue. The cranial border should be below the head of the clavicle at the insertion of the second rib. Caudal border is defined by the loss of breast tissue. Medial border is at the edge of the sternum and should not cross midline. Lateral border is defined by the midaxillary line but is dependent on ptosis of the breast tissue. Anterior border is the skin or a few millimeters from the surface of the skin (for dose reporting) and the posterior border is the pectoralis muscles and muscles of the chest wall. The volume should not include these muscles or the ribs |
| Lumpectomy cavity | Seroma, surgical clips, and notable differences in the glandular breast tissue should be included. Comparison to the contralateral breast may be useful particularly when fluid and/or surgical clips are not present. All imaging studies should be reviewed prior to planning to assist in delineating this volume. This volume should not extend outside of the breast tissue |
| Lumpectomy CTV[a] | Lumpectomy cavity with a 1.0–1.5 cm expansion. This volume should not extend outside of the body or into the pectoralis muscles and/or muscles of the chest wall |
| Lumpectomy PTV[a] | Lumpectomy CTV with a margin based on setup uncertainty and predicted patient motion (generally 0.5–1.0 cm). This volume may extend outside of the patient surface and into the pectoralis muscles and/or muscles of the chest wall. Adjustments to this volume may be necessary for dose reporting purposes |

[a]For APBI only; for whole-breast irradiation, the lumpectomy cavity alone is the target for boost

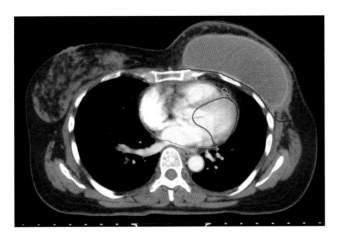

**Fig. 1** Cardiac contours including the left ventricle, left anterior descending artery, and heart

≤3 mm. Some physicians prefer to place a wire around the breast tissue, while others may prefer to place a wire 2 cm under the breast tissue to assist with determination of the lower border. Most landmarks can be determined on CT scan and also seen on digitally reconstructed radiographs (DRR). The seroma can usually be identified on CT, but a wire on the incision *may* be helpful in determining seroma location. Caution should be taken, however, as incisions do not always correlate well with seromas and is often placed some distance away from the site of the breast cancer for cosmetic reasons. All glandular breast tissue and OARs should be contoured (Fig. 2). The physician or dosimetrist then determines tangent fields. These fields should encompass all breast tissue, collimated to be parallel with the chest wall. Gantry angles, collimation, and multileaf collimator (MLC) or cerrobend blocks can be used to best avoid heart

and lung while treating the breast tissue and being careful to give an adequate margin for the seroma. After choosing and approving tangent fields, compensation for homogeneity is addressed. Some centers use wedges for compensation. Another option that may require more work on the part of the dosimetrist, but will provide better compensation and allow for more efficient delivery in the treatment room, is MLC field segment compensation. The concept is to reduce the dose in high-dose regions by adding an additional field or two that block the high-dose regions but do not reduce the dose coverage to the remainder of the breast and the resection site. MLCs are added to the field edges including any already determined blocking (i.e., heart block) and the energy of the beams should remain the same. To do this, each field is copied and named as a subfield. The dose is displayed in BEV windows and the high-dose areas noted and displayed alone (Fig. 3). This beam is then modified using the MLC leaf positions to cover this isodose volume. The number of monitor units for each of these fields is usually very small. Typically 2–4 subfields are necessary to reduce hot spots to less than 8 %. Another option is to use intensity-modulated radiation therapy (IMRT). IMRT uses inverse planning optimizing plans through a software system that takes constraints and desires for treatment plan and runs multiple iterations of treatment plans until the "best" treatment plan is achieved. This process is less labor intensive for dosimetry and results in a very homogeneous plan; however, it is more expensive.

For left-sided breast cancer patients, an increasingly used technique is breath hold. This technique involves the patient taking a deep inspiration and holding for a short time (30 s to 1 min). This allows for displacement of the heart from the chest wall and often allows for better breast/chest wall

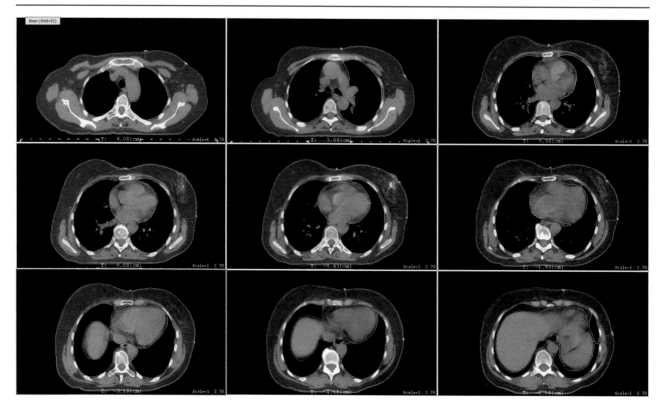

**Fig. 2** Axial images in the supine position for a woman with left-sided stage I breast cancer

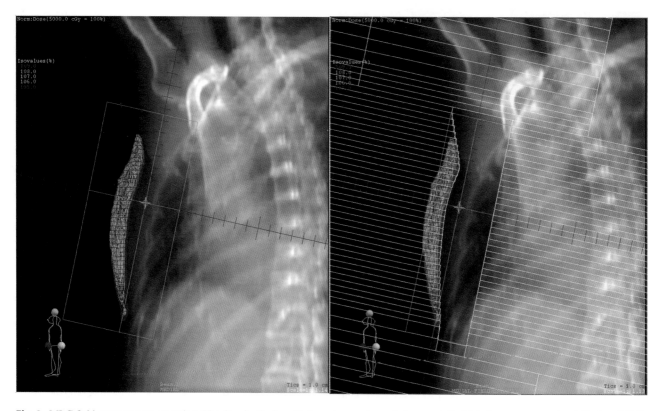

**Fig. 3** MLC field segment compensation. The dose is displayed in beam's eye view windows and the high-dose areas noted and displayed. This beam is then modified using the MLC leaf positions to cover this isodose volume

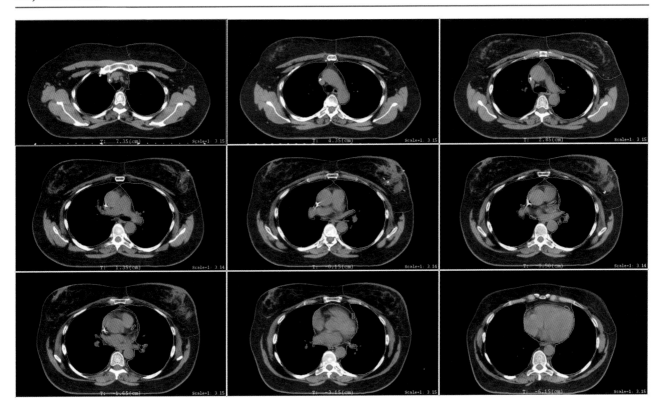

**Fig. 4** Axial images in the supine position demonstrating breath-hold technique. This patient takes a deep inspiration during planning and treatment. This results in displacement of the heart from the chest wall and increases the distance from the breast to the heart

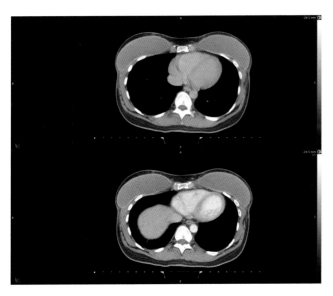

**Fig. 5** This figure demonstrates a case for which breath hold was ineffective. (**a**) Breath-hold scan, (**b**) free breathing scan

coverage with improved cardiac sparing (Fig. 4). The technique is helpful for many, but not ideal for all patients. For some patients, no improvement is seen (Fig. 5). Other patients may find it too stressful to be responsible for maintaining this position. It must be verified that patients are consistently

taking a deep breath as simulated at the time of treatment planning. The use of a feedback system, such as ABC breath hold or respiratory gating may be used to assist in reproducibility. Vision RT has also been studied as a method of verification.

## 6 Prone Positioning

Patients with pendulous breasts and/or tumor bed in close proximity to the chest wall and critical structures (heart/lung) may benefit from prone positioning. Prone breast positioning minimizes inframammary desquamation and reduces the separation for large-breasted women resulting in a more homogeneous dose distribution with lower/less hot spots. Avoidance of the heart is also a benefit seen for many women, but not all.

For prone positioning, patient selection is important. The prone position will not be comfortable for all patients and reproducibility can be more challenging. It is crucial that the patient is relatively comfortable to allow for a position that can be reproduced on a daily basis. Patients with orthopedic injuries to the back or neck may not be ideal candidates for prone positioning. Many breast patients have had breast MRIs in the prone position. It may be useful to inquire about their comfort during this study to assess how well they will tolerate the prone position. In addition, depending on the breast board used, it is possible that the patient will be too

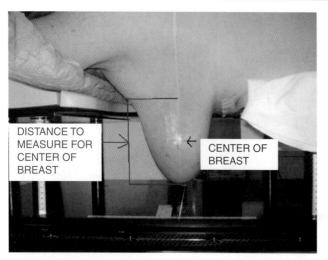

**Fig. 6** Prone breast radiation positioning. It is important that the breast fall into the opening evenly. Radiopaque marker on the center of the breast may be useful for isocenter definition and reproducibility

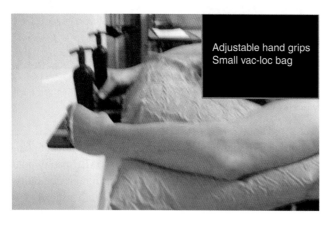

**Fig. 7** Prone breast radiation positioning. The use of small Vac-Lok bag and arm grips may be helpful for reproducibility

large to obtain necessary CT images. The breast board lifts the patient higher than the regular CT table and it may not be possible to capture the patient's entire body, even with a wide-bore CT.

At our institution, we place radiopaque markers on the patient prior to the CT simulation. While the patient is supine, the physician places markers for the superior border of the breast field just lateral to the head of the clavicle, at midline, and 2 cm inferior to the breast tissue. After the patient is positioned prone, midaxillary and breast radiopaque markers are placed (Fig. 6).

To help with reproducibility, a small blue Vac-Lok bag may be placed on the prone breast board where the patient's head and arms would fall when they lay down. The patient is then placed in the prone position on the board with both arms above the head. Patients can hold onto poles to assist

with reproducibility. Once the patient is in a comfortable position, the air is removed out of the Vac-Lok bag (Fig. 7). We recommend having the patient turn her head toward the direction of the affected breast. This helps to minimize over-rotation towards the affected breast and into the opening of the board. A good hand position should help keep both elbows on the board, minimize skin folds in the axilla, and keep arms comfortable. A wedge under the patient's ankles may improve comfort and setup reproducibility.

The breast tissue should fall through the center of the opening evenly. The breast must be completely in the opening so all the breast tissue is below the breast board insert. This will cause some rotation of the body toward the affected breast. Before scanning, attempt to clinically straighten the spine. Scouts may be helpful to ensure the patient is as straight as possible. The isocenter should be placed at the level of the breast radiopaque marker ~3 cm from the medial skin surface. CT images should be obtained at a slice thickness of $\leq 3$ mm. Breast contour will appear different compared with supine contours as the breast tissue falls forward (Fig. 8). Tangent fields with MLC field compensation as described above are used to create a homogeneous plan.

## 7 APBI

APBI can be delivered in the supine or prone position. Reproducibility is very important for these patients to ensure the lumpectomy cavity plus an adequate margin receive full prescription dose. The seroma, surgical clips, and notable differences in the glandular breast tissue should be included for the lumpectomy cavity. Comparison to the contralateral breast may be useful particularly when fluid and/or surgical clips are not present. All imaging studies should be reviewed prior to planning. The CTV for APBI should include the lumpectomy cavity with a 1.0–1.5 cm expansion. This volume should not extend outside of the body or into the pectoralis muscles, ribs, or muscles of the chest wall. PTV will vary based on institutional setup error. Standard PTV margins for ABPI are typically 1.5 cm. The ratio for PTV to breast volume should be <1:3. The PTV should not cross midline into the contralateral breast. OARs include the heart, lung, LAD, and left ventricle. A technique using mini-tangents and an en face electron field is preferred at our institution. The majority of the dose is delivered through photon mini-tangent fields, and approximately 20 % is delivered through the electron field (Figs. 9 and 10). Additional techniques include the delivery of APBI in the prone position with mini-tangents only and the use of multiple noncoplanar photon fields.

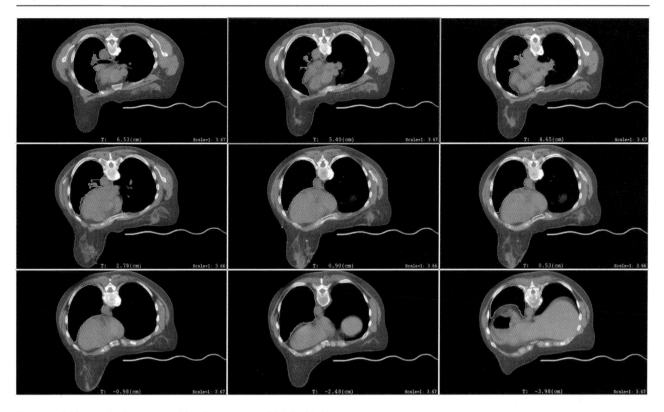

**Fig. 8** Axial images in the prone position for a woman with left-sided breast cancer

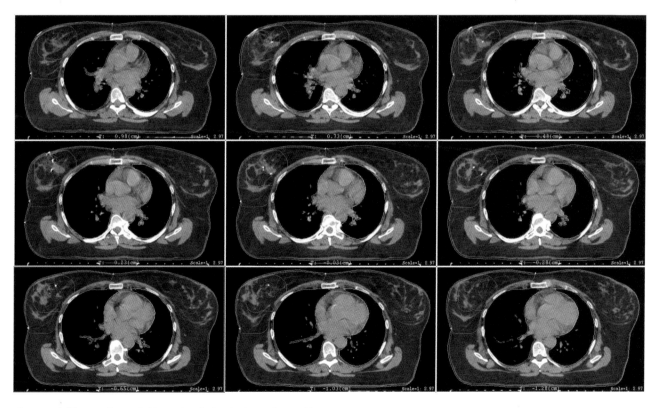

**Fig. 9** Axial images for partial breast irradiation in the supine position

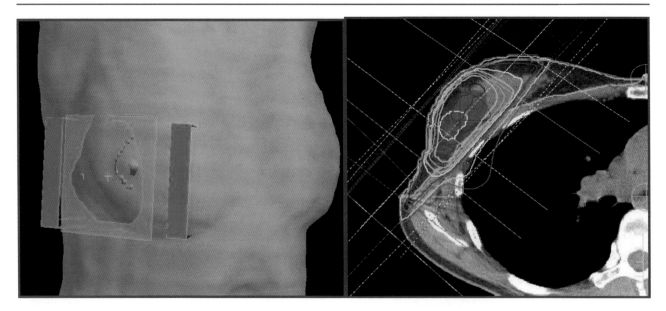

**Fig. 10** Representative beam angles and plan for APBI with mini-tangents and electron field

# References

Ciervide R, Dhage S, Guth A et al (2012) Five year outcome of 145 patients with ductal carcinoma in situ (DCIS) after accelerated breast radiotherapy. Int J Radiat Oncol Biol Phys 83:e159–e164

Fisher B, Dignam J, Wolmark N et al (1998) Lumpectomy and radiation therapy for the treatment of intraductal breast cancer: findings from National Surgical Adjuvant Breast and Bowel Project B-17. J Clin Oncol 16:441–452

Fisher B, Anderson S, Bryant J et al (2002) Twenty-year follow-up of a randomized trial comparing total mastectomy, lumpectomy, and lumpectomy plus irradiation for the treatment of invasive breast cancer. N Engl J Med 347:1233–1241

Hathout L, Hijal T, Theberge V et al (2013) Hypofractionated radiation therapy for breast ductal carcinoma in situ. Int J Radiat Oncol Biol Phys 87:1058–1063

Smith BD, Arthur DW, Buchholz TA et al (2009) Accelerated partial breast irradiation consensus statement from the American Society for Radiation Oncology (ASTRO). J Am Coll Surg 209:269–277

Whelan TJ, Pignol JP, Levine MN et al (2010) Long-term results of hypofractionated radiation therapy for breast cancer. N Engl J Med 362:513–520

# Locally Advanced Breast Cancer

Alice Ho, Ase Ballangrud, Guang Li, Kate Krause,
Chun Siu, and Simon N. Powell

## Contents

A. Ho, MD, MBA (✉) • S.N. Powell, MD, PhD
Department of Radiation Oncology,
Memorial Sloan-Kettering Cancer Center,
New York, NY, USA
e-mail: hoa1234@mskcc.org

A. Ballangrud
Memorial Sloan Kettering, NY, NY

G. Li
Department of Medical Physics,
Memorial Sloan Kettering, NY, NY

K. Krause
Department of Radiation Onoclogy,
Memorial Sloan Kettering, NY, NY

C. Siu
Department of Radiation Onoclogy,
Memorial Sloan Kettering, NY, NY

## 1   General Principles of Target Delineation

- Patients undergo CT simulation in the treatment position with both arms extended above their head using an Alpha Cradle or breast board immobilization; IV contrast is not necessary.
- In cases where the patient has an intact breast, wires are placed around the borders of the breast on the patient's skin prior to scanning.
- Patients are scanned from the cricoid through 5 cm below the clinically marked inferior port edge. The entire lung must be included.
- PTV is defined as any breast tissue or chest wall, ipsilateral level I–III axillary lymph nodes, ipsilateral supraclavicular lymph nodes, ipsilateral interpectoral lymph nodes, and ipsilateral internal mammary lymph nodes.
- A bolus of 3–5 mm is used daily over the chest wall or breast (Table 1).

Table 1   Suggested target volumes at the gross disease region

| Target volumes | Definition and description |
| --- | --- |
| CTV | Breast tissue or chest wall as defined by RTOG Breast Cancer Atlas[1], ipsilateral regional lymph nodes[2], interconnecting lymphatic drainage routes, and chest wall musculature/skin determined to be at risk for microscopic disease |
| PTV | A margin of 3–5 mm medially, 5–10 mm laterally, 3–5 mm posteriorly, and 5–10 mm superiorly, inferiorly, and anteriorly (to include the skin surface) will be added to the CTV. The amount of lung can be trimmed per physician discretion |

N.Y. Lee et al. (eds.), *Target Volume Delineation for Conformal and Intensity-Modulated Radiation Therapy*,
Medical Radiology. Radiation Oncology, DOI: 10.1007/174_2014_990, © Springer International Publishing Switzerland 2014
Published Online: 31 October 2014

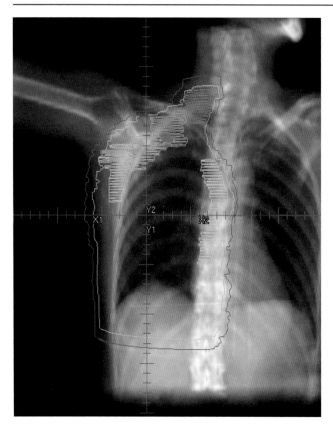

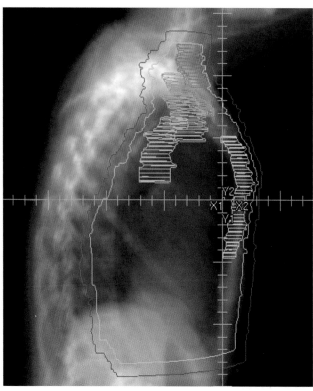

**Fig. 1** Coronal view. *Red* PTV, *light orange* CTV, *blue* level I lymph nodes, *light purple* level II lymph nodes, *dark orange* level III lymph nodes, *green* supraclavicular lymph nodes, *yellow green* internal mammary nodes (IMN)

**Fig. 2** Sagittal view. *Red* PTV, *light orange* CTV, *blue* level I lymph nodes, *light purple* level II lymph nodes, *dark orange* level III lymph nodes, *green* supraclavicular lymph nodes, *yellow green* internal mammary nodes (IMN)

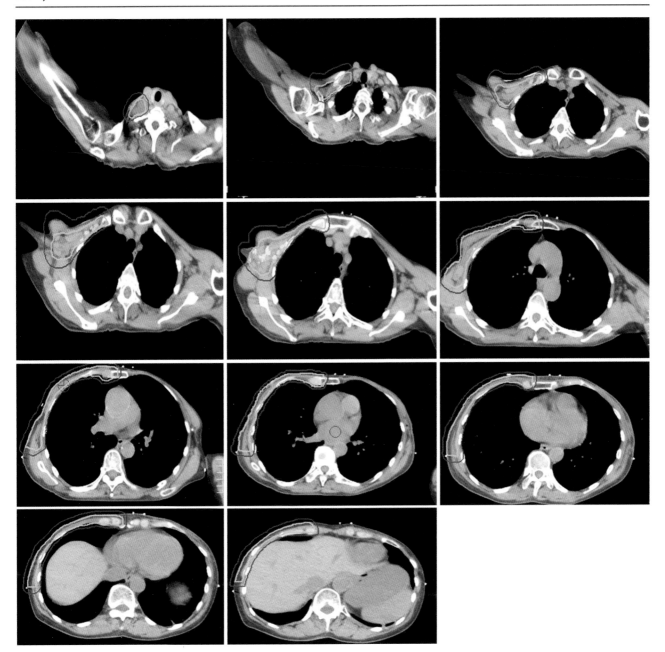

**Fig. 3** Axial slices in the cranial to caudal direction

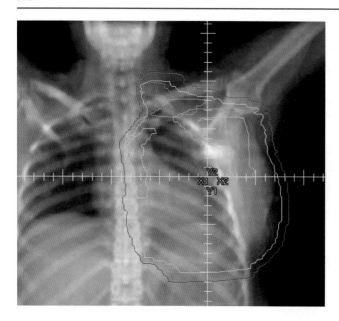

**Fig. 4** Coronal view: *red* PTV, *light orange* CTV, *blue* level I lymph nodes, *light purple* level II lymph nodes, *dark orange* level III lymph nodes, *green* supraclavicular lymph nodes, *yellow green* internal mammary nodes (IMN), *yellow* heart, *dark purple* contralateral breast

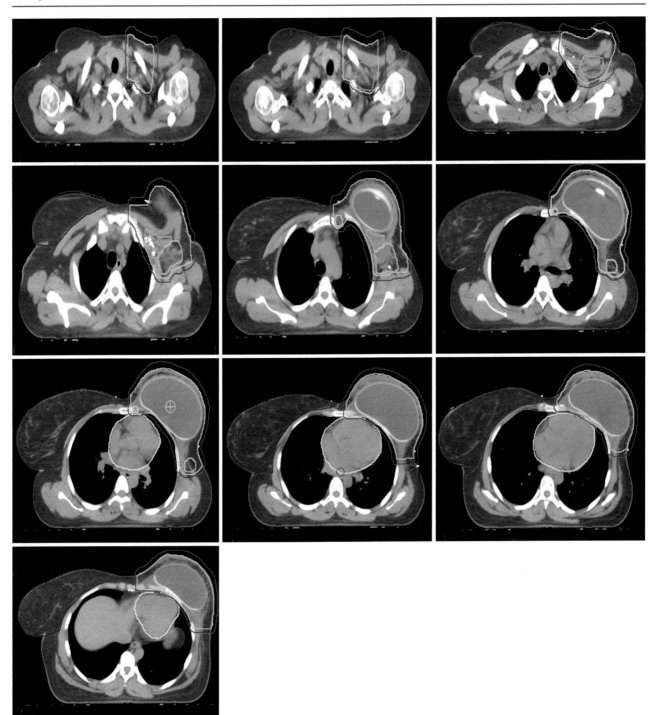

**Fig. 5** Axial slices in the cranial to caudal direction

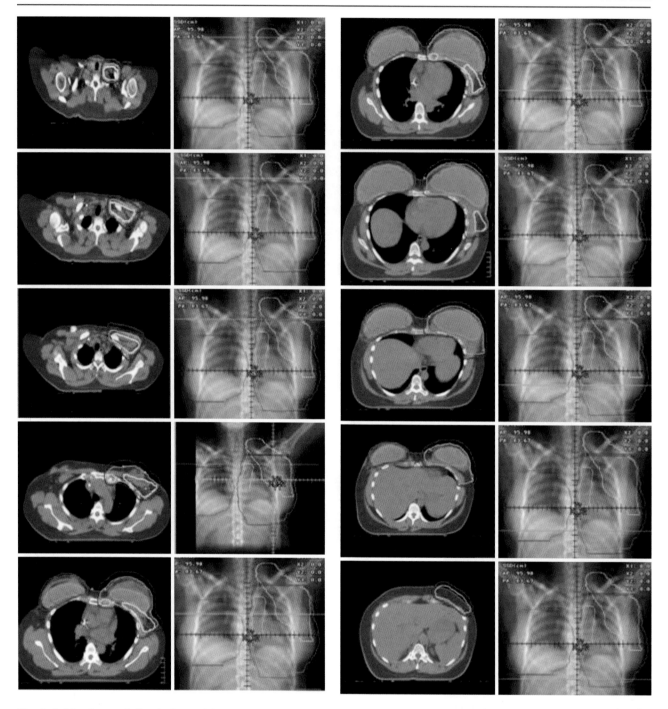

**Fig. 6** Axial and coronal slices in the cranial to caudal direction: *red* PTV; *light orange* CTV; *yellow* level I, II, and III and supraclavicular lymph nodes; *yellow green* internal mammary nodes (IMN); *pink* contralateral implant; *purple* the superior border of daily bolus

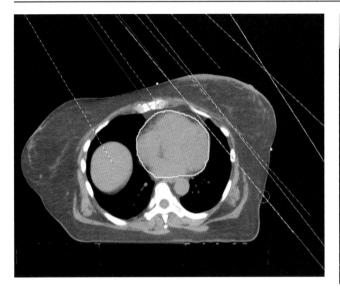

**Fig. 7** Axial view of three beams: a medial en face electron beam (*red*) matched to two lateral opposing tangent fields (*blue* and *green*)

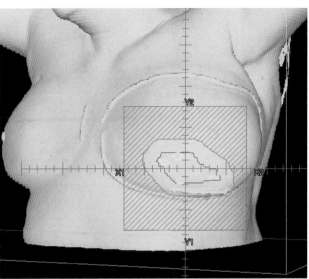

**Fig. 9** 3D view of a boost to the tumor bed: An en face electron field with a custom cutout (*blue*) encompasses the tumor bed (*maroon*), clips (*light green*), and lumpectomy scar (*gray*)

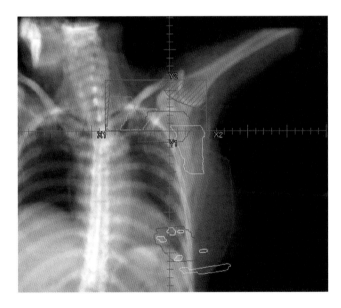

**Fig. 8** Coronal view of supraclavicular field and lymph node targets

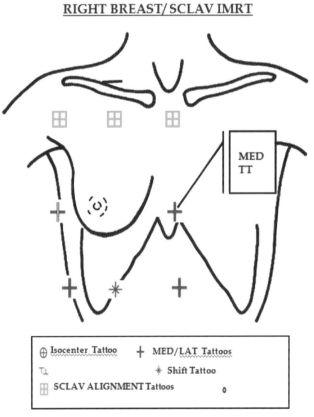

**Fig. 10** *Daily* setup tattoos in a patient receiving multi-beam breast IMRT. A diagram for right breast IMRT patient setup. The medial tattoo (MED TT) is the starting point for isocenter shift

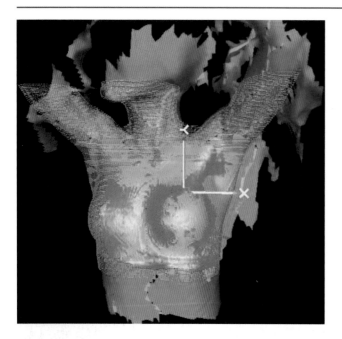

**Fig. 11** *Align* RT for daily setup verification. An example of a breast IMRT patient setup in a patient with left-sided breast cancer, using AlignRT surface images to align with the external contour of simulation CT image as the reference. The solid pink area is the region of interest (ROI) on the CT contour and the green surface is the setup surface image acquired at treatment. The arm, chin, and neck region are aligned well with the ROI surface

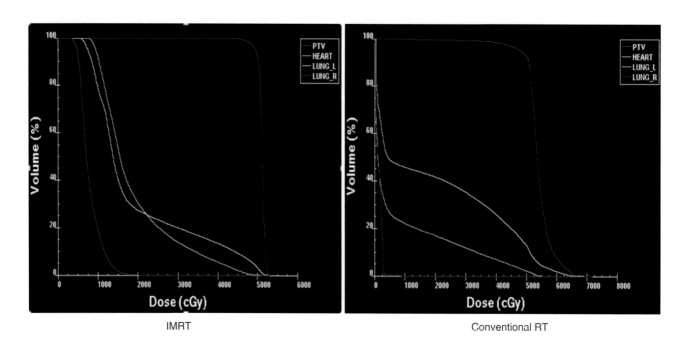

**Fig. 12** Dose-volume histograms of a conventional RT versus an 8-field IMRT treatment plan

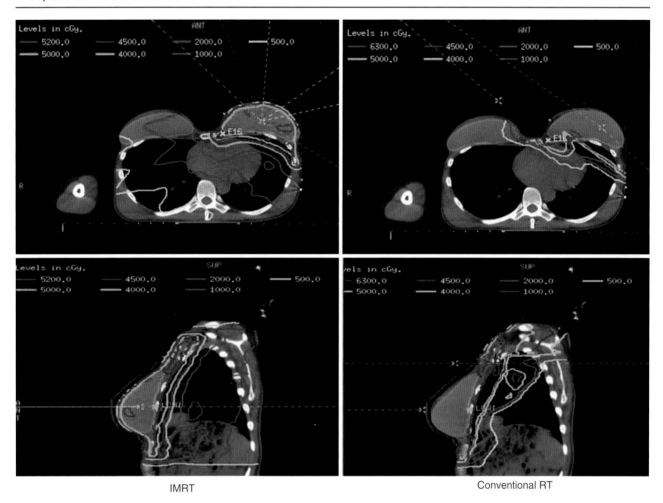

**Fig. 13** Axial and sagittal views of isodose lines in a conventional RT versus an 8-field IMRT treatment plan

## 2 Simulation and Setup Verification

The radiotherapy treatment planning process starts at the time of simulation, where the patient position is set to the anticipated position for treatment planning. The rule of thumb for patient positioning includes (1) easy access by radiation beams without passing through unnecessary normal tissue or causing collision with the gantry, couch, or patient; (2) a comfortable position with an immobilization device that enables the patient to lie still in supine position during treatment; and (3) a reproducible approach with body tattoos, body-couch index, and image guidance to facilitate patient setup at treatments. A three-dimensional (3D) computed tomography (CT) image of a patient at the treatment position will be acquired, which is essential for 3D or intensity-modulated radiotherapy (IMRT) planning (Leibel et al. 2002; Aird and Conway 2002). Additional imaging modalities may be prescribed and acquired to enhance the visualization of a tumor and surrounding normal tissues and to facilitate tumor delineation and localization, including positron emission tomography (PET)/CT, magnetic resonance imaging (MRI), or respiratory-correlated 4DCT images.

At Memorial Sloan Kettering Cancer Center, a simulation for breast IMRT treatment requires that the patient lies in supine position on a breast board (CIVICO Medical Solutions, Kalona, Iowa) or a body mold, with the torso tilted upward with 5°–10° and both arms up. A clinician places wire markers around the breast or implant and on the surgical scar. Patient alignment is checked with scout radiograph images, followed by CT scanning with a field of view from the chin to about 5 cm inferior to the marked breast tissue. It is essential to ensure that the entirety of both lungs is included in the simulation scan, so that a lung DVH (dose-volume histogram) may be subsequently constructed at the treatment planning stage. Patients are scanned in free breathing on a helical CT scanner (BigBore Brilliance, Philips Healthcare, Andover, MA). After the treatment isocenter is localized on the reconstructed CT image, the room laser is used to mark the patient with bi-angulation tattoos at the medial and lateral sides on the supraclavicular line, inferior treatment boarder and midline in between, as shown in Fig. 10. Three tattoos on the supraclavicular match line, two on the midline, and two on inferior boarder. These seven tattoos are used to straighten out the patient body at daily treatment to reproduce the simulation position. An additional tattoo is marked to reflect the lateral shift to the isocenter from the medial tattoo (which is also used to define the superior-inferior (SI) and vertical shifts to the isocenter – the tattoo is indicating the lateral shift only). The source-skin distance (SSD) at the medial tattoo and the isocenter will be checked before and after isocenter shift from the medial tattoo. A simulation document is written and checked by two simulation therapists, including the board tilt, bottom stop position, arm rest indexing, knee support size, as well as the coordinates of the isocenter, which again will be checked by a planner. A detailed setup instruction is also checked by the simulation therapists before releasing to the physics team for IMRT planning.

## 2.1 Simulation for Breast Boost

For patients with an intact breast receiving a boost to the lumpectomy cavity, the same simulation CT image can be used to select electron boost beam angle, aperture, energy, and customized bolus. The boost beam is often en face (Fig. 9). Dose is prescribed to the 90 % isodose line, based on hand calculation. The boost treatment is delivered sequentially following IMRT to the breast and regional lymph nodes. The boost treatment does not require IGRT and is verified with conventional setup.

## 3 Treatment Delivery

After the treatment plan has been generated, approved, and checked, the IMRT treatment plan is ready to be delivered. At MSKCC, an image-guided radiotherapy (IGRT) patient setup is utilized with optical surface imaging (AlignRT, VisionRT Ltd, London, UK) to align on the skin surface. Alternatively, if AlignRT is not available, orthogonal 2D kilovoltage (2DkV) imaging (OBI, Varian Medical Systems, Inc, Palo Alto, CA) is employed to align on the rib bones. The planner prepares AlignRT setup reference images with an appropriate region of interest (ROI) using the external contour from simulation CT image for surface alignment and/or two orthogonal digitally reconstructed radiograph (DRR) images for 2DkV alignment on bony structure.

At MSKCC, an IGRT patient setup is always preceded by conventional setup using the skin tattoos, which provides a reliable estimate of the treatment position (Li et al. 2012). Similar to the free breathing simulation, no respiratory gating or motion management is performed during IGRT setup.

The 8 tattoo marks (3 on the supraclavicular line, 2 on medial and 2 on the lateral side, and one ISO-shift tattoo on the inferior border, Fig. 10) will be used to check axial alignment on the medial three tattoos, body rotation on the lateral two tattoos, as well as the isocenter localization using the setup shifts in reference to the mediastinum tattoo and ISO-shift tattoo. After the isocenter is positioned, the source-to-skin distance (SSD) is checked comparing with the measurement on simulation CT image.

## 3.1 AlignRT

The first option of IGRT method is optical surface imaging using AlignRT. This imaging modality uses video-based stereoscopic image capturing, triangulation algorithm for 3D surface reconstruction, and fast surface registration for alignment with the simulation CT reference surface (Fig. 11). AlignRT provides multiple advantages over x-ray imaging, including non-ionization radiation source, real-time performance, large field of view, and 3D surface for (breast) skin matching. It enables capture of 3D surface images at 1–3 frames per second, provides real-time surface registration, and adjusts the couch position interactively using registration shift as guidance. The registration produces 6° of freedom (DOF), including body rotations for adjustment of the patient manually or using 6D couch. All of these actions occur inside the treatment room without leaving the room and closing the treatment room door. It also permits checking of the arm and chin positions and the reproducibility of their simulation positions. In addition, the alignment of the ipsilateral arm is important to minimize the breast deformation due to different muscle stretching in patients with intact breast tissue (Bert et al. 2006). This will reduce the deformation of breast tissue, improving the surface alignment for setup. This is an important advantage of AlignRT, since axillary and supraclavicular nodes are targeted in patients with locally advanced breast cancer. At MSKCC, we have developed a two-step breast setup procedure, in which the arm and chin alignments are first checked and corrected by moving the arm and chin, and then the breast tissue is aligned with couch shifts to the isocenter. Currently, if any of the three translational shifts is greater than 5 mm from the conventional setup position, then the procedure requires 2DkV imaging to verify setup alignment using bony landmarks.

## 3.2 2D Kilovoltage Imaging

Daily 2DkV can be also prescribed for IGRT setup according to the breast IMRT protocol. A pair of LAO (45°) and RAO (135°) for the left breast and a pair of RL (270°) and PA (180°) for the right breast will be used for 2DkV setup. In bony alignment, the ipsilateral and anterior rib cage will be aligned using DRR images from the simulation CT as the reference. The advantage of x-ray alignment is to use internal bony landmarks (rib bones), which lie adjacent to the breast and are relatively rigid, with only a small range of respiratory motion (usually less than 5 mm). However, the use of 2D radiographic images does not facilitate accurate verification of the arm and chin positions, which are checked at the conventional setup without IGRT verification.

Because AlignRT uses 3D skin surface for alignment and 2DkV uses 2D bony projections for alignment, they often provide slightly different results in terms of couch shift. Historically, x-ray imaging is an established clinical standard, so when there is considerable discrepancy (>5 mm) between conventional setup and AlignRT-guided setup, the 2DkV method serves as a clinical standard. Because 7–9 beam fields are usually employed in an IMRT plan, accurate imaging of the entire breast is critical for optimal plan delivery (Goddu et al. 2009a). Therefore, unlike a tangent plan where only chest wall alignment is critical, the skin alignment is also important to deliver the planned dose distribution to the IMRT patients for proper dose coverage. From our clinical experience with AlignRT setup, it works well for breast cancer patient of average body habitus. Women with obese habituses and/or multiple skin folds may be subject to large deformation with AlignRT – the deformation leads to registration problems in AlignRT. In supine conditions, breast tissue deformation almost always occurs and cannot be corrected effectively and definitively. Using AlignRT, however, the tissue deformation caused by stretching of the chest wall can be minimized by reproducing the ipsi arm position at the treatment – a step that is often omitted from 2DkV setup. In addition, the body rotation is also critical since it alters the relative position of the breast on the ellipsoidal rib case, particularly in a woman with a large breast and small rib cage. Because of tissue deformation, the surface registration accuracy is not as good as in rigid anatomy, such as the head (in head and neck cancer patients) (Schoffel et al. 2007; Li et al. 2011), leading to at least 3–5 mm of setup uncertainty. The dosimetric consequences of setup errors have been reported to be anisotropic, with the most error-sensitive region occurring at the chest wall with sharp dose falloff (Goddu et al. 2009a).

In the current IGRT setup procedure, body rotation cannot be corrected using a regular treatment couch that has only 3 or 4 DOF, unless manual adjustment of patient position is performed or a 6 DOF treatment couch with 3 rotational adjustments is used (yaw, along the vertical axis; roll, along the longitudinal axis; and pitch, along the lateral axis). Body rotation can be seen from both AlignRT and 2DkV images, while AlignRT quantifies the rotation in 6 DOF. Rotation and translation are sometimes tangled, because only partial surface of the subject is used as the ROI for alignment, and the limited surface of interest is subject to deformation. In a breast IMRT patient setup, body rotation is controlled within 3° in any direction; otherwise, therapists will manually adjust the patient to improve alignment.

# 4 Treatment Planning

## 4.1 Conventional 3D Conformal Planning

The standard radiation treatment technique for the chest wall or reconstructed breasts is parallel-opposed tangential fields. The supraclavicular and axillary nodes are typically treated by an anterior oblique photon field matched to the tangential fields (Fig. 8). Inclusion of IMN in the target can be accomplished either by using wider tangential fields or by matching a medial electron field to the medial tangential designed to cover the IMNs (Fig. 6). In attempting to cover the target tissues, these conventional treatment techniques can result in high dose to a significant volume of the lung and heart, whereas the normal tissue outside of the tangential fields is spared. These radiation plans may constitute high-dose inhomogeneity due to the opposing tangential fields and the matching of radiation fields (Klein et al. 1994; van der Laan et al. 2005; Severin et al. 2003; Chui et al. 2005).

## 4.2 IMRT Treatment Planning

To date, several experiences utilizing multiple beam IMRT fields, TomoTherapy, or volumetric modulated arc therapy (VMAT) have been reported (Jagsi et al. 2010; Goddu et al. 2009b; Jin et al. 2013). These planning techniques differ from the conventional techniques by using multiple intensity-modulated fields or arcs in order to improve dose homogeneity and target coverage. These new treatment approaches introduce regions of low-dose radiation to areas that are normally spared when using the conventional techniques, such as the contralateral lung. A comparison of dose-volume histograms (DVH) of a patient treated with conventional radiation techniques (tangents and a medial electron strip) but in whom a hypothetical 8-field IMRT plan was generated is shown in Fig. 12. The axial and sagittal views of the isodose lines of both plans (Fig. 13) demonstrate that there is improved coverage of the chest wall with the IMRT plan. In contrast, the conventional treatment demonstrates a "cold triangle" or lack of coverage of the chest wall, corresponding to where the electron strip matches the tangent beams. As would be expected with a plan utilizing multiple beams, a greater volume of the heart and lung are receiving low dose from the IMRT plan, with the 500 cGy isodose line including the entire ipsilateral hemithorax. The clinical significance of low dose to the normal organs is not well established at this time, and dose constraints for these organs (detailed below) were met with both plans. The DVHs of both plans demonstrate that compared to conventional RT plan, the IMRT plan has lower hot spots for the PTV, a lower V20 to the ipsilateral lung, and lastly, a slightly higher V25 to the heart, although still meeting the dosimetric goal of V25<25 %. The dose to the contralateral lung is higher than would be expected with a conventional RT plan; however, it met the dose constraint of V20<8 %.

IMRT treatment plans are generated using 8–10 fields equally spaced about 30° apart in an arc from close to a posterior entry to and medial anterior oblique field, not entering through the contralateral breast. The superior jaw is closed for posterior oblique fields to avoid entering through the shoulder area and to reduce the effect of possible position inaccuracy. The superior part of the PTV will then be treated with 4–5 anterior oblique fields. All IMRT fields are delivered with 6 MV photons. A 3 mm custom bolus is used to increase the skin dose over the chest wall.

The treatment plans were optimized to generate plans that met the MSKCC dosimetric criteria for breast IMRT, using a prescription dose of 50 Gy in 25 fractions. It is important to note that these parameters are guidelines that are subject to ongoing refinement at MSKCC, as we gain increasing experience with IMRT treatment planning and delivery. Furthermore, consideration of the unique clinical needs of the patient is an essential component of IMRT plan evaluation.

**MSKCC dosimetric planning guidelines for breast IMRT**

| | |
|---|---|
| PTV D05 | ≤110 % |
| Ipsilateral lung V20Gy | ≤30 % |
| Ipsilateral lung Dmean | ≤22 Gy |
| Contralateral lung V20Gy | ≤8 % |
| Heart V25Gy | ≤25 % |
| Heart Dmean | ≤20 Gy |
| Heart Dmax | ≤53 Gy |
| Contralateral breast Dmean | <5 Gy |
| Thyroid Dmean | <20 Gy |
| Esophagus Dmax | <50 Gy |
| Brachial plexus Dmax | <53 Gy |

## Suggested Reading

Dijkema IM, Hofman P, Raaijmakers CP et al (2004) Locoregional conformal radiotherapy of the breast: delineation of the regional lymph node clinical target volumes in treatment position. Radiother Oncol 71:287–295

White J, Tai A, Arthur D et al (2011) Breast cancer atlas for radiation therapy planning: consensus definitions. Radiat Ther Oncol Group. http://www.rtog.org/CoreLab/ContouringAtlases/BreastCancerAtlas.aspx

## References

Aird EG, Conway J (2002) CT simulation for radiotherapy treatment planning. Br J Radiol 75:937–949

Bert C, Metheany KG, Doppke KP, Taghian AG, Powell SN, Chen GT (2006) Clinical experience with a 3D surface patient setup system for alignment of partial-breast irradiation patients. Int J Radiat Oncol Biol Phys 64:1265–1274

Chui CS, Hong L, McCormick B (2005) Intensity-modulated radiotherapy technique for three-field breast treatment. Int J Radiat Oncol Biol Phys 62(4):1217–1223

Goddu SM, Yaddanapudi S, Pechenaya OL, Chaudhari SR, Klein EE, Khullar D, El Naqa I, Mutic S, Wahab S, Santanam L, Zoberi I, Low DA (2009a) Dosimetric consequences of uncorrected setup errors in helical tomotherapy treatments of breast-cancer patients. Radiother Oncol 93:64–70

Goddu SM, Chaudhari S, Mamalui-Hunter M, Pechenaya OL, Pratt D, Mutic S, Zoberi I, Jeswani S, Powell SN, Low DA (2009b) Helical tomotherapy planning for left-sided breast cancer patients with positive lymph nodes: comparison to conventional multiport breast technique. Int J Radiat Oncol Biol Phys 73(4):1243–1251

Jagsi R, Moran J, Marsh R, Masi K, Griffith KA, Pierce LJ (2010) Evaluation of four techniques using intensity-modulated radiation therapy for comprehensive locoregional irradiation of breast cancer. Int J Radiat Oncol Biol Phys 78(5):1594–1603

Jin GH, Chen LX, Deng XW, Liu XW, Huang Y, Huang XB (2013) A comparative dosimetric study for treating left-sided breast cancer for small breast size using five different radiotherapy techniques: conventional tangential field, filed-in-filed, tangential-IMRT, multibeam IMRT and VMAT. Radiat Oncol 8:89

Klein EE, Taylor M, Michaletz-Lorenz M, Zoeller D, Umfleet W (1994) A mono isocentric technique for breast and regional nodal therapy using dual asymmetric jaws. Int J Radiat Oncol Biol Phys 28(3):753–760

Leibel SA, Fuks Z, Zelefsky MJ, Wolden SL, Rosenzweig KE, Alektiar KM, Hunt MA, Yorke ED, Hong LX, Amols HI, Burman CM, Jackson A, Mageras GS, LoSasso T, Happersett L, Spirou SV, Chui CS, Ling CC (2002) Intensity-modulated radiotherapy. Cancer J 8:164–176

Li G, Ballangrud A, Kuo LC, Kang H, Kirov A, Lovelock M, Yamada Y, Mechalakos J, Amols H (2011) Motion monitoring for cranial frameless stereotactic radiosurgery using video-based three-dimensional optical surface imaging. Med Phys 38:3981–3994

Li G, Mageras G, Dong L, Mohan R (2012) Image-guided radiation therapy. In: Khan FM, Gerbi BJ (eds) Treatment planning in radiation oncology. Lippincott Williams & Wilkins, Philadelphia, pp 229–258

Schoffel PJ, Harms W, Sroka-Perez G, Schlegel W, Karger CP (2007) Accuracy of a commercial optical 3D surface imaging system for realignment of patients for radiotherapy of the thorax. Phys Med Biol 52:3949–3963

Severin D, Connors S, Thompson H, Rathee S, Stavrev P, Hanson J (2003) Breast radiotherapy with inclusion of internal mammary nodes: a comparison of techniques with three-dimensional planning. Int J Radiat Oncol Biol Phys 55(3):633–644

van der Laan HP, Dolsma WV, van't Veld AA, Bijl HP, Langendijk JA (2005) Comparison of normal tissue dose with three-dimensional conformal techniques for breast cancer irradiation including the internal mammary nodes. Int J Radiat Oncol Biol Phys 63(5):1522–1530, Epub 2005 Jul 5

# Locally Advanced Non-Small Cell Lung Cancer and Small Cell Lung Cancer

Daniel Gomez, Peter Balter, and Zhongxing Liao

## Contents

D. Gomez (✉) • P. Balter • Z. Liao
Department of Radiation Oncology,
MD Anderson Cancer Center, Houston, TX, USA
e-mail: DGomez@mdanderson.org; zliao@mdanderson.org

## 1 Anatomy and Patterns of Spread

- Carcinomas of the lung originate from the pulmonary parenchyma or the tracheobronchial tree. The latter consists of the trachea, which subdivides into the main bronchi and lobar bronchi bilaterally.
- The lung is surrounded by the pleura (visceral and parietal), with a potential space between the two layers.
- The mediastinum lies in the central region of the thorax and contains the heart, great vessels, thymus, esophagus, and regional lymph node levels. The regional lymph nodes extend superiorly-inferiorly from the supraclavicular region to the diaphragm. Several classification schemes have been devised to describe the lymph node regions, the most widely used of which in North America and Europe is the American Thoracic Society lymph node map with the Mountain-Dresler modification (MD-ATS) (Mountain and Dresler 1997) (Fig. 1).
- The pattern of spread for a primary lung malignancy is typically through the regional lymph nodes (levels N1-N3) and then distantly, with the most common distant sites being the brain, adrenal gland, bone, contralateral lung, liver, and pericardium. However, almost any organ can be potentially involved with disease, and many tumors spread distantly without first demonstrating evidence of regional involvement.
- Both non-small cell lung cancer (NSCLC) and small cell lung cancer (SCLC) utilize the American Joint Committee on Cancer TNM staging system and have a predilection for distant spread. Differences between these two diseases with regard to presentation at diagnosis and patterns of spread include:
  - NSCLC frequently presents with a primary malignancy, while SCLC often is only detectable in the mediastinum at diagnosis.

N.Y. Lee et al. (eds.), *Target Volume Delineation for Conformal and Intensity-Modulated Radiation Therapy*,
Medical Radiology. Radiation Oncology, DOI: 10.1007/174_2014_976, © Springer International Publishing Switzerland 2014
Published Online: 6 November 2014

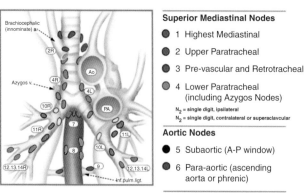

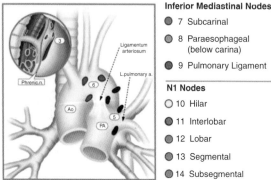

**Superior Mediastinal Nodes**

● 1  Highest Mediastinal

● 2  Upper Paratracheal

● 3  Pre-vascular and Retrotracheal

◉ 4  Lower Paratracheal
     (including Azygos Nodes)

N2 = single digit, ipsilateral
N3 = single digit, contralateral or superaclavcular

**Aortic Nodes**

● 5  Subaortic (A-P window)

● 6  Para-aortic (ascending
     aorta or phrenic)

**Inferior Mediastinal Nodes**

● 7  Subcarinal

● 8  Paraesophageal
     (below carina)

● 9  Pulmonary Ligament

**N1 Nodes**

○ 10  Hilar

◉ 11  Interlobar

◉ 12  Lobar

● 13  Segmental

◉ 14  Subsegmental

**Fig. 1** Mountain-Dresler lymph node staging system (from Mountain and Dresler (1997), with permission)

– SCLC more frequently presents with bulky mediastinal disease. Within the NSCLC subtype, squamous cell carcinoma more commonly presents in this manner.

## 2 Diagnostic Workup Relevant for Target Volume Delineation

- Target volume delineation for NSCLC is dependent on the following studies: computed tomography (CT) scan of the chest with contrast, positron emission tomography (PET)/CT imaging, and, particularly in the case of NSCLC, comprehensive mediastinal evaluation, either with mediastinoscopy or endobronchial ultrasound (EBUS).
- On CT scan with contrast, we consider lymph nodes measuring at least 1 cm in shortest diameter are to be positive radiographically for malignant involvement.
- It has been found that with regard to tumor contouring, PET imaging provides novel information in up to 20 % of patients when compared to CT scan alone, and with upstaging occurring in approximately 15–30 % of patients

(Nawara et al. 2012; Bradley et al. 2004), and that this modality can also be used to distinguish atelectasis from tumor.

- PET/CT scan is used in combination for imaging delineation. PET/CT scan provides a high level of sensitivity, and CT scan with contrast can be used to delineate involved lymph nodes from surrounding vasculature.
- PET/CT scans have been found to have false-positive rates of involved lymph nodes of up to 30 %, depending on the patient population (De Ruysscher et al. 2012; De Ruysscher 2011), and therefore, histologic confirmation for the purposes of target delineation should be obtained when possible, particularly if positivity will substantially affect the dose to normal structures (e.g., contralateral lymph nodes).
- In addition, background avidity in normal thoracic tissues (lung, esophagus, aorta) can vary greatly between structures (Chen et al. 2013), indicating that this background uptake should also be taken into account with treatment planning (Fig. 2).

## 3 Simulation and Daily Localization

- Patients are typically immobilized with their arms over their head to maximize the number of potential beam angles. The upper body cradle extends inferiorly to provide immobilization through the thorax.
- CT simulations are performed with a slice thickness of 2.5–3 mm. Intravenous contrast can be considered when necessary to differentiate tumor involvement from mediastinal structures such as the vasculature.
- Four-dimensional (4D) CT scans are acquired, to account for internal motion. When the magnitude of respiratory motion is ≥1 cm and regular, patients are treated with a "free-breathing" approach, in which they breathe regularly during treatment. If irregular or motion >1 cm, then respiratory management is considered, either deep breath hold (inspiratory or expiratory) or respiratory gating, in which radiation is delivered at specific periods of the breathing cycle. Both techniques have been shown to be beneficial in reducing target volumes for tumors that have substantial motion (Muirhead et al. 2010; Underberg et al. 2005).
- For patients to tolerate the deep breath hold technique, they need to be able to maintain the appropriate position in the respiratory cycle for at least 15 s, which is difficult for a significant percentage of patients with lung cancer.
- The 4D CT scan range typically extends from at least the thoracic inlet to the inferior portion of the diaphragm.

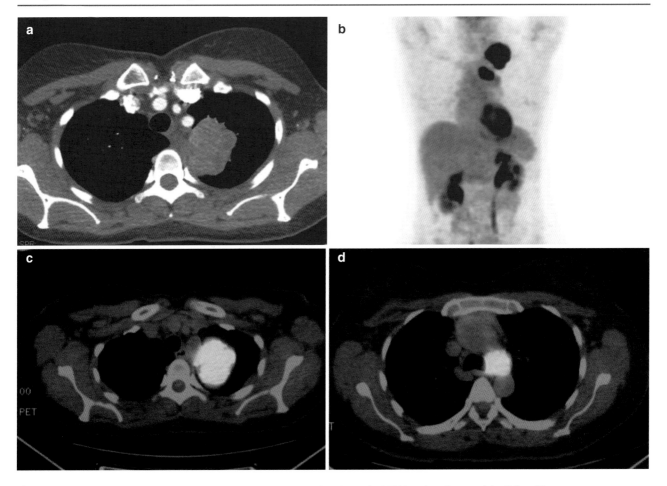

**Fig. 2** PET/CT imaging of a locally advanced NSCLC. (**a**) CT imaging alone, (**b**) PET imaging alone, and (**c, d**) fused images

- Image fusion with PET/CT scans is recommended when feasible, particularly in cases with atelectasis or when directly adjacent to critical structures. Our iCTV-to-PTV margin is 5 mm if daily kV imaging is used and 3 mm for daily CBCT.
- Image registration and fusion applications with MRI and PET scans should be used to help in the delineation of target volumes, especially for regions of interest encompassing the GTV, skull base, brainstem, and optic chiasm. The GTV and CTV and normal tissues should be outlined on all CT slices in which the structures exist.
- At our institution, we routinely utilize daily kV imaging and weekly CT scan alignment for localization (cone-beam CT scan or CT scan on rails). Daily CT scan localization is utilized when more precise localization is necessary (e.g., tumors adjacent to the spinal cord), when the size of the tumor is rapidly changing, or when

bony landmarks are not representative of internal anatomy. Prior studies have shown that with daily kV imaging, interfractional variation is approximately 5 mm (Nelson et al. 2008) and, with CBCT, can be reduced to approximately 3 mm. These are thus the margins that are utilized at our institution (Borst et al. 2007).

## 4 Target Volume Delineation and Treatment Planning

- When conformal techniques are utilized and the treating physician has performed a comprehensive evaluation of disease involvement, an involved field approach is used for target volume delineation in NSCLC, due to the published low likelihood of disease recurrence in elective lymph nodes (Rosenzweig et al. 2001, 2007). An involved field technique plus inclusion of the ipsilateral hilum is also now recommended in the Radiation Therapy Oncology Group's (RTOG's) recent randomized trial examining the effect of dose on survival (RTOG 0538).

- Accounting for respiratory motion is critical in treatment planning. After assessing respiratory motion at the time of simulation, the standard International Commission of Radiological Units and Measurements (ICRU) volumes are as follows:
  - Gross tumor volume (GTV) – gross disease, including primary tumor and lymph nodes.
  - Clinical target volume (CTV) – gross disease + region at risk for microscopic spread. In the setting of NSCLC in which an involved nodal technique is used, this volume often includes the remainder of the involved lymph node *station*. For example, in the case of an involved subcarinal lymph node, the node would be covered in the iGTV and then expanded and the entire subcarinal nodal station also encompassed in the iCTV. This volume is also edited to respect anatomical boundaries (taken off of bones, arteries, etc.). Margins for microscopic disease of 0.5–1.0 cm for either microscopic disease are generally considered acceptable, though studies establishing the extent of microscopic spread beyond that visualized on CT scan have been published in the setting of NSCLC (Giraud et al. 2000) but not SCLC.
  - Internal target volume (ITV) – clinical target volume + respiratory motion.
  - Planning target volume (PTV) – ITV + daily setup variation. At our institution, we utilize daily imaging for all patients being treated with locally advanced disease.
- At our institution, we frequently utilize a slight variation on standard treatment volumes, in which the GTV, rather than the CTV, is expanded to account for respiratory motion. One advantage to this technique from a practical standpoint is that it is often easier to assess motion on simulation imaging when evaluating the discrete tumor volume of the GTV if one exists. That is, when evaluating motion on the CTV, this region may consist of an anatomical space such as a lymph node region, leading to a less precise estimate of the true motion of the target volume. The target contours defined using this method are as follows:
  - GTV – gross disease
  - Internal gross tumor volume (iGTV) – gross disease with motion, as measured on the 4D simulation CT scan
  - Internal clinical target volume (iCTV) – iGTV expanded to encompass microscopic disease and for involved lymph nodes, consideration of the remainder of the involved lymph node *station*
  - PTV – iCTV plus a margin to account for daily setup variation

- These techniques are compared in Fig. 3 and yield an almost identical PTV. The generation of an iGTV can lead to slightly smaller volumes due to expansion of the GTV, rather than the CTV, for microscopic motion. However, this difference is very minor, and at our institution, we have observed similar to improved rates of locoregional control in locally advanced NSCLC using this approach (Liao et al. 2010).
- Target volumes are delineated on the maximal projection image, to ensure adequate coverage. Normal structure contours are defined on the "average" image set.
- For patients who have undergone induction chemotherapy with a reduction in tumor size, our guidelines are as follows:
  - Parenchymal lesions: target post-chemotherapeutic volume with GTV; coverage of pre-chemotherapeutic volume with CTV is at physician's discretion.
  - Involved lymph nodes: post-chemotherapy volume covered with GTV, entire nodal station (superior-inferior extent) covered with CTV.

## 5 Case Examples: Locally Advanced NSCLC and SCLC

- Margins utilized are as follows: GTV to CTV = 8 mm and CTV to PTV = 5 mm. Daily kV imaging is utilized, with weekly CBCT imaging to ensure concordance with bony anatomy.
- CTV shaved off of the vessels, esophagus, and bone. Extension into the chest wall is considered for lesions directly adjacent to this structure.
- While involved nodal techniques are typically utilized, elective coverage of the ipsilateral hilum can be considered when there is involvement of the primary tumor and mediastinal lymph nodes, particularly in central tumors.
- With SCC, GTV-to-CTV margins of 6 mm can be utilized (vs. 8 mm in adenocarcinoma), based on a prior pathologic study showing that this margin can encompass histologic extension from radiographic findings in 95 % of tumors (Giraud et al. 2000).
- Tumors located in the superior portion of the lung typically have reduced motion compared to inferior tumors in closer proximity to the diaphragm. Similarly, larger tumors have been shown to have reduced motion during breathing.
- With apical tumors, the brachial plexus should be contoured and constrained accordingly.
- Lung windows should be utilized for parenchymal lesions and abdominal windows for the mediastinal lymph nodes.

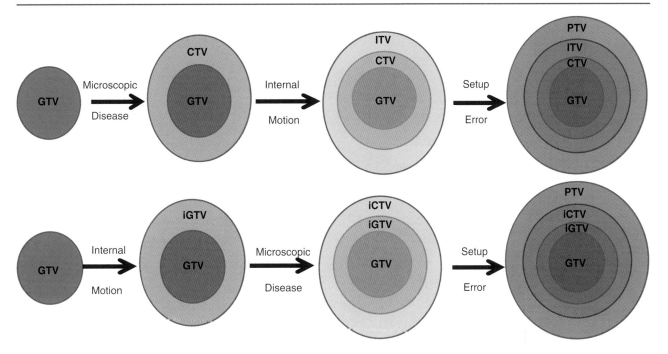

**Fig. 3** Two different methods of target delineation, accounting for respiratory motion. (*Top*) Standard volumes that take into account tumor motion, with ICRU definitions. (*Bottom*) Variation used at MDACC in select patients

- For apical tumors, contouring of the brachial plexus and attention to dose constraints is necessary.
- For high supraclavicular/low cervical tumors, contouring of the larynx may also be indicated.
- For patients with bilateral hilar involvement, the hila can be contoured individually, though sparing central structures in the subcarinal region is difficult in this scenario.
- As SCLC is more likely to present with bulky disease, it may be difficult to avoid the inclusion of the esophagus in the treatment volumes, particularly in the case of large-volume subcarinal lymphadenopathy.
- Involved field techniques, incorporation of tumor motion, and guidelines for delineating target volumes based on available imaging (GTV, CTV, ITV) do not differ between locally advanced NSCLC and SCLC.
- GTV-to-CTV margins of 0.5–1.0 cm are considered acceptable.
- Coverage of the ipsilateral hilum should be considered, as outlined in protocol RTOG 0538.

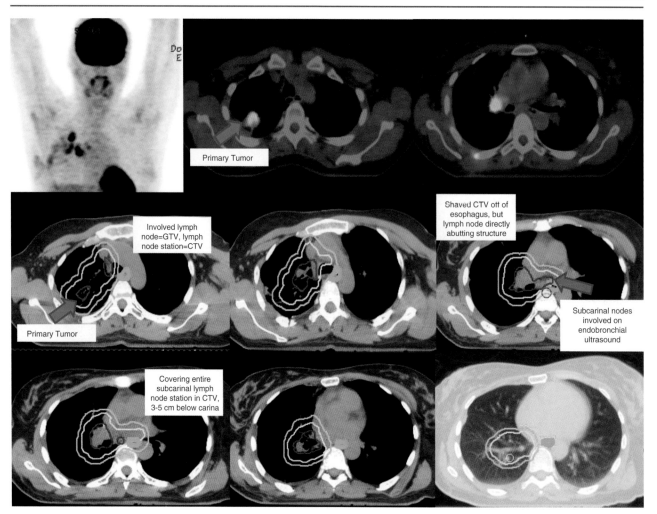

**Fig. 4** A 52-year-old woman with h/o stage T2N2M0 adenocarcinoma of the right upper lobe, with multistation lymph node involvement. The patient received 66 Gy in 33 fractions with radiation therapy and received concurrent chemotherapy (*red*, GTV; *beige*, CTV; *blue*, PTV; *green*, esophagus). Involved lymph node=GTV; lymph node station=CTV. Shaved CTV off of esophagus, but lymph node directly abutting structure

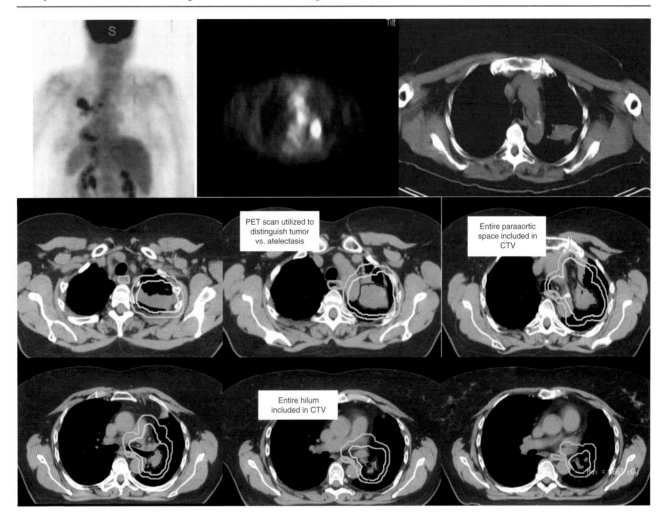

**Fig. 5** A 69-year-old woman with a history of T3N2M0 squamous cell carcinoma of the left upper lobe. The patient received concurrent chemoradiation to a total dose of 70 Gy in 35 fractions with concurrent chemotherapy (*red*, iGTV; *beige*, iCTV; *blue*, PTV)

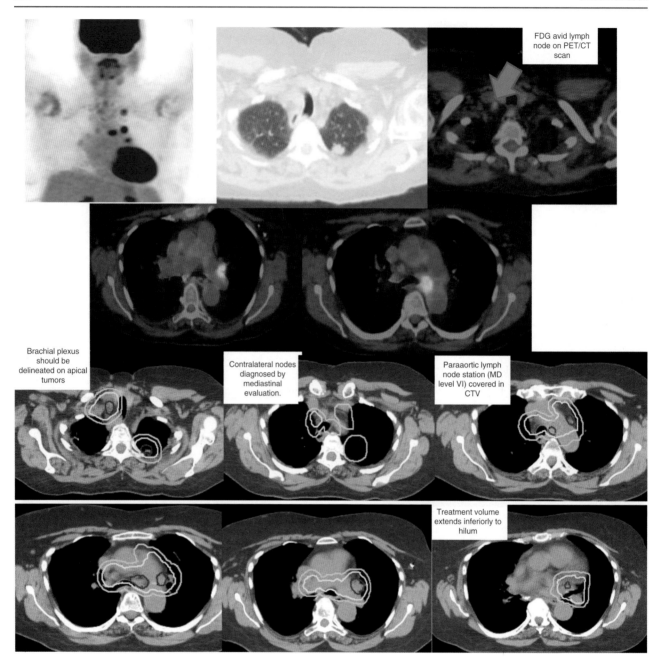

**Fig. 6** A 78-year-old woman with a history of T1N3M0 adenocarcinoma of the left upper lobe, with contralateral lymph nodes diagnosed on mediastinal evaluation, referred for chemoradiation. The patient received a total dose of 60 Gy in 30 fractions with concurrent chemotherapy (*red*, iGTV; *beige*, iCTV; *blue*, PTV)

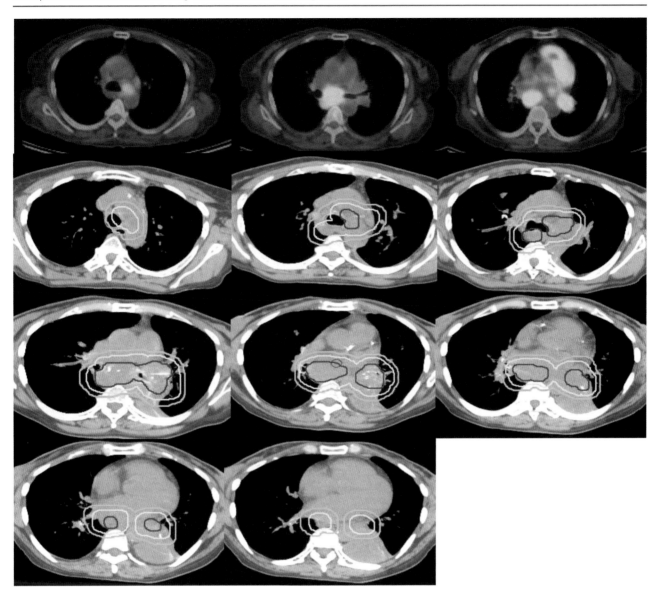

**Fig. 7** A 57-year-old woman with history of 3.5 cm left lower lobe mass in continuity with the hilum, with FDG avid left paratracheal/AP window and subcarinal lymph nodes also involved with malignancy. The patient received a total dose of 66 Gy in 33 fractions with concurrent chemotherapy (*red*, iGTV; *beige*, iCTV; *blue*, PTV)

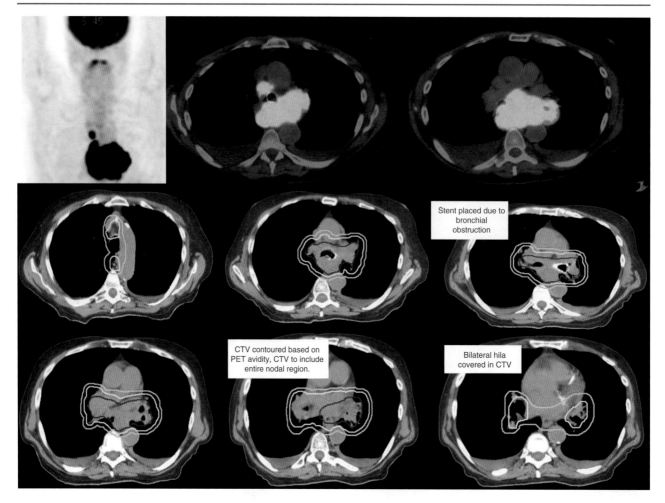

**Fig. 8** A 65-year-old man with a history of limited-stage small cell lung cancer (SCLC) (TXN3M0, with the pleural effusions being negative for malignancy), with bulky mediastinal involvement. The patient had bronchial obstruction and therefore underwent stent placement. He was then referred for definitive chemoradiation (*red*, iGTV; *beige*, iCTV; *blue*, PTV)

## Bibliography/Suggested Reading

Borst GR, Sonke JJ, Betgen A, Remeijer P, van Herk M, Lebesque JV (2007) Kilo-voltage cone-beam computed tomography setup measurements for lung cancer patients; first clinical results and comparison with electronic portal-imaging device. Int J Radiat Oncol Biol Phys 68:555–561

Bradley J, Thorstad WL, Mutic S et al (2004) Impact of FDG-PET on radiation therapy volume delineation in non-small-cell lung cancer. Int J Radiat Oncol Biol Phys 59:78–86

Chen GH, Yao ZF, Fan XW et al (2013) Variation in background intensity affects PET-based gross tumor volume delineation in non-small-cell lung cancer: the need for individualized information. Radiother Oncol 109:71–76

De Ruysscher D (2011) PET-CT in radiotherapy for lung cancer. Methods Mol Biol 727:53–58

De Ruysscher D, Nestle U, Jeraj R, Macmanus M (2012) PET scans in radiotherapy planning of lung cancer. Lung Cancer 75:141–145

Giraud P, Antoine M, Larrouy A et al (2000) Evaluation of microscopic tumor extension in non-small-cell lung cancer for three-dimensional conformal radiotherapy planning. Int J Radiat Oncol Biol Phys 48:1015–1024

Liao ZX, Komaki RR, Thames HD Jr et al (2010) Influence of technologic advances on outcomes in patients with unresectable, locally advanced non-small-cell lung cancer receiving concomitant chemoradiotherapy. Int J Radiat Oncol Biol Phys 76:775–781

Mountain CF, Dresler CM (1997) Regional lymph node classification for lung cancer staging. Chest 111:1718–1723

Muirhead R, Featherstone C, Duffton A, Moore K, McNee S (2010) The potential clinical benefit of respiratory gated radiotherapy (RGRT) in non-small cell lung cancer (NSCLC). Radiother Oncol 95(2):172–177

Nawara C, Rendl G, Wurstbauer K et al (2012) The impact of PET and PET/CT on treatment planning and prognosis of patients with NSCLC treated with radiation therapy. Q J Nucl Med Mol Imaging 56:191–201

Nelson C, Balter P, Morice RC et al (2008) A technique for reducing patient setup uncertainties by aligning and verifying daily positioning of a moving tumor using implanted fiducials. J Appl Clin Med Phys 9:2766

Rosenzweig KE, Sim SE, Mychalczak B, Braban LE, Schindelheim R, Leibel SA (2001) Elective nodal irradiation in the treatment of non-small-cell lung cancer with three-dimensional conformal radiation therapy. Int J Radiat Oncol Biol Phys 50:681–685

Rosenzweig KE, Sura S, Jackson A, Yorke E (2007) Involved-field radiation therapy for inoperable non small-cell lung cancer. J Clin Oncol 25:5557–5561

Underberg RW, Lagerwaard FJ, Slotman BJ, Cuijpers JP, Senan S (2005) Benefit of respiration-gated stereotactic radiotherapy for stage I lung cancer: an analysis of 4DCT datasets. Int J Radiat Oncol Biol Phys 62:554–560

# Stereotactic Ablative Body Radiation (SABR) and Postoperative Radiation in Non-Small Cell Lung Cancer (NSCLC)

Daniel Gomez, Peter Balter, and Zhongxing Liao

## Contents

D. Gomez (✉) • P. Balter • Z. Liao
Division of Radiation Oncology, University of Texas MD
Anderson Cancer Center,
Houston TX 77030
e-mail: dgomez@mdanderson.org

## 1   Anatomy and Patterns of Spread

- Carcinomas of the lung originate from the pulmonary parenchyma or the tracheobronchial tree. The latter consists of the trachea, which subdivides into the main bronchi and lobar bronchi bilaterally.

- The lung is surrounded by the pleura (visceral and parietal), with a potential space between the two layers.

- The mediastinum lies in the central region of the thorax and contains the heart, great vessels, thymus, esophagus, and regional lymph node levels. The regional lymph nodes extend superiorly and inferiorly from the supraclavicular region to the diaphragm. Several classification schemes have been devised to describe the lymph node regions, the most widely used of which in North America and Europe is the American Thoracic Society lymph node map with the Mountain-Dresler modification (MD-ATS) (Mountain and Dresler 1997).

- Several computed tomography (CT)-based atlases of mediastinal lymph nodes have been published, an excellent example of which was published by investigators at the University of Michigan and delineates lymph nodes level 1–11 (Chapet et al. 2005) (Fig. 1 and Table 1).

- The pattern of spread for a primary lung malignancy is typically through the regional lymph nodes (levels N1–N3) and then distantly, with the most common distant sites being the brain, adrenal gland, bone, contralateral lung, liver, and pericardium. However, almost any organ can be potentially involved with disease, and many tumors spread distantly without first demonstrating evidence of regional involvement.

N.Y. Lee et al. (eds.), *Target Volume Delineation for Conformal and Intensity-Modulated Radiation Therapy*,
Medical Radiology. Radiation Oncology, DOI: 10.1007/174_2014_994, © Springer International Publishing Switzerland 2014
Published Online: 1 November 2014

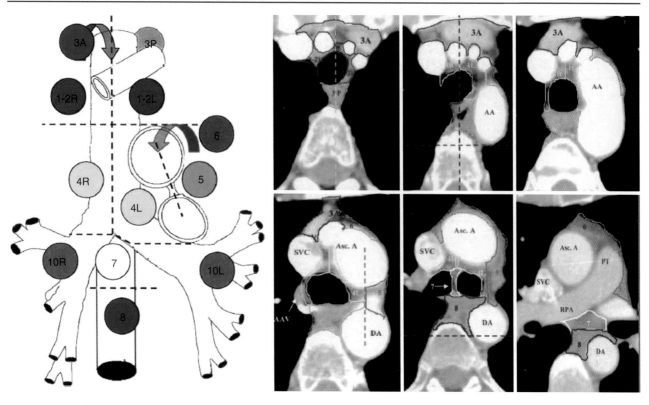

**Fig. 1** Mediastinal lymph node station atlas (taken from Chapet et al., 2005)

**Table 1** Description of mediastinal lymph node levels based on anatomical boundaries (permission pending) (Chapet et al. 2005)

| Station | Description |
|---|---|
| 1R: Highest mediastinal nodes | Nodes lying above horizontal line at upper rim of bracheocephalic (left innominate) vein where it ascends to left, crossing in front of trachea at its midline |
| 2R and 2L: Upper paratracheal nod | Nodes lying above horizontal line drawn tangential to upper margin of aortic arch and below inferior boundary of station 1 nodes |
| 3: Prevascular nodes and retrotracheal nod | Prevascular and retrotracheal nodes may be designed 3A and 3P; midline nodes are considered to be ipsilateral |
| 4R and 4L: Right and left lower paratracheal nodes | Lower paratracheal nodes on right lie to right of midline of trachea between horizontal line drawn tangential to upper margin of aortic arch and line extending across right main bronchus, and contained within mediastinal pleural envelope; lower paratracheal nodes on left lie to left of midline of trachea between horizontal line drawn tangential to upper margin of aortic arch and line extending across left main bronchus at level of upper margin of left upper lobe bronchus, medial to ligamentum arteriosum and contained within mediastinal pleural envelope |
| 5: Subaortic (aortic–pulmonary window) | Subaortic nodes are lateral to ligamentum arteriosum or aorta or left pulmonary artery and proximal to first branch of left pulmonary artery and lie within mediastinum pleural envelope |
| 6: Paraaortic nodes | Nodes lying anterior and lateral to ascending aorta and aortic arch or innominate artery beneath line tangential to upper margin of aortic arch |
| 7: Subcarinal nodes | Nodes lying caudal to carina of trachea but not associated with lower lobe bronchi or arteries within lung |
| 8: Paraeosphageal nodes | Nodes lying adjacent to wall of esophagus and to right or left of midline, excluding subcarinal nodes |
| 10: Hilar nodes | Proximal lobar nodes, distal to mediastinal pleural reflection and nodes adjacent to bronchus intermedius on right; radiographically, hilar shadow may be created by enlargement of both hilar and interlobar nodes |
| 11: Interlobar nodes | Nodes lying between lobar bronchi |

## 2 Diagnostic Workup Relevant for Target Volume Delineation

- *SABR*
  - SABR is primarily utilized for stage T1–T2, node-negative tumors.
  - The goal of the workup for early-stage lesions treated with SABR is thus to rule out locally advanced or metastatic disease. This staging approach therefore includes computed tomography (CT) scan of the chest and positron emission tomography (PET)/CT study. Magnetic resonance imaging (MRI) of the brain is also recommended for patients with T2 disease or higher. Mediastinal evaluation should be considered in all patients, particularly those with stage T2 disease or higher or in centrally located lesions.
- *PORT*
  - Postoperative radiation therapy is indicated in the following circumstances:
    - R1 and R2 resections.
    - N2 or N3 lymph node positivity, diagnosed prior to surgical resection or histologically from the surgical specimen.
    - Prior studies have also supported the use of PORT in the following circumstances: close margins, extracapsular extension, multiple N1 positivity, a high ratio of positive lymph nodes to resected lymph nodes, incomplete mediastinal evaluation, and operative assessment indicating a high risk for residual disease (Urban et al. 2013; Osarogiagbon and Yu 2012; Lopez Guerra et al. 2013).
  - Given these indications for PORT, the following studies should be utilized to aid in target utilization:
    - Preoperative CT scan of the chest with contrast and PET/CT scan.
    - Preoperative mediastinal evaluation.
    - Operative report, to include a) extent of lung resection and mediastinal lymph node dissection, b) description of tumor extent operatively, and c) concern for residual disease and potential placement of clips in those regions.
    - Pathology report, to include a) margin status and location of positive margins (e.g., bronchial stump, parenchymal margins), b) number and stations of lymph nodes sampled, and c) lymph node stations involved with malignancy.
    - Postoperative imaging (PET/CT scan or CT scan of the chest). In the immediate postoperative period (2–3 months), increased uptake on PET/CT scan often represents postoperative changes. However, particularly if there is an operative concern for residual disease, postoperative imaging can assist in identifying regions of concern for consideration of a boost dose.

## 3 Simulation and Daily Localization

- *SABR*
  - *Immobilization* – Various immobilization systems are available for SABR. Early SABR used body frame systems that were designed to allow the patient to be imaged in a different room than the treatment was taking place, analogous to the head frame used in SRS. These include the BodyFix™ and Body Pro-Lock™ systems which also provided abdominal compression devices. With the advent of in-room CT, modified upper body cradles could be used as final volumetric imaging was now being done in the treatment room. SABR immobilization devices typically provide greater support than those utilized in standard fractionation regimens. Figure 2 demonstrates an example of an upper body cradle utilized for SABR (Fig. 2a) vs. that in conventional fractionation (Fig. 2b).
  - *Simulation* – CT simulations are performed with a slice thickness of 2.5–3 mm. Four-dimensional (4D) CT scans are acquired, to account for internal motion. Intravenous contrast can be considered when necessary to differentiate tumor involvement from mediastinal structures such as the vasculature, and this should be done on a traditional fast helical CT immediately after the 4DCT without moving the patient. When the magnitude of respiratory motion is less than 1 cm and regular, patients are typically treated with a "free-breathing" approach, in which they breathe regularly during a treatment designed to cover the entire track of the tumor motion. If irregular or motion >1 cm, then respiratory management is considered, either breath hold at deep inspiration or at expiration or free-breathing respiratory gating in which radiation is delivered at specific periods of the breathing cycle. Any gating technique should include daily imaging that can verify the gating level each day. Both breath-hold and free-breathing gating techniques have been shown to be beneficial in reducing target volumes for tumors that have substantial motion (Muirhead et al. 2010; Underberg et al. 2005). Deep inspiration breath hold has been shown to reduce overall lung dose by expanding the healthy lung away from the tumor, but for patients to this, they need to be able to maintain the appropriate position in the respiratory cycle for at least 15 s, which is difficult for a significant percentage of patients with lung cancer. They also need to be able to reproduce the location of the tumor on successive breath holds as verified by repeated breath-hold CTs;

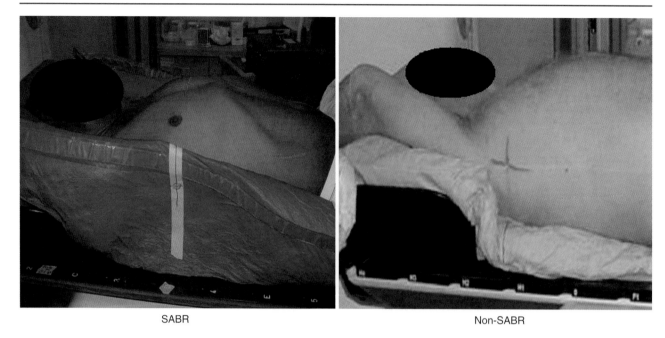

SABR                                                                        Non-SABR

**Fig. 2** Differences between an SABR and non-SABR bag. The SBRT holds an actual impression of the patient and provides more support, is generally longer, and provides an area for fiducial placement. A conventional bag is not adequate for setup or immobilization for SABR

this may be added by video feedback or an occlusion value system such as that found in the ABC device.

– Daily Localization – Daily volumetric imaging is used during treatment (cone-beam CT scan, CT on rails). The daily imaging must be performed in a way consistent with the delivery method, e.g., free-breathing CBCT for free-breathing patients, breath-hold CT for breath-hold patients, or dynamically gated CT for free-breathing gated patients. If volumetric imaging is not available, then fiducial implants can be placed to provide more accurate localization, though this fiducial placement should be correlated with bony anatomy and with each other daily to assess for interfraction migration.

- *PORT*

  – *Immobilization* – Conventional fractionation upper body cradles with arms over the head are utilized (Fig. 2b).

  – *Simulation* – CT simulations are performed with a slice thickness of 2.5–3 mm. 4D CT simulations are again recommended, with measurement of target motion and respiratory management if the target motion is >1 cm. The 4D CT scan range typically extends from at least the thoracic inlet to the inferior portion of the diaphragm. This scan should be inclusive of the involved lymph nodes on imaging and histologically.

  – *Daily Localization* – Daily kV imaging is typically utilized with consideration of weekly volumetric imaging in a subgroup of patients, to confirm that the bony alignment is concordant with the underlying anatomical target.

## 4 Target Volume Delineation and Treatment Planning

- *SABR*

  – *Image Fusion* – Image fusion with PET/CT scans can be useful for SABR treatments, particularly if there is surrounding atelectasis.

  – *Target Volumes* – Gross tumor volume (GTV) with tumor motion taken into account for free-breathing treatments. The motion is taken from the 4DCT for gated treatments, and it is taken from the gated images with a margin for the patient-specific uncertainty in the gating. In this context, the GTV is equivalent to the internal target volume (ITV) (i.e., not enlarged for presumed microscopic extension). The ITV is then expanded to create the planning target volume (PTV). The GTV to PTV expansion is then 0.5 cm. These guidelines are consistent with those described in protocol RTOG 0915.

  – *Radiation Dosing Regimens* – Fractionation regimens from 1 to 10 fractions have been explored, and dose constraints for organs at risk vary based on the number of fractions utilized (www.nccn.org).

    - For peripheral lesions, outside of the "no-fly zone," 1–4 fraction regimens are commonly used. Commonly used regimens include 20 Gy × 3 fractions and 12.5 Gy × 4 fractions. For central lesions, regimens of 4–10 fractions have been explored. RTOG 0813 assessed the safety and efficacy of a dose-escalation regimen in a seamless phase I/II design, beginning at 10 Gy × 5 fractions and increasing to 12 Gy × 5 fractions. The study is closed and the results are pending.

– *Dose-Volume Constraints* – Dose-volume constraints are based on the number of fractions utilized. Please see the National Comprehensive Cancer Network guidelines for specific constraints at various fraction regimens (www.nccn.org). In addition, a chest wall dose of V30-V35<50 cc is utilized with <5 fraction regimens at our institution based on multiple studies showing that this constraint is correlated with chest wall pain (Welsh et al. 2011; Mutter et al. 2012). Diabetes mellitus and obesity may also be risk factors for this toxicity.

• **PORT**

– *Image Fusion* – If a PET/CT scan is obtained postoperatively, then residual inflammatory effects can be present with increased avidity, and inclusion of these regions should be discussed with the operating surgeon and in the context of the histologic and preoperative imaging findings.

– *Target Volumes*

• *Positive margins or gross disease (R1 and R2 resections)* – The region of positive margins or gross disease, as discussed with the operating surgeon. Clips may also be placed in the appropriate region. In the case of potential gross disease, postoperative imaging can assist in elucidating this region.

– If gross disease is present, we recommend GTV to CTV margins of 6–8 mm.

• *Negative margins with N2–N3 positivity (R0 resection)* – Historically, the CTV volume has included the bilateral mediastinum and ipsilateral hilum/bronchial stump in the setting of N2 disease, regardless of the site of disease. With the advent of more sensitive imaging techniques and radiation modalities that increase conformality, there is a trend towards smaller volumes. This target has included either *involved nodal regions plus the bronchial stump* or *high-risk draining lymph node regions plus the bronchial stump*. For the latter, one common approach is the "one-up, one-down" contouring technique (e.g., one lymph node station below, one above on the ipsilateral side). The ongoing LungArt trial, which examines the role of PORT in N2 disease, utilizes this general technique, with the recommendations varying by the laterality of the primary tumor due to differences in nodal drainage (Spoelstra et al. 2010) (Table 2).

• In summary, there is heterogeneity among physicians in PORT volumes, and possible approaches include:

– Whole mediastinum – Bilateral mediastinum and ipsilateral bronchial stump; exclude

**Table 2** Delineation of target volumes for PORT in the LungART study (permission pending)

| Surgically involved mediastinal nodes | LN stations to be included in the CTV |
| --- | --- |
| 1–2R | 1–2R, 4R, 7, 10R. Maximal upper limit: 1 cm above sternal notch but homolateral subclavicular node station may be treated if needed. Maximal lower limit: 4 cm below the carina[a] |
| 1–2L | 1-2L, 4L, 7, 10L. Maximal upper limit: 1 cm above the sternal notch but homolateral subclavicular node station may be treated if needed. Maximal lower limit: 4 cm below the carina[a] |
| 3 (Right-sided tumor) | 3, 4L, 7, 10R. Maximal upper limit: 1 cm above the sternal notch. Maximal lower limit: 4 cm below the carina[a] |
| 3 (Left-sided tumor) | 3, 4L, 7, 10L. Maximal upper limit: 1 cm above the sternal notch. Maximal lower limit: 4 cm below the carina[a] |
| 4R | 2R, 4R, 7, 10R. Maximal upper limit: sternal notch. Maximal lower limit: 4 cm below the carina[a] |
| 4L | 2L, 4L, 7, 10L. Maximal upper limit: sternal notch. Maximal lower limit: 4 cm below the carina[a] |
| 5 | 2L, 4L, 5, 6, 7. Maximal upper limit: top of aortic arch. Maximal lower limit: 4 cm below the carina[a] |
| 6 | 2L, 4L, 5, 6, 7. Maximal upper limit: sternal notch. Maximal lower limit: 4 cm below the carina[a] |
| 7 (Right-sided tumor) | 4R. Maximal upper limit: top of aortic arch. Maximal lower limit: 5 cm below the carina[a] |
| 7 (Left-sided tumor) | 4L, 5, 6, 7. Maximal upper limit: top of aortic arch. Maximal lower limit: 5 cm below the carina[a] |
| 8 (Right-sided tumor) | 4R, 7, 8. Maximal upper limit: top of aortic arch. The lower limit should be the gastroesophageal junction |
| 8 (Left-sided tumor) | 4L, 5, 6, 7, 8. Maximal upper limit: top of aortic arch. The lower limit should be the gastroesophageal junction |

*Abbreviations*: *LN* lymph node, *CTV* clinical target volume
[a]Unless other nodes are involved

contralateral hilum and supraclavicular lymph nodes unless involved.

– High-risk nodal volumes – The "one-up, one-down" technique on the ipsilateral side plus the bronchial stump, or per the guidelines of the LungART study. Contralateral lymph nodes are only covered if involved prior to or at the time of surgery or suspicious on postoperative imaging.

– Involved nodal regions plus the bronchial stump – Only those nodal stations involved with disease on imaging or histologically.

**Table 3** Differences in treatment between PORT and SABR

| Characteristic | SABR | PORT |
|---|---|---|
| Diagnostic workup for target delineation | 1. CT scan chest with contrast<br>2. PET/CT scan<br>3. Mediastinal evaluation to confirm N0 disease | 1. Preoperative CT scan chest with contrast<br>2. Preoperative PET/CT scan<br>3. Preoperative mediastinal evaluation<br>4. Operative report<br>5. Operative pathology report |
| Simulation immobilization | Stereotactic body frame or cradle with high level of immobilization (higher level than with PORT or conventionally fractionated RT due to larger fraction size) | Upper body cradle with immobilization |
| Simulation motion assessment | 4D CT simulation (recommended) *or* abdominal compression | 4D CT simulation |
| Target definition | GTV with motion = CTV<br>GTV/CTV + 5 mm = PTV | GTV – if gross residual disease present<br>CTV – (1) whole mediastinum, (2) high-risk nodal fields (e.g., LungART), (3) involved nodal regions, all with bronchial stump<br>PTV – CTV + 5 mm |
| Radiation dosing regimen | Peripherally located lesions – 1–4 fraction regimens (examples are 20 Gy × 3 fractions, 12.5 Gy × 4 fractions)<br>Centrally located lesions (within the "no-fly" zone) – 5–10 fraction regimens (examples are 10 Gy × 5 fractions, 7 Gy × 10 fractions) | Microscopic disease only – 1.8–2.0 Gy fractions to 50–54 Gy<br>Positive microscopic margins – 1.8–2.0 Gy fractions to 54–60 Gy<br>Gross residual disease – 1.8–2.0 Gy to 60–70 Gy |
| Concurrent chemotherapy | No | Can be considered for positive margins or gross residual disease |
| Daily localization | Daily volumetric imaging (e.g., cone-beam CT scan, CT scan on rails) | Daily kV imaging, consider weekly volumetric imaging for unique cases |

Again, contralateral lymph nodes are only covered if involved prior to or at the time of surgery or suspicious on postoperative imaging.

- It is important to note that no prospective trials have compared these treatment volumes with regard to toxicity and efficacy. Thus, all techniques could be considered acceptable, though many institutions are shifting away from whole mediastinal fields and towards more conformal volumes. There is general agreement that the bronchial stump should be included regardless of treatment volume.
- We recommend CTV to PTV margins of 5 mm with daily kV imaging, though the margin can be reduced to 3 mm if volumetric imaging is used, for unique cases such as tumor volumes encroaching on a critical structure, or bulky disease that may change with treatment.
- Variations in treatment volumes for less-established indications for PORT, such as extracapsular extension, lymphovascular invasion, and

high ratio of lymph node involvement, have not been established.
- Radiation Dosing Regimens – Standard doses after complete resection are 50–54 Gy in 1.8–2.0 Gy fractions. Higher doses can be considered for positive margins (60 Gy) and gross residual disease (60–70 Gy). Concurrent chemotherapy can also be considered for gross disease or positive margins at the treating physician's discretion.
- *Dose-Volume Constraints* – Standard fractionation dose constraints are used. Some normal tissue constraints at our institution are mean lung dose < 20 Gy, V20 > 35 %, mean esophagus dose < 34 Gy, and maximum spinal cord dose < 45 Gy.
- Key characteristics of radiation technique for PORT vs. SABR are outlined in Table 3.

## 5 Case Examples – SABR (Figs. 3–4)

- The GTV adjusted for motion is expanded by 5 mm for the PTV, with no shaving off of critical structures.

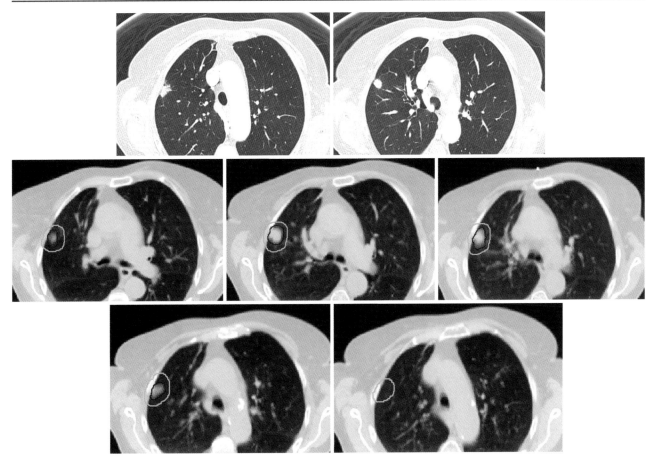

**Fig. 3** Involved lymph node = GTV, lymph node station = CTV shaved CTV off of esophagus, but lymph node directly abutting structure of a 68-year-old man with a history of stage T1N0M0 medically inoperable

SCC of the *right upper lobe*, being treated with SABR to a dose of 50 Gy in 4 fractions (*red* = GTV with motion, *blue* = PTV)

- The lesion is close to the chest wall, such that there will inevitably be dose to this structure. A chest wall constraint of V30-35 < 35 cc for < 5 fraction regimens is a threshold that can be used to minimize the risk of chest wall discomfort.
- Dose constraints for 4-fraction regimens utilized at our institution are as follows: MLD $\leq 6$ Gy, lung V20 $\leq 12$ %, bronchial tree maximum dose $\leq 38$ Gy, bronchial tree V35 $\leq 1$ cm$^3$, major vessels maximum dose $\leq 56$ Gy, maximum esophagus dose $\leq 35$ Gy, esophagus V30 $\leq 1$ cm$^3$, and maximum brachial plexus dose $\leq 35$ Gy.
- To distinguish tumor spiculations from bronchioles, it is necessary to follow the bronchial tree to attempt to follow them distally.
- There remains variation in treatment practice on the most appropriate method to cover tumor spiculations. At our institution, spiculations are covered in their entirety with the GTV in the majority of cases.

## 6    Case Examples - PORT (Figs. 5–6)

- The high risk nodal region in this case covers the following lymph node stations: 2L, 4L, 5, 6, and 7, with the superior-inferior extension being from the sternal notch to 4 cm below the carina (as described in Table 2).
- Clips are placed at the bronchial stump and should be included in the treatment volume.
- The pretracheal nodes can be covered in both fields, but in the high-risk nodal field, the volume can extend to midline superior to the carina.

## Suggested Reading

National Comprehensive Cancer Network Guidelines – www.nccn.org

RTOG 0813 – www.rtog.org

RTOG 0915 – www.rtog.org

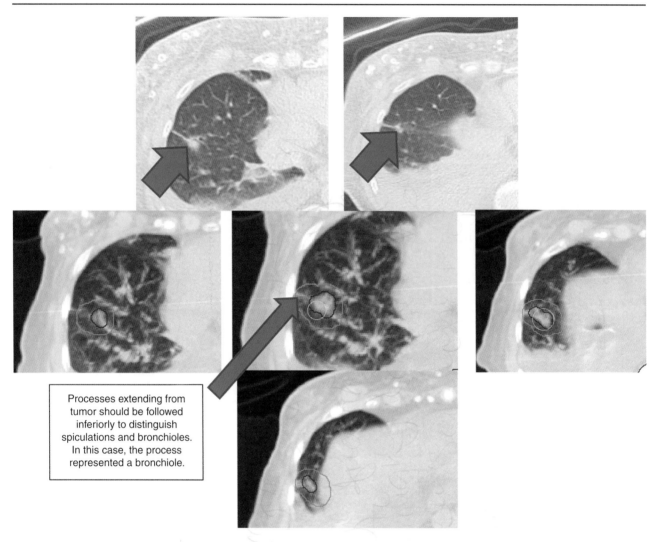

Processes extending from tumor should be followed inferiorly to distinguish spiculations and bronchioles. In this case, the process represented a bronchiole.

**Fig. 4** A 72-year-old man with a history of stage T1N0M0 medically inoperable adenocarcinoma of the *right upper lobe*, receiving SABR to 50 Gy in 4 fractions (*red*=GTV with motion, *orange*=PTV)

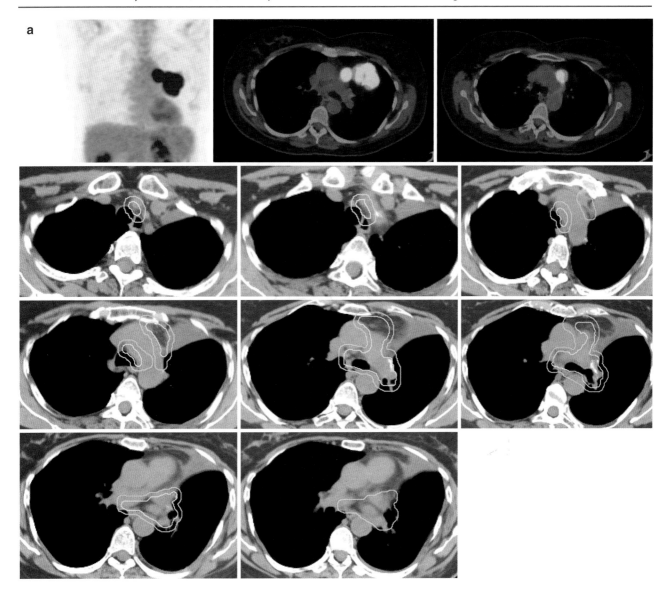

**Fig. 5** (**a**, **b**) A 56-year-old man with a history of stage T3N2M0 adenocarcinoma of the *left upper lobe*, who underwent induction chemotherapy and lobectomy with mediastinal nodal dissection. Pathology demonstrated 2/3 para-aortic lymph nodes involved with disease, with 0/13 other lymph nodes involved. All margins were negative for disease. Figure (**a**) represents a "high-risk nodal level" volume, as specified per LungArt, and (**b**) represents a whole mediastinal volume (bilateral mediastinum and bronchial stump) (*beige* = CTV, *blue* = PTV)

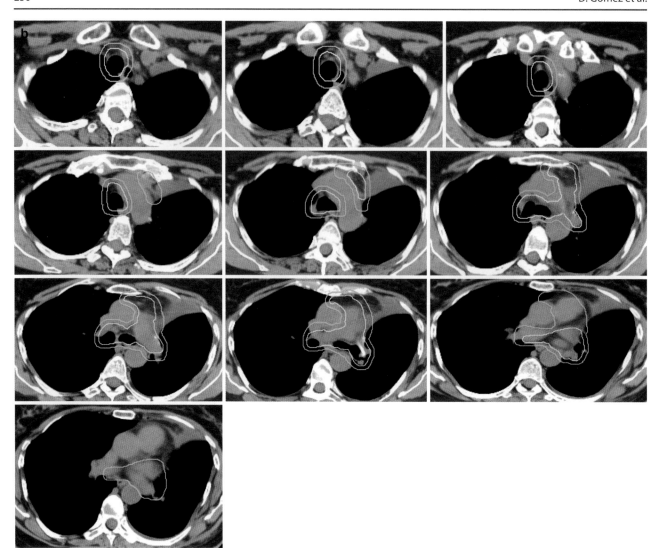

**Fig.5** (continued)

## Bibliography

Chapet O, Kong FM, Quint LE et al (2005) CT-based definition of thoracic lymph node stations: an atlas from the University of Michigan. Int J Radiat Oncol Biol Phys 63:170–178

Lopez Guerra JL, Gomez DR, Lin SH et al (2013) Risk factors for local and regional recurrence in patients with resected N0-N1 non-small-cell lung cancer, with implications for patient selection for adjuvant radiation therapy. Ann Oncol 24:67–74

Mountain CF, Dresler CM (1997) Regional lymph node classification for lung cancer staging. Chest 111:1718–1723

Muirhead R, Featherstone C, Duffton A, Moore K, McNee S (2010) The potential clinical benefit of respiratory gated radiotherapy (RGRT) in non-small cell lung cancer (NSCLC). Radiother Oncol 95(2):172–177

Mutter RW, Liu F, Abreu A, Yorke E, Jackson A, Rosenzweig KE (2012) Dose-volume parameters predict for the development of chest wall pain after stereotactic body radiation for lung cancer. Int J Radiat Oncol Biol Phys 82:1783–1790

Osarogiagbon RU, Yu X (2012) Mediastinal lymph node examination and survival in resected early-stage non-small-cell lung cancer in the surveillance, epidemiology, and end results database. J Thorac Oncol 7:1798–1806

Spoelstra FO, Senan S, Le Pechoux C et al (2010) Variations in target volume definition for postoperative radiotherapy in stage III non-small-cell lung cancer: analysis of an international contouring study. Int J Radiat Oncol Biol Phys 76:1106–1113

Underberg RW, Lagerwaard FJ, Slotman BJ, Cuijpers JP, Senan S (2005) Benefit of respiration-gated stereotactic radiotherapy for stage I lung cancer: an analysis of 4DCT datasets. Int J Radiat Oncol Biol Phys 62:554–560

Urban D, Bar J, Solomon B, Ball D (2013) Lymph node ratio may predict the benefit of postoperative radiotherapy in non-small-cell lung cancer. J Thorac Oncol 8:940–946

Welsh J, Thomas J, Shah D et al (2011) Obesity increases the risk of chest wall pain from thoracic stereotactic body radiation therapy. Int J Radiat Oncol Biol Phys 81:91–96

# Part IV

# Gastrointestinal Tract

# Esophageal Cancer

Jason Chia-Hsien Cheng, Feng-Ming Hsu, Abraham J. Wu,
and Lisa A. Kachnic

## Contents

J.C.-H. Cheng, MD, PhD (✉)
Graduate Institute of Oncology, National Taiwan University
College of Medicine, Taipei, Taiwan

Division of Radiation Oncology, Department of Oncology,
National Taiwan University Hospital, Taipei, Taiwan
e-mail: jasoncheng@ntu.edu.tw

F.-M. Hsu, MD
Division of Radiation Oncology, Department of Oncology,
National Taiwan University Hospital, Taipei, Taiwan

A.J. Wu, MD
Department of Radiation Oncology, Memorial Sloan-Kettering
Cancer Center, New York, NY, USA

L.A. Kachnic, MD
Department of Radiation Oncology, Boston Medical Center,
Boston University School of Medicine, Boston, MA, USA
e-mail: lisa.kachnic@bmc.org

## 1 General Principles of Planning and Target Delineation

- *Evaluation.* Patients should have complete evaluations including contrast-enhanced computed tomography (CT) of the neck, chest, and abdomen, esophagogastroduodenoscopy (EGD), endoscopic ultrasound (EUS), whole-body fluorodeoxyglucose (FDG) positron emission tomography (PET)/CT, and bronchoscopy for upper- and middle-third lesions. Upper gastrointestinal series (barium swallow) is recommended if EGD or EUS study is incomplete due to severe luminal obstruction. These studies help the treating physician in determining disease extension and allow accurate target volume delineation for esophageal cancer.
- *Technique.* CT-based treatment planning utilizing conformal techniques is recommended for esophageal cancer. Both three-dimensional conformal radiation therapy (3DCRT) and intensity-modulated radiation therapy (IMRT) can be used to generate an evaluable dose–volume histogram (DVH) with a setup of multiple beam angles. Special consideration is required in beam angle arrangement to reduce the pulmonary and cardiac toxicity following chemoradiation (Hong et al. 2007). It is necessary to understand the anatomy of the neck, mediastinum, and upper abdomen. The RTOG contouring atlases are great references in delineating normal organs (Kong et al. 2013).
- *Immobilization.* Patients should be adequately immobilized according to the location of esophageal cancer. For tumor(s) located at the cervical or upper-third thoracic esophagus, patients should ideally be immobilized with head–neck–shoulder thermoplastic shells. For tumor(s) located at the thoracic esophagus or esophagogastric junction (EGJ), patients should ideally be immobilized with their arms above their head in a vacuum bag. Four-dimensional (4D) CT simulation can be considered for the tumors located at the distal esophagus or EGJ. Patients with tumors involving the

N.Y. Lee et al. (eds.), *Target Volume Delineation for Conformal and Intensity-Modulated Radiation Therapy*,
Medical Radiology. Radiation Oncology, DOI: 10.1007/174_2014_998, © Springer International Publishing Switzerland 2014
Published Online: 22 October 2014

**Table 1** Summary of guidelines for contouring esophageal cancer

| Tumor location | Definition | GTV to CTV margin | CTV to PTV margin | Elective nodal coverage | Dose |
|---|---|---|---|---|---|
| Upper esophagus | Above carina | Primary: 3~5 cm longitudinally; 0.5~1 cm circumferentially<br><br>Involved lymph node: 0.5~1 cm in all directions | No IGRT: 0.5~1.0 cm<br><br>IGRT: 0.5 cm | Periesophageal, mediastinal, supraclavicular | Neoadjuvant: 40~50.4 Gy in 1.8~2 Gy per fraction<br><br>Definitive: 50.4 Gy (up to 66 Gy for tumor at cervical esophagus) in 1.8~2 Gy per fraction |
| Lower esophagus | Below carina | Same as upper esophagus | Same as upper esophagus | Periesophageal, mediastinal, perigastric, celiac | Neoadjuvant: 40~50.4 Gy in 1.8~2 Gy per fraction<br>Definitive: 50.4 Gy in 1.8~2 Gy per fraction |

lower-third thoracic esophagus or EGJ should be advised to be nil per os (NPO) for at least 2–4 h prior to simulation and with each treatment so as to limit differences in gastric filling and displacement, which may affect dose distribution on a day-to-day basis. In addition, intravenous contrast can be considered at simulation to better identify vascular structures and delineate nodal targets.

- For contouring purposes, esophageal malignancies (squamous cell carcinoma or adenocarcinoma) are divided anatomically into two separate regions: upper esophagus tumors (tumors above carina, including the cervical esophagus) and lower esophagus tumors (tumors below carina, including EGJ). Tumors that originate in the lower-third thoracic esophagus extending to upper-third thoracic esophagus, or vice versa, can follow the contouring guidelines of both subsets (Table 1).

- In all esophageal malignancies, the entire esophagus from cricoid cartilage to EGJ and bilateral lungs should be contoured for proper DVH analysis. In upper esophagus tumors, the brachial plexus, larynx, and spinal cord should be contoured. In lower esophagus tumors, the heart, liver, stomach, duodenum, bilateral kidneys, and spinal cord should be delineated.

- The gross tumor volume (GTV) consists of primary esophageal tumor (the greatest extension on CT, EUS, or FDG-PET) and involved lymph nodes. Lymph nodes with biopsy proof, increased FDG uptake, or enlarged short-axis diameter are delineated as GTV. The EUS can be used to better classify small paraesophageal lymph nodes that are difficult to classify on CT or FDG-PET scan.

- Standard GTV to clinical target volume (CTV) expansions for the primary tumor are 3–5 cm in the longitudinal direction and 0.5–1 cm in the circumferential direction. The larger margins are applied in the longitudinal direction to account for submucosal spread (Gao et al. 2007). For involved lymph nodes, a 0.5–1-cm margin to all directions can be utilized. The CTV can be shaved off normal structures accordingly to respect anatomical boundaries. These margins can be adjusted based on the treating physician's confidence about the disease extension (Figs. 1, 2, and 3).

- There is no consensus about elective nodal coverage for esophageal cancer (Qiao et al. 2008; Hsu et al. 2011). Generally, in upper esophagus tumors, periesophageal, mediastinal, and supraclavicular lymphatics should be considered elective nodal regions. In lower esophagus tumors, periesophageal, mediastinal, perigastric, and celiac lymphatics should be considered elective nodal regions (Figs. 4 and 5).

- Tumor location, motion management technique, image guidance utilization, and institutional-defined setup errors should be considered to generate proper margins for the planning target volume (PTV). Typically, a 0.5-cm CTV to PTV margin can be applied when daily kilovoltage (kv) image guidance is used. In the absence of daily kv imaging guidance, a margin of 0.5–1.0 cm can be applied to ensure adequate dose coverage to the CTV.

**Fig.** **1** Locally advanced (cT3N1M0) esophageal squamous cell carcinoma of middle esophagus with paraesophageal lymphadenopathy. The primary tumor was located at 25–32 cm below incisors. A representative FDG-PET image is shown to facilitate GTV (in *red*) contouring. 4-cm longitudinal and 0.5- to 1-cm circumferential margins were added for the CTV (in *green*) of the primary tumor. The bilateral supraclavicular lymphatics were covered electively in the presence of upper paraesophageal lymph node metastasis

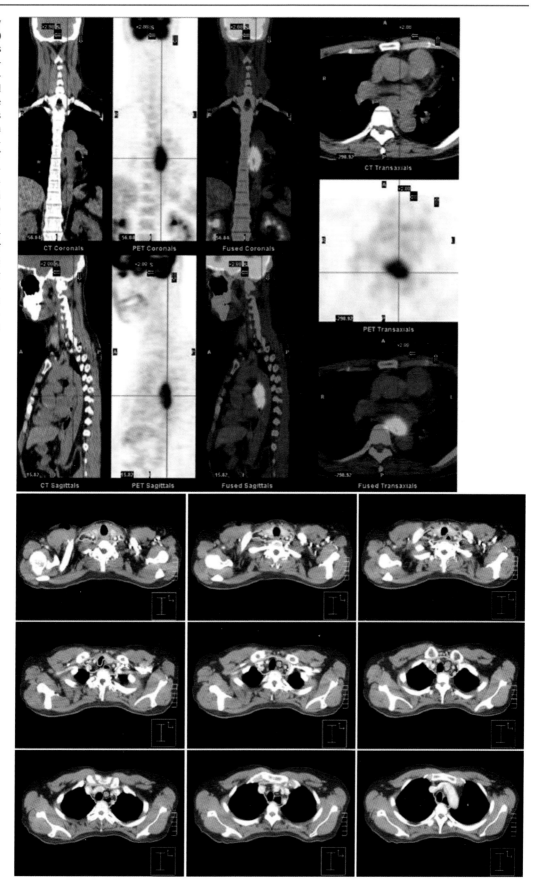

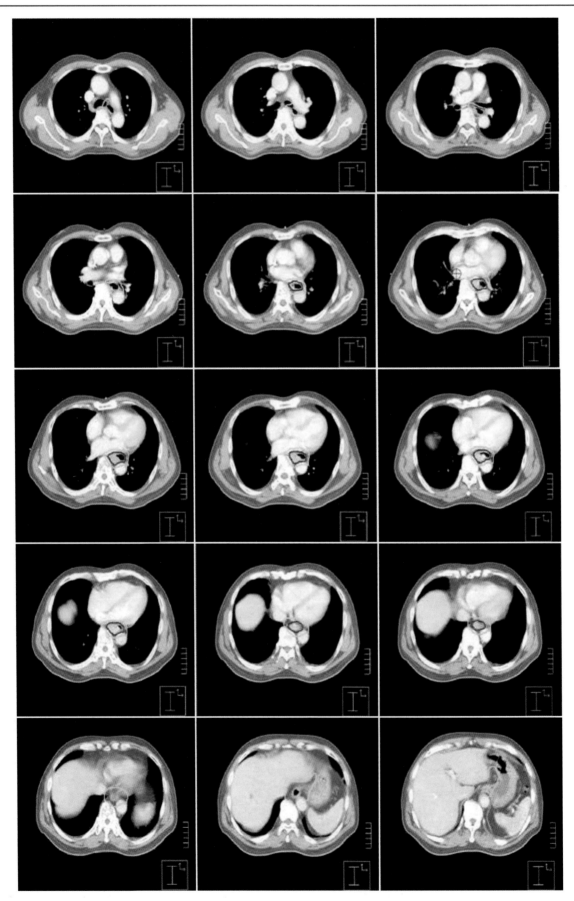

**Fig. 2** Locally advanced (cT3N0M0) esophageal squamous cell carcinoma of lower esophagus. The primary tumor (in *red*) was located at 32–38 cm below incisors. 4-cm longitudinal and 0.5- to 1-cm circumferential margins were added to create the CTV plus elective nodal coverage including perigastric and celiac lymphatics (in *green*)

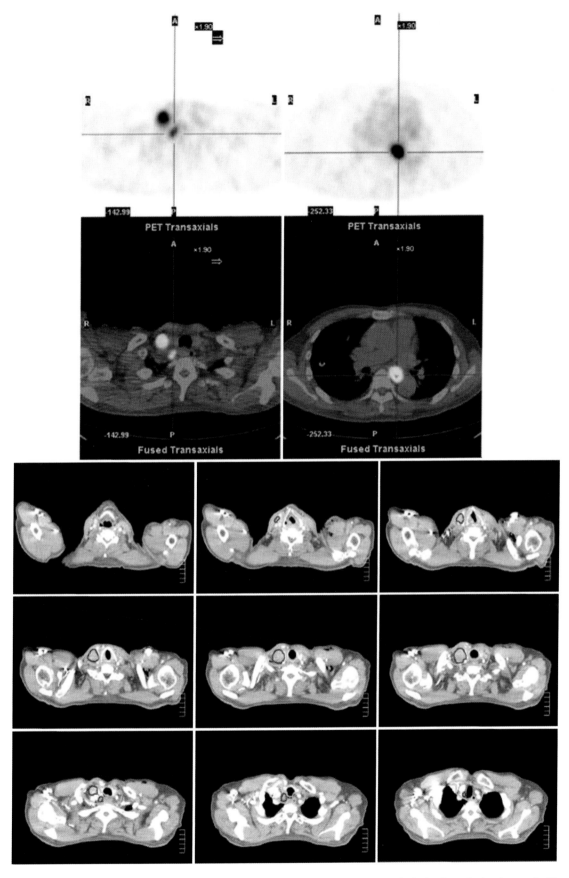

**Fig. 3** Locally advanced (cT3N1M0) esophageal squamous cell carcinoma of middle esophagus with left supraclavicular lymphadenopathy. The primary tumor was located at 30–37 cm below incisors. A representative FDG-PET image is shown to facilitate GTV (in *red*) contour-ing. The bilateral supraclavicular (superior border to cricoid cartilage) and left level III lymphatics were included in the CTV (in *green*). The posterior neck lymphatics (level V) were omitted

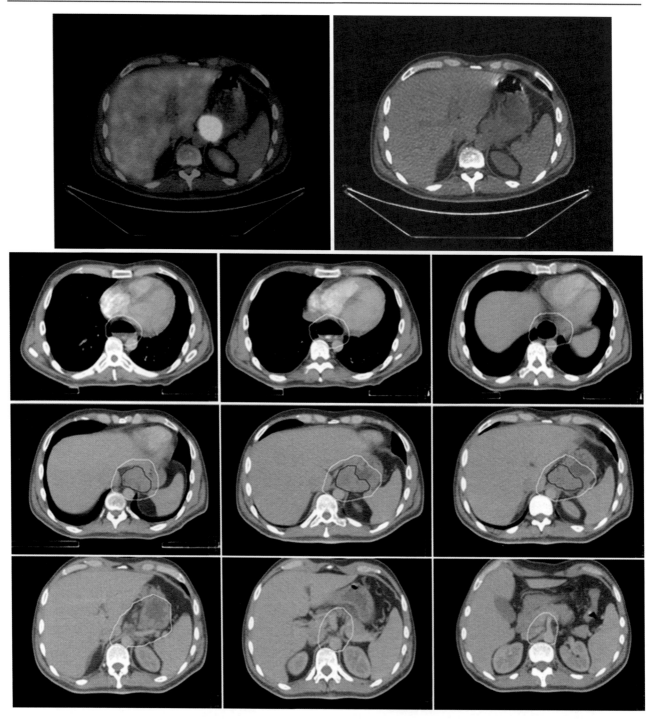

**Fig. 4** Locally advanced esophagogastric junction (EGJ) adenocarcinoma, stage T3N0, Siewert type II, with significant involvement of the gastric cardia. The esophagus is distended due to tumor obstruction. Perigastric and celiac lymphatics were included in the CTV (in *yellow*). A representative PET/CT image is shown to facilitate GTV contouring (in *red*)

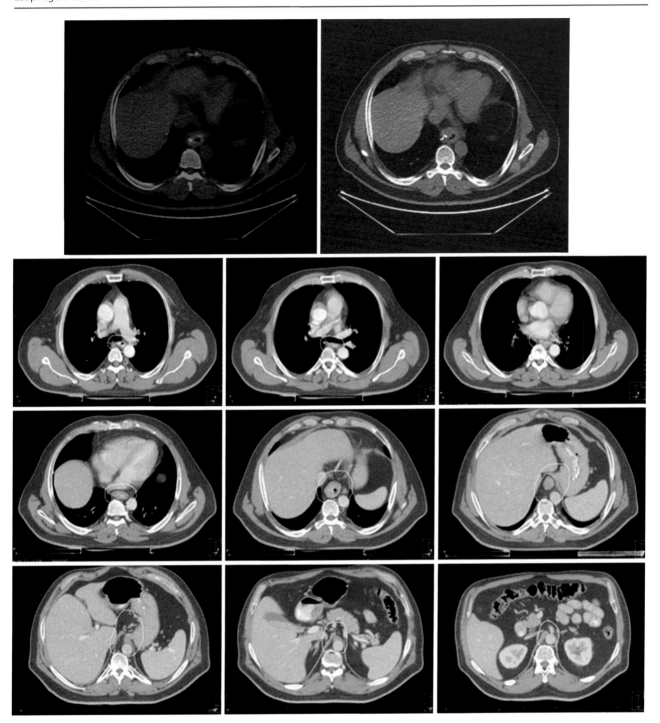

**Fig. 5** T3N1 adenocarcinoma of the distal esophagus. The mass extended from 35 to 39 cm from the incisors but did not cross the EGJ. Mildly FDG-avid perigastric lymph nodes were noted on PET/CT scan. The perigastric and celiac nodes were included in the CTV (in *yellow*). A representative PET/CT image is shown to facilitate GTV contouring (in *red*)

## References and Suggested Reading

Gao XS, Qiao X, Wu F, Cao L, Meng X, Dong Z, Wang X, Gao G, Wu TT, Komaki R et al (2007) Pathological analysis of clinical target volume margin for radiotherapy in patients with esophageal and gastroesophageal junction carcinoma. Int J Radiat Oncol Biol Phys 67(2):389–396

Hong TS, Crowley EM, Killoran J, Mamon HJ (2007) Considerations in treatment planning for esophageal cancer. Semin Radiat Oncol 17(1):53–61

Hsu FM, Lee JM, Huang PM, Lin CC, Hsu CH, Tsai YC, Lee YC, Cheng JC (2011) Retrospective analysis of outcome differences in preoperative concurrent chemoradiation with or without elective nodal irradiation for esophageal squamous cell carcinoma. Int J Radiat Oncol Biol Phys 81(4):e593–e599

Kong FM, Quint L, Machtay M, Bradley J (2013) Atlases for organs at risk (OARs) in thoracic radiation therapy. http://www.rtog.org/CoreLab/ContouringAtlases/LungAtlas.aspx

Qiao XY, Wang W, Zhou ZG, Gao XS, Chang JY (2008) Comparison of efficacy of regional and extensive clinical target volumes in post-operative radiotherapy for esophageal squamous cell carcinoma. Int J Radiat Oncol Biol Phys 70(2):396–402

# Gastric Cancer

Jeremy Tey and Jiade J. Lu

## Contents

J. Tey, MD
Department of Radiation Oncology,
National University Cancer Institute, Singapore (NCIS),
National University Health System (NUHS),
1E Kent Ridge Road, NUHS Tower Block Level 7,
Singapore 119228, Singapore
e-mail: Jeremy_Tey@nuhs.edu.sg

J.J. Lu, MD, MBA (✉)
Shanghai Proton and Heavy Ion Center (SPHIC),
4365 Kangxin Road, Pudong, Shanghai 201321, China
e-mail: jiade.lu@sphic.org.cn

## 1   Anatomy and Patterns of Spread

- The stomach begins at the gastrooesophageal junction and ends at the pylorus. The greater curvature forms the left and convex border of the stomach, and the lesser curvature forms the right and concave border of the stomach (Fig. 1a). It is divided into four parts: the cardia, fundus, body and antrum. The gastric wall is divided into five layers: mucosa, submucosa, muscularis externa, subserosa and serosa.
- The stomach is covered with peritoneum and is closely related to the left lobe of the liver, spleen, left adrenal gland, superior portion of the left kidney, pancreas, transverse colon and major blood vessels including the coeliac axis and superior mesenteric artery (Fig. 1b).
- Probability of gastric carcinoma varies according to the primary location: ~35 % of tumours arise from the gastroesophageal junction, cardia and fundus. ~25 % of tumours arise from the body. ~40 % of tumours arise from the antrum and distal stomach.
- Local extension
  - The tumour can invade locally with direct involvement of the liver, duodenum, pancreas, transverse colon, omentum and diaphragm.
  - Proximal tumours may spread upwards to involve the oesophagus.
  - Perineural invasion can occur.
- Regional lymph node metastases (Fig. 2, Table 1)

N.Y. Lee et al. (eds.), *Target Volume Delineation for Conformal and Intensity-Modulated Radiation Therapy,*
Medical Radiology. Radiation Oncology, DOI: 10.1007/174_2014_991, © Springer International Publishing Switzerland 2014
Published Online: 4 November 2014

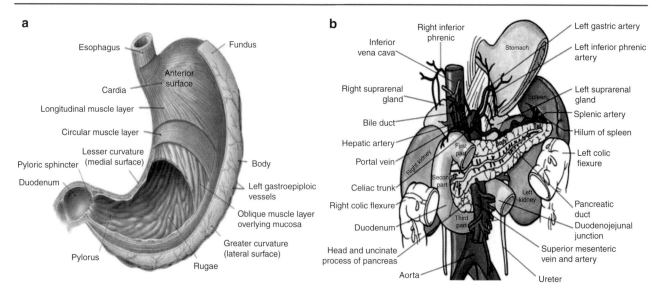

**Fig. 1** Regions of stomach (**a**) and relations of the stomach (**b**)

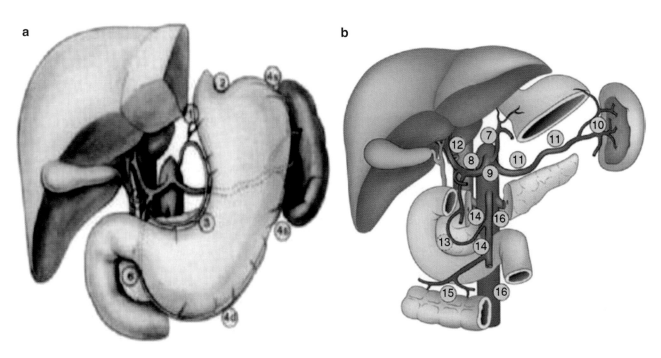

**Fig. 2** Lymph node groups surrounding the stomach

**Table 1** Lymph node stations commonly involved in gastric cancer (Japanese Research Society for the Study of Gastric Cancer (JRSGC))

| | |
|---|---|
| 1. Right cardial nodes | 9. Nodes along the coeliac axis |
| 2. Left cardial nodes | 10. Nodes at the splenic hilus |
| 3. Nodes along the lesser curvature | 11. Nodes along the splenic artery |
| 4. Nodes along the greater curvature | 12. Nodes in the hepatoduodenal ligament |
| 5. Suprapyloric nodes | 13. Nodes at the posterior aspect of the pancreatic head |
| 6. Infrapyloric nodes | 14. Nodes at the root of the mesenterium |
| 7. Nodes along left gastric artery | 15. Nodes in the mesocolon of the transverse colon |
| 8. Nodes along the common hepatic artery | 16. Para-aortic lymph nodes |

*Source*: Figure and table adapted from Hartgrink and Van De Velde (2005). Used with permission from Wiley Inc.

- Lymph node involvement is seen in up to 80 % of cases at diagnosis.
- Lymph node involvement depends on the origin of primary disease.
- Proximal/gastrooesophageal junction tumours may spread to lower paraoesophageal lymph nodes.
- Tumours of the body can involve all nodal sites.
- Tumours of the distal stomach/antrum may involve periduodenal and porta hepatis lymph nodes.

- Preoperative CT scans should be reviewed to identify the location of primary tumour and involved regional lymphatics.
- Consider preradiation quantitative renal perfusion study to evaluate relative bilateral renal function.
- Postoperative diagnostic CT scan with oral and intravenous contrast is required with the identification of the following:
    - Oesophagus and gastric remnant
    - Anastomosis (gastrojejunal, oesophagojejunal)
    - Duodenal stump
    - Porta hepatis
    - Splenic hilum
    - Pancreas
    - Coeliac artery and superior mesenteric artery
- The type of surgery performed depends on the location of tumour, histology pattern (Fig. 3).

## 2    Diagnostic Workup Relevant for Target Volume Delineation

- Prior to radiotherapy planning, it is imperative to review surgical and pathology reports and discuss with the surgeon to identify the areas considered to be the highest risk for recurrence; the type of operation, i.e. total vs. partial gastrectomy, needs to be noted.

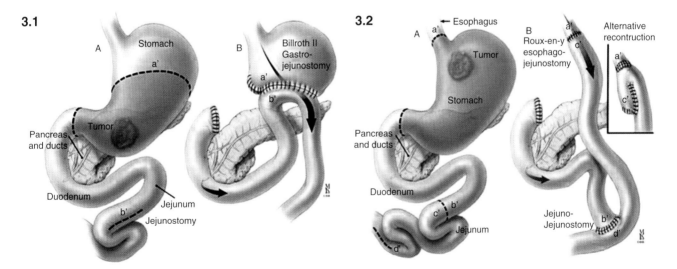

**Fig. 3** Types of gastric cancer surgery. 3.1 (**a**) Subtotal gastrectomy, (**b**) Bilroth II anastomosis. 3.2 (**a**) Total gastrectomy, (**b**) Roux-en-Y esophagojejunostomy

## 3    General Principles of Planning and Target Delineation for Adjuvant Radiation for Adenocarcinomas of the Gastrooesophageal Junction and the Stomach

- Patients should fast for 2–3 h before CT simulation and before treatments to ensure an empty stomach and enhance daily treatment reproducibility.
- Radiotherapy planning CT scans of 3–5 mm thickness should be obtained with the patient in the supine position with arms overhead, from top of the diaphragm (for stomach) or carina (for tumour of GE junction or cardia) to the bottom of L4.
- Immobilisation with a Vac-Lok is recommended for treatment with IMRT.
- Intravenous contrast is preferred to demonstrate blood vessels and guide clinical target volume (CTV) delineation, particularly for lymph nodes; preoperative CT scans should be used to aid identification of preoperative tumour volume and nodal groups to be treated.
- CTV for adjuvant radiation therapy for gastric cancer depends on the position of the primary disease as well as the status of lymph node metastasis. Suggested target volumes for CTV coverage depending on subsite are detailed in Tables 2, 3, 4, 5 and 6.
- Three areas must be identified as CTV for adjuvant radiotherapy: the gastric tumour bed, the anastomosis or stumps and the regional lymphatics.
- In addition, the hepatogastric ligament should preferably be treated in all cases as it is at high risk of recurrence. It represents the part of the lesser omentum that runs between the lesser curvature of the stomach and liver and contains the left and right gastric nodes that are not always completely removed at surgery.
- The benefits of intensity modulated radiotherapy (IMRT) have been suggested by many publications. If used,

**Table 2** Target volume definition and description

| Target volumes | Definition and description |
| --- | --- |
| GTV | Gross residual disease defined by CT imaging and surgical findings |
| PTV (residual disease) | GTV/positive margins + 1.5 cm. Cone down boost after 45 Gy to a total dose of 50.4 to 54Gy in 1.8Gy/fraction |
| $CTV_{45}$ | Coverage of nodal groups according to subsite (see Table xx). Also includes remnant stomach, anastomosis (gastrojejunal, oesophagojejunal), duodenal stump |
| $PTV_{45}$ | $CTV_{45}$ + 1 cm margin. A larger margin may be required for organ motion and setup uncertainties |

**Table 3** General considerations for clinical target volume

| Target volumes | Definition and description |
| --- | --- |
| Duodenal stump | Should preferably be covered in patients who have had a partial gastrectomy for distal/antral tumours |
|  | Should not be covered in patients with proximal/cardia tumours who have had a total gastrectomy |
| Anastomosis | Gastrojejunal anastomosis (partial gastrectomy for tumours of the distal stomach) |
|  | Oesophagojejunal anastomosis (total gastrectomy for tumours of proximal stomach or GE junction) should be treated |
| Para-aortic nodes | Should be included for the entire length of the CTV |
| Paraoesophageal nodes | A 4 cm margin of the oesophagus should be included in the clinical target volume for tumours of the gastrooesophageal junction |

**Table 4** Recommended nodal coverage depending on the site of primary tumour in the stomach: *oesophagogastric junction*

| Origin and stage (AJCC 7th edition) | Remaining stomach | Tumour bed volumes[a] | Nodal volume |
| --- | --- | --- | --- |
| EG junction | If allows exclusion of 2/3 of the right kidney | T stage dependent | N stage dependent |
| T3N0, invasion of subserosa, especially posterior wall | Variable, dependent on surg-path findings[b] | Medial left hemidiaphragm; adjacent body of pancreas | None or PG, PEN[c] |
| T4aN0 | Variable, dependent on surg-path findings[b] | Medial left hemidiaphragm; adjacent body of pancreas | None or PG, PEN, MN, CN[c] |
| T4bN0 | Preferable but dependent on surg-path findings[b] | As for T4aN0 plus sites of adherence with 3–5 cm margin | Nodes related to sites of adherence +/– PG, PEN, MN, CN |
| T1-3 N+ | Preferable | Not indicated for T1-2, as above for T3 | PEN, MN, prox PG, CN |
| T4a/bN+ | Preferable | As for T4a/bN0 | As for T1–T3 N+ and T4bN0 |

Modified from Gunderson and Tepper (2007)

*PG* perigastric, *CN* coeliac, *PEN* perioesophageal, *MN* mediastinal

[a]Use preoperative imaging (CT, barium swallow), surgical clips and postoperative imaging (CT, barium swallow)

[b]For tumours with >5 cm margins confirmed pathologically, treatment of residual stomach is optional, especially if this would result in substantial increase in normal tissue morbidity

[c]Optional node inclusion for T3–T4a N0 lesions if adequate surgical node dissection (D2) and at least 10–15 nodes are examined pathologically

**Table 5** Recommended nodal coverage depending on the site of primary tumour in the stomach: *body/middle third of the stomach*

| Site of primary and TN stage | Remaining stomach | Tumour bed volumes[a] | Nodal volume |
|---|---|---|---|
| Body/middle third of the stomach | Yes, but spare 2/3 one kidney | T stage dependent | N stage dependent, spare 2/3 of one kidney |
| T3N0, especially posterior wall | Yes | Body of pancreas (+/− tail) | None or PG<br>Optional: CN, SplN, SplNs, HNpd, PHN[b] |
| T4aN0 | Yes | Body of pancreas (+/− tail) | None or perigastric<br>Optional: CN, SplN, SplNs, HNpd, PHN[b] |
| T4bN0 | Yes | As for T4aN0 plus sites of adherence with 3–5 cm margin | Nodes related to sites of adherence +/−<br>PG, SplNs, SplN, HNpd, CN, PHN |
| T1–T3 N+ | Yes | Not indicated for T1–T2, as above for T3 | PG, CN, SplN, SplNs, HNpd, PHN |
| T4a/bN+ | Yes | As for T4a/bN0 | As for T1–T3 N+ and T4bN0 |

Modified from Gunderson and Tepper (2007)

*PG* perigastric, *CN* coeliac, *SplN* splenic, *SplNs* suprapancreatic, *PHN* porta hepatis, *HNpd* pancreaticoduodenal, *PEN* perioesophageal, *MN* mediastinal

[a]Use preoperative imaging (CT, barium swallow), surgical clips and postoperative imaging (CT, barium swallow)

[b]Optional node inclusion for T3–T4a N0 lesions if adequate surgical node dissection (D2) and at least 10–15 nodes are examined pathologically

**Table 6** Recommended nodal coverage depending on the site of primary tumour in the stomach: *cardia/proximal third of the stomach* (**prox**) *and antrum/pylorus/distal third of the stomach* (**distal**)

| Origin and stage (AJCC 7th edition) | Remaining stomach | Tumour bed volumes[a] | Nodal volume |
|---|---|---|---|
| Cardia/proximal third of the stomach | Preferred, but spare 2/3 of one kidney (usually right) | T category dependent | N classification dependent |
| Antrum/distal third of the stomach | Yes, but spare 2/3 of one kidney (usually left) | | |
| T3N0, | Variable, dependent on surgical pathological findings[b] | *Prox*: medial left hemidiaphragm, adjacent body of pancreas (+/− tail)<br>*Distal*: head of pancreas (+/− body), 1st and 2nd part of the duodenum | *Prox*: none or PG[c]<br><br>*Distal*: none or PG<br>Optional: CN, SplNs, HNpd, PHN[c] |
| T4aN0 | Variable, dependent on surgical pathological findings[b] | *Prox*: medial left hemidiaphragm, adjacent body of pancreas (+/− tail)<br>*Distal*: head of pancreas (+/− body), 1st and 2nd part of the duodenum | *Prox*: none or PG; optional: PEN, MN, CN[c]<br><br>*Distal*: none or PG;<br>Optional: CN, SplNs, HNpd, PHN[c] |
| T4bN0 | Prox: variable, dependent on surgical pathological finding[b]<br>Distal: preferable, dependent on surgical pathological finding[b] | As for T4aN0 plus sites of adherence with 3–5 cm margin | *Prox*: nodes related to sites of adherence +/− PG, PEN, MN, CN<br>*Distal*: nodes related to sites of adherence +/− PG, SplNs, HNpd, CN, PHN |
| T1–T3 N+ | Preferable | Not indicated for T1–T2, as above for T3 | *Prox*: PEN, CN, SplN, SplNs, +/− PEN, MN, HNpd, PHN[d]<br>*Distal*: PG, CN, HNpd, PHN, SplNs<br>Optional: splenic hilum |
| T4a/bN+ | Preferable | As for T4a/bN0 | As for T1–T3 N+ and T4bN0 |

Modified from Gunderson and Tepper (2007)

*PG* perigastric, *CN* coeliac, *SplN* splenic, *SplNs* suprapancreatic, *PHN* porta hepatis, *HNpd* pancreaticoduodenal, *PEN* perioesophageal, *MN* mediastinal

[a]Use preoperative imaging (CT, barium swallow), surgical clips and postoperative imaging (CT, barium swallow)

[b]For tumours with >5 cm margins confirmed pathologically, treatment of residual stomach is not necessary, especially if this would result in substantial increase in normal tissue morbidity

[c]Optional node inclusion for T3–T4a N0 lesions if adequate surgical node dissection (D2) and at least 10–15 nodes are examined pathologically

[d]Pancreaticoduodenal and porta hepatis nodes are at low risk of nodal positivity is minimal (1–2 positive nodes with 10–15 examined) and this region does not need to be irradiated. Perioesophageal and mediastinal nodes are at risk if there is oesophageal extension

tumour bed and subclinical target volumes including lymphatic draining regions should be delineated.

- Planning target volume (PTV): CTV + margin considering organ motion and setup uncertainties. A minimum expansion of 1 cm is suggested.
- A total dose of 45Gy in 25 fractions is recommended for adjuvant radiotherapy with concurrent chemotherapy, using high-energy (≥6MV) photons. Boosts to 50.4–54Gy for positive margins or residual disease should be

given, if doses to surrounding critical organs are within tolerance (Figs. 4, 5, 6 and 7).

## 4    Plan Assessment

- In advanced cases, we typically prioritise normal structure constraints, specifically the brainstem, spinal cord and optic chiasm over full coverage of the tumour.

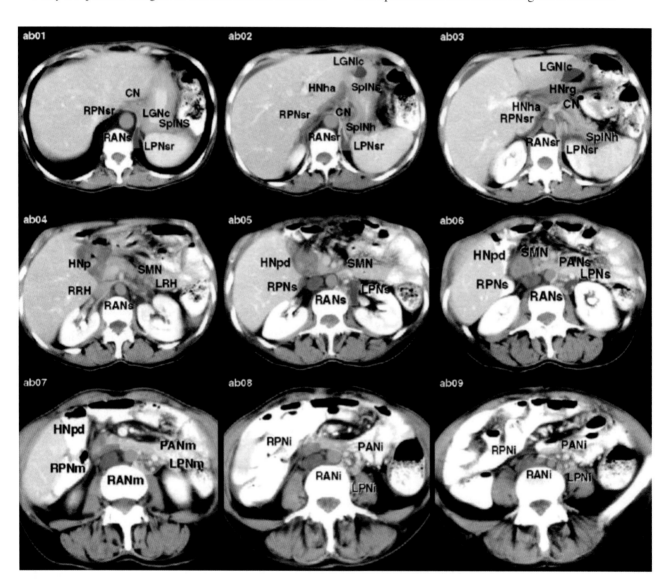

**Fig. 4** Nodal distribution for adjuvant radiotherapy for gastric cancer. Lymph node groups commonly involved in gastric cancer on CT images. *CN* coeliac, *SMN* superior mesenteric, *RRH* right renal hilum, *LRH* left renal hilum, *HNpd* hepatic nodes (pancreaticoduodenum), *HNp* hepatic nodes (pyloric), *HNha* hepatic nodes (hepatic artery), *HNrg* hepatic nodes (right gastroepiploic), *LPN* left para-aortic nodes, *RPN* right para-aortic nodes, *RAN* retroaortic nodes, *PAN* preaortic nodes, *SpINs* splenic nodes, *SpINh* splenic nodes (hilar), *LGN* left gastric nodes, *LGNIc* left gastric nodes(gastropancreatic), *sr* suprarenal, *s* superior, *m* middle, *i* inferior (Adapted from Martinez-Monge et al. (1999). Used with permission from RSNA)

**Fig. 5** Clinical target volumes for a patient with T1N1M0 adenocarcinoma of the gastric cardia post total gastrectomy

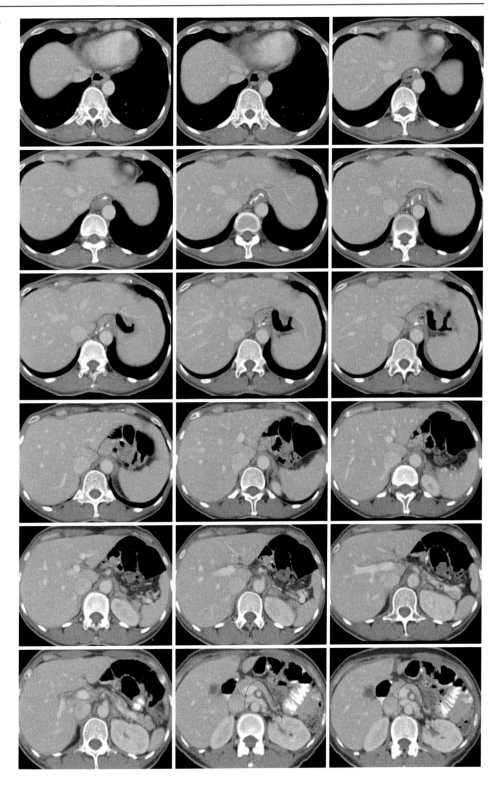

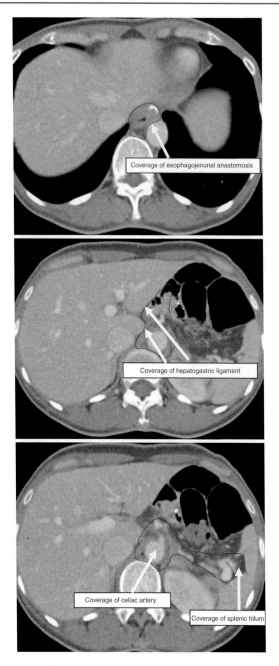

**Fig. 5** (continued)

**Fig. 6** Clinical target volumes for a patient with T3N3M0 adenocarcinoma of the gastric body post distal gastrectomy

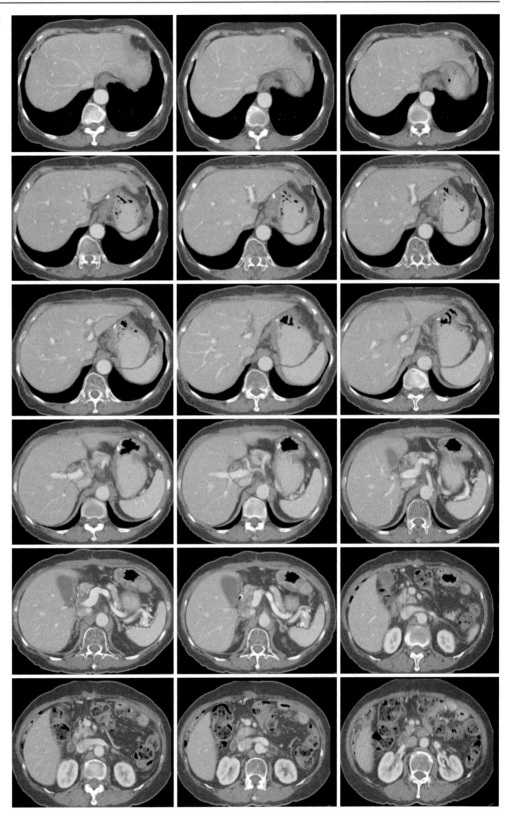

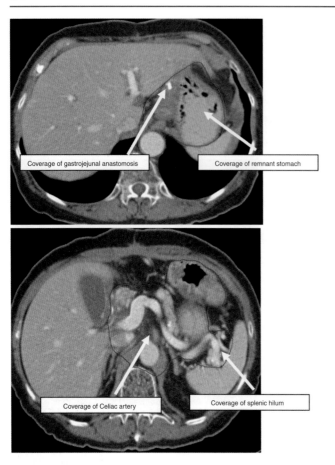

**Fig. 6** (continued)

**Fig. 7** Clinical target volumes for a patient with T2N1M0 adenocarcinoma of the antrum/pylorus post distal gastrectomy

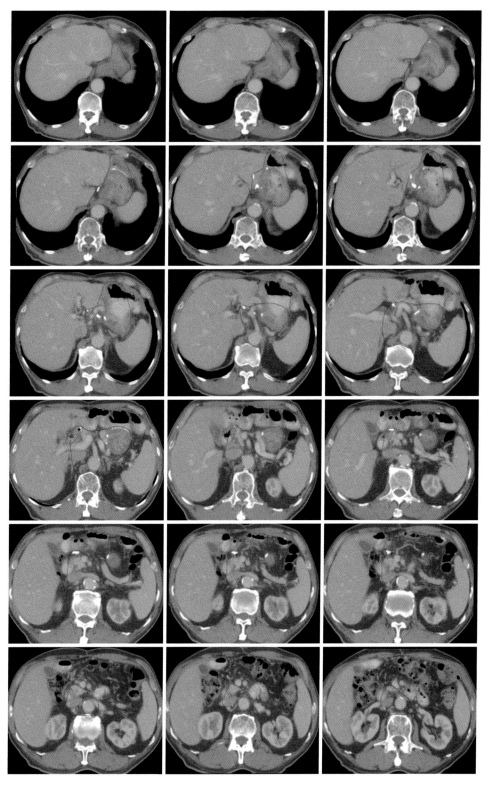

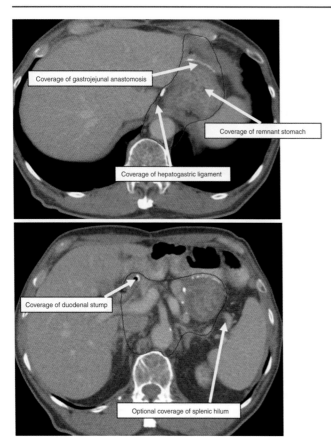

**Fig. 7** (continued)

- Ideally, at least 95 % of the volume of $PTV_{45}$ should receive 45 Gy. In addition, the dose to 100 % of the $PTV_{45}$ should be $\geq 42.75$ Gy.
- Critical normal structures surrounding the CTV need to be outlined for dose constraints (Table 7). These structures include the spinal cord, liver, small intestines, heart and bilateral kidneys.

**Table 7** Dose limitations of OAR in radiation therapy for upper abdominal malignancies

| OAR | Dose limitation | End point | Rate (%) |
|---|---|---|---|
| Spinal cord | $D_{max} = 50$ | Myelopathy | 0.2 |
|  | $D_{max} = 60$ |  | 6 |
|  | $D_{max} = 69$ |  | 50 |
| Whole liver[a] | Mean dose 30–32 | Classical RILD | <5 |
|  | Mean dose <42 |  | <50 |
| Small intestine[b] | V45 < 195 cc (entire potential space within the peritoneal cavity) | Grade ≥3 acute toxicity | <10 |
| Heart | Mean dose <26 (pericardium) | Pericarditis | <15 |
|  | V30 < 46 % (pericardium) | Long-term cardiac mortality | <15 |
|  | V25 < 10 % (whole heart) |  | <1 |
| Bilateral whole kidneys | Mean dose <15–18 | Clinically relevant renal dysfunction | <5 |
|  | Mean dose <28 |  | <50 |

*Source*: Marks et al. (2010)

$D_{max}$ maximum dose, *RILD* radiation-induced liver dysfunction, $V_n$ volume receiving $n$ Gray

[a]Patients with no pre-existing liver disease or hepatocellular carcinoma

[b]Entire potential space within the peritoneal cavity

## Suggested Reading

Defining the target volume for post-op radiotherapy after D2 dissection by CT based vessel-guided delineation (2013). Radiother Oncol 108(1):72–77

Nam et al (2008) A new suggestion for the radiation target volume after a subtotal gastrectomy in patients with stomach cancer. Int J Radiat Oncol Biol Phys 71(2):448–455

Radiation treatment parameters in the adjuvant postoperative therapy of gastric cancer (2002). Semin Radiat Oncol 12(2):187–195

Wo et al (2013) Gastric lymph node contouring atlas: a tool to aid clinical target volume definition in 3-dimensional treatment for gastric cancer. Pract Radiat Oncol 3:e1–e9

## References

Gunderson LL, Tepper JE (eds) (2007) Clinical radiation oncology, 2nd edn. Philadelphia, Churchill Livingstone/Elsevier

Hartgrink HH, Van De Velde CJH (2005) Status of extended lymph node dissection. J Surg Oncol 90:153–165

Marks LB et al (2010) Use of normal tissue complication probability models in the clinic. Int J Radiat Oncol Biol Phys 76(3):S10–S19

Martinez-Monge R, Fernandez PS, Gupta N et al (1999) Cross-sectional nodal atlas: a tool for the definition of clinical target volumes in three-dimensional radiation therapy planning. Radiology 211:815–82

# Pancreatic Adenocarcinoma

Paul B. Romesser, Michael R. Folkert,
and Karyn A. Goodman

## Contents

## 1   Anatomy and Patterns of Spread

- The pancreas, a retroperitoneal organ that performs a range of both endocrine and exocrine functions, lies within the curve of the first, second, and third parts of the duodenum (i.e., the C loop) and extends across the posterior abdominal wall behind the stomach to the splenic hilum. It is divided into four parts (head, neck, body, and tail) and one accessory lobe, the uncinate process (Fig. 1) (Strandring 2005).

- The majority of pancreatic adenocarcinomas arise in the head of the pancreas, which lies anterior and to the right side of the vertebral column and adjacent to the first part of the duodenum. Tumors arising here tend to be identified earlier than those in the body or tail because they obstruct the distal common bile duct and often present with painless jaundice (most common), a dilated gallbladder (Courvoisier's sign), or less commonly with cholangitis (Niederhuber et al. 2014).

- The boundary between the head and neck of the pancreas is marked anteriorly by a groove for the gastroduodenal artery and posteriorly by a deep groove from the union of the superior mesenteric and splenic veins, which form the portal vein (Strandring 2005).

- The body of the pancreas is the largest part of the gland and is located to the left of the superior mesenteric vein (SMV), extending to the left border of the aorta. The pancreatic tail extends from the left border of the aorta to the splenic hilum and lies between the layers of the splenorenal ligaments. The splenic vein forms a shallow groove on the posterior border of the gland (Strandring 2005).

- The accessory lobe of the pancreas, or uncinate process, extends from the inferior lateral end of the head of the gland. It is an anatomically and embryonically distinct portion of the gland, and as a result it lies posterior to the superior mesenteric vessels. Inflammation of the pancreas can result in compression of the superior mesenteric artery (SMA) and SMV between the uncinate process and the neck of the pancreas. Tumors of the uncinate process may not cause obstruction of the common bile duct, but rather can compress

P.B. Romesser, MD • M.R. Folkert, MD, PhD
K.A. Goodman, MD, MS (✉)
Department of Radiation Oncology, Memorial Sloan Kettering
Cancer Center, New York, NY, USA
e-mail: goodmank@mskcc.org

N.Y. Lee et al. (eds.), *Target Volume Delineation for Conformal and Intensity-Modulated Radiation Therapy*,
Medical Radiology. Radiation Oncology, DOI: 10.1007/174_2014_977, © Springer International Publishing Switzerland 2014
Published Online: 22 October 2014

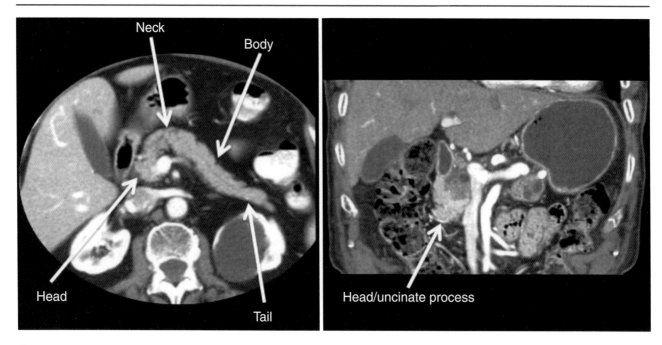

**Fig. 1** Pancreas anatomy (Image courtesy of Corrine Winston, MD)

the third portion of the duodenum or, rarely, result in thrombosis of the SMA or SMV.

- Given the exocrine function of the pancreas, some tumors can present with signs/symptoms of enzyme insufficiency (i.e., malabsorption, increased flatulence, fatty stools, weight loss, and ascities). Diabetes can also be a presenting symptom given the endocrine function of the gland.
- The main pancreatic duct, the duct of Wirsung, lies within the substance of the gland with increasing caliber as it approaches the ampulla in the descending duodenum (papilla of Vater). A separate accessory duct, the duct of Santorini, drains the lower part of the head and uncinate process and usually enters the duodenum at a minor papilla approximately 2 cm proximal to the major papilla of Vater. The main and accessory ducts have anatomic variability, but in many adults the main pancreatic duct merges with the common bile duct proximal to the papilla of Vater (Strandring 2005).
- Sympathetic innervation of the pancreas originates from the 6th to the 10th thoracic spinal segments. Parasympathetic innervation is from the posterior vagus nerve and the parasympathetic celiac plexus. Referred pain from the pancreas is poorly localizing, but often described as a dull deep abdominal or middle back pain (Niederhuber et al. 2014).
  - Pain at time of diagnosis has been correlated with a worse prognosis as it is usually indicative of locally advanced disease or perineural invasion.
- The pancreas has a rich arterial supply. The head and neck of the pancreas are supplied from the superior and inferior pancreaticoduodenal arteries. which arise from the celiac trunk and SMA, respectively. Venous drainage is predominantly through the splenic vein. Given their intimate

proximity to the pancreas, the SMA and SMV are most commonly involved. Vascular invasion is a critical factor to consider when assessing the surgical resectability of the tumor (Niederhuber et al. 2014).

- Lymph node involvement is the strongest predictor for survival. The first echelon nodes include the pancreaticoduodenal, suprapancreatic, pyloric, and splenic hilar (if lateralized body or tail tumor) lymph nodes. Second echelon nodes include the celiac nodes, porta hepatis, and superior mesenteric and para-aortic nodes.
- The majority of patients (>85 %) present with locally advanced or metastatic disease. Given the location of the gland in the retroperitoneum, the most common sites of local invasion include the duodenum, SMV, portal vein, SMA, stomach, liver, and gallbladder.
- The liver is the most common site of metastasis as venous drainage of the pancreas is predominantly through the portal system. Peritoneal metastases are also common. The lung is the most common site of metastatic disease outside the abdomen. Brain and bone metastases are uncommon.
- Local control in pancreatic adenocarcinoma is important, as approximately 30 % of patients die from the significant morbidity associated with locally advanced disease (Iacobuzio-Donahue et al. 2009).

## 2     Diagnostic Workup Relevant for Target Volume Delineation

- In addition to physical examination, adequate imaging studies should be obtained for diagnosis, staging, and planning. Unless contraindicated (renal disease/allergy), all patients should undergo a computed tomography (CT)-angiogram pancreas protocol. Alternatively, MRI may be considered if an iodinated contrast allergy is present. Positron-emission tomography (PET)/CT may be considered, but its contribution to target delineation has not been fully characterized.

- CT-angiogram pancreas protocol often includes a non-contrast phase plus arterial, pancreatic parenchymal, and portal-venous phases of contrast enhancement with thin cuts (3 mm or less) through the abdomen. Multiplanar reconstruction is preferred (Network NCC 2013).
  - This technique allows precise visualization of the relationship of the primary tumor to the mesenteric vasculature as well as detection of metastatic deposits as small as 3–5 mm (Network NCC 2013).
- In patients with localized disease, an endoscopic ultrasonography (EUS) should be considered to help evaluate resectability and obtain tissue to confirm diagnosis.
  - EUS-directed fine-needle aspiration (FNA) is preferable to a CT-guided FNA because of improved diagnostic yield, safety, and a potentially lower risk of peritoneal seeding compared with percutaneous approaches (Network NCC 2013).
- Borderline resectable and unresectable patients with obstructive jaundice should undergo biliary stenting prior to initiating radiation therapy planning, preferably with a metal wall stent.
- Laboratory workup should include complete blood count, carcinoembryonic antigen, CA19-9, glucose, amylase, lipase, bilirubin, alkaline phosphatase, lactate dehydrogenase, and liver function tests.
  - Pretreatment CA19-9 <90 U/mL has been correlated with improved overall survival (Berger et al. 2008).

# 3 Pancreatic Cancer Staging

- An American Joint Committee on Cancer (AJCC) TNM staging exists for pancreatic exocrine cancer; however, the most commonly used classification is based on resectability and evidence of metastatic disease (Edge et al. 2010). Pancreatic tumors are largely categorized into three groups: (1) resectable; (2) locally advanced, non-metastatic; and (3) metastatic. More recently, tumors that are considered "borderline resectable" have been defined by several groups; however, this remains a less well-characterized subset.
- Criteria for resectability vary by institution and surgical technique/experience:
  - Tumors considered localized and clearly resectable should demonstrate the following: (1) no distant metastases, (2) no radiographic evidence of SMV or portal vein distortion, and (3) clear fat plane around the celiac axis, hepatic axis, and SMA. Splenic vein involvement is permissible (Network NCC 2013; Callery et al. 2009).
  - Tumors considered to be borderline resectable have the following: (1) no distant metastases; (2) venous involvement of the SMV or portal vein with distortion or narrowing of the vein or occlusion of the vein with suitable vessel proximal and distal, allowing for safe resection and replacement; (3) gastroduodenal artery encasement up to the hepatic artery with either short-segment encasement or direct abutment of the hepatic artery, without extension to the celiac axis; and (4) tumor abutment of the celiac axis or SMA not to exceed greater than 180° of circumference of the vessel wall (Network NCC 2013; Callery et al. 2009).
  - Unresectable disease is usually characterized by one or more of the following features: (1) distant metastasis or extensive peripancreatic lymph node involvement, (2) encasement or occlusion of the SMV or SMV/portal confluence, and (3) direct involvement of the SMA, inferior vena cava, aorta, or celiac axis (Network NCC 2013; Callery et al. 2009).

# 4 Locally Advanced, Unresectable Pancreatic Adenocarcinoma

## 4.1 General Points

- While radiation therapy remains controversial, it is often considered the only definitive option for patients with locally advanced unresectable pancreatic adenocarcinoma.
- The principles of radiotherapy in patients undergoing neoadjuvant and definitive radiation are similar.
- Intensity-modulated radiation therapy (IMRT) is becoming the standard technique for definitive or neoadjuvant radiation therapy for locally advanced and borderline resectable pancreatic adenocarcinoma and is preferred over three-dimensional chemoradiation therapy (3D-CRT), given that it is associated with less treatment-related toxicity (decreased nausea, vomiting, and diarrhea) (Yovino et al. 2011).
- Depending on patient anatomy and tumor location, treatment recommendations can include conventionally fractionated IMRT or stereotactic body radiation therapy (SBRT).
  - Ideal candidates for SBRT are those with tumors <5 cm without abutment of adjacent critical organs such as the stomach, liver, non-duodenal small bowel, and large bowel.

## 5 Conventionally Fractionated Chemoradiation Therapy for Unresectable Pancreatic Adenocarcinoma

### 5.1 Simulation and Daily Localization

- Motion management should be considered for patients being treated with definitive chemoradiation for locally advanced unresectable pancreatic adenocarcinoma given the significant tumor and normal tissue motion with respiration.
- Motion management may be addressed by several techniques, including respiratory gating, breath hold (active breathing control [ABC]), respiratory tracking, or abdominal compression.
- For patients treated with motion-management techniques, fiducial markers should be placed prior to simulation (preferably at least 5 days prior to simulation due to the possibility of migration) to assist in motion management using percutaneous, intraoperative, or endoscopic techniques.
- CT simulation with oral and IV contrast (unless contraindicated) should be performed to help guide the gross tumor volume (GTV) target as well as lymph node coverage.
  - Patients are generally asked not to eat any large meals 2–3 h prior to simulation and treatment to avoid significant interfraction variation in stomach distention.
- Arms should be above the head in the alpha cradle, with oral and IV contrast.
  - Planning scan should be obtained using pancreatic protocol (minimum of 3 mm cuts) with a scan from carina to iliac crest.
  - If using respiratory gating or breath-hold technique for motion management, the planning scan should be performed during a breath hold at end expiration using voice coaching.
  - For patients treated with respiratory gating or without a specific motion-management technique, a four-dimensional (4D) CT is necessary to evaluate the degree of tumor motion. The motion can be accounted for with an internal target volume or can guide the gating interval for patients undergoing respiratory gating.
- Typical anatomic landmarks that can help in guiding clinical target volume (CTV) delineation include:
  - Pancreas generally lying at L1–L2
  - Celiac axis generally lying at T12
  - SMA generally lying at L1

### 5.2 Target Volume Delineation and Treatment Planning

- The GTV is contoured on the treatment-planning expiratory phase CT after reviewing the diagnostic CT, respiratory-correlated 4D-CT, pancreas protocol CT, PET-CT, and/or MR abdomen if applicable.
- The CTV includes a 1 cm expansion off the GTV and should encompass all relevant nodal regions (Table 1).
- Lymph node coverage
  - Head/neck/proximal body lesions
    - Pancreaticoduodenal, suprapancreatic, porta hepatis, celiac, superior mesenteric, and para-aortic lymph nodes at the level of the tumor and/or celiac axis/SMA

**Table 1** Target volumes

| Target volumes | Definition and description |
|---|---|
| GTV | Consists of the hypodense area in the pancreas, if visible, corresponding to biopsy-proven disease, and any positive lymph nodes visualized on diagnostic pancreatic protocol CT, parenchyma, or portal-venous phase. The tumor may be isointense with the normal pancreas, and it may be difficult to distinguish the tumor boundaries. In addition, pancreatic tumors tend to be highly infiltrative, and extrapancreatic spread may appear as soft tissue encasement of the adjacent vessels or even just soft tissue stranding in the abdominal fat. Consultation with a diagnostic radiologist may aid in determining the extent of the GTV (GTV should be contoured on the IV-contrast planning scan in the end-expiration phase) |
| CTV | The CTV encompasses all relevant nodal regions including the porta hepatis, celiac/SMA, and PA/RP lymph nodes approximately from the top of T11 to bottom of L2, but may often be smaller than this and should be adjusted based on location of primary tumor; the superior–inferior extent is primarily determined by overlapping coverage of the appropriate nodal regions and tumor location. The CTV should also include areas of subclinical direct tumor extension. In general, the GTV is also expanded by 1 cm; this expansion is then added to the nodal CTV |
| PTV | Expansion on the CTV by 5 mm (receives 5,040 cGy in 180 cGy fractions) |
| PTV boost | Expansion on the GTV by 3–5 mm margin, shrinking the margin to <3 mm to minimize overlap with the duodenum. Note that this is an integrated boost guideline based on Memorial Sloan Kettering Cancer Center standard practice, and the PTV boost receives 5,600 cGy in 200 cGy fractions |

- Distal body/tail lesions
  - Pancreaticoduodenal, suprapancreatic, splenic hilar, celiac, superior mesenteric, and para-aortic lymph nodes at the level of the tumor and celiac axis/SMA
- If using respiratory gating, plan on expiratory breath-hold scan first and assess the motion of implanted fiducial markers with 4D-CT scan.
  - Adjust CTV and planning target volume (PTV) for motion >5 mm, whereas if tumor motion on 4D-CT is <5 mm, no change in volumes is needed.
  - Delivery of treatment with respiratory gating usually occurs during end expiration (30–70 % respiratory phases, where 50 % represents end expiration using the Varian Real-Time Position Management (RPM) system (Varian Medical Systems, Inc. Palo Alto, CA, USA)) (Figs. 2 and 3).

## 5.3 Plan Assessment

**Table 2** Intensity-modulated radiation therapy: normal tissue dose constraints

| Organ at risk | Constraints |
|---|---|
| Liver | Mean dose <25 Gy, V20<30 % |
| Kidney | V18<33 %, V15<30 % (each kidney evaluated separately) |
| Cord | $D_{max}$ <40 Gy |
| Stomach | Mean dose <30 Gy (stomach excluding PTV) |
| Small bowel | $D_{max}$ =prescription dose, D5% <45 Gy (bowel is contoured 2 cm superior and inferior to PTV) |
| Duodenum | $D_{max}$ < global maximum dose, D5% <54 Gy |
| Heart | V15<30 %, mean dose <30 Gy |

Based on guidelines presently used at Memorial Sloan Kettering Cancer Center
*PTV* planning target volume

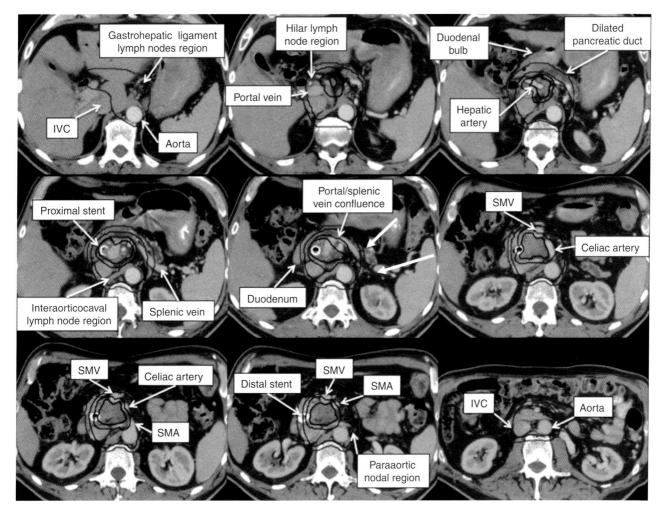

**Fig. 2** A patient with T4N0 unresectable pancreatic adenocarcinoma with a 5 cm mass in the pancreatic head, extensive compression of the main portal vein, encasement of the common hepatic and gastroduodenal arteries, and abutment of the celiac, proper hepatic, and superior mesenteric artery. Patient was simulated with 4DCT, with 2.5 mm slice thickness on each slice. GTV is in *red*, CTV is in *blue*, PTV5040 is in *green*, and PTV5600 is in *pink*. Please note that these are representative slices, and not all slices are included. *IVC* inferior vena cava, *SMA* superior mesenteric artery, *SMV* superior mesenteric vein

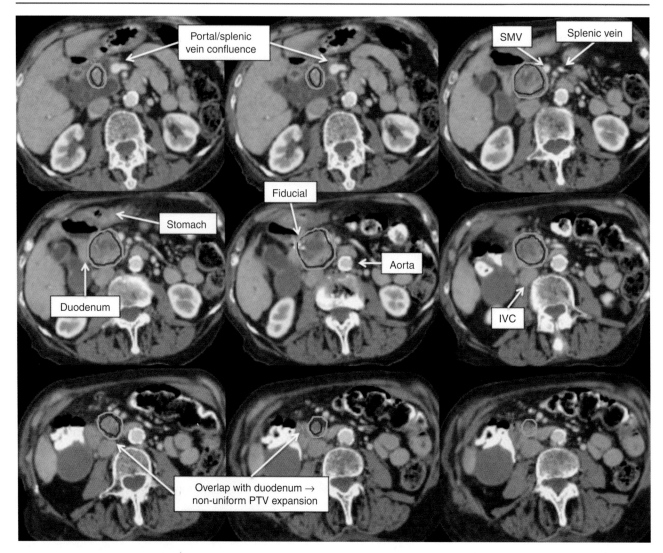

**Fig. 3** A patient with T3N0 borderline resectable pancreatic adenocarcinoma with a 3.1 cm mass in the inferior pancreatic head and uncinate process obstructing the pancreatic duct and common bile duct. The tumor contacted the superior mesenteric vein with 120-° involvement at the level of the first jejunal branch. The tumor also contacted the gastric antrum and the first and second parts of the duodenum. The patient underwent a CT simulation, with 2 mm slice thickness, with abdominal compression. GTV is in red and PTV 3,300 cGy is in green. Please note that these are representative slices, and not all slices are included. *IVC* inferior vena cava, *SMV* superior mesenteric vein

## 6 Stereotactic Body Radiotherapy for Unresectable Pancreatic Adenocarcinoma

### 6.1 Simulation and Daily Localization

- Fiducial markers should be placed prior to simulation, preferably at least 5 days prior to simulation, to assist in motion management using percutaneous, intraoperative, or endoscopic techniques.
- Motion management may be addressed using respiratory gating, breath hold (ABC), respiratory tracking, or abdominal compression.
- In patients being planned for abdominal compression, fluoroscopic evaluation of tumor motion and patient tolerance is recommended prior to simulation.

- Pre-abdominal compression fluoroscopy should be used to evaluate tumor motion with regular breathing.
- The abdominal compression belt should be insufflated until the tumor motion is less than 5 mm.
- Tattoos are placed on the patient to note the belt position and allow reproducible setup.
- The belt size, belt location, belt girth, and belt pressure should be recorded to facilitate reproducible setup.
- If discomfort and anxiety render the patient unable to tolerate abdominal compression, alternative motion-management techniques such as respiratory gating, breath hold, or respiratory tracking should be employed.
  - It is important to note that the use of image-guided techniques for SBRT will prolong patient time on

the treatment table and will likely be significantly longer than for conventionally fractionated chemoradiation therapy. As such, the patient's ability to tolerate setup and immobilization is of critical importance.

- PET-CT simulation with IV contrast (unless contraindicated) should be performed to help guide the GTV target delineation as well as design lymph node coverage.
  - Arms should be above the head in the alpha cradle, with oral and IV contrast (generally 100 cm$^3$ Omnipaque), 4D-CT pancreatic protocol with scan from carina to iliac crest.
    - We generally recommend 2 mm slice thickness for SBRT plans.
  - The abdominal compression belt should be in place and insufflated to the appropriate pressure to ensure accuracy of treatment planning.
  - Patients are generally asked not to eat any large meals 2–3 h prior to simulation and treatment, though if getting a PET-CT simulation, they should have nothing by mouth for 6 h prior to scan per PET protocol.
- The CT simulation images will be used throughout the treatment course as the reference images to which the daily cone-beam CT is compared. The reproducibility of the abdominal compression belt is critical to ensure the accuracy of the treatment plan. Even a 3 cm change in separation can result in significant changes in dose delivery.

## 6.2 Target Volume Delineation and Treatment Planning

- The GTV is contoured on the treatment-planning CT after reviewing the diagnostic CT, respiratory-correlated 4D-CT, pancreas protocol CT, PET-CT, and/or MR abdomen as applicable.
  - Maximum standardized uptake value (SUV$_{max}$) has been demonstrated to correlate with overall and progression-free survival in patients undergoing SBRT for locally advanced pancreatic adenocarcinoma (Schellenberg et al. 2010).
- The GTV will be expanded 3–5 mm to a final PTV, except if the margin results in expansion into the duodenum or stomach; it is permitted to limit the margin expansion at these critical structures to avoid overlap.
- Contours of the fiducial makers with a 3 mm uniform expansion for target localization on applicable image sets should be generated for use in patient setup on treatment.
- The duodenum is contoured as an independent organ at risk, and the small bowel organ at risk only includes the jejunum and ileum.
  - After 25 Gy×1, grade 2–4 duodenal toxicity approached 30 % at 12 months with a median time of

6.3 months from end of RT to observed duodenal toxicity. Retrospective review correlated the duodenal V10–V25 and D$_{max}$ with duodenal toxicity (Murphy et al. 2010).

- At Memorial Sloan Kettering Cancer Center, we generally treat to 33 Gy in 6.6 Gy fractions every other day, with the dose prescribed to the isodose line that completely surrounds the PTV.
  - There are no established standards for SBRT dose and fractionation. Dose and fractionation schedules reported in the literature range from 25 Gy in 1 fraction to 30 Gy in 3 fractions.
  - As toxicity is still a major concern associated with SBRT, we have adopted a less aggressive dose and fractionation schedule with good results and acceptable toxicity in a phase II multi-institutional trial (Dholakia et al. 2013).
- For LINAC-based treatment, the use of IMRT is strongly preferred with 6–12 coplanar fields or volumetric modulated arc therapy. Forward planning with noncoplanar beam arrangement is permissible for patients treated with Cyberknife.

**Table 3** Target volumes

| Target volumes | Definition and description |
|---|---|
| GTV | Consists of the hypodense area and fluorodeoxyglucose-avid disease corresponding to biopsy-proven disease in the pancreas visualized on diagnostic pancreatic protocol CT and arterial phase (contoured on expiration phase planning CT) |
| CTV | None |
| PTV | Expansion on the GTV by 2–3 mm with a nonuniform expansion to prevent overlap of the PTV with the stomach or duodenum |

**Table 4** Stereotactic body radiotherapy: normal tissue dose constraints

| Organ at risk | Constraints |
|---|---|
| Liver | V12 < 50 % |
| Kidney | V12 < 25 % (both kidneys combined) |
| Cord | V8 < 1 cm$^3$ |
| Stomach | V33 < 1 cm$^3$, V20 < 3 cm$^3$, V15 < 9 cm$^3$, V12 < 50 % |
| Duodenum | V33 < 1 cm$^3$, V20 < 3 cm$^3$, V15 < 9 cm$^3$, V12 < 50 % |
| Bowel not duodenum | V20 < 5 cm$^3$ (bowel is contoured 2 cm superior and inferior to PTV) |

Based on guidelines presently used at Memorial Sloan Kettering Cancer Center
*PTV* planning target volume

## 6.3 Plan Assessment

- No more than 1 cm$^3$ of PTV can receive >130 % prescription dose, and greater than 90 % of PTV should receive 100 % of prescription dose.

## 7 Adjuvant (Postoperative) Chemoradiation for Resectable Pancreatic Adenocarcinoma

### 7.1 General Points

- While the role of adjuvant therapy remains debated, many centers, including ours, favor adjuvant CRT. Our general approach is for adjuvant chemotherapy followed by restaging, as approximately 30 % of patients will develop metastatic disease in this period. In patients with no evidence of metastases, we generally recommend adjuvant CRT. Given the controversy surrounding adjuvant treatment recommendations and conflicting studies, we generally prefer to treat these patients on protocol.

### 7.2 Simulation and Daily Localization

- Ensure placement of operative clips, which may be used to assist in motion management.
- If gross recurrent disease is present, consider referral for fiducial marker placement prior to simulation.
- Motion management may be addressed using respiratory gating, breath hold (ABC), respiratory tracking, or abdominal compression.
- CT simulation with oral and IV contrast (unless contraindicated) should be performed to help guide the GTV target as well as lymph node coverage.
  - Arms should be above the head in the alpha cradle, with oral and IV contrast (generally 100 cm$^3$ Omnipaque), 4D-CT pancreatic protocol, with 3 mm slice thickness, with scan from carina to iliac crest.
  - If using respiratory gating, plan on end-expiration scan and assess motion of surgical clips and/or implanted fiducial markers with 4D-CT scan.

### 7.3 General Principles of Planning and Target Delineation

- IMRT has become a standard technique for delivery of adjuvant radiation therapy for pancreatic adenocarcinoma in the postoperative setting (Yovino et al. 2011).
- A common site for positive surgical margins and local recurrence is the retroperitoneal/uncinate/SMV margin.
- Preoperative imaging should be obtained to facilitate contouring of the tumor bed; in addition, postoperative imaging is used to evaluate the surgical bed. Nonmetastatic patients with recurrent disease are considered for a boost, either as an integrated boost with IMRT dose painting or as a cone-down field.

### 7.4 Target Volume Delineation and Treatment Planning

- Generally there is no GTV, unless the patient has recurrent disease.
- The CTV is the area with the highest likelihood for residual subclinical tumor. The goal is to identify an area that can be safely treated with radiotherapy without resulting in a treatment volume that includes an excessive amount of normal organs at risk.
- It is imperative to review the preoperative imaging, operative notes, and surgical pathology report at the time of treatment planning.
- Comprehensive guidelines for the contouring of adjuvant pancreatic adenocarcinoma have been published by the Radiation Therapy Oncology Group (RTOG) (Goodman et al. 2012).
- For the pancreaticojejunostomy or pancreaticogastrostomy, refer to operative notes to confirm their presence and assist in identification on the postoperative planning CT. The hepaticojejunostomy, SMA, and celiac artery, aorta, portal vein, and preoperative tumor bed should be identified on the planning CT. The pancreaticojejunostomy usually is readily identified by following the pancreatic remnant medially and anteriorly until the junction with the jejunal loop is noted; a similar technique can be used to identify the pancreaticogastrostomy if present. The hepaticojejunostomy may be more difficult to identify, but by following air in the biliary tree to the common hepatic duct or common bile duct remnant to the jejunal loop, or by following the portal vein out of the liver to the jejunal loop region, the hepaticojejunostomy can often be identified. The goal is to identify the junction of the common bile duct remnant and the jejunal loop, not to include the entire hepatic hilum or a large volume of jejunum.
- The RTOG contouring guidelines, summarized in Table 5, provide specific expansions on these normal structures with the goal of creating a CTV that includes the high-risk pancreatic bed and high-risk lymph node regions including the para-aorta, celiac, superior mesenteric, and porta hepatis lymph nodes. In patients with pancreatic body/tail tumors, the splenic hilar remnant is covered in lieu of the porta hepatis (Goodman et al. 2012).
- The significance of surgical clips placed intraoperatively can vary. At times clips are placed for purposes of delineating areas of concern intraoperatively. These should be included in the CTV if there is documentation in the operative report (or via direct communication with the operating surgeon) that these were intentionally placed to aid in treatment planning (Figs. 4, 5, and 6).

**Table 5** Target volumes

| Target volumes | Definition and description |
|---|---|
| GTV (if applicable) | Positive lymph nodes and/or positive margin region (based on operative report and pathology report) visualized on pancreatic protocol planning CT scan (arterial phase, contour on expiration phase if using 4DCT), or any targetable residual and/or recurrent disease |
| CTV | The CTV includes the para-aortic nodes (Ao), pancreaticojejunostomy (PJ), portal vein segment (PV), superior mesenteric artery (SMA), celiac artery (CA), and the postoperative bed (Postop) |
| | Ao extends from the top of the uppermost PV, CA, or SMA slice to the bottom of L2 or L3 if there is a low-lying tumor |
| | PJ usually is identified by following the pancreatic remnant medially and anteriorly until the junction with the jejunal loop is noted |
| | PV is the portion of the vein running anterior and medial to the IVC and stops prior to the confluence of the SMV or splenic vein |
| | SMA is the proximal 2.5–3.0 cm of the vessel |
| | CA is the most proximal 1.0–1.5 cm of the vessel |
| | Postop is the area occupied by the tumor on preoperative scans |
| | Ao is expanded 2.5 cm to the right, 1 cm to the left, 0.2 cm posteriorly, and 2 cm anteriorly; PJ, PV, SMA, CA, and Postop are generally expanded by 1 cm; these two expansions are then added to make the CTV, which is then adjusted to ensure coverage of the draining nodal regions while limiting overlap with the kidneys |
| | *Special case*: the above guidelines are for pancreatic head lesions; in the setting of a tail lesion, the porta hepatis can be omitted |
| PTV5040 | Expansion on the CTV by 5 mm (receives 5040 cGy in 180 cGy fractions) |
| PTV boost (if applicable) | Expansion on the GTV by a 3–5 mm margin (receives 5,600 cGy in 200 cGy fractions via integrated boost at MSKCC), minimize overlap with bowel |

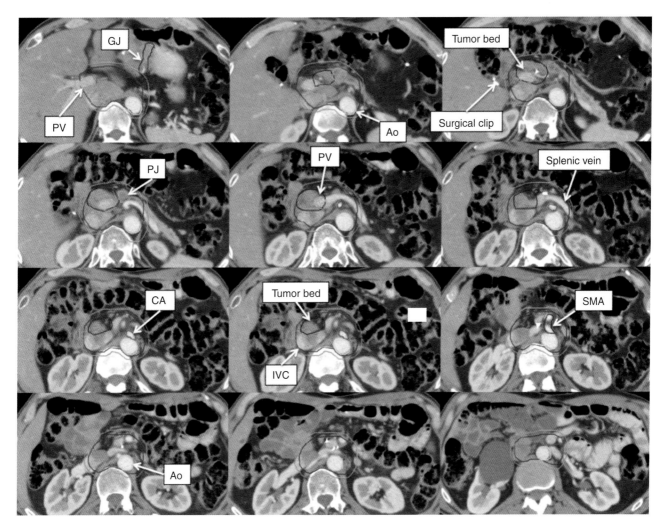

**Fig. 4** Postoperative case: a patient with pT1N1 resected pancreatic adenocarcinoma with a 1.8 cm lesion in the head of the pancreas, positive distal surgical margin, and 3/13 nodes positive for involvement. Images below show PTV in *green*, CTV in *blue*, and postoperative bed in *red*. Relevant structures including the pancreaticojejunostomy (*PJ*), aorta (*Ao*), celiac artery (*CA*), superior mesenteric artery (*SMA*), gastrojejunostomy (*GJ*), and portal vein (*PV*) are labeled. The GJ should not be included in the CTV. Please note that these are representative slices, and not all slices are included. *IVC* inferior vena cava, *SMA* superior mesenteric artery

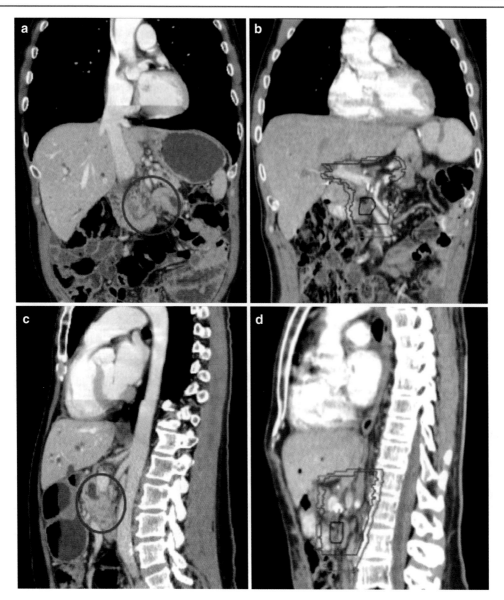

**Fig. 5** Postoperative case, example of low-lying tumor: a patient with pT3N1 resected pancreatic adenocarcinoma with a 2.3 cm lesion in the head/uncinate, close <1 mm margins posteriorly and inferiorly, and 14/25 nodes positive for involvement. (**a**) Coronal preoperative CT with tumor marked in *red*; (**b**) coronal planning images with PTV in *green*, CTV in *blue*, and postoperative bed in *red*; (**c**) sagittal preoperative CT with tumor marked in *red*; (**d**) sagittal planning images with PTV in *green*, CTV in *blue*, and postoperative bed in *red*; (**e**) axial preoperative CT with tumor marked in *red*; (**f–h**) axial planning images with PTV in *green*, CTV in *blue*, and postoperative bed in *red*

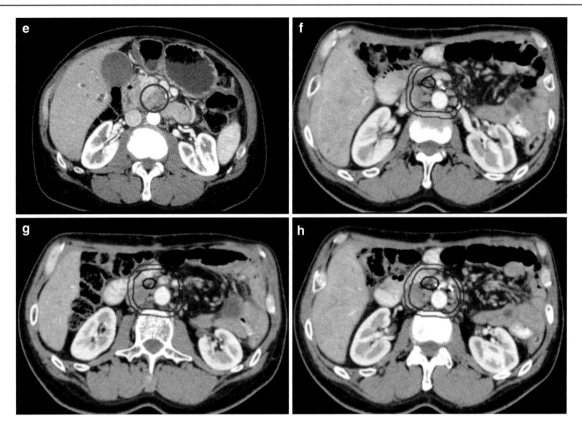

**Fig. 5** (continued)

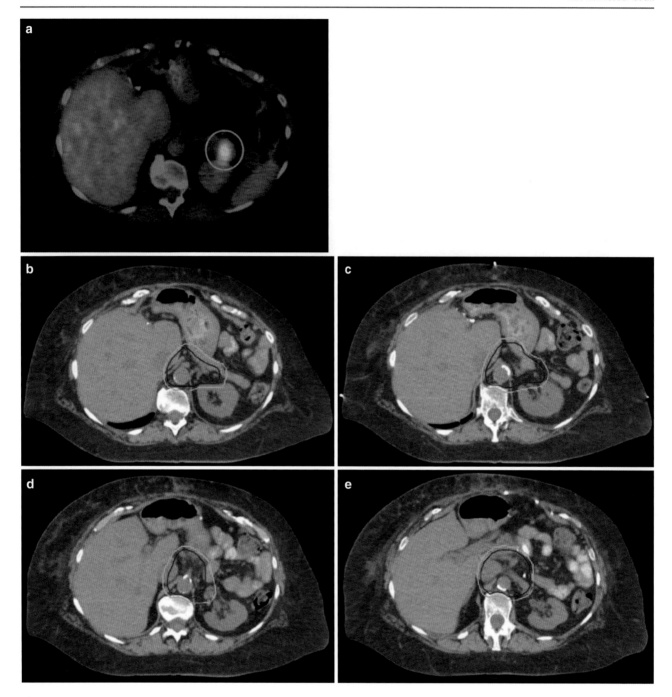

**Fig. 6** Postoperative case, example of a distal pancreatic cancer: a patient with stage IIA (pT3N0) pancreatic adenocarcinoma, 2.5 cm lesion in pancreatic tail with+PNI/VI and negative margins, 0/9 nodes involved. (**a**) Preoperative positron-emission tomography-computed tomography (PET–CT) scan showing fluorodeoxyglucose-avid pancreatic tail lesion; (**b–e**) planning images show PTV in *green*, CTV in *blue*, showing coverage of postoperative bed, splenic hilar lymph nodes, para-aortic nodes, and celiac/SMA nodes. Note that this patient was unable to receive iodinated contrast due to allergy, so the disease was characterized with PET; comparison of this patient's vessels to the patients shown in II.2 and II.1 illustrates the importance of IV contrast in defining the vessels on which the CTV is based

## 7.5 Plan Assessment

**Table 6** Intensity-modulated radiation therapy: normal tissue dose constraints

| Organ at risk | Constraints |
|---|---|
| Liver | Mean dose <25 Gy, V20<30 % |
| Kidney | V18<33 %, V15<30 % (each kidney evaluated separately) |
| Cord | $D_{max}$ <45 Gy |
| Stomach | $D_{max}$ <54 Gy, mean dose <30 Gy |
| Bowel | $D_{max}$ <54 Gy, D15% <45 Gy (bowel is contoured 2 cm superior and inferior to PTV) |
| Heart | V30<20 %, mean dose <30 Gy |

Based on guidelines presently used at Memorial Sloan Kettering Cancer Center and Radiation Therapy Oncology Group (RTOG) 0848

## Suggested Reading

Goodman KA, Regine WF, Dawson LA et al (2012) Radiation Therapy Oncology Group consensus panel guidelines for the delineation of the clinical target volume in the postoperative treatment of pancreatic head cancer. Int J Radiat Oncol Biol Phys 83:901–908

Yovino S, Poppe M, Jabbour S et al (2011) Intensity-modulated radiation therapy significantly improves acute gastrointestinal toxicity in pancreatic and ampullary cancers. Int J Radiat Oncol Biol Phys 79:158–162

## References

Berger AC, Garcia M Jr, Hoffman JP et al (2008) Postresection CA 19–9 predicts overall survival in patients with pancreatic cancer treated with adjuvant chemoradiation: a prospective validation by RTOG 9704. J Clin Oncol 26:5918–5922

Callery MP, Chang KJ, Fishman EK et al (2009) Pretreatment assessment of resectable and borderline resectable pancreatic cancer: expert consensus statement. Ann Surg Oncol 16:1727–1733

Dholakia AS, Chang DT, Goodman KA et al (2013) A phase II multicenter study to evaluate gemcitabine and fractionated stereotactic body radiotherapy for locally advanced pancreatic adenocarcinoma. Accepted for oral presentation at the ASTRO annual meeting, Atlanta, GA.

Edge SB, Byrd DR, Compton CC et al (eds) (2010) AJCC cancer staging manual, 7th edn. Springer, Chicago

Goodman KA, Regine WF, Dawson LA et al (2012) Radiation Therapy Oncology Group consensus panel guidelines for the delineation of the clinical target volume in the postoperative treatment of pancreatic head cancer. Int J Radiat Oncol Biol Phys 83:901–908

Iacobuzio-Donahue CA, Fu B, Yachida S et al (2009) DPC4 gene status of the primary carcinoma correlates with patterns of failure in patients with pancreatic cancer. J Clin Oncol 27:1806–1813

Murphy JD, Christman-Skieller C, Kim J et al (2010) A dosimetric model of duodenal toxicity after stereotactic body radiotherapy for pancreatic cancer. Int J Radiat Oncol Biol Phys 78:1420–1426

National Comprehensive Cancer (NCC) Network (2013) NCCN Clinical Practice Guidelines in Oncology: Pancreatic Adenocarcinoma Verison 1.2013

Niederhuber JE, Armitage JO, Doroshow JH et al (eds) (2014) Abeloff's clinical oncology. Elsevier/Churchill Livingstone, Philadelphia

Schellenberg D, Quon A, Minn AY et al (2010) 18Fluorodeoxyglucose PET is prognostic of progression-free and overall survival in locally advanced pancreas cancer treated with stereotactic radiotherapy. Int J Radiat Oncol Biol Phys 77:1420–1425

Strandring S (ed) (2005) Gray's anatomy: the anatomical basis of clinical practice, 39th edn. Elsevier/Churchill Livingstone, New York

Yovino S, Poppe M, Jabbour S et al (2011) Intensity-modulated radiation therapy significantly improves acute gastrointestinal toxicity in pancreatic and ampullary cancers. Int J Radiat Oncol Biol Phys 79:158–162

# Hepatocellular Carcinoma and Cholangiocarcinoma

Jason Chia-Hsien Cheng, Chia-Chun Wang,
Inigo San Miguel, and Laura A. Dawson

## Contents

J.C.-H. Cheng, MD, PhD (✉)
Graduate Institute of Oncology,
National Taiwan University College of Medicine,
Taipei, Taiwan

Division of Radiation Oncology, Department of Oncology,
National Taiwan University Hospital, Taipei, Taiwan
e-mail: jasoncheng@ntu.edu.tw

C.-C. Wang, MD (✉)
Division of Radiation Oncology, Department of Oncology,
National Taiwan University Hospital, Taipei, Taiwan
e-mail: chiachun@ntuh.gov.tw

I.S. Miguel, MD • L.A. Dawson, MD, FRCPC
Department of Radiation Oncology,
Princess Margaret Cancer Centre, University of Toronto,
Toronto, ON, Canada

# 1    Hepatocellular Carcinoma

## 1.1    General Principles of Planning and Target Delineation

- Three-dimensional conformal radiation therapy (3DCRT) has been the standard technique for hepatocellular carcinoma (HCC). Intensity-modulated radiation therapy (IMRT) may be useful to improve target coverage and for normal organ sparing, especially in the setting of unusually shaped target volumes. More recently, stereotactic body radiation therapy (SBRT) has been increasingly used. Individualized prescription doses are commonly used due to variable liver volume irradiation and proximity to luminal gastrointestinal tissues.

- In addition to a history and physical exam, laboratory examinations, a liver function assessment, and imaging studies should be obtained for diagnosis, staging, and planning. Patients should undergo a contrast-enhanced (preferably triphasic [arterial, portal-venous, and delayed phases]) computed tomography (CT) scan of the liver, with 3–5 mm slice thickness. Multiphase dynamic magnetic resonance imaging (MRI) scans can be used if CT contrast is contraindicated. Additionally, MRI scans may be complimentary to CT scans for target delineation. 18F-fluorodeoxyglucose (18F-FDG) positron emission tomography (PET) images may be helpful in localizing the viable tumor(s) of individual cases such as patients with recurrent tumor(s) at previous lipiodol retention and/or radiofrequency ablation areas.

- Half-body or whole-body immobilization with respiratory control is needed for better reproducibility. Devices

N.Y. Lee et al. (eds.), *Target Volume Delineation for Conformal and Intensity-Modulated Radiation Therapy*,
Medical Radiology. Radiation Oncology, DOI: 10.1007/174_2014_978, © Springer International Publishing Switzerland 2014
Published Online: 4 November 2014

such as a vacuum bag or chest board may be used to immobilize a patient, preferably with arms up, during simulation and used throughout the course of treatment. This will enable reproducibility and allow spatial freedom of beam directions. The systems for respiratory coordination should be made of materials not attenuating radiation doses and should not interfere with the gantry positions that may be required for coplanar and noncoplanar beams.

- Respiratory motion management using a number of techniques is frequently needed to minimize imaging artifacts from changes in liver position due to breathing (e.g., active breath hold, abdominal compression). Delineation of target volumes is most often done on multiphasic, multimodality imaging, obtained in breath hold (i.e., similar to diagnostic imaging for HCC). Image-guided radiation therapy (IGRT) is required to account for changes in the liver position day to day. In patients who cannot tolerate active breath control, the use of abdominal compression devices with four-dimensional computed tomography (4DCT) provides information about internal organ motion and can compensate for liver position changes. Gated treatment may also be useful for patients that cannot tolerate breath control.

- CT simulation with IV contrast to obtain multiphase imaging is required. This should be obtained with the patient in the treatment position. Fusion of the different phase imaging and/or diagnostic images will aid in the delineation of the gross tumor volume (GTV). Usually the viable HCC is best visualized (brightest) on the arterial-phase CT scan, with less enhancement seen relative to the liver on venous- and delayed-phase imaging. Tumor invasion into the vascular structures (e.g., portal vein or inferior vena cava) is often best observed on either portal-venous- or delayed-venous-phase CT scans.

- Suggested target volumes for gross disease (GTV) and, in certain circumstances, clinical target volumes (CTV) for high-risk regions are detailed in Table 1 (CTV-macroscopic and CTV-microscopic) (Figs. 1, 2, 3, 4 and 5).

**Table 1** Suggest target volumes at the GTV and CTV regions

| Target volumes | Definition and description |
| --- | --- |
| GTV | Liver tumor: intrahepatic enhancing tumor on arterial-phase contrast CT with washout on venous- or delayed-phase CT |
| | Lipiodol-retaining tumor: lipiodol (white) contiguous to the enhancing tumor[d] |
| | Vascular tumor thrombus: arterial enhancing thrombus with washout on venous-phase CT |
| CTVmacroscopic[a] (optional according to clinical indication/protocol) | Liver tumor: the intrahepatic enhancing tumor on arterial-phase contrast CT |
| | Lipiodol-retaining tumor: TACE zone contiguous to the enhancing tumor included in GTV |
| | Enhancing tumor vascular thrombus |
| CTVmicroscopic (elective)[b] (optional according to clinical indication/protocol) | 3–5 mm margin around intrahepatic GTV[c] |
| | 2–3 mm margin around the tumor thrombus GTV within the vessel |
| | Bland thrombus adjacent to tumor thrombus GTV |
| | Radiofrequency ablation zone adjacent to the GTV |
| | TACE zone not directly adjacent to the GTV |
| | CTV should not cross natural barriers such as the surface of the liver |
| PTV | CTV (or GTV) + 5–20 mm (may be asymmetric), depending on immobilization and respiration control. The internal organ motion and the setup error form the basis of this margin. Four-dimensional computed tomography (4DCT) acquired from all respiratory phases may help define PTV and cover the extent of internal organ motion |

[a]Macroscopic/gross GTV. For example, to be treated to 39–54 Gy in 5 to 6 fractions. Note that the "safe" dose may need to be reduced if limited by normal tissues

[b]Elective/microscopic CTV (optional according to clinical indication/protocol). For example, to be treated to 27.5–30 Gy in 5 to 6 fractions

[c]The additional margin around the intrahepatic HCC may be treated to macroscopic/higher doses if safe

[d]18F-fluorodeoxyglucose (18F-FDG) positron emission tomography (PET) images may be helpful in the individual cases to localize the recurrent tumor(s) at lipiodol retention and/or radiofrequency ablation areas. Note that motion may lead to inaccurate GTV based on PET alone, and PET should only be used together with IV contrast CT and/or MRI

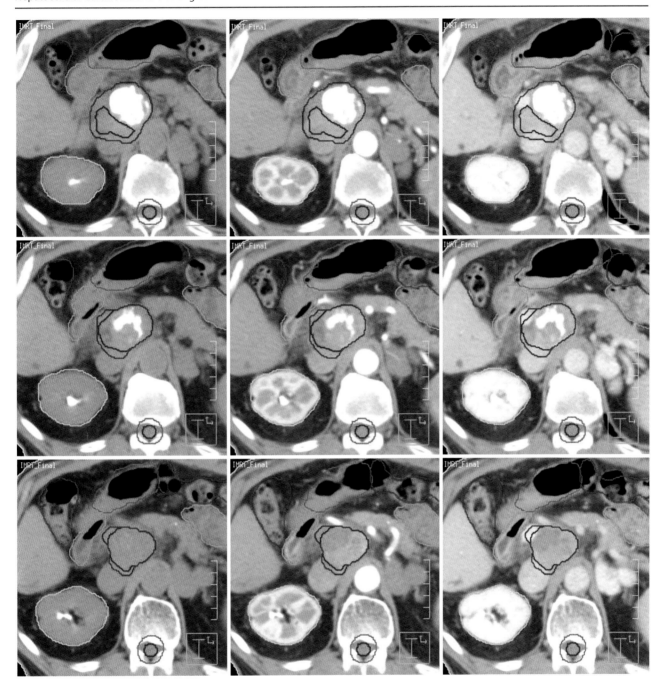

**Fig. 1** Transcatheter arterial chemoembolization (TACE) refractory hepatocellular carcinoma at the caudate lobe with viable tumor around the lipiodol. Selected slices from triphasic contrast-enhanced computed tomography simulation (from *left to right*: no contrast, arterial, and portal-venous phases), acquired by using active breath coordination for liver immobilization. The gross tumor volume (GTV) was shown in *purple*, and the clinical target volume (CTV) was shown in *red*

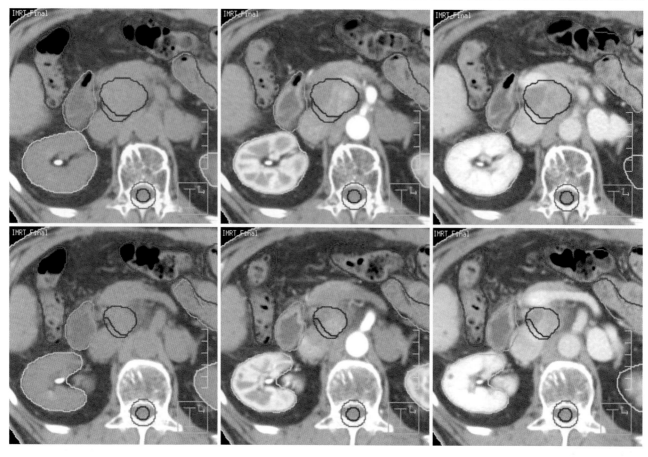

**Fig. 1** (continued)

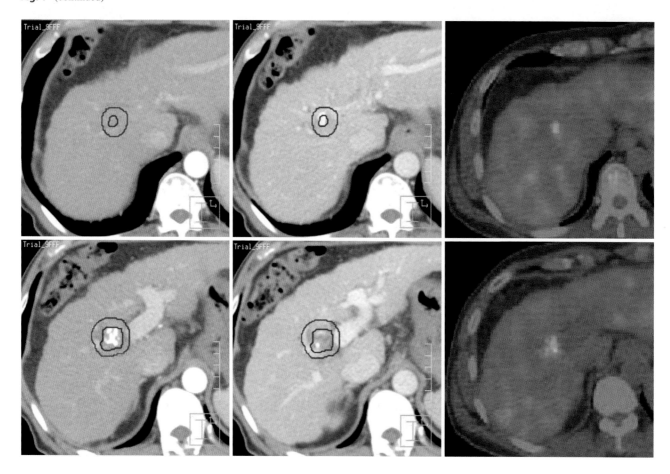

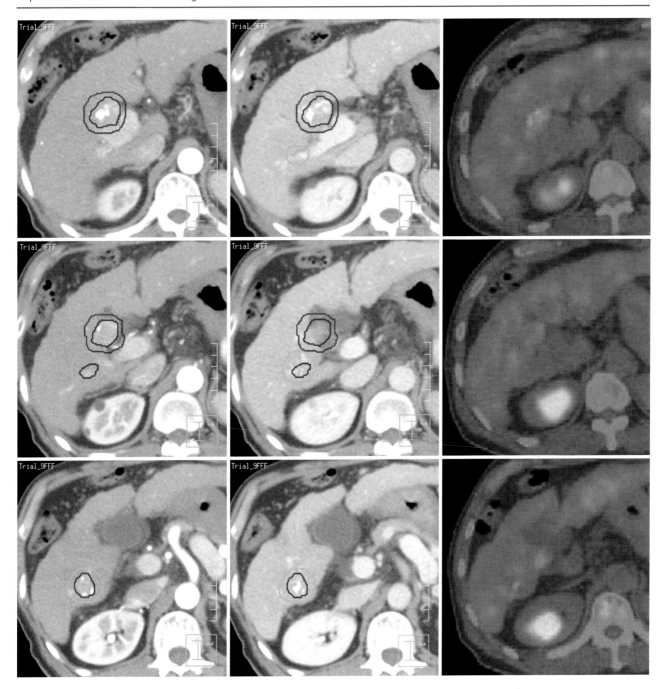

**Fig. 2** (continued)

**Fig. 2** Two viable tumors with partial lipiodol retention were found at S5/S8 and S5. The gross tumor volumes (GTVs) were shown in *purple* and *blue*, while the clinical target volumes (CTVs) were shown in *red* and *sky blue*, respectively. 18 F-fluorodeoxyglucose (18 F-FDG) positron emission tomography (PET) images were useful in delineating the viable tumor part. From *left to right*: arterial-phase computed tomography (CT) scan, portal-venous-phase CT scan, and PET

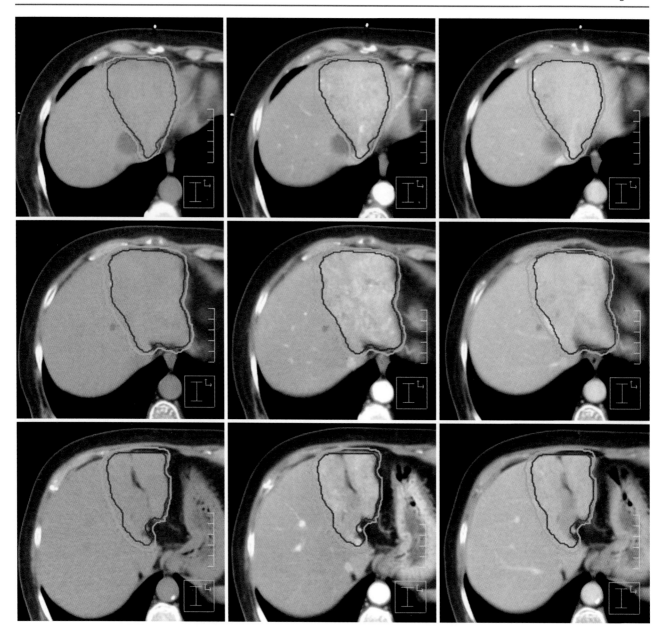

**Fig. 3** Infiltrative tumors occupying the left hepatic lobe were demonstrated with the tumor thrombi in the left portal vein (PV) and toward the right PV. The gross tumor volume (GTV) was shown in *red*, and the clinical target volume (CTV) was shown in *green*

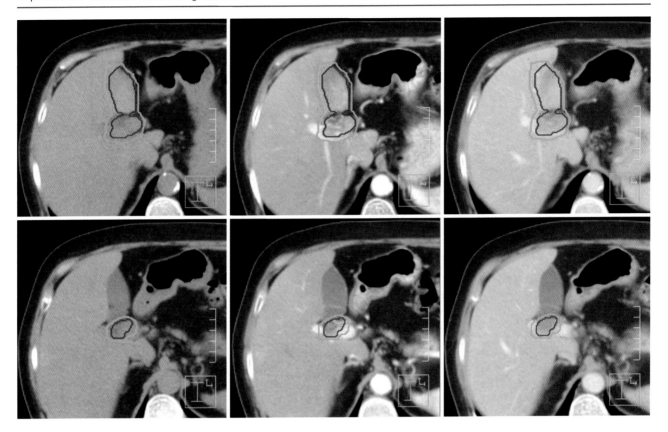

**Fig. 3** (continued)

Arterial CT        Venous CT        Venous MR

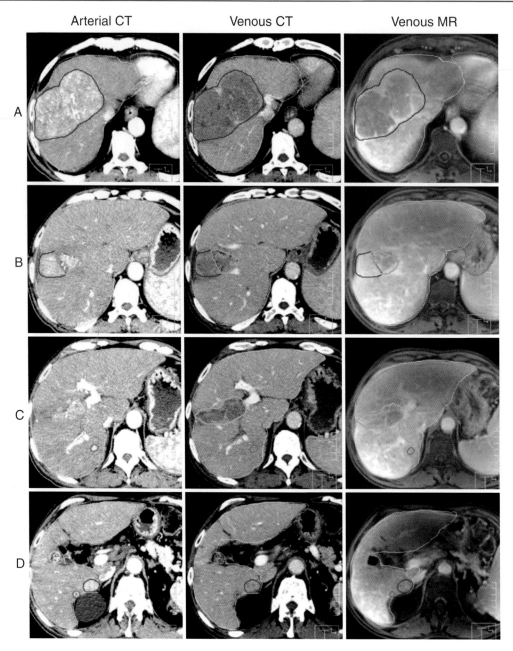

**Fig. 4** Multifocal HCC with tumor thrombosis involving the anterior segmental branch of the right portal vein, contoured as per RTOG1112 (https://www.ctsu.org). Contours are based on arterial-phase CT (*first column*), venous-phase CT (*second column*), and venous-phase MR (*third column*). Three hepatic parenchyma GTVs (GTVp) are shown in shades of *red*. The vascular tumor thrombus (GTVv) is shown in *green* in rows (**B**) and (**C**). There was no extra GTV to CTV margin. https://www.ctsu.org

Arterial CT          Venous CT          MR

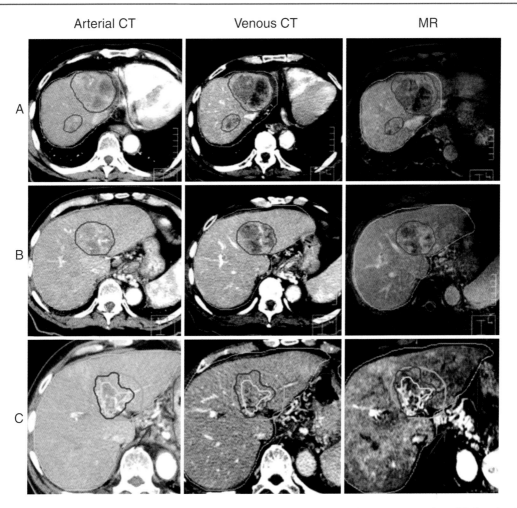

**Fig. 5** Biopsy-proven multifocal HCC with tumor thrombus in the left portal vein, contoured as per RTOG1112[1] https://www.ctsu.org. The HCC does not show classic enhancement in arterial-phase CT imaging (*first column*), but does demonstrate classic washout in venous-phase CT (*second column*) and venous-phase MR (*third column*). Parenchymal HCC GTVs are shown in *red*, and vascular HCC thrombus is shown in *green* (*row C*). Varices secondary to portal hypertension are shown with *red arrows* (*row C*). There was no extra GTV to CTV margin. In row C, the blue contour represents the PTV and the green is the covering iso-dose. https://www.ctsu.org

## 2    Intrahepatic Cholangiocarcinoma

### 2.1    General Principles of Planning and Target Delineation

- Radiation therapy is used in the definitive treatment for unresectable tumors and in the adjuvant treatment for resectable disease. Although the role of adjuvant radiotherapy remains controversial, it may be considered for patients with certain adverse risk factors such as involved resection margins.
- Three-dimensional conformal radiation therapy (3DCRT) or intensity-modulated radiation therapy (IMRT) should be used for treating cholangiocarcinoma. IMRT may have better dosimetric and clinical results. Stereotactic body radiation therapy (SBRT) for cholangiocarcinoma is under investigation. Image-guided radiation therapy (IGRT) is required to account for setup error and internal organ motion between fractionated treatments.
- Half-body or whole-body immobilization with respiratory motion management is needed for daily reproducibility. Acceptable techniques for respiratory

motion management include active breath hold, abdominal compression, four-dimensional computed tomography (4DCT), and gating.

- Delineation of target volumes is most often done with contrast-enhanced CT simulation images. This should be obtained with the patient in the treatment position and with the same respiratory motion management technique used during treatment. Fusion of different phase imaging modalities including magnetic resonance imaging (MRI) can help delineate the gross tumor volume (GTV).
- Cholangiocarcinoma frequently invades surrounding tissue directly. Lymph node metastasis in the porta hepatis, pancreaticoduodenal, common hepatic, and celiac regions has been reported, with an incidence up to 50–60 %. Tumors located at the perihilar area have a higher risk of lymph node metastasis.
- Suggested target volumes for gross disease (GTV) and high-risk regions (clinical target volume (CTV)-microscopic with/without CTV-lymphatics) are detailed in Table 2 (Figs. 6 and 7).

**Table 2**  Suggest target volumes at the GTV and CTV regions

| Target volumes | Definition and description |
|---|---|
| GTV (used in the definitive treatment) | Tumor shown on contrast-enhanced CT scan or magnetic resonance imaging (MRI) better with 18F-fluorodeoxyglucose (18F-FDG) positron emission tomography (PET) to delineate the tumor extent |
| CTV-microscopic | This CTV should not cross natural barriers such as the surface of the liver |
|  | (Used in the definitive treatment) GTV + 5~8 mm margin, with biliary system |
|  | (Used in the adjuvant treatment) tumor bed with possible extension to focal biliary system |
| CTV-lymphatics | May include the porta hepatis, pancreaticoduodenal, common hepatic, and celiac regions (strong consensus on including portal lymphatics electively, with more variability depending on the individual case for other nodal regions) |
| PTV | CTV + 5–20 mm (may be asymmetric), depending on immobilization and respiration control. The internal organ motion and the setup error form the basis of this margin. Four-dimensional computed tomography (4DCT) acquired from all respiratory phases may help define PTV and cover the extent of internal organ motion |

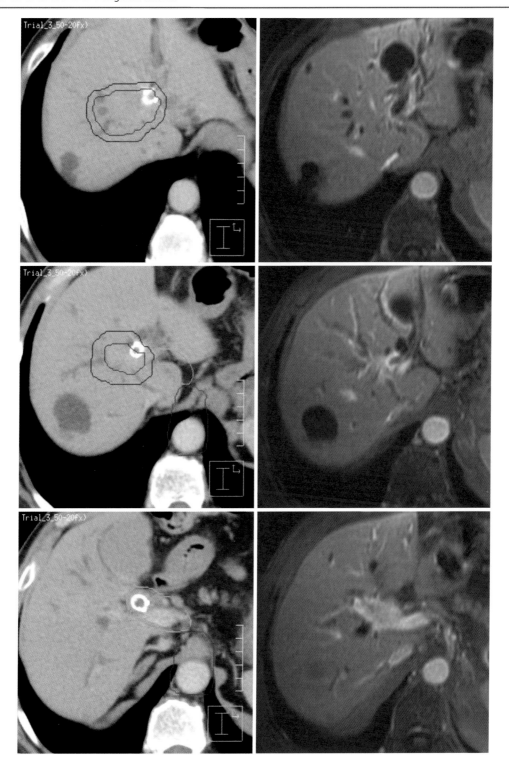

**Fig. 6** Infiltrative cholangiocarcinoma at the hepatic hilum, status post biliary stenting. The gross tumor volume (GTV) was shown in *red*, and the clinical target volume (CTV) was shown in *blue*. CTV-elective included the porta hepatis (shown in *green)* and the celiac region (shown in *purple*). Magnetic resonance imaging (MRI) images were helpful in delineating the tumor

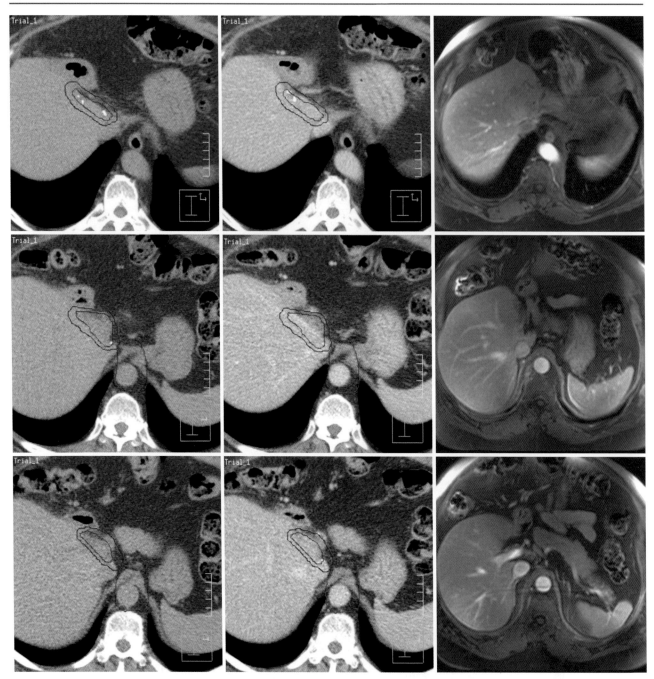

**Fig. 7** Adjuvant radiotherapy planned for an intrahepatic cholangio-carcinoma, status post left hepatectomy (S1,S2,S3,S4), pT2bNx, with involved parenchymal margin. The tumor bed was shown in *red*, and the clinical target volume (CTV) was shown in *blue*. CTV-elective included the porta hepatis (shown in *green*) and the celiac region (shown in *purple*). Magnetic resonance imaging (MRI) showed the original tumor location before surgery. From *left to right*: (**a**) non-contrast computed tomography (CT) scan, contrast-enhanced CT scan, and MRI. (**b**) non-contrast CT scan and contrast-enhanced CT scan

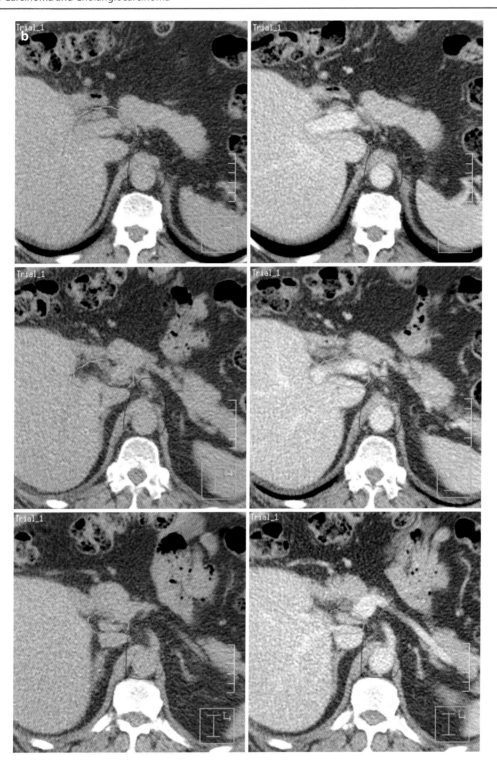

**Fig. 7** (continued)

## Further Reading

Bi AH et al (2010) Impact factors for microinvasion in intrahepatic cholangiocarcinoma: a possible system for defining clinical target volume. Int J Radiat Oncol Biol Phys 78:1427–1436

Cheng JC et al (2000) Local radiotherapy with or without transcatheter arterial chemoembolization for patients with unresectable hepatocellular carcinoma. Int J Radiat Oncol Biol Phys 47:435–442

Todoroki T et al (2000) Benefits of adjuvant radiotherapy after radical resection of locally advanced main hepatic duct carcinoma. Int J Radiat Oncol Biol Phys 46:581–587

Tse RV et al (2008) Phase I study of individualized stereotactic radiotherapy for hepatocellular carcinoma and intrahepatic cholangiocarcinoma. J Clin Oncol 26:657–664

Tsuji T et al (2001) Lymphatic spreading pattern of intrahepatic cholangiocarcinoma. Surgery 129:401–407

Wang NH et al (2010) Impact factors for microinvasion in patients with hepatocellular carcinoma: possible application to the definition of clinical tumor volume. Int J Radiat Oncol Biol Phys 76:467–476

# Rectal Cancer

Jose G. Bazan, Albert C. Koong, and Daniel T. Chang

## Contents

J.G. Bazan, MD • A.C. Koong, MD, PhD • D.T. Chang, MD (✉)
Department of Radiation Oncology, Stanford University,
875 Blake Wilbur Drive, Stanford, CA 94305, USA
e-mail: dtchang@stanford.edu; jose.bazan2@osumc.edu

## 1   Anatomy and Patterns of Spread

- The rectum is approximately 15 cm long and is divided into upper, middle, and lower thirds based on the distance from the anal verge.
- The arterial supply to the rectum comes from the superior, middle, and inferior rectal arteries, which are branches of the inferior mesenteric artery.
- The venous drainage of the upper rectum via the superior rectal vein has connections with the inferior mesenteric vein and eventually into the portal venous system. The middle and inferior rectal veins drain into the internal iliac vein leading to the inferior vena cava. Rectal cancer can therefore have distant metastatic spread to both the liver and the lungs.
- Lymph nodes at risk include the perirectal, presacral, and internal iliac (hypogastric) nodes. Involvement of the external iliac nodes is uncommon except for tumors that invade adjacent structures (e.g., bladder, cervix, prostate). Spread to the inguinal nodes is also unlikely except for distal rectal tumors that extend inferiorly into the anal canal below the dentate line.

## 2   Diagnostic Workup Relevant for Target Volume Delineation

- Physical examination is an important part of the staging and planning process. For tumors that are palpable, attention should be paid to how far the tumor begins from the anal verge. The mobility of the tumor should also be noted. Early tumors (T1-2) are typically mobile. Tumors that have penetrated through the muscularis propria into the perirectal tissue (T3) feel tethered, while tumors that invade adjacent structures such as the pelvic sidewall (T4) will feel firm and fixed. Careful attention should also be placed on sphincter function.

N.Y. Lee et al. (eds.), *Target Volume Delineation for Conformal and Intensity-Modulated Radiation Therapy*,
Medical Radiology. Radiation Oncology, DOI: 10.1007/174_2014_979, © Springer International Publishing Switzerland 2014
Published Online: 11 October 2014

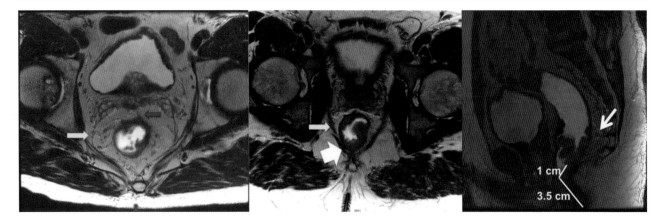

**Fig. 1** Axial T2 sequence without fat suppression for staging of rectal cancer. The mesorectal fat surrounds the rectum and is enclosed within the mesorectal fascia (*yellow arrows*). In the *left panel*, the tumor was staged as an early T3 tumor with minimal invasion into the perirectal fat. The distance from the mesorectal fascia is more than 1 cm (*red arrow*). In the *middle panel*, a more extensive example of a T3 tumor is shown with a tumor that approaches within 2 mm of the mesorectal fascia (*large white arrow*). In the *right panel*, a sagittal view is shown. A mesorectal lymph node is visible (*thin white arrow*). The estimated distance of the tumor from the anal verge is 4.5 cm

- The standard imaging studies include CT of the pelvis with contrast to assess the primary tumor and the status of the regional lymph nodes.
- Rigid sigmoidoscopy is used to directly visualize the lesion, to obtain an estimate of the size of the lesion, to obtain biopsy, and to accurately measure the distance from the anal verge. A colonoscopy should also be performed to visualize the entire colon and ensure that synchronous lesions are not present. For low-lying tumors, direct visualization is necessary to determine the relationship to the dentate line since the dentate line is not palpable.
- Endorectal ultrasound (EUS) is used to determine the depth of invasion of the primary tumor as well as to assess the lymph node status. EUS overstages or understages the true T stage in approximately 20 % of cases.
- MRI is becoming a standard part of the preoperative staging workup to determine invasion of tumor into the mesorectal fat (T3) and into adjacent organs (T4), to assess lymph node status, verify distance from the anal verge, and to assess operability with negative margins. Examples can be seen in Fig. 1.
- Rectal tumors are well visualized on PET, so PET/CT is also becoming a standard part of staging and planning to help delineate the extent of gross disease (Fig. 2). However, areas of low uptake on PET should not supercede physical exam findings or abnormalities seen on CT.

## 3    Simulation and Daily Localization

- Most patients that are to be treated with standard 3D conformal radiotherapy are simulated in the prone position with the use of a belly board for anterior displacement of the bowel. However, if IMRT is planned, then we recommend that the patient be simulated in the supine position in a body mold or other immobilization device to ensure more accurate setup reproducibility. A radiopaque marker should be placed on the anus.
- CT simulation with ≤3 mm thickness with IV contrast should be performed to delineate the pelvic blood vessels and gross tumor volume. The use of oral contrast may be helpful to identify the small bowel, which is an important organ at risk. If PET/CT is available, a PET/CT fusion should be obtained to aid in target volume delineation. For patients that underwent preoperative MRI, MR fusion could also aide with treatment planning.
- Bladder filling/emptying may be considered, especially if IMRT is used. A full bladder may keep bowel from migrating into the pelvis. An empty bladder may be more reproducible.
- We recommend daily orthogonal kilovoltage images and weekly cone beam CT scans (to assess soft tissue) to verify alignment during treatment. Cone beam CTs may be done more frequently if there is significant variation in bladder and/or rectal filling.

## 4    Target Volume Delineation and Treatment Planning

- Conventional 3D conformal radiotherapy for rectal cancer involves a PA field and two opposed lateral fields (Figs. 3 and 4).
- Traditional borders for the PA field are *superior*, L5/S1 interspace; *inferior*, the inferior edge of the obturator foramen or 3 cm below the GTV, whichever is more distal; and *lateral*, 1.5–2 cm beyond the pelvic brim.

- Borders for the lateral fields include *superior*, same as PA field; *inferior*, same as PA field; *anterior*, posterior margin of the pubic symphysis (bony landmark for internal iliac nodes) for T3 disease or at least 1 cm anterior to the anterior edge of the pubic symphysis (bony landmark for external iliac nodes) for T4 disease; and *posterior*, 1–1.5 cm posterior to the posterior edge of the bony sacrum.
- With the use of CT-based planning, the borders described above can be modified to ensure adequate coverage of the planning target volumes (PTV). Target volumes including gross tumor volume (GTV), clinical target volumes (CTV), and the PTV should be delineated on every applicable slice of the planning CT.
- The primary gross tumor volume (GTV-P) is defined as all gross disease on physical examination and imaging.
- The nodal GTV (GTV-N) includes all visible perirectal, mesorectal, and involved iliac lymph nodes. Include any lymph node in bout as GTV-N in the absence of a biopsy.

- The high-risk CTV (CTV-HR) should include the GTV with a minimum of 1.5–2-cm superior and inferior margin as well as the entire rectum, mesorectum, and presacral space. Additional details are given in Table 1.
- The standard-risk CTV (CTV-SR) should cover the entire mesorectum and bilateral internal iliac lymph nodes for T3 tumors. The CTV-SR should also include the bilateral external iliac nodes for patients with T4 tumors with anterior organ involvement. Additional details are found in Table 1.
- Target volume delineation in the postoperative setting is similar to the preoperative setting. However, in the case of an abdominoperineal resection, the entire surgical bed extending inferiorly to the level of the perineal scar needs to be included. Additional details are given in Table 2.
- The RTOG anorectal contouring atlas (Myerson et al. 2009) provides a detailed consensus contouring descriptions of three elective CTVs that should be considered in patients with rectal and anal cancers. CTV-A includes the perirectal, presacral, and internal iliac regions and should

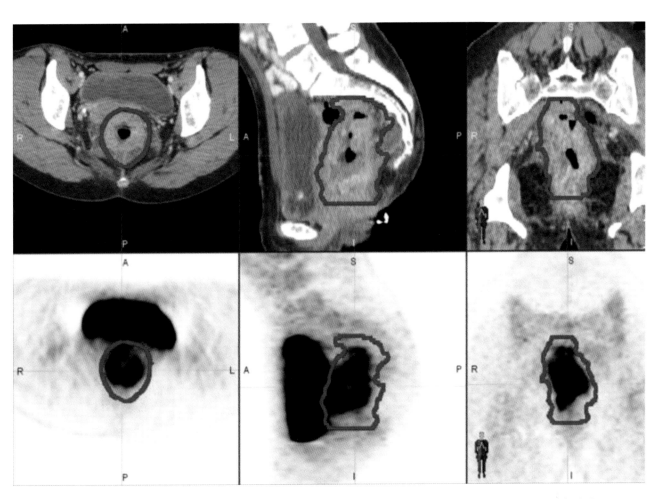

**Fig. 2** A patient with T4N0 rectal adenocarcinoma (invasion into the cervix). GTV: These panels illustrate the utility of PET in target volume delineation. In the *upper panel*, the GTV (*red*) is seen on representative axial, sagittal, and coronal images, respectively, on both the treatment planning CT and PET. The *lower panel* shows additional axial slices

**Fig. 2** (continued)

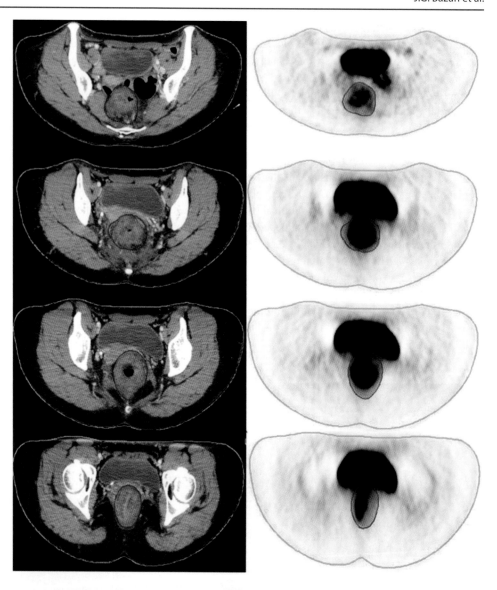

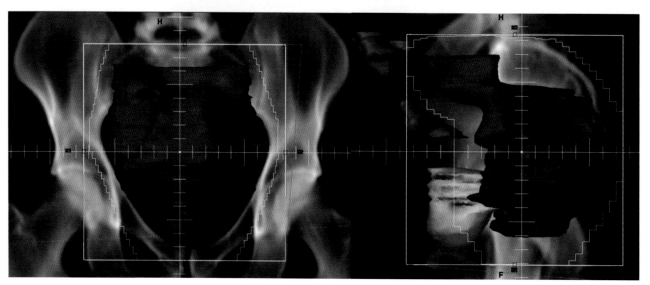

**Fig. 3** Standard fields used for a T3N1 rectal cancer receiving preoperative chemoradiation, PA (*left panel*) and left lateral (*right panel*). The CTV-SR is shown in *red*. The patient was simulated in prone in a belly board allowing the small bowel (shown in *purple*) to fall anteriorly away from the CTV. The bladder is shown in *yellow*

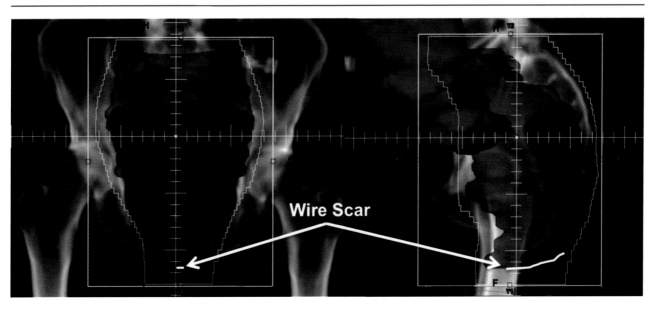

**Fig. 4** Standard fields used for a T3N2a rectal cancer receiving postoperative chemoradiation following an APR. PA (*left panel*) and left lateral (*right panel*). The CTV-SR is shown in *red*. The field includes the perineal scar. The patient was simulated in prone in a belly board allowing the small bowel (shown in *purple*) to fall anteriorly away from the CTV. Note that more small bowel is in the pelvis in the postoperative setting

**Table 1** Suggested target volumes for gross and microscopic disease in the preoperative setting

| Target volumes | Definition and description |
|---|---|
| GTV (gross tumor volume) | Primary (GTV-P): all gross disease on physical examination and imaging |
| | Regional nodes (GTV-N): all visible perirectal and involved iliac nodes; include any lymph node in doubt as GTV in the absence of a biopsy |
| CTV-high risk (CTV-HR) | CTV-HR should cover the GTV-P and GTV-N with 1.5–2-cm margin expansion superiorly and inferiorly, but excluding the uninvolved bone, muscle, or air. This volume should include the entire rectum, mesorectum, and presacral space axially at these levels. A 1–2-cm margin around gross tumor invasion into adjacent organs should be added. Coverage of the entire presacral space and mesorectum should be strongly considered. Any visible mesorectal nodes on CT and PET should also be included |
| | To cover the iliac lymphatics, a 0.7-cm margin around the iliac vessels should be drawn (excluding the muscle and bone) (Myerson et al. 2009; Taylor et al. 2005) |
| | To cover the external iliac nodes, an additional 1-cm margin anterolaterally around the vessels is needed. Any adjacent small nodes should be included (Myerson et al. 2009; Taylor et al. 2005) |
| | Anteriorly, a margin of 1–1.5 cm should be added into bladder to account for changes in bladder and rectal filling (Myerson et al. 2009; Daly et al. 2011) |
| | A 1.8-cm-wide volume between the external and internal iliac vessels is needed to cover the obturator nodes (Taylor et al. 2005) |
| CTV-standard risk (CTV-SR) | Should cover the entire mesorectum and right and left internal iliac lymph nodes for T3 tumors. The right and left external iliac lymph nodes for T4 tumors with anterior organ involvement should also be included |
| | A 1–2-cm margin in adjacent organs with gross tumor invasion should be added for T4 lesions |
| | Superiorly, the entire rectum and mesorectum should be included (usually up to L5/S1) and at least 2-cm margin superior to gross disease, whichever is most cephalad |
| | Inferiorly, the CTV should extend to the pelvic floor or at least 2 cm below the gross disease, whichever is most caudad |
| | To cover the iliac lymphatics, a 0.7-cm margin around the internal iliac vessels should be drawn (excluding the muscle and bone) (Myerson et al. 2009; Taylor et al. 2005) |
| | To cover the external iliac nodes (for T4 lesions), an additional 1-cm margin anterolaterally around the vessels is needed. Any adjacent small nodes should be included (Myerson et al. 2009; Taylor et al. 2005) |
| | Anteriorly, a margin of 1–1.5 cm should be added into bladder to account for changes in bladder and rectal filling (Myerson et al. 2009; Daly et al. 2011) |
| | A 1.8-cm-wide volume between the external and internal iliac vessels is needed to cover the obturator nodes (Taylor et al. 2005) |
| Planning target volume (PTV) | Each CTV should be expanded by 0.5–1 cm, depending on the physician's comfort level with setup accuracy, frequency of imaging, and the use of IGRT |

**Table 2** Suggested target volumes in the postoperative setting

| Target volumes | Definition and description |
|---|---|
| CTV (positive margin or gross disease) | Should include the area of known microscopically involved margin or macroscopic residual disease plus a 1–2-cm margin, but exclude the uninvolved bone, muscle, or air |
| CTV-high risk (CTV-HR) | Should include the entire remaining rectum (if applicable), mesorectal bed, and presacral space axially at these levels but exclude uninvolved bone, muscle, or air. Coverage of the entire presacral space and mesorectum should be considered |
| CTV-standard risk (CTV-SR) | Should cover the entire mesorectum and right and left internal iliac lymph nodes for T3 tumors. The right and left external iliac lymph nodes for T4 tumors with anterior organ involvement should also be included |
| | Superiorly, the entire remaining rectum and mesorectum should be included (usually up to L5/S1) and at least 1-cm margin superior to the anastomosis, whichever is most cephalad |
| | Inferiorly, the CTV should extend to the pelvic floor or at least 1 cm below the anastomosis or rectal stump, whichever is most caudad. If patient is status post an abdominoperineal resection, the surgical bed extending down to the perineal scar should be included. The scar should be outlined with a radiopaque marker. |
| | To cover the iliac lymphatics, a 0.7-cm margin around the internal iliac vessels should be drawn (excluding muscle and bone) (Myerson et al. 2009; Taylor et al. 2005) |
| | To cover the external iliac nodes (for T4 lesions), an additional 1-cm margin anterolaterally around the vessels is needed. Any adjacent small nodes should be included (Myerson et al. 2009; Taylor et al. 2005) |
| | Anteriorly, a margin of 1–1.5 cm should be added into bladder to account for changes in bladder and rectal filling (Myerson et al. 2009; Daly et al. 2011) |
| | A 1.8-cm-wide volume between the external and internal iliac vessels is needed to cover the obturator nodes (Taylor et al. 2005) |
| | For tumors that extend inferiorly to or inferior to the dentate line, the bilateral inguinal nodes should be included |
| Planning target volume (PTV) | Each CTV should be expanded by 0.5–1 cm, depending on the physician's comfort level with setup accuracy, frequency of imaging, and the use of IGRT |

**Table 3** Description of the borders of CTV-A in the RTOG anorectal contouring atlas

| Clinical target volume | Key highlights |
|---|---|
| CTV-A: Lower pelvis | *Inferior*: inferior border should be 2 cm below gross disease. Should include the entire mesorectum down to the pelvic floor |
| | *Lateral*: Does not need to extend more than a few millimeters beyond the levator muscles unless there is tumor extension into the ischiorectal fossa. For T4 tumors, should include 1–2-cm margin around identified areas of invasion |
| CTV-A (mid-pelvis) | Includes the rectum, mesorectum, internal iliac region, and margin for bladder variability |
| | *Posterolateral*: Extends to the pelvic sidewall muscles or bone (when muscles are absent) |
| | *Anterior*: At least 1 cm into the posterior bladder. Should also include at least the posterior portion of the internal obturator vessels |
| | Recommend 7–8-mm margin in the soft tissue around the internal iliac vessels. CTV should be trimmed off the uninvolved muscle and bone |
| CTV-A (upper pelvis) | *Superior (perirectal component)*: Should be at the rectosigmoid junction or at least 2 cm proximal to macroscopic disease in the rectum/perirectal nodes, whichever is most superior. The entire length of the rectum should be included |
| | *Superior (nodal coverage)*: Should be at the bifurcation of the common iliac vessels into the external/internal iliacs |
| | *Anterior*: At midline, should extend at least 1 cm anterior the sacrum for adequate coverage of the presacral nodes |
| | Recommend 7–8-mm margin in the soft tissue around the internal iliac vessels. CTV should be trimmed off the uninvolved muscle and bone |

be covered in all patients with rectal cancer. CTV-B includes the external iliac nodes (covered only in rectal cancer cases with T4 disease or for primary rectal tumors that extend inferiorly into the distal anal canal). CTV-C includes the inguinal region (should be considered in rectal cancer cases that extend into the distal anal canal). A detailed description of CTV-A is given in Table 3.

- The Australasian GI Trials Group atlas (Ng et al. 2012) describes seven elective regions to be considered when treating anal cancer: mesorectum, presacral space, internal iliac nodes, ischiorectal fossa, obturator nodes, external iliac nodes, and inguinal nodes. Table 4 is a summary of the definition of these regions.

**Table 4** Description of the borders used in defining the elective nodal regions from the Australasian GI Trials Group contouring atlas (Ng et al. 2012)

| | Mesorectum | Presacral space | Internal iliac nodes | Ischiorectal fossa | Obturator nodes | External iliac nodes | Inguinal nodes |
|---|---|---|---|---|---|---|---|
| Cranial | Rectosigmoid junction | Sacral promontory (L5/S1) interspace | Bifurcation of the common iliac artery (L5/S1) | Apex formed by the levator ani, g. maximus, obturator internus | 3–5 mm cranial to the obturator canal | Bifurcation of the common iliac artery | Level where ext. iliac a. leaves bony pelvis to become femoral artery |
| Caudal | Anorectal junction (levators fuse with external sphincter) | Inferior edge of coccyx | Level of the obturator canal or level where there is no space between the obturator internus and midline organs | Anal verge | Obturator canal, where the obturator artery has exited the pelvis | Between the roof of acetabulum and superior pubic rami | Lower edge of the ischial tuberosities |
| Posterior | Presacral space | Position at the anterior border of the sacral bone; should include sacral hollow | N/A | Transverse plane joining the anterior edge of the medial walls of the gluteus maximus muscle | Internal iliac nodes | Internal iliac nodes | Muscle boundaries |
| Anterior | Males: penile bulb and prostate in lower pelvis, SV, and bladder Females: bladder, vagina, cervix, uterus Internal margin of 10 mm added to anterior mesorectal border on slices containing bladder, SV, or uterus for variation | 10 mm anterior to the sacral border encompassing any lymph nodes | Obturator internus mm or bone in the lower pelvis; in the upper pelvis, 7-mm margin around the internal iliac vessels | Level where the obturator internus, levator ani, and sphincter muscle fuse; inferiorly, at least 10–20 mm anterior to sphincter muscles | Anterior extent of obturator internus | 7-mm margin anterior to the external iliac vessels | Minimum 2-cm margin on the inguinal vessels |
| Lateral | Lower pelvis = medial edge of levator ani; upper pelvis = internal iliac nodes | Sacroiliac joints | Medial edge of muscle or bone | Ischial tuberosity, muscles | Obturator internus | Iliopsoas muscle | Medial edge of the sartorius or iliopsoas |
| Medial | N/A | N/A | Mesorectum and presacral space in the lower pelvis; 7-mm margin around the vessel in the upper pelvis | N/A | Bladder | Bladder or 7-mm margin around the vessel | 10–20-mm margin around the femoral vessels |

- There are multiple techniques and methods of dose prescription for rectal cancer. In the preoperative setting, the most common prescription dose is 1.8 Gy/fraction to 45 Gy to the PTV-SR and 1.8 Gy/fraction to 50.4 Gy to the PTV-HR.
- Figure 5 shows a case of a T3N1 rectal cancer receiving preoperative chemoradiation.
- Figure 6 shows a case of a T4N0 rectal cancer receiving preoperative chemoradiation.

- Figure 7 shows a case of a T3N2a rectal cancer status post abdominoperineal resection receiving postoperative chemoradiation.
- Conventional technique uses opposing lateral fields with a PA field. An example is shown in Figs. 3 and 4.
- With IMRT, simultaneous integrated boosts can be considered. Table 5 lists several suggested dose and fractionation schemes for various settings.
- Alternatively with short-course radiotherapy, the PTV-SR would receive 25 Gy at 5 Gy/fraction.

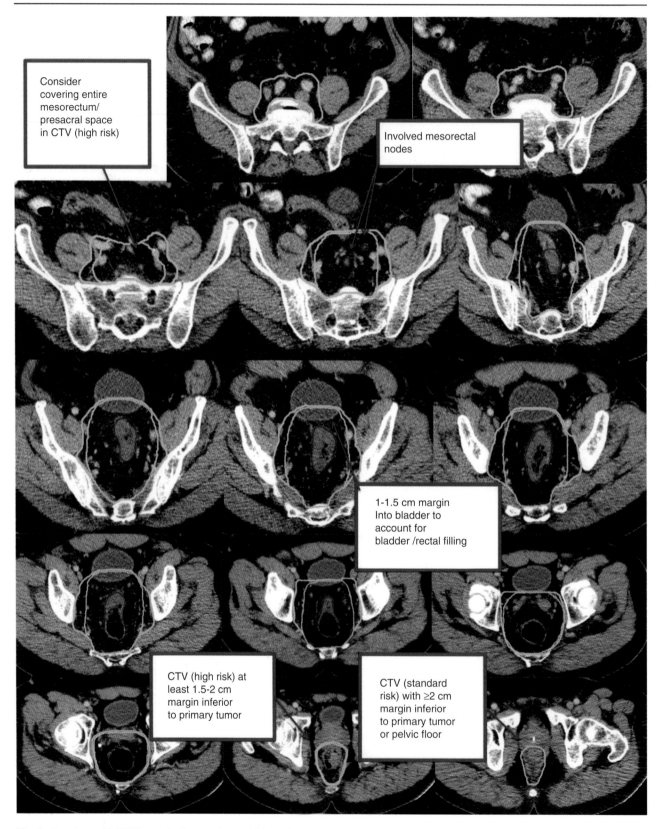

**Fig. 5** A patient with T3N1 rectal adenocarcinoma. This patient was simulated prone (note the anterior displacement of the small bowel) with PET/CT simulation with 2.5 mm thickness on each slice. CTV (standard risk, *cyan*), CTV (high risk, *orange*), and GTV (*red, shaded*) are shown. Note that these are representative slices and not all slices are contoured. Also, the patient was simulated prone, but the CT images are rotated 180° for viewer orientation

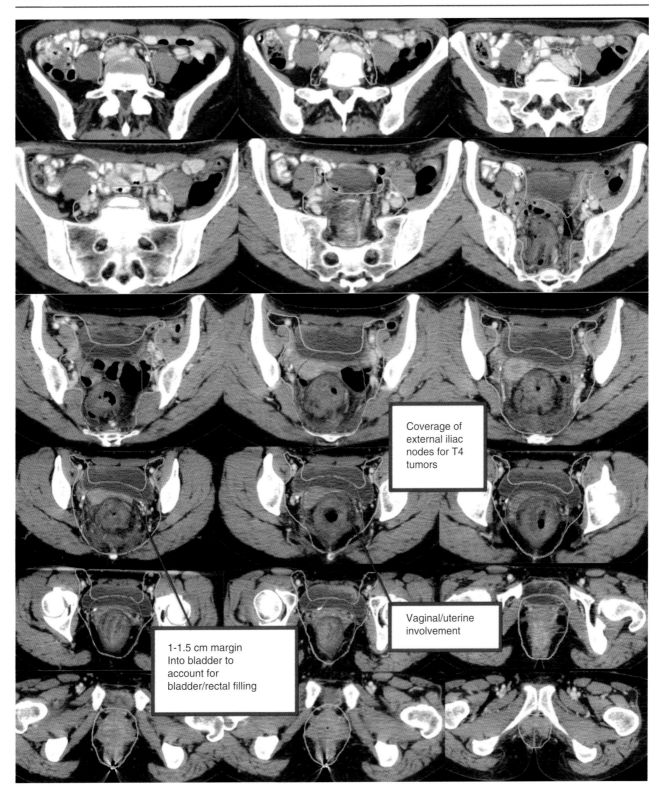

**Fig. 6** A patient with T4N0 rectal adenocarcinoma (invasion into the cervix). Axial slices showing CTV (standard risk, *cyan*) in relation to the CTV (high risk, *orange*) and GTV (*red, shaded*). Note that in this case, the CTV (standard risk) covers the external iliac nodal region due to the T4 disease. Also note that these are representative slices and not all slices are contoured

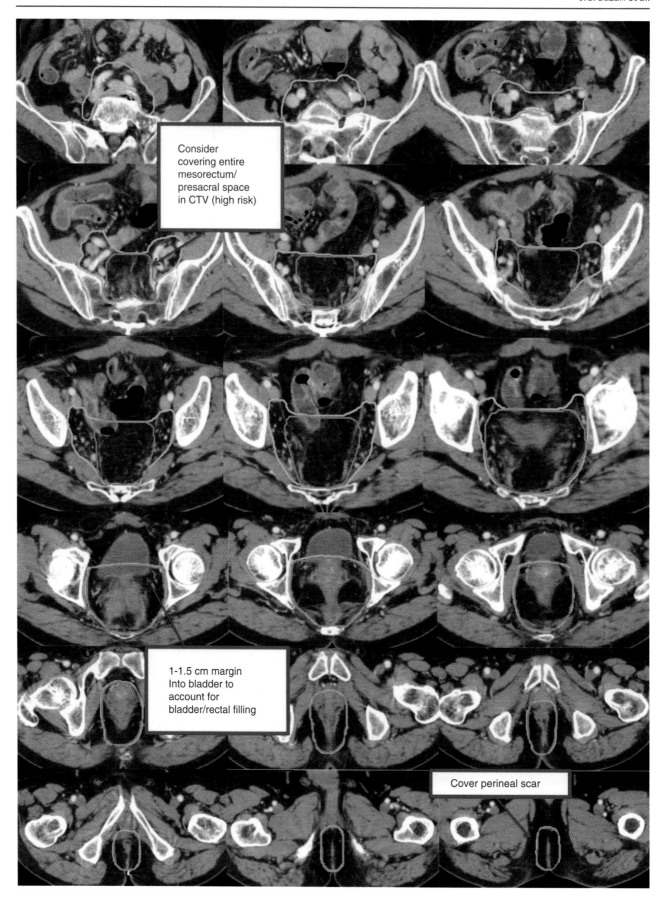

Consider
covering entire
mesorectum/
presacral space
in CTV (high risk)

1-1.5 cm margin
Into bladder to
account for
bladder/rectal filling

Cover perineal scar

**Table 5** Suggested dose and fractionation methods for rectal cancer

|  | PTV-HR | PTV-SR |
|---|---|---|
| Preoperative T3 or T1-2 N+ | 50.4 Gy at 1.8 Gy/fx, OR | 45 Gy at 1.8 Gy/fx, OR |
|  | 50 Gy at 2 Gy/fx (SIB) | 45 Gy at 1.8 Gy/fx (SIB) |
| Preoperative T4 any N | 54–55.8 Gy at 1.8 Gy/fx, OR | 45 Gy at 1.8 Gy/fx, OR |
|  | 54 Gy at 2 Gy/fx (SIB) | 45.9 Gy at 1.7 Gy/fx (SIB) |
| Preoperative (short course) T3-4 or N+ |  | 25 Gy at 5 Gy/fx |
| Postoperative (negative margins) | 54–55.8 Gy at 1.8 Gy/fx, OR | 45 Gy at 1.8 Gy/fx |
|  | 54 Gy at 2 Gy/fx (SB) | 45.9 Gy at 1.7 Gy/fx (SIB) |
| Postoperative (gross disease or positive margin) | 54–59.4 Gy at 1.8 Gy/fx, OR | 45 Gy at 1.8 Gy/fx, OR |
|  | 54–60 Gy at 2 Gy/fx (SIB) | 45.9 Gy at 1.7 Gy/fx (SIB) |

*Abbreviations*: *fx* fraction, *SIB* simultaneous integrated boost

## 4.1 Plan Assessment

- Ideally, at least 95 % of each PTV should receive 100 % of the prescription dose. In addition, the maximum dose in the PTV should be <110 %.
- When evaluating plans with a sequential boost to the gross disease, each individual plan should be scrutinized before the "plan sum" to assess for areas that may be over- or underdosed.
- The organs at risk include the small bowel, large bowel, bladder, femoral heads, iliac crest, and external genitalia. Uniform consensus guidelines for contouring the small and large bowel, bladder, and femoral heads are available from an RTOG consensus panel (Gay et al. 2012). Suggested dose constraints from QUANTEC (Marks et al. 2010) and RTOG 0822 (Garofalo et al. 2014) are shown in Table 6.

**Table 6** Dose constraints for organs at risk

| Organ at risk | Constraints |
|---|---|
| Small bowel | **QUANTEC** |
|  | V15Gy < 120 cc (individual loops) |
|  | V45Gy < 195 cc (entire potential space within peritoneal cavity) |
|  | **RTOG 0822** |
|  | V35Gy < 180 cc |
|  | V40Gy < 100 cc |
|  | V45 Gy < 65 cc |
|  | Dmax < 50 Gy |
| Bladder | **QUANTEC** |
|  | Dmax < 65 Gy |
|  | V65Gy < 50 % |
|  | **RTOG 0822** |
|  | V40Gy < 40 % |
|  | V45Gy < 15 % |
|  | Dmax < 50 Gy |
| Femoral heads | **RTOG 0822** |
|  | V40Gy < 40 % |
|  | V45Gy < 25 % |
|  | Dmax < 50 Gy |

## Suggested Reading

Dutch TME trial (van Gijn et al. 2011): Established that preoperative short-course radiotherapy improved local control over total mesorectal excision alone.

German rectal cancer trial (Sauer et al. 2004, 2012): Established that preoperative chemoradiation had superior local control and improved toxicity compared with postoperative chemoradiation in patients with locally advanced rectal cancer.

Medical Research Council trial (Sebag-Montefiore et al. 2009): Established that preoperative short-course radiotherapy improved local control compared with the selective use of postoperative chemoradiation.

Polish trial (Bujko et al. 2006): Randomized trial showing no difference in outcome or toxicity between preoperative short-course radiotherapy and long-course chemoradiation.

Trans-Tasman Radiation Oncology Group (TROG) trial 01.04 (Ngan et al. 2012): Randomized trial showing no difference in outcome or toxicity between preoperative short-course radiotherapy and long-course chemoradiation.

Contouring resources: RTOG anorectal guidelines (Myerson et al. 2009) (target volumes), Taylor et al. (2005) (pelvic nodal delineation), and RTOG pelvic normal tissue panel (Gay et al. 2012).

**Fig. 7** A patient with pathologic T3N2a rectal adenocarcinoma. This patient underwent an abdominoperineal resection (APR) without neoadjuvant chemoradiotherapy. The primary tumor extended from 2 to 5 cm from the anal verge. The patient was simulated prone with CT with slices of 2.5 mm thickness. CTV (standard risk, *cyan*) and CTV (high risk, *orange*) are shown. In this case, due to the absence of small bowel near the postoperative bed, the total dose was 55.8 Gy. However, if a portion of bowel was near the boost volume, the dose could be reduced. Note that these are representative slices and not all slices are contoured. Also, the patient was simulated prone but the CT images are rotated 180° for viewer orientation

# References

Bujko K, Nowacki MP, Nasierowska-Guttmejer A, Michalski W, Bebenek M, Kryj M (2006) Long-term results of a randomized trial comparing preoperative short-course radiotherapy with preoperative conventionally fractionated chemoradiation for rectal cancer. Br J Surg 93(10):1215–1223

Daly ME, Murphy JD, Mok E, Christman-Skieller C, Koong AC, Chang DT (2011) Rectal and bladder deformation and displacement during preoperative radiotherapy for rectal cancer: are current margin guidelines adequate for conformal therapy? Pract Radiat Oncol 1(2):85–94

Garofalo MC, Hong T, Bendell J et al (2014) RTOG 0822: a phase II evaluation of preoperative chemoradiotherapy utilizing intensity modulated radiation therapy (IMRT) in combination with capecitabine and oxaliplatin for patients with locally advanced rectal cancer. http://www.rtog.org/ClinicalTrials/ProtocolTable/StudyDetails.aspx?study=0822. Accessed 31 Jan 2014

Gay HA, Barthold HJ, O'Meara E et al (2012) Pelvic normal tissue contouring guidelines for radiation therapy: a Radiation Therapy Oncology Group consensus panel atlas. Int J Radiat Oncol Biol Phys 83(3):e353–e362

Marks LB, Yorke ED, Jackson A et al (2010) Use of normal tissue complication probability models in the clinic. Int J Radiat Oncol Biol Phys 76(3 Suppl):S10–S19

Myerson RJ, Garofalo MC, El Naqa I et al (2009) Elective clinical target volumes for conformal therapy in anorectal cancer: a radiation therapy oncology group consensus panel contouring atlas. Int J Radiat Oncol Biol Phys 74(3):824–830

Ng M, Leong T, Chander S et al (2012) Australasian Gastrointestinal Trials Group (AGITG) contouring atlas and planning guidelines for intensity-modulated radiotherapy in anal cancer. Int J Radiat Oncol Biol Phys 83(5):1455–1462

Ngan SY, Burmeister B, Fisher RJ et al (2012) Randomized trial of short-course radiotherapy versus long-course chemoradiation comparing rates of local recurrence in patients with T3 rectal cancer: Trans-Tasman Radiation Oncology Group trial 01.04. J Clin Oncol 30(31):3827–3833

Sauer R, Becker H, Hohenberger W et al (2004) Preoperative versus postoperative chemoradiotherapy for rectal cancer. N Engl J Med 351(17):1731–1740

Sauer R, Liersch T, Merkel S et al (2012) Preoperative versus postoperative chemoradiotherapy for locally advanced rectal cancer: results of the German CAO/ARO/AIO-94 randomized phase III trial after a median follow-up of 11 years. J Clin Oncol 30(16):1926–1933

Sebag-Montefiore D, Stephens RJ, Steele R et al (2009) Preoperative radiotherapy versus selective postoperative chemoradiotherapy in patients with rectal cancer (MRC CR07 and NCIC-CTG C016): a multicentre, randomised trial. Lancet 373(9666):811–820

Taylor A, Rockall AG, Reznek RH, Powell ME (2005) Mapping pelvic lymph nodes: guidelines for delineation in intensity-modulated radiotherapy. Int J Radiat Oncol Biol Phys 63(5):1604–1612

van Gijn W, Marijnen CA, Nagtegaal ID et al (2011) Preoperative radiotherapy combined with total mesorectal excision for resectable rectal cancer: 12-year follow-up of the multicentre, randomised controlled TME trial. Lancet Oncol 12(6):575–582

# Anal Canal Cancer

Jose G. Bazan, Albert C. Koong, and Daniel T. Cang

## Contents

J.G. Bazan, MD
Department of Radiation Oncology,
Arthur G. James Cancer Hospital&Solove Research Institute,
The Ohio State University,
300 West 10th Avenue, Columbus, OH 43210, USA
e-mail: jose.bazan2@osumc.edu

A.C. Koong, MD, PhD • D.T. Chang, MD (✉)
Department of Radiation Oncology,
Stanford University, 875 Blake Wilbur Drive,
Stanford, CA 94305, USA
e-mail: dtchang@stanford.edu

## 1   Anatomy and Patterns of Spread

- The anal canal is about 4 cm in length and extends from the anorectal ring (palpable border of anal sphincter and puborectalis muscle) superiorly to the anal verge distally.
- The anal verge is the junction of the nonkeratinized squamous epithelium of the distal anal canal and the keratinized hair-bearing skin.
- Embryologically, the dentate line (or pectinate line) is formed by the junction of the endoderm superiorly and the ectoderm inferiorly, leading to important differences in both histology and lymphatic drainage between the mucosa proximal and distal.
- The dentate line is a histologic landmark that demarcates the transition from the columnar epithelium of the proximal anal canal to the squamous epithelium of the distal anal canal.
- The primary draining lymphatics include the perirectal, internal iliac (hypogastric), and superficial inguinal lymph nodes, and the pattern of drainage depends on the location of the primary tumor within the anal canal as depicted in Table 1.
- Nearly 20 % of patients present with involved nodes at the time of diagnosis.

## 2   Diagnostic Workup Relevant for Target Volume Delineation

- Physical examination is an important part of the staging and planning process and should include detailed assessment of the characteristics of the primary tumor (size, anal sphincter competence, invasion of adjacent structures) as well as an assessment of inguinal lymph nodes.
- Lymph nodes in the inguinal region that are suspicious but borderline should be biopsied (nearly 50 % of suspicious nodes are related to reactive hyperplasia).
- Standard imaging includes CT or MRI of the pelvis to assess the primary tumor and status of the regional lymph

**Table 1** Lymphatic drainage of the anal canal

| Location of primary tumor | Draining lymphatics |
|---|---|
| Distal anal canal, perianal skin, and anal verge | Superficial inguinal lymph nodes |
| | Femoral nodes |
| | External iliac nodes |
| Anal canal just proximal to dentate line | Internal pudendal |
| | Hypogastric |
| | Obturator nodes |
| | Inferior and middle hemorrhoidal |
| Proximal anal canal | Perirectal |
| | Superior hemorrhoidal |

nodes. CT of the chest and abdomen completes the metastatic workup.

- These tumors can be well visualized on PET, so PET/CT is becoming a standard part of staging and recommended for planning to help delineate extent of gross disease (Fig. 1).
- Areas of low uptake on PET should not supersede physical exam findings or abnormalities seen on CT.

## 3    Simulation and Daily Localization

- The patient can be simulated in the supine position in a body mold or other immobilization device to ensure reproducibility. Prone position with the use of a belly board can be used to allow for anterior displacement of the bowel, but setup reproducibility is more variable and using bolus or additional electron fields to supplement dose to the inguinal regions would not be possible. A radiopaque marker should be placed on the anus.
- CT simulation using ≤3 mm thickness with IV contrast should be performed to delineate the pelvic blood vessels and gross tumor volume (GTV). If PET/CT is available, a PET/CT fusion should be obtained to aid in target volume delineation. MRI may also be useful.
- Bladder filling/emptying should be considered. A full bladder may keep bowel from migrating into the pelvis. An empty bladder may be more reproducible.
- We recommend daily orthogonal kilovoltage images and weekly cone beam CT scans (to assess soft tissue) to verify alignment during treatment. Cone beam CTs may be done more frequently if there is significant variation in bladder and/or rectal filling.

## 4    Target Volume Delineation and Treatment Planning

- Conventional radiation therapy for anal canal cancers is complex due to the need to irradiate the groins as well as the pelvis. The "thunderbird" technique was the most common

method used to treat anal cancer. An example of the thunderbird technique compared to an IMRT plan is shown in Fig. 2. In the thunderbird technique, a wide AP field is used to encompass the inguinal lymph nodes. The PA field is narrowed to exclude the inguinal lymph nodes so that the femoral heads are also excluded. An additional boost field must therefore be used to supplement dose to the inguinal regions. This can be accomplished with either photons (with a skin match or a deep match) or electrons. A more detailed description of these thunderbird technique variations is described by Gilroy et al. (2004). Figure 2 shows a standard dose distribution of a photon/electron thunderbird technique.

- RTOG 0529 (Kachnic et al. 2013) has established the feasibility of IMRT in a multi-institution setting and demonstrated lower rates of grade 2 or higher dermatologic toxicity and lower rates of grade 3 or higher gastrointestinal or genitourinary toxicity when compared to historical controls in the RTOG 98-11 (Ajani et al. 2008) trial.
- The primary gross tumor volume (GTV-P) is defined as all gross disease on physical examination and imaging.
- The nodal GTV (GTV-N) includes all nodes that are ≥1.5 cm, PET positive, or biopsy proven. In the absence of biopsy, any clinically or radiographically suspicious lymph nodes should be included in the GTV-N.
- The high-risk clinical target volume (CTV-HR) should include the entire mesorectum, the bilateral internal iliac nodes inferior to the inferior-most level of the sacroiliac joint, and the inguinal or external iliac lymphatics if the inguinal nodes are involved. Additional details are given in Table 2.
- The low-risk CTV (CTV-LR) should include the uninvolved inguinal, external iliac, and internal iliac nodes superior to the inferiormost level of the sacroiliac joint.
- Figure 3 shows a case example of a T2N0 anal cancer.
- Figure 4 shows a case example of a T3N3 anal cancer.
- Detailed contouring atlases available include the RTOG anorectal contouring atlas (Myerson et al. 2009) and the Australasian GI Trials Group Atlas (Ng et al. 2012).
- The RTOG anorectal contouring atlas (Myerson et al. 2009) describes 3 CTV regions that should be included for all patients with anal canal cancer. CTV-A includes the perirectal, presacral, and internal iliac regions. CTV-B includes the external iliac nodes. CTV-C includes the inguinal region. Table 3 provides a more detailed description of these regions.

### 4.1    Plan Assessment

- Ideally, at least 95 % of each PTV should receive 100 % of the prescription dose. In addition, the maximum dose in the PTV should not exceed 10 %.
- The Australasian GI Trials Group Atlas (Ng et al. 2012) describes seven elective regions to be considered when

**Fig. 1** An example of how PET can help delineate GTV. The GTV (*red*) is seen on representative axial, sagittal, and coronal images, respectively, on both the treatment planning CT and PET in the *upper panels*. Additional representative axial slices are shown below in the *lower panels*

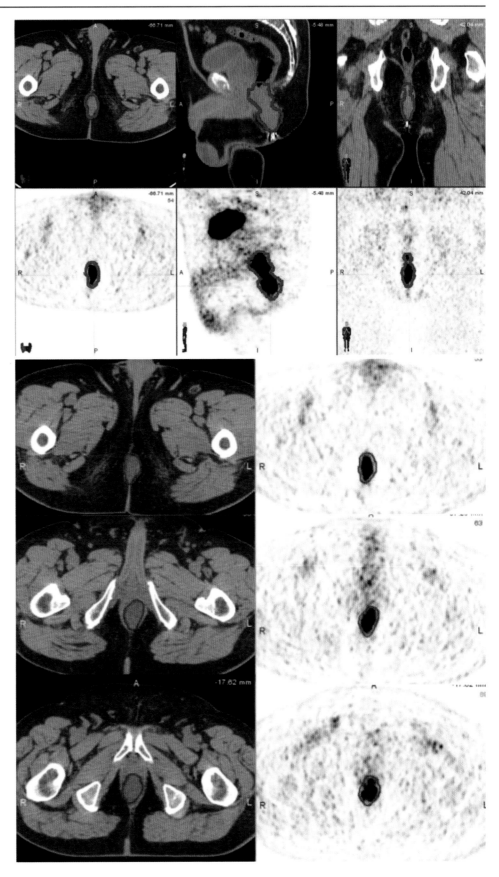

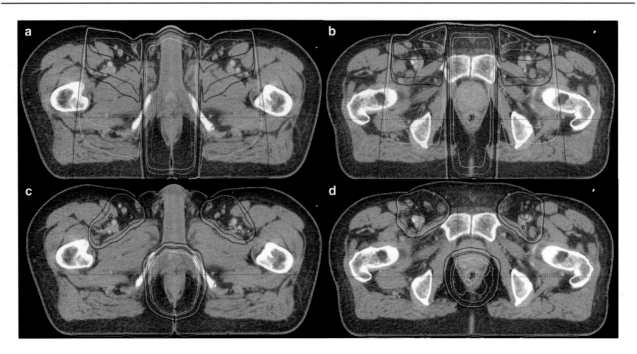

**Fig. 2** Comparison of a photon/electron thunderbird technique (panel **a** and **b**) and intensity-modulated radiotherapy (panel **c** and **d**)

**Table 2** Suggested target volumes for gross and microscopic disease

| Target volumes | Definition and description |
|---|---|
| GTV (gross tumor volume) | Primary (GTV-P): all gross disease on physical examination and imaging |
| | Regional nodes (GTV-N): all nodes ≥1.5 cm, PET-positive, or biopsy proven include any lymph node in doubt as GTV in the absence of a biopsy |
| Clinical target volume (CTV) gross disease | CTV-P should cover the GTV-P with 1.5–2.5 cm margin expansion but excluding uninvolved bone, muscle, or air. The CTV-N should cover the GTV-N with a 1.0–1.5 cm margin but excluding uninvolved bone, muscle or air |
| CTV-high risk (CTV-HR) | Should cover the entire mesorectum, the right and left internal iliac lymph nodes inferior to the inferior-most level of the sacroiliac joint, and the inguinal or external iliac lymphatics if the inguinal nodes are uninvolved |
| | To cover the iliac lymphatics, a 0.7-cm margin around the iliac vessels should be drawn (excluding muscle and bone) (Myerson et al. 2009; Taylor et al. 2005) |
| | To cover the external iliac nodes, an additional 1 cm margin anterolaterally around the vessels is needed. Any adjacent small nodes should be included (Myerson et al. 2009; Taylor et al. 2005) |
| | Anteriorly, a margin of 1–1.5 cm should be added into the bladder to account for changes in the bladder and rectal filling (Myerson et al. 2009; Daly et al. 2011) |
| | A 1.8-cm wide volume between the external and internal iliac vessels is needed to cover the obturator nodes (Taylor et al. 2005) |
| CTV-low risk (CTV-LR) | Should include the uninvolved inguinal, external iliac, and internal iliac nodes superior to the inferior-most level of the sacroiliac joint |
| | To cover the iliac lymphatics, a 0.7-cm margin around the iliac vessels should be drawn (excluding muscle and bone) (Myerson et al. 2009; Taylor et al. 2005) |
| | To cover the external iliac nodes, an additional 1 cm margin anterolaterally around the vessels is needed. Any adjacent small nodes should be included (Myerson et al. 2009; Taylor et al. 2005) |
| | Anteriorly, a margin of 1–1.5 cm should be added into bladder to account for changes in the bladder and rectal filling (Myerson et al. 2009; Daly et al. 2011) |
| | A 1.8-cm wide volume between the external and internal iliac vessels is needed to cover the obturator nodes (Taylor et al. 2005) |
| Planning target volume (PTV) | Each CTV should be expanded by 0.5–1 cm, depending on the physician's comfort level with setup accuracy, frequency of imaging, and the use of IGRT |

**Fig. 3** (**a**) A patient with T2N0 anal canal cancer. This patient was simulated supine using PET/CT simulation with a 2.5 mm thickness on each slice. CTV is shown. Note that these are representative slices and not all slices are included. CTV (low risk, *cyan*), CTV (high risk, *orange*), CTV (gross disease, *green*), and GTV (*red*, *shaded*) are shown. (**b**) Enhanced view of the lower pelvis showing CTV (low risk, *blue*), CTV (high risk, *orange*), CTV (gross disease, *green*), and GTV (*red*, *shaded*)

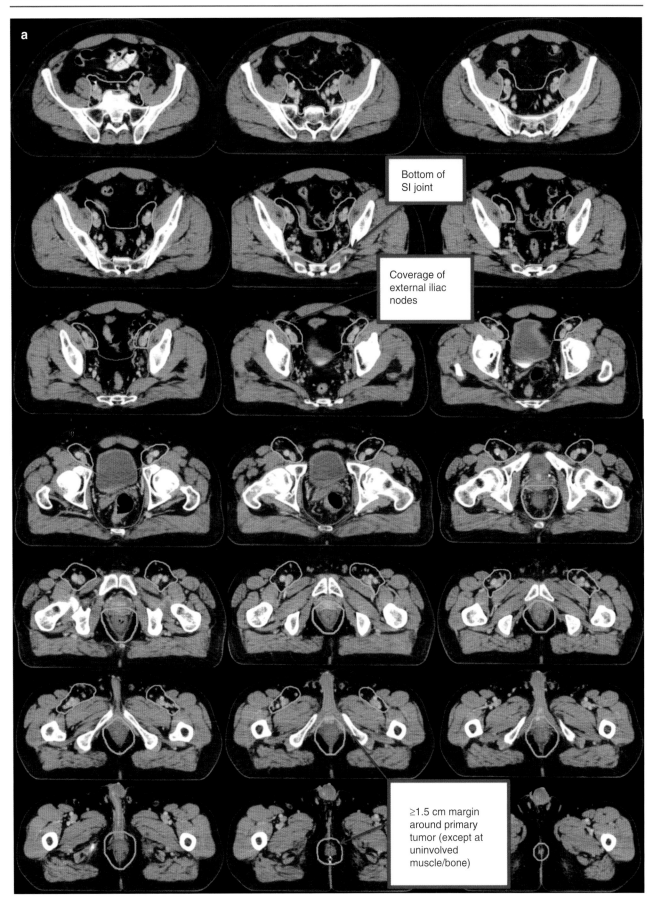

Bottom of SI joint

Coverage of external iliac nodes

≥1.5 cm margin around primary tumor (except at uninvolved muscle/bone)

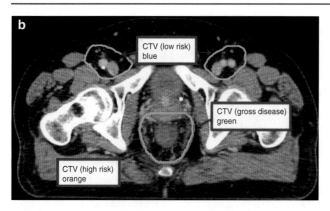

CTV (low risk) blue

CTV (gross disease) green

CTV (high risk) orange

**Fig. 3** (continued)

treating anal cancer: the mesorectum, presacral space, internal iliac nodes, ischiorectal fossa, obturator nodes, external iliac nodes, and inguinal nodes. Table 4 is a summary of the definition of these regions.

- There are multiple techniques and methods of dose prescription for anal cancer, and the exact dose and fractionation will vary based on which technique is used. The current recommendations are based on the treatment plan used in RTOG 98-11 (Ajani et al. 2008) (see Table 5).
- When evaluating plans with a sequential boost to the gross disease, each individual plan should be scrutinized before the "Plan Sum" to assess for areas that may be over- or underdosed.

- The organs at risk include the small bowel, large bowel, bladder, femoral heads, iliac crest, and external genitalia. Uniform consensus guidelines for contouring the small and large bowel, bladder, and femoral heads are available from an RTOG consensus panel (Gay et al. 2012). Suggested dose constraints from QUANTEC (Marks et al. 2010) and RTOG 0529 (Kachnic et al. 2013) are listed in Table 6.
- Pelvic bone marrow is emerging as an important organ at risk with respect to minimizing acute hematologic toxicity in patients receiving concurrent chemoradiotherapy for anal cancer (Bazan et al. 2012, 2013; Mell et al. 2008). Currently, the pelvic bones serve as a surrogate for the pelvic bone marrow. Delineation of the pelvic bone marrow structure is described by Mell et al. (2006). The pelvic bone marrow consists of 3 subsites: the lumbosacral spine, the ilium, and the lower pelvis.
- We suggest that potential dose constraints for the pelvic bone marrow should include mean dose< 28 Gy, V10< 90 %, and V20< 75 %. However, these constraints have not been validated prospectively and should not supersede other planning objectives. The lumbosacral spine may be the most active subsite of the entire pelvic bone marrow structure (Bazan et al. 2012, 2013; Rose et al. 2012), and limiting dose to this site may be sufficient to reduce hematologic toxicity.

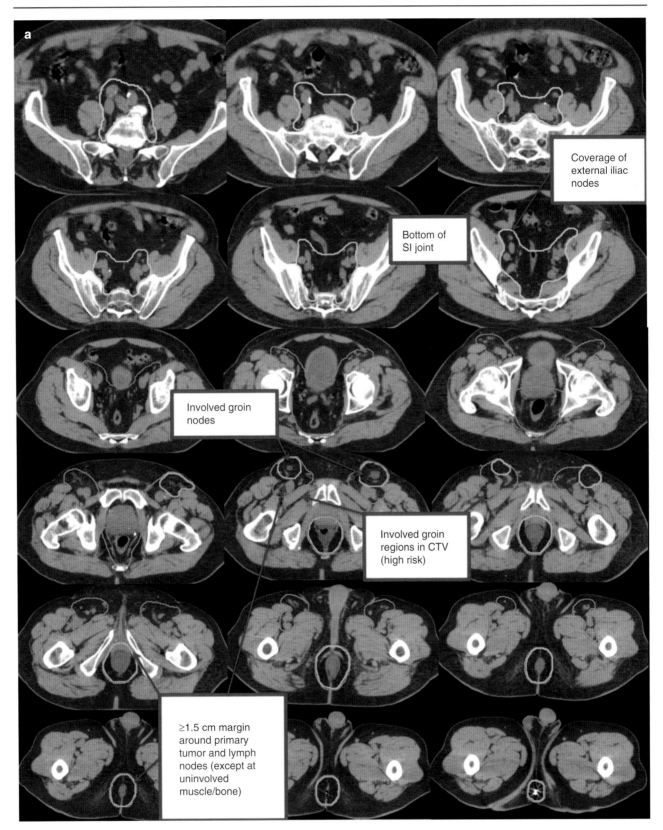

**Fig. 4** (**a**) A patient with T3N3 anal canal cancer with bilateral inguinal lymph node involvement. This patient was simulated supine using PET/CT simulation with a 2.5 mm thickness on each slice. CTV (low risk, *cyan*), CTV (high risk, *orange*), CTV (gross disease, *green*), and GTV (*red*, *shaded*) are shown. Note that these are representative slices and not all slices are included. (**b**) Enhanced view of the lower pelvis showing CTV (high risk, *orange*), CTV (gross disease, *green*), and GTV (*red*, *shaded*)

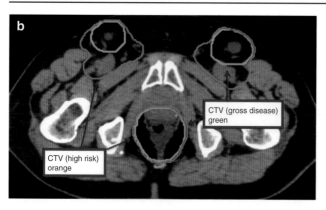

**Fig. 4** (continued)

**Table 3** Elective nodal regions described in RTOG anorectal contouring atlas (Myerson et al. 2009)

| Clinical target volume | Key highlights |
|---|---|
| CTV-A (perirectal, presacral, internal iliac regions) | Lower pelvis: The inferior border should be 2 cm below gross disease. Should include the entire mesorectum. Does not need to extend more than a few millimeters beyond the levator muscles |
| | Mid-pelvis: Includes the internal iliac region. Posterior and lateral margins should extend to pelvic sidewall muscle or bone. Recommends at least 1 cm anteriorly into the bladder |
| | Upper pelvis: The most superior extent should be at the bifurcation of the common iliac vessels (approximate bony landmark: the sacral promontory). At midline, CTVA should extend at least 1 cm anterior to the sacrum |
| | Recommend 7–8 mm margin in soft tissue around the iliac vessels, but at least 1 cm anteriorly, especially if vessels or small nodes are seen in this area. CTV should be trimmed off uninvolved muscle and bone |
| CTV-B (external iliac region) | The border between the inguinal and external iliac region is somewhat arbitrary. The consensus was that the border should be set at the level of the inferior extent of the internal obturator vessels (bony landmark: the upper edge of the superior pubic rami) |
| | Recommend 7–8 mm margin in soft tissue around the iliac vessels, but at least 1 cm anteriorly, especially if vessels or small nodes are seen in this area. CTV should be trimmed off uninvolved muscle and bone |
| CTV-C (inguinal region) | The most inferior extent should be 2 cm below the saphenous/femoral junction |

**Table 4** Description of the borders used in defining the elective nodal regions from the Australasian GI Trials Group Contouring Atlas (Ng et al. 2012)

| | Mesorectum | Presacral space | Internal iliac nodes | Ischiorectal fossa | Obturator nodes | External iliac nodes | Inguinal nodes |
|---|---|---|---|---|---|---|---|
| Cranial | Rectosigmoid junction | Sacral promontory (L5/S1) interspace | Bifurcation of common iliac artery (L5/S1) | Apex formed by levator ani, g. maximus, obturator internus | 3–5 mm cranial to obturator canal | Bifurcation of common iliac artery | Level where ext. iliac a. leaves bony pelvis to become femoral artery |
| Caudal | Anorectal junction (levators fuse with external sphincter) | Inferior edge of coccyx | Level of obturator canal or level where there is no space between obturator internus and midline organs | Anal verge | Obturator canal, where obturator artery has exited the pelvis | Between roof of acetabulum and superior pubic rami | Lower edge of ischial tuberosities |
| Posterior | Presacral space | Position at anterior border of sacral bone; should include sacral hollow | N/A | Transverse plane joining anterior edge of medial walls of the gluteus maximus muscle | Internal iliac nodes | Internal iliac nodes | Muscle boundaries |
| Anterior | Males: penile bulb and prostate in the lower pelvis, SV, and bladder Females: bladder Internal margin of 10 mm added to anterior mesorectal border on slices containing bladder | 10 mm anterior to the sacral border encompassing any lymph nodes | Obturator internus mm or bone in the lower pelvis; in upper pelvis, 7 mm margin around the internal iliac vessels | Level where obturator internus, levator ani, and sphincter muscle fuse; inferiorly, at least 10–20 mm anterior to sphincter muscles | Anterior extent of obturator internus | 7 mm margin anterior to the external iliac vessels | Minimum 2 cm margin on the inguinal vessels |
| Lateral | Lower pelvis = medial edge of levator ani; upper pelvis = internal iliac nodes | Sacroiliac joints | Medial edge of muscle or bone | Ischial tuberosity, muscles | Obturator internus | Iliopsoas muscle | Medial edge of sartorius or iliopsoas |
| Medial | N/A | N/A | Mesorectum and presacral space in the lower pelvis; 7 mm margin around vessel in the upper pelvis | N/A | Bladder | Bladder or 7 mm margin around vessel | 10–20 mm margin around the femoral vessels |

**Table 5** Suggested dose and fractionation schemes for anal canal cancer

| Target volume | RTOG 98-11 (Ajani et al. 2008) | RTOG 0529/trans-Australian |
|---|---|---|
| CTV-P | T1N0: 45–50.4 Gy at 1.8 Gy/fraction | T1N0: not included |
| | T2N0: 50.4 Gy at 1.8 Gy/fx | T2N0: 50.4 Gy at 1.8 Gy/fx |
| | N+ or T3-T4: 54–59.4 Gy at 1.8 Gy/fx | N+ or T3-T4: 54 Gy at 1.8 Gy/fx |
| CTV-N | 54–59.4 Gy at 1.8 Gy/fx | 50.4 Gy at 1.68 Gy/fx if node ≤ 3 cm |
| | | 54 Gy at 1.8 Gy/fx if node > 3 cm |
| CTV-HR | 45 Gy at 1.8 Gy/fx | T2N0: 42 Gy at 1.5 Gy/fx |
| | | T2N+ or T3-T4: 45 Gy at 1.5 Gy/fx |
| CTV-LR | 30.6–36 Gy at 1.8 Gy/fx (alternatively 40 Gy at 1.6 Gy/fx may be used if using IMRT) | RTOG 0529 does not differentiate between high- and low-risk regions, so this region should receive the same dose as CTV-HR |

**Table 6** Dose constraints for organs at risk

| Organ at risk | Constraints |
|---|---|
| Small bowel | **QUANTEC** |
| | V15Gy < 120 cc (individual loops) |
| | V45Gy < 195 cc (entire potential space within peritoneal cavity) |
| | **RTOG 0529** |
| | V30Gy < 200 cc |
| | V35Gy < 150 cc |
| | V45Gy < 20 cc |
| | Dmax < 50Gy |
| Large bowel | **RTOG 0529** |
| | V30Gy < 200 cc (Kachnic et al. 2013) |
| | V35Gy < 150 cc (Kachnic et al. 2013) |
| | V45Gy < 20 cc (Kachnic et al. 2013) |
| Bladder | **QUANTEC** |
| | Dmax < 65 Gy (Marks et al. 2010) |
| | V65Gy < 50 % (Marks et al. 2010) |
| | **RTOG 0529** |
| | V35Gy < 50 % (Kachnic et al. 2013) |
| | V40Gy < 35 %(Kachnic et al. 2013) |
| | V50Gy < 5 % (Kachnic et al. 2013) |
| Femoral heads | **RTOG 0529** |
| | V30Gy < 50 % (Kachnic et al. 2013) |
| | V40Gy < 35 % (Kachnic et al. 2013) |
| | V44Gy < 5 % (Kachnic et al. 2013) |
| Iliac crest | **RTOG 0529** |
| | V30Gy < 50 % (Kachnic et al. 2013) |
| | V40Gy < 35 % (Kachnic et al. 2013) |
| | V50Gy < 5 % (Kachnic et al. 2013) |
| External genitalia | **RTOG 0529** |
| | V20Gy < 50 % (Kachnic et al. 2013) |
| | V30Gy < 35 % (Kachnic et al. 2013) |
| | V40Gy < 5 % (Kachnic et al. 2013) |

## Suggested Reading

UKCCCR ACT I (UKCCCR Anal Cancer Trial Working Party 1996) and EORTC (Bartelink et al. 1997) Trials: Established that concurrent chemoradiotherapy is superior to radiotherapy alone.

RTOG 87-04 (Flam et al. 1996): Established that mitomycin-C is a necessary component of concurrent chemoradiation.

RTOG 98-11 (Ajani et al. 2008; Gunderson et al. 2012): Demonstrated that induction cisplatin-based chemotherapy followed by concurrent cisplatin-based chemoradiotherapy is inferior to concurrent mitomycin-C based chemoradiotherapy. Long-term update showed that overall survival is compromised by induction chemotherapy (Gunderson et al. 2012).

UKCCCR ACT II Trial (James et al. 2013): Randomized head-to-head comparison of mitomycin-C-based chemoradiotherapy versus cisplatin-based chemotherapy.

RTOG 0529 (Kachnic et al. 2013): Demonstrated prospectively that IMRT is feasible and less toxic when compared to the mitomycin-C arm of RTOG 98-11.

Contouring resources: RTOG anorectal guidelines (Myerson et al. 2009) (target volumes), Australasian GI Trials Group (Ng et al. 2012) (target volumes), Taylor et al. (2005) (pelvic nodal delineation), and RTOG pelvic normal tissue panel (Gay et al. 2012).

## References

Ajani JA, Winter KA, Gunderson LL et al (2008) Fluorouracil, mitomycin, and radiotherapy vs fluorouracil, cisplatin, and radiotherapy for carcinoma of the anal canal: a randomized controlled trial. JAMA 299(16):1914–1921

Bartelink H, Roelofsen F, Eschwege F et al (1997) Concomitant radiotherapy and chemotherapy is superior to radiotherapy alone in the treatment of locally advanced anal cancer: results of a phase III randomized trial of the European Organization for Research and Treatment of Cancer Radiotherapy and Gastrointestinal Cooperative Groups. J Clin Oncol 15(5):2040–2049

Bazan JG, Luxton G, Mok EC, Koong AC, Chang DT (2012) Normal tissue complication probability modeling of acute hematologic toxicity in patients treated with intensity-modulated radiation therapy for squamous cell carcinoma of the anal canal. Int J Radiat Oncol Biol Phys 84(3):700–706

Bazan JG, Luxton G, Kozak MM et al (2013) Impact of chemotherapy on normal tissue complication probability models of acute hematologic toxicity in patients receiving pelvic intensity modulated radiation therapy. Int J Radiat Oncol Biol Phys 87(5):983–991

Daly ME, Murphy JD, Mok E, Christman-Skieller C, Koong AC, Chang DT (2011) Rectal and bladder deformation and displacement during preoperative radiotherapy for rectal cancer: are current margin guidelines adequate for conformal therapy? Pract Radiat Oncol 1(2):85–94

Epidermoid anal cancer: results from the UKCCCR randomised trial of radiotherapy alone versus radiotherapy, 5-fluorouracil, and mitomycin. UKCCCR Anal Cancer Trial Working Party. UK Co-ordinating Committee on Cancer Research (1996) Lancet 348(9034): 1049–1054

Flam M, John M, Pajak TF et al (1996) Role of mitomycin in combination with fluorouracil and radiotherapy, and of salvage chemoradiation in the definitive nonsurgical treatment of epidermoid carcinoma of the anal canal: results of a phase III randomized intergroup study. J Clin Oncol 14(9):2527–2539

Gay HA, Barthold HJ, O'Meara E et al (2012) Pelvic normal tissue contouring guidelines for radiation therapy: a Radiation Therapy Oncology Group consensus panel atlas. Int J Radiat Oncol Biol Phys 83(3):e353–e362

Gilroy JS, Amdur RJ, Louis DA, Li JG, Mendenhall WM (2004) Irradiating the groin nodes without breaking a leg: a comparison of techniques for groin node irradiation. Med Dosim 29(4): 258–264

Gunderson LL, Winter KA, Ajani JA et al (2012) Long-term update of US GI intergroup RTOG 98-11 phase III trial for anal carcinoma: survival, relapse, and colostomy failure with concurrent chemoradiation involving fluorouracil/mitomycin versus fluorouracil/cisplatin. J Clin Oncol 30(35):4344–4351

James RD, Glynne-Jones R, Meadows HM et al (2013) Mitomycin or cisplatin chemoradiation with or without maintenance chemotherapy for treatment of squamous-cell carcinoma of the anus (ACT II): a randomised, phase 3, open-label, 2 x 2 factorial trial. Lancet Oncol 14(6):516–524

Kachnic LA, Winter K, Myerson RJ et al (2013) RTOG 0529: a phase 2 evaluation of dose-painted intensity modulated radiation therapy in combination with 5-fluorouracil and mitomycin-C for the reduction of acute morbidity in carcinoma of the anal canal. Int J Radiat Oncol Biol Phys 86(1):27–33

Marks LB, Yorke ED, Jackson A et al (2010) Use of normal tissue complication probability models in the clinic. Int J Radiat Oncol Biol Phys 76(3 Suppl):S10–S19

Mell LK, Kochanski JD, Roeske JC et al (2006) Dosimetric predictors of acute hematologic toxicity in cervical cancer patients treated with concurrent cisplatin and intensity-modulated pelvic radiotherapy. Int J Radiat Oncol Biol Phys 66(5):1356–1365

Mell LK, Schomas DA, Salama JK et al (2008) Association between bone marrow dosimetric parameters and acute hematologic toxicity in anal cancer patients treated with concurrent chemotherapy and intensity-modulated radiotherapy. Int J Radiat Oncol Biol Phys 70(5):1431–1437

Myerson RJ, Garofalo MC, El Naqa I et al (2009) Elective clinical target volumes for conformal therapy in anorectal cancer: a radiation therapy oncology group consensus panel contouring atlas. Int J Radiat Oncol Biol Phys 74(3):824–830

Ng M, Leong T, Chander S et al (2012) Australasian Gastrointestinal Trials Group (AGITG) contouring atlas and planning guidelines for intensity-modulated radiotherapy in anal cancer. Int J Radiat Oncol Biol Phys 83(5):1455–1462

Rose BS, Liang Y, Lau SK et al (2012) Correlation between radiation dose to (1)(8)F-FDG-PET defined active bone marrow subregions and acute hematologic toxicity in cervical cancer patients treated with chemoradiotherapy. Int J Radiat Oncol Biol Phys 83(4): 1185–1191

Taylor A, Rockall AG, Reznek RH, Powell ME (2005) Mapping pelvic lymph nodes: guidelines for delineation in intensity-modulated radiotherapy. Int J Radiat Oncol Biol Phys 63(5):1604–1612

# Part V

# Gynecological Tract

# Cervical Cancer

Daniel R. Simpson, Anthony J. Paravati,
Catheryn M. Yashar, Loren K. Mell, and Arno J. Mundt

## Contents

D.R. Simpson, MD (✉) • A.J. Paravati, MD MBA
C.M. Yashar, MD • L.K. Mell, MD • A.J. Mundt, MD
Department of Radiation Medicine and Applied Sciences,
University of California San Diego, La Jolla, CA, USA
e-mail: drsimpson@ucsd.edu

## 1    Anatomy and Patterns of Spread

- The cervix is the inferior portion of the uterus that is bound superiorly by the lower uterine segment and it protrudes into the upper vagina. The cervix is conical in shape and typically measures $3 \times 3$ cm.
- The portion of the cervix that protrudes into the upper vagina is referred to as the ectocervix. The ectocervix has a central opening referred to as the external cervical os that extends superiorly to become the endocervical canal and terminates at the internal cervical os to become the endometrial canal.
- The endocervix is lined by columnar epithelium, while the ectocervix is covered by squamous epithelium. The region where these two epithelial layers meet is referred to as the squamocolumnar junction (SCJ).
- The cervix is attached to the lateral pelvic wall by a pair of ligaments at the base of the broad ligament referred to as the cardinal ligaments. This ligament contains the uterine arteries and veins. The uterine arteries pass over the ureters on each side in close proximity to the cervix.
- The cervix drains into the paracervical lymph nodes which then drain into the obturator, internal iliac, and external iliac lymph nodes followed by the common iliac and para-aortic lymph nodes.
- Most cervical malignancies arise in the mucosa of the SCJ and invade into the underlying cervical stroma.
- Lesions can be exophytic or endophytic and spread by direct extension to the uterine fundus, surrounding vaginal fornices, parametrial tissues, pelvic sidewalls, rectum, and vagina.
- Paracervical extension depends on tumor size, depth of stromal invasion, and the presence of lymphovascular invasion.
- Regional lymphatic spread typically follows a stepwise pattern by spreading to the pelvic lymph nodes before the para-aortic lymph nodes.
- Patients with lesions involving the distal vagina are at risk for inguinal lymph node metastases.
- The incidence of pelvic and para-aortic lymph node involvement varies by stage (Table 1) as well as tumor size

N.Y. Lee et al. (eds.), *Target Volume Delineation for Conformal and Intensity-Modulated Radiation Therapy*,
Medical Radiology. Radiation Oncology, DOI: 10.1007/174_2014_995, © Springer International Publishing Switzerland 2014
Published Online: 20 September 2014

**Table 1** Incidence of pelvic and para-aortic nodal metastases by stage (Berman et al. 1984; Delgado et al. 1989; Hoskins 1988; Lagasse et al. 1980; Lee et al. 1989)

| FIGO stage | I | II | III |
|---|---|---|---|
| Pelvic nodes (%) | 15 | 30 | 50 |
| Para-aortic nodes (%) | 5 | 20 | 30 |

*FIGO* International Federation of Gynecology and Obstetrics

and depth of invasion (Berman et al. 1984; Delgado et al. 1989; Hoskins 1988; Lagasse et al. 1980; Lee et al. 1989).

- The most common sites of hematogenous spread are the lungs, mediastinum, supraclavicular fossae, bones, and liver.

## 2 Diagnostic Workup Relevant for Target Volume Delineation

- Patients with a diagnosis of invasive cervical cancer should have a thorough physical examination including pelvic exam as well as evaluation of the inguinal and supraclavicular lymph nodes.
- During the pelvic exam, special attention should be given to evaluation of the vaginal vault, rectovaginal septum, and bilateral parametria and sidewalls. Exam under anesthesia is indicated if patient discomfort prohibits a thorough examination.
- Patients suspected to have urinary bladder or rectal involvement should undergo cystoscopy or rectosigmoidoscopy.
- Magnetic resonance imaging (MRI) of the pelvis with intravenous contrast is helpful for determination of tumor extension into surrounding soft tissues and delineation of tumor during treatment planning (Fig. 1). MRI has been shown to be superior to CT and physical examination for determining size and extent of tumor invasion (Mitchell et al. 2006).
- A computed tomography (CT) scan with contrast or positron-emission tomography (PET) scan is recommended for the evaluation of draining lymph nodes. PET scans are preferable if available, as they offer higher sensitivity and specificity than CT (Grigsby et al. 2001).

## 3 Simulation and Daily Localization

- Patients may be set up in either a supine position or prone position for simulation. Prone positioning requires use of a belly board to allow setup reproducibility. Prone positioning allows the small bowel to fall out of the pelvis.
- If intensity-modulated radiotherapy (IMRT) is going to be used, a supine position with a customized immobilization

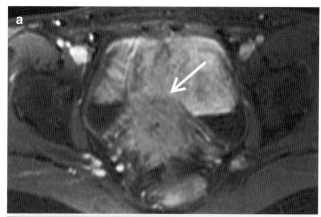
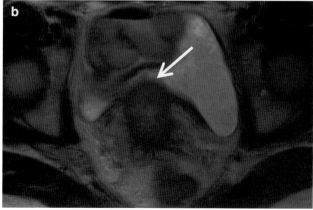

**Fig. 1** Magnetic resonance imaging in a patient with a stage IVA cervical tumor with posterior bladder wall invasion (*arrow*) on axial contrast-enhanced T1 (**a**) and T2 (**b**) sequences

cradle should be employed to minimize treatment setup error.

- CT simulation should be done with ≤3 mm slice thickness. Intravenous contrast is helpful for blood vessel delineation and should be used at the time of simulation unless medically contraindicated.
- In cases of vaginal involvement, a radiopaque marker should be placed at the caudal extent of the tumor and consideration should be made for fiducial markers in the cervix.
- The degree of bladder and rectal fullness should be made to duplicate that which is anticipated for daily treatment, i.e., if the patient is instructed to maintain a full bladder for treatment, she should be simulated as such. It is recommended to use a consistent bladder filling state (e.g., always full or always empty) for simulation and treatment. An enema may be applied at the discretion of the physician.
- Patients should undergo at least weekly imaging with megavoltage portal, kilovoltage imaging, or cone beam CT (CBCT) to verify treatment setup. Patients being

treated with IMRT should undergo image guidance with at least weekly CBCT.

## 4 Target Volume Delineation and Treatment Planning

- Suggested target volumes for the clinical target volume (CTV) based on guidelines from Radiation Therapy Oncology Group, the Gyn IMRT consortium, and the Japan Clinical Oncology Group (Lim et al. 2011; Small et al. 2008; Toita et al. 2011) are shown for both intact (Fig. 2) and postoperative (Fig. 3) cases.
- The CTV should be divided into three subregions: CTV1, CTV2, and CTV3.
- CTV1 should include the gross tumor volume (GTV), cervix, and entire uterus for intact patients or 3 cm of the proximal vaginal cuff for postoperative patients.
- CTV2 should extend 2 cm below the most inferior extent of vaginal disease.
- CTV3 will include the common, external, and internal iliac and presacral lymph nodes with a 7 mm margin around the vessels and any additional visible lymph nodes, lymphoceles, or pertinent surgical clips.
- CTV3 should not extend into adjacent bowel, bone, or muscle.
- The upper border of the CTV3 should not extend above the aortic bifurcation and should begin no lower than the level of the inferior border of the L4–5 interspace.
- The presacral nodes should be contoured until the superior border of the S3 vertebral body or the origin of the piriformis muscle is reached.
- The external iliac nodes should be contoured until the external iliac vessels exit from the pelvis (approximated by the appearance of the femoral heads).
- In cases with distal one-third vaginal involvement, the inguinal nodes will be contoured continuously from the external iliac nodes to 2 cm caudal to the saphenous/femoral junction.
- If para-aortic nodes are involved, an "extended-field" technique should be used by extending the cranial border of CTV3 superiorly to encompass involved nodes. The superior border should be chosen at the discretion of the treating physician.
- Each CTV should be expanded differentially to form PTV1, PTV2, and PTV3 (Table 2). The three PTVs will then be combined to form $PTV_{sum}$.
- An additional boost of 5–15 Gy may be added for gross nodal disease or parametrial involvement at the discretion of the treating physician.

## 5 External Beam Plan Assessment

- Ideally, at least 95 % of the PTV should receive 100 % of the prescription dose, and $\geq$99 % of the PTV will receive $\geq$90 % of the prescription dose.
- The dose maximum should occur within the PTV and dose areas >100 % of the prescription dose outside of the PTV should be minimized.
- Organs at risk (OAR) include the bowel, rectum, bone marrow, bladder, and femoral heads (Fig. 4). Table 3 provides details for delineation of OARs. The dose constraints for these structures are outlined in Table 4.
- The bowel should be contoured as the entire peritoneal space encompassing the bowel such that the superoinferior boundaries extend 1.5 cm superior to the caudal aspect of the PTV and inferiorly to the rectosigmoid junction. In the anterior-posterior direction, the bowel should be delineated from the anterior abdominal wall to the most posterior extent of bowel. The bilateral bowel edges serve as the left-right boundaries.

## 6 Image-Guided Brachytherapy Target Volume Delineation and Treatment Planning

- Image-guided brachytherapy (IGBT) volumes (Fig. 5) are adapted from the published experience and recommendations from the Groupe Européen de Curiethérapie and the European Society for Radiotherapy & Oncology (GEC-ESTRO) (Haie-Meder et al. 2005; Potter et al. 2006).
- An MRI should be obtained immediately prior to or at the time of brachytherapy implantation with an MR-compatible applicator.
- The planning CT should be fused to the MRI using rigid registration along the brachytherapy applicator.
- The gross tumor volume (GTV) is defined as all known gross disease determined from CT, MRI, and clinical information.
- The high-risk CTV (HRCTV) is defined as the GTV plus the entire cervix and any presumed extra cervical tumor extension at the time of brachytherapy
- The HRCTV should be contoured using a combination of the axial, coronal, and sagittal slices of the CT scan as well as a fused T2-weighted MRI (Fig. 6) and any relevant clinical examination findings.
- The HRCTV should be contoured prior to planning each implant to account for daily changes in anatomy.
- Table 5 shows the different fractionation schedules for high-dose-rate brachytherapy based on the guidelines from the American Brachytherapy Society (Viswanathan et al. 2012).

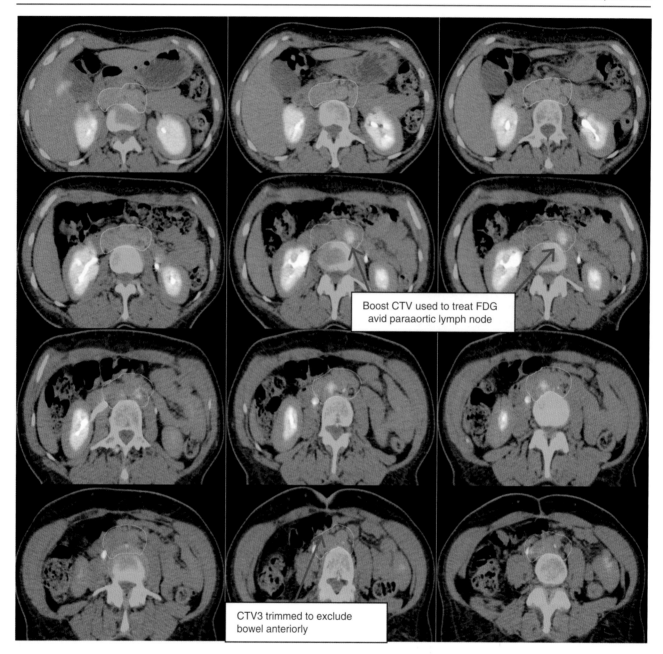

Boost CTV used to treat FDG
avid paraaortic lymph node

CTV3 trimmed to exclude
bowel anteriorly

**Fig. 2** A patient with International Federation of Gynecology and Obstetrics (FIGO) stage IIIB (American Joint Committee on Cancer stage T3bN1M1) cervical carcinoma with para-aortic nodal metastases who underwent definitive extended-field intensity-modulated radiation therapy and concomitant cis-platinum. Three clinical target volumes (CTV) are shown: (CTV1) (*blue*), CTV2 (*red*), CTV3 (*yellow*) and boost volume (*green*) on a positron-emission tomography/computed tomography simulation. Please note that these are representative slices and not all slices are included. *FDG* fluorodeoxyglucose

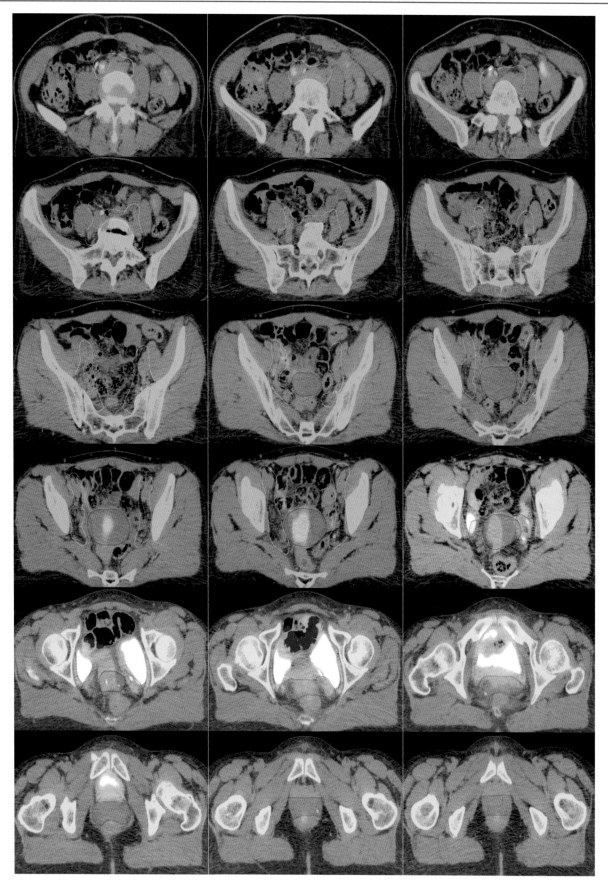

**Fig. 2** (continued)

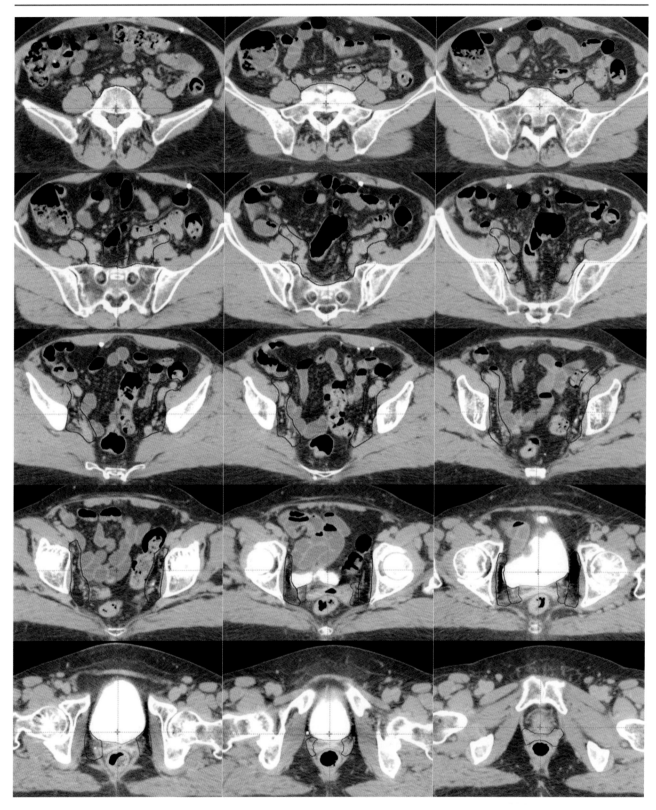

**Fig. 3** A patient with International Federation of Gynecology and Obstetric (FIGO) stage IB1 cervical cancer who underwent a radical hysterectomy and pelvic lymphadenectomy. Pathology revealed deep cervical stromal invasion as well as 3 of 15 positive nodes. She was treated with adjuvant intensity-modulated pelvic radiation therapy and concomitant cis-platinum. Three clinical target volumes (CTV) are shown: $CTV_1$ (*green*), $CTV_2$ (*blue*), and $CTV_3$ (*red*)

**Table 2** Suggested target volumes

| Target volumes | Definition[a] | Planning volumes[b] | Definition[c] |
|---|---|---|---|
| CTV1 | Gross tumor, cervix, and uterus or vaginal cuff. | PTV1 | CTV1 + 15 mm |
| CTV2 | Parametria and superior third to half of the vagina | PTV2 | CTV2 + 10 mm |
| CTV3 | Common, external, and internal iliac and presacral lymph nodes | PTV3 | CTV3 + 7 mm |

*CTV* clinical target volume, *PTV* planning target volume

[a]Based on guidelines from Radiation Therapy Oncology Group, the Gyn IMRT consortium, and the Japan Clinical Oncology Group (Lim et al. 2011; Small et al. 2008; Toita et al. 2011)

[b]PTVs 1–3 are combined to form PTV$_{sum}$, which receives 1.8 Gy/fraction to 45 Gy over 25 fractions for intact cases or 1.8 Gy/fraction to 50.4 Gy over 28 fractions for postoperative cases

[c]Based on work from Khan et al. (2012)

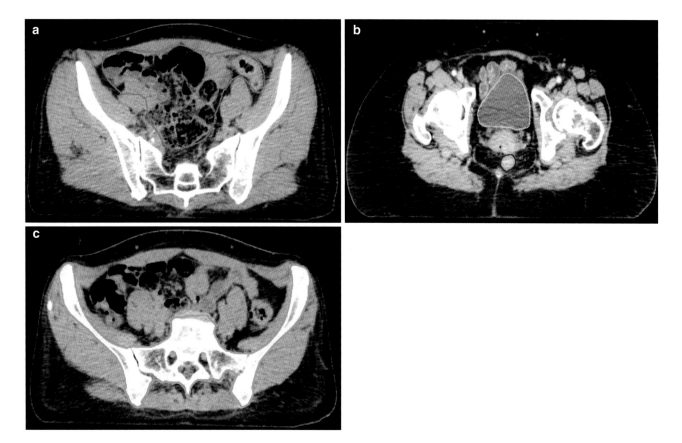

**Fig. 4** Contours for organs at risk including bowel (**a**, *orange*), rectum (**b**, *brown*), bladder (**b**, *yellow*), and bone marrow (**c**, *green*) on representative computed tomography slices

**Table 3** Organs at risk

| Organ | Definition and description |
|---|---|
| Bowel | Outermost loops of bowel from the level of the L4–5 interspace to the sigmoid flexure |
| | Includes the sigmoid colon and ascending/descending colon present in the pelvis |
| | In women with intact cervical cancer, bowel loops posterior to the uterus in the lower pelvis within the PTV are not included |
| Rectum | Defined by the outer rectal wall from the level of the sigmoid flexure to the anus |
| Bladder | Defined by the outer bladder wall |
| Bone marrow | The pelvic bones serve as a surrogate for the pelvic bone marrow. Regions included are the os coxae, L5 vertebral body, entire sacrum, acetabulae, and proximal femora superior extent: superior border of L5 or the iliac crest (whichever is more superior) |
| | Inferior extent: ischial tuberosities |
| Femoral heads | Entire femoral head excluding the femoral neck |

*PTV* planning target volume

## 7    Brachytherapy Plan Assessment

- The D90 (dose to 90 % of the HRCTV) should be equal to or higher than the prescription dose.
- Organs at risk including the bladder, rectum, and sigmoid colon should be contoured at the time of each brachytherapy implant.

- HDR dose should be converted to 2-Gy equivalent doses (EQD2) using the linear quadratic model ($\alpha/\beta = 10$ for HRCTV and $\alpha/\beta = 3$ for OARs) and the total combined IMRT and summed brachytherapy doses should be calculated and recorded.
- Total EQD2 doses to 2 cc for the rectum, sigmoid, and bladder should be kept below 75, 75, and 85 Gy, respectively.

**Table 4**  Intensity-modulated radiation therapy: normal dose constraints

| Structures | Constraints |
|---|---|
| Bowel | Volume receiving >45 Gy ($V_{45}$) $\leq$ 250 cc; maximum dose <115 % |
| Rectum | Maximum dose <115 % |
| Bone marrow | $V_{10} < 90$ %; $V_{20} < 75$ % |
| Bladder | Maximum dose <115 % |
| Femoral head | Maximum dose <115 % |
| Spinal cord | Maximum dose <45 Gy |

$V_x$ volume receiving "X" Gy
Constraints presently used at the University of California, San Diego

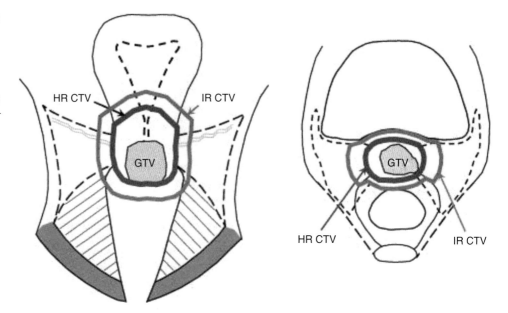

**Fig. 5**  Suggested image-guided brachytherapy target volumes from the Groupe Européen de Curiethérapie and the European Society for Radiotherapy & Oncology (Haie-Meder et al. 2005). *HRCTV* high-risk clinical target volume, *IRCTV* intermediate-risk clinical target volume, *GTV* gross tumor volume (Used with permission)

**Fig. 6** A patient with International Federation of Gynecology and Obstetrics (FIGO) stage IB2 cervical cancer being treated with image-guided brachytherapy using a tandem and ovoid high-dose-rate applicator following the completion of intensity-modulated radiotherapy and concomitant cis-platinum. Target delineation for a patient with axial (**a**) and sagittal images (**b**) of the planning computed tomography (*left*) and fused magnetic resonance imaging (*right*) are shown below. The high-risk clinical target volume is outlined in *red*

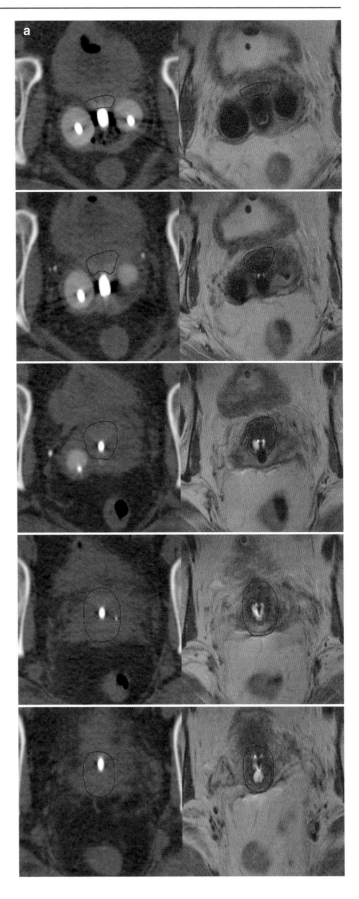

**Fig. 6** (continued)

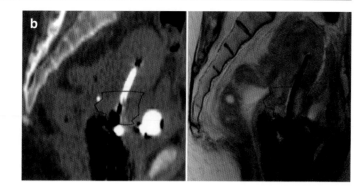

**Table 5** Dose fractionation schedules for high-dose-rate brachytherapy

| Fractionation | EQD2[a] (Gy) to HRCTV |
|---|---|
| 4×7 Gy | 83.9 |
| 5×6 Gy | 84.3 |
| 6×5 Gy | 81.8 |
| 5×5.5 Gy | 79.8 |

EQD2: high-dose-rate brachytherapy dose converted to 2-Gy equivalent doses

*HRCTV* high-risk clinical target volume

Adapted from guidelines from the American Brachytherapy Society (Viswanathan et al. 2012)

[a]Following 45 Gy of external beam radiotherapy in 1.8 Gy fractions

# References

Berman ML, Keys H, Creasman W et al (1984) Survival and patterns of recurrence in cervical cancer metastatic to periaortic lymph nodes (a Gynecologic Oncology Group study). Gynecol Oncol 19:8–16

Delgado G, Bundy BN, Fowler WC Jr et al (1989) A prospective surgical pathological study of stage I squamous carcinoma of the cervix: a Gynecologic Oncology Group Study. Gynecol Oncol 35:314–320

Grigsby PW, Siegel BA, Dehdashti F (2001) Lymph node staging by positron emission tomography in patients with carcinoma of the cervix. J Clin Oncol 19:3745–3749

Haie-Meder C, Potter R, Van Limbergen E et al (2005) Recommendations from Gynaecological (GYN) GEC-ESTRO Working Group (I): concepts and terms in 3D image based 3D treatment planning in cervix cancer brachytherapy with emphasis on MRI assessment of GTV and CTV. Radiother Oncol 74:235–245

Hoskins WJ (1988) Prognostic factors for risk of recurrence in stages Ib and IIa cervical cancer. Baillieres Clin Obstet Gynaecol 2:817–828

Khan A, Jensen LG, Sun S et al (2012) Optimized planning target volume for intact cervical cancer. Int J Radiat Oncol Biol Phys 83:1500–1505

Lagasse LD, Creasman WT, Shingleton HM et al (1980) Results and complications of operative staging in cervical cancer: experience of the Gynecologic Oncology Group. Gynecol Oncol 9:90–98

Lee YN, Wang KL, Lin MH et al (1989) Radical hysterectomy with pelvic lymph node dissection for treatment of cervical cancer: a clinical review of 954 cases. Gynecol Oncol 32:135–142

Lim K, Small W Jr, Portelance L et al (2011) Consensus guidelines for delineation of clinical target volume for intensity-modulated pelvic radiotherapy for the definitive treatment of cervix cancer. Int J Radiat Oncol Biol Phys 79:348–355

Mitchell DG, Snyder B, Coakley F et al (2006) Early invasive cervical cancer: tumor delineation by magnetic resonance imaging, computed tomography, and clinical examination, verified by pathologic results, in the ACRIN 6651/GOG 183 Intergroup Study. J Clin Oncol 24:5687–5694

Potter R, Haie-Meder C, Van Limbergen E et al (2006) Recommendations from gynaecological (GYN) GEC ESTRO working group (II): concepts and terms in 3D image-based treatment planning in cervix cancer brachytherapy-3D dose volume parameters and aspects of 3D image-based anatomy, radiation physics, radiobiology. Radiother Oncol 78:67–77

Small W Jr, Mell LK, Anderson P et al (2008) Consensus guidelines for delineation of clinical target volume for intensity-modulated pelvic radiotherapy in postoperative treatment of endometrial and cervical cancer. Int J Radiat Oncol Biol Phys 71:428–434

Toita T, Ohno T, Kaneyasu Y et al (2011) A consensus-based guideline defining clinical target volume for primary disease in external beam radiotherapy for intact uterine cervical cancer. Jpn J Clin Oncol 41:1119–1126

Viswanathan AN, Beriwal S, De Los Santos JF et al (2012) American Brachytherapy Society consensus guidelines for locally advanced carcinoma of the cervix. Part II: high-dose-rate brachytherapy. Brachytherapy 11:47–52

# Uterine Cancer

Anthony J. Paravati, Daniel R. Simpson,
Catheryn M. Yashar, Loren K. Mell, and Arno J. Mundt

## Contents

- Intensity-modulated radiation therapy (IMRT) is becoming increasingly popular in treatment of gynecologic malignancies, particularly in patients with cervical and endometrial cancers (Mell and Mundt 2008; Mell et al. 2003).
- IMRT is appealing in endometrial cancer patients undergoing postoperative pelvic radiotherapy (RT) to reduce the volume of small bowel irradiated and thus the risk of acute and chronic toxicities (Yang et al. 2010; Heron et al. 2003).
- Endometrial cancer patients treated with postoperative pelvic IMRT have had low rates of toxicities and high rates of pelvic control. Long-term outcome data, however, remain limited in this setting.
- Target delineation is an essential component of IMRT treatment in endometrial cancer patients. Consensus guidelines have been published (Small et al. 2008; Toita et al. 2011; Nag et al. 2000) and have been used in the Radiation Therapy Oncology Group (RTOG) 0921 Phase II trial.
- All endometrial cancer patients should undergo a complete history and physical examination including a pelvic exam as part of initial diagnosis and staging. Standard radiographic workup in these patients includes a computed tomography (CT) scan to assess the extent of local disease involvement and sites of extrauterine spread.
- Treatment consists of upfront surgery (total abdominal hysterectomy and bilateral salpingo-oophorectomy) when possible. Radiation therapy is used postoperatively in women with high-risk pathologic features including deep myometrial invasion, cervical stromal extension, high-grade disease, and regional lymph node involvement (Keys et al. 2004; Naumann and Coleman 2007).
- Traditionally, most endometrial cancer patients undergoing adjuvant RT received pelvic irradiation. However, select patients undergoing surgical staging who are found to have negative nodes may undergo vaginal brachytherapy alone (Nout et al. 2010).

A.J. Paravati, MD, MBA • D.R. Simpson, MD
C.M. Yashar, MD • L.K. Mell, MD • A.J. Mundt, MD (✉)
Department of Radiation Medicine and Applied Sciences,
University of California, San Diego, La Jolla, CA, USA
e-mail: amundt@ucsd.edu

N.Y. Lee et al. (eds.), *Target Volume Delineation for Conformal and Intensity-Modulated Radiation Therapy*,
Medical Radiology. Radiation Oncology, DOI: 10.1007/174_2014_996, © Springer International Publishing Switzerland 2014
Published Online: 20 September 2014

# 1    Anatomy and Patterns of Spread

- The uterus is a pelvic organ bordered anteriorly by the bladder and posteriorly by the rectum. It is covered by peritoneal reflections and is divided into the fundus, isthmus, and cervix.
- The uterine wall consists of an outer smooth muscle layer (the myometrium) and an inner layer of glandular epithelium (endometrium).
- The uterus is supported by five ligaments: broad, round, cardinal, uterosacral, and vesicouterine.
- The uterus is attached at the cervix to the lateral pelvic wall by a pair of ligaments at the base of the broad ligament referred to as the cardinal ligaments which contain arteries, veins, and lymphatics. The uterine arteries pass over the ureters on each side in close proximity to the cervix.
- Most uterine malignancies arise in the epithelium and are adenocarcinomas of endometrioid subtype.
- Lesions may extend locally in either longitudinal or radial growth patterns. Longitudinal growth may result in local extension along the endometrial surface to either the lower uterine segment or cervix inferiorly or the fallopian tubes superolaterally.
- The uterine myometrium drains into a rich subserosal lymphatic network which joins into larger lymphatic channels before exiting the uterus.
- Lymphatics of the fundus drain toward the adnexa and infundibulopelvic ligaments; the lymphatics of the middle and lower uterus drain into the base of the broad ligament toward the pelvic sidewall.
- The nodal areas at risk in uterine cancer patients include the obturator, external iliac, internal iliac, common iliac, and para-aortic lymph nodes.
- Lesions involving the uterine fundus can spread directly to the para-aortic lymph nodes.
- The incidence of pelvic and para-aortic lymph node involvement varies according to risk categories (low, medium, and high) as defined in Gynecologic Oncology Group (GOG) 33 study (Table 1) as well as tumor size and depth of invasion (Creasman et al. 1987).
- The most common sites of hematogenous spread are lungs, mediastinum, supraclavicular fossae, bones, and liver.

# 2    Diagnostic Workup Relevant for Target Volume Delineation

- Patients with a diagnosis of endometrial cancer should have a thorough physical examination including pelvic exam as well as evaluation of the inguinal and supraclavicular lymph nodes.
- During the pelvic exam, special attention should be given to evaluation of the vaginal vault, rectovaginal septum,

**Table 1** Incidence of nodal metastases by risk category (low, no invasion or grade I disease with invasion; medium, all other; high, grade 3 or outer third invasion) in GOG 33

|             | Pelvic lymph nodes (%) | Para-aortic lymph nodes (%) |
|-------------|------------------------|------------------------------|
| Low risk    | <5                     | <5                           |
| Medium risk | 5–10                   | <5                           |
| High risk   | >10                    | >10                          |

Adapted from Creasman et al. (1987)
*GOG* Gynecologic Oncology Group

and bilateral parametria and sidewalls. Exam under anesthesia is indicated if patient discomfort prohibits a thorough examination.
- Patients often undergo transvaginal ultrasound for assessment of postmenopausal bleeding (Smith-Bindman et al. 1998).
- Pelvic CT with oral and intravenous contrast could be considered for evaluation of the extent of the endometrial tumor.
- On CT, endometrial carcinoma typically appears as a hypodense mass relative to the surrounding myometrium. It may appear as a diffuse, circumscribed, vegetative, or polypoidal mass within the uterine cavity.
  - If myometrial invasion is seen, it usually implies involvement of more than one-third to one-half of myometrial thickness.
  - Involvement of the cervix is visualized on CT as cervical enlargement >3.5 cm in diameter with heterogeneous low-attenuation areas within the fibromuscular stroma.
  - Parametrial or sidewall extension is seen by the loss of periureteral fat in the former and <3 mm of intervening fat between the soft tissue mass and the pelvic sidewall in the latter.
- Dynamic contrast-enhanced magnetic resonance imaging (MRI) is the optimal method for detecting cervix invasion (Fig. 1) and myometrial invasion with an accuracy of 85–93 % (Frei et al. 2000).
- The sensitivity of MRI in detecting lymph node metastasis is 27–66 % and the specificity is 73–94 % in surgically staged patients (Kitajima et al. 2011). However, PET is preferable if available. The sensitivity and specificity of PET for assessing regional lymph node metastases have been shown to range from 50 to 100 % and 87 % to 100, respectively (Kitajima et al. 2011).

# 3    Simulation and Daily Localization

- Patients may be simulated in either a supine position or prone position. Prone positioning requires use of a belly board to allow setup reproducibility.
- Endometrial cancer patients undergoing pelvic IMRT are typically simulated in the supine position. Immobilization

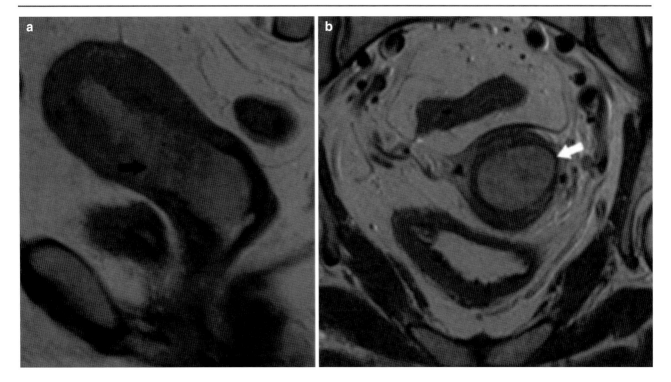

**Fig. 1** Magnetic resonance imaging (MRI) of endometrial cancer growing into the endocervical canal: (**a**) sagittal and (**b**) axial T2-weight sequences demonstrate thinning of the low signal intensity cervical stroma (*white arrow*) which suggests cervical stroma invasion (Image adapted from Imaging of Endometrial and Cervical Cancer by Patel et al. (2010))

**Table 2** Suggested target volumes used in endometrial cancer patients undergoing postoperative pelvic IMRT

| Target volume | Definition and description |
| --- | --- |
| GTV | Visible disease on imaging and/or physical exam |
| CTV$_1$ | Vaginal cuff |
| | Include any fat and soft tissue anterior and posterior to the vaginal cuff between the bladder and rectum |
| CTV$_2$ | Paravaginal/parametrial tissues, proximal vagina (excluding the cuff) |
| CTV$_3$ | Includes common iliac,[a] external, and internal iliac nodal regions |
| | In patients with cervical stromal involvement, the presacral region is also included |
| | The common iliac and external and internal iliac regions are defined by including the pelvic vessels plus a 7-mm expansion (excluding bone, muscle, and bowel) as well as all suspicious lymph nodes, lymphoceles, and pertinent surgical clips |
| | Soft tissues between the internal and external iliac vessels along the pelvic sidewall are included |
| | The presacral area consists of the soft tissues anterior (minimum 1.0 cm) to the S1–S2 vertebrae |
| | Upper extent: 7 mm inferior to L4–5 interspace |
| | Lower extent: superior aspect of femoral head (lower extent of external iliacs) and paravaginal tissues at level of vaginal cuff (lower extent of internal iliacs) |
| PTV$_1$ | CTV$_1$ + 15 mm |
| PTV$_2$ | CTV$_2$ + 10 mm |
| PTV$_3$ | CTV$_3$ + 7 mm |

The final PTV is then generated by the union of the PTV$_1$, PTV$_2$, and PTV$_3$: PTV = PTV$_1$ $\bigcup$ PTV$_2$ $\bigcup$ PTV$_3$
*IMRT* intensity-modulated radiation therapy, *GTV* gross tumor volume, *CTV* clinical target volume, *PTV* planning target volume
[a]To the level of L4–L5 which will not include the entire common iliac nodal region in many patients

with a customized cradle should be employed to minimize treatment setup error.
• Patients should be simulated with a comfortably full bladder. At some centers, two scans are performed (full bladder and empty bladder) and the two scans are fused to generate an integrated target volume (ITV).
• CT simulation should be done with ≤3 mm slice thickness. Intravenous contrast is helpful for blood vessel delineation.

- In cases of vaginal involvement, a radiopaque marker should be placed at the caudal extent of the tumor.
- Patients should undergo at least weekly imaging with megavoltage (MV) portal, kilovoltage (kV) imaging, or cone beam CT (CBCT) to verify treatment setup. Patients being treated with IMRT should undergo image guidance, preferably with daily imaging.

## 4 Target Volume Delineation and Treatment Planning

- Suggested postoperative clinical target volumes (CTV) are detailed in Table 2 and are based on guidelines from Radiation Therapy Oncology Group (RTOG) and the Gynecologic IMRT Consortium (Small et al. 2008).
- The CTV is divided into three subregions: $CTV_1$, $CTV_2$, and $CTV_3$.
- In the intact/palliative patient $CTV_1$ should include the entire uterus. $CTV_2$ should include the paravaginal/parametrial tissues as in the postoperative setting plus 3 cm of the proximal vagina. $CTV_3$ is the same as in the postoperative setting.
- In patients with distal one-third vaginal involvement, the inguinal nodes should be contoured continuously from the external iliac nodes to 2 cm caudad to the saphenous/femoral junction.
- If para-aortic nodes are involved, an extended field technique should be used by extending the cranial border of $CTV_3$ superiorly to encompass involved nodes. The superior border should be chosen at the discretion of the treating physician.
- Each CTV should be expanded differentially to form $PTV_1$, $PTV_2$, and $PTV_3$ (Table 2). These three PTVs are then combined to form $PTV_{sum}$.
- An additional boost of 5–15 Gy may be added for gross nodal disease or parametrial involvement at the discretion of the treating physician. This many be done sequentially or by an integrated boost (Figs. 2, 3, 4, and 5).

## 5 External Beam Plan Assessment

- Ideally, at least 95 % of the PTV should receive 100 % of the prescription dose, and ≥99 % of the PTV should receive ≥90 % of the prescription dose.
- The dose maximum should occur within the PTV and dose areas >100 % of the prescription dose outside of the PTV should be minimized.
- Organs at risk (OAR) include the bowel, rectum, bone marrow, bladder, and femoral heads (Fig. 6). Table 3 provides details for delineation of OARs. The dose constraints for these structures are outlined in Table 4.
- The bowel should be contoured as the entire peritoneal space encompassing the bowel such that the superior-

inferior boundaries extend 1.5 cm superior to the caudal aspect of the PTV and inferiorly to the rectosigmoid junction. In the anterior-posterior direction, the bowel should be delineated from the anterior abdominal wall to the most posterior extent of bowel. The bilateral bowel edges serve as the left-right boundaries.

## 6 Endometrial Brachytherapy

- Brachytherapy is often an integral component of treatment for endometrial carcinoma in both the postoperative and intact setting. Guidelines are provided from the published experience and recommendations of American Brachytherapy Society (ABS) and the Groupe Europeen de Curietherapie–European Society for Therapeutic Radiology and Oncology (GEC-ESTRO) (Nag et al. 2000).
- After placement of the brachytherapy device, a method of localization such as a portable x-ray or conventional radiotherapy CT simulation is indicated.
- In the intact setting CT, MRI, and/or ultrasound should be employed to determine uterine wall thickness. Additionally, MRI provides information regarding the depth of myometrial or cervical invasion.
- If an MRI is obtained, the planning CT should be fused to the MRI using rigid registration along the brachytherapy applicator.
- When using a fixed geometry applicator such as a cylinder in the postoperative setting, localization radiographs are not required for treatments subsequent to the first fraction.
- HDR applicators for inoperable primary endometrial carcinoma are as in cervical carcinoma and include tandem and ovoids, tandem and ring, and tandem and cylinder.
- When treating the vaginal cuff with HDR brachytherapy, it is imperative for the vaginal mucosa to be in contact with the applicator surface and that the cylinder is apposed to the apex without intervening air or fluid to have effective dose distribution.
- Table 5 shows the dose and fractionation schedules for HDR brachytherapy based on the guidelines from the ABS for HDR alone as adjuvant treatment of postoperative endometrial cancer.
- The ABS recommends treating the proximal 3–5 cm of the vagina for endometrial carcinoma and consideration of treatment of the full length of the vagina for serous and clear cell histologies
- HDR treatment of recurrences at the vaginal cuff should generally follow pelvic EBRT
  - According to ABS recommendations, intracavitary brachytherapy should be used only for non-bulky recurrences with thickness <0.5 cm after completion of EBRT.

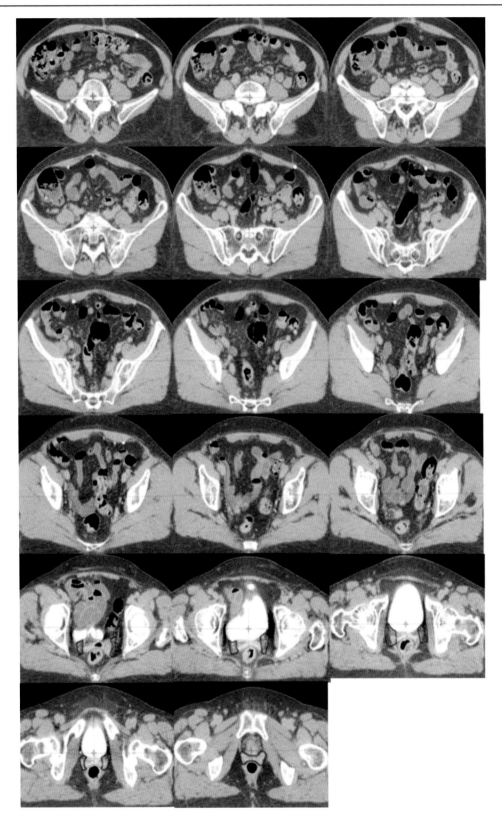

**Fig. 2** A patient with stage IB grade 3 endometrial cancer who underwent a total abdominal hysterectomy and bilateral salpingo-oophorectomy (TAH BSO) with sampling of the pelvic lymph nodes. Pathology revealed deep (>1/2) myometrial invasion of a grade 3 tumor with extensive angiolymphatic invasion. Disease was limited to the fundus with no involvement of the lower uterine segment or cervix. Zero of 5 pelvic nodes were involved with tumor. She was treated with adjuvant intensity-modulated pelvic radiation therapy. Three clinical target volumes (CTV) are shown: CTV1 (*green*) consists of the vaginal cuff, CTV2 (*blue*) includes the paravaginal/parametrial tissues and proximal vagina (excluding the cuff), and CTV3 (*red*) consists of the common iliac, external, and internal iliac lymph nodes

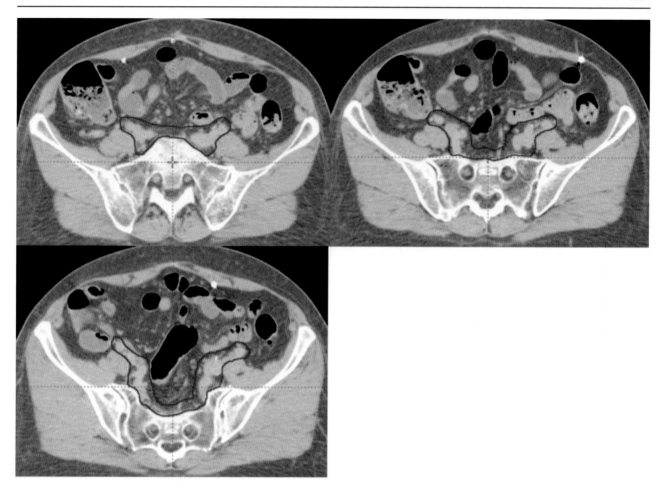

**Fig. 3** The clinical target volume-3 (CTV₃) (*orange*) is modified in endometrial cancer patients with cervical stromal invasion to include the pre-sacral region

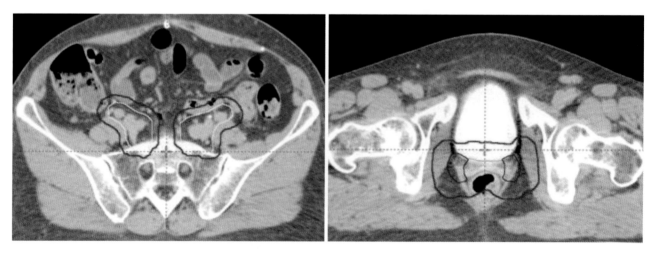

**Fig. 4** Three separate planning target volumes (PTV) are generated in the postoperative endometrial cancer patient described in Fig. 2 (see Table 2). The final PTV used for treatment planning is generated by combining PTV₁, PTV₂, and PTV₃. The resultant PTV (*red*) is shown in the figure encompassing CTV₁ (*green*), CTV₂, and CTV₃ (*yellow*)

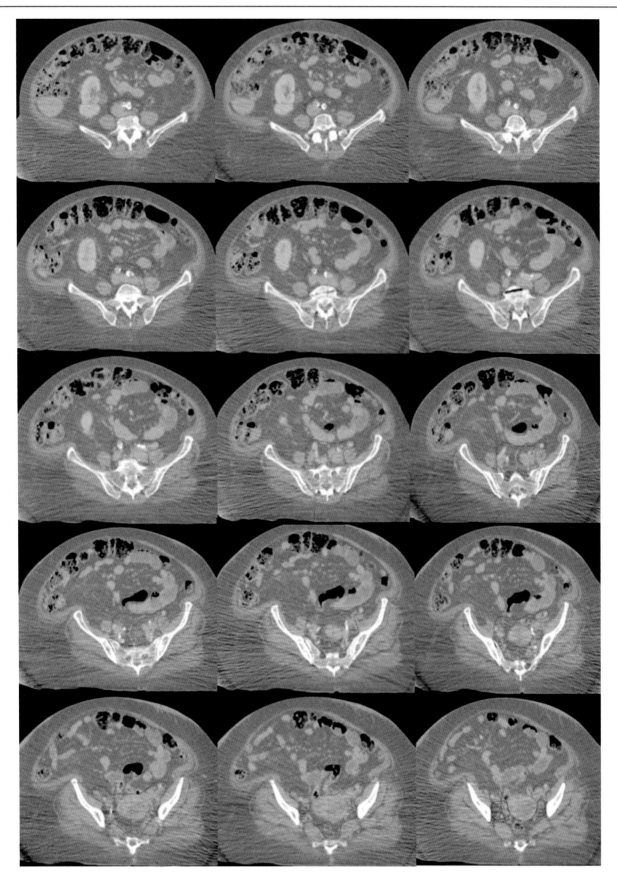

**Fig. 5** Target delineation of $CTV_1$ (*green*), $CTV_2$ (*blue*), and $CTV_3$ (*red*) on a CT simulation in a 65-year-old woman with multiple comorbidities with high-grade medically inoperable stage IIIC uterine carcinoma

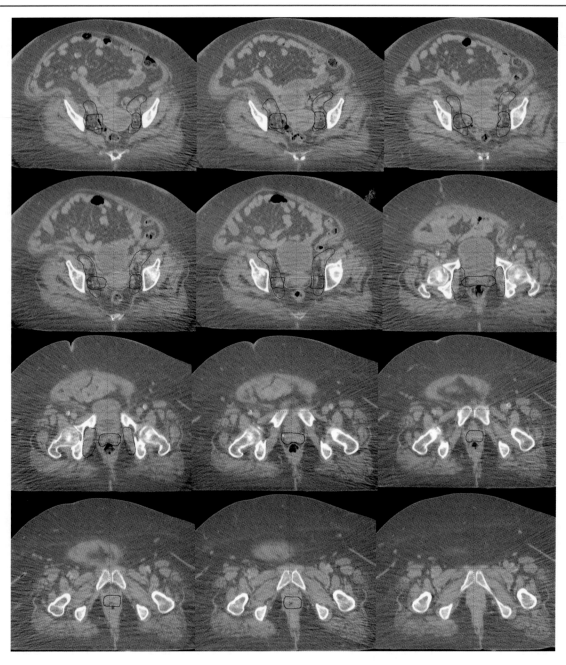

**Fig. 5** (continued)

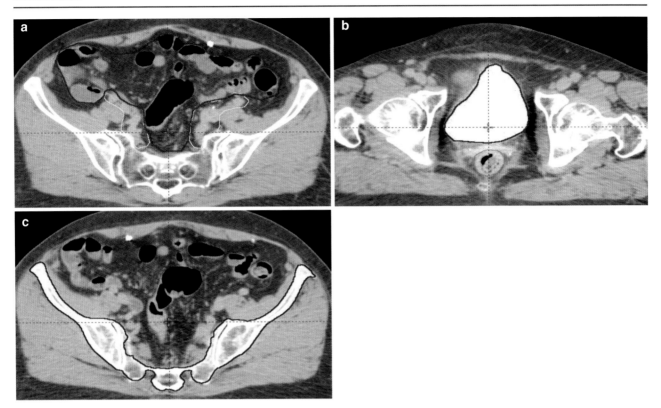

**Fig. 6** Contours for organs at risk including bowel (**a**, *red*), rectum (**b**, *brown*), bladder (**b**, *red*), and bone marrow (**c**, *blue*) on representative computed tomography slices. Clinical target volume 3 (CTV₃) is also depicted

**Table 3** Organs at risk

| Organ | Definition and description |
|---|---|
| Bowel | Outermost loops of bowel from the level of the L4–5 interspace to the sigmoid flexure |
| | Includes the sigmoid colon and ascending/descending colon present in the pelvis |
| | In the intact/palliative setting bowel loops posterior to the uterus in the lower pelvis within the PTV are not included |
| Rectum | Defined by the outer rectal wall from the level of the sigmoid flexure to the anus |
| Bladder | Defined by the outer bladder wall |
| Bone marrow | The pelvic bones serve as a surrogate for the pelvic bone marrow. Regions included are the os coxae, L5 vertebral body, entire sacrum, acetabulae, and proximal femora |
| | Superior extent: superior border of L5 or the iliac crest (whichever is more superior) |
| | Inferior extent: ischial tuberosities |
| Femoral heads | Entire femoral head excluding the femoral neck |

*PTV* planning target volume

**Table 4** Intensity-modulated radiation therapy: normal dose constraints

| Structures | Constraints |
|---|---|
| Bowel | Volume receiving >45 Gy ($V_{45}$) ≤ 250 cc; maximum dose <115 % |
| Rectum | Maximum dose <115 % |
| Bone marrow | $V_{10}$<90 %; $V_{20}$<75 % |
| Bladder | Maximum dose<115 % |
| Femoral head | Maximum dose <115 % |
| Spinal cord | Maximum dose <45 Gy |

$V_x$ volume receiving "X" Gy
Constraints presently used at the University of California, San Diego

**Table 5** Dose-fractionation schedules for high-dose-rate brachytherapy alone for adjuvant treatment of endometrial cancer in the postoperative setting

| Fractionation | Dose-specific point | Equiv. dose for late effects |
|---|---|---|
| 3×10.5 Gy | Vaginal surface | 45.6 |
| 4×8.8 Gy | Vaginal surface | 45.1 |
| 5×7.5 Gy | Vaginal surface | 43.3 |
| 3×7.0 Gy | 0.5 cm depth | 23.2 |
| 4×5.5 Gy | 0.5 cm depth | 21.1 |
| 5×4.7 Gy | 0.5 cm depth | 20.7 |

Adapted from guidelines from the American Brachytherapy Society (Nag et al. 2000)

– Interstitial brachytherapy should be offered for recurrences with thickness >0.5 cm after EBRT.
– Table 6 shows the suggested HDR doses after EBRT to 45 Gy.
- HDR treatment in the intact setting should also follow EBRT in many cases. However, bachytherapy alone may be appropriate in patients with low risk disease and/or for patients for whom EBRT may present unacceptable morbidity.
- Tables 7 and 8 show the dose and fractionation schedules for treatment with brachytherapy alone and brachytherapy in combination with EBRT for intact endometrial cancer.
- The target volume is the entire uterus, cervix, and proximal 3–5 cm of the vagina.
  – At the level of the vagina, the dose distribution should be optimized to deliver the prescribed dose to a depth of 0.5 cm unless treating to the surface.
  – As above, it is ideal for treatment planning to include image guidance to ensure the entire uterine serosa and vaginal wall are enclosed within the prescription dose.

**Table 6** Dose-fractionation schedules for high-dose-rate brachytherapy following EBRT to 45 Gy in 1.8 Gy daily fractions for adjuvant treatment of endometrial cancer

| Fractionation | Dose-specification point | Equivalent dose for tumor effects | Equiv. dose for late effects |
|---|---|---|---|
| 2×5.5 Gy | 0.5 cm depth | 58.5 | 53.7 |
| 3×4.0 Gy | 0.5 cm depth | 58.3 | 52.9 |
| 2×8.0 Gy | Vaginal surface | 68.3 | 62.5 |
| 3×6.0 Gy | Vaginal surface | 68.3 | 61.3 |

Adapted from guidelines from the American Brachytherapy Society (Nag et al. 2000)

**Table 7** Dose-fractionation schedules for high-dose-rate brachytherapy following EBRT to 45 Gy in 1.8 Gy daily fractions for treatment of vaginal cuff recurrences from endometrial cancer

| Fractionation | Dose-specification point | Equivalent dose for tumor effects | Equiv. dose for late effects |
|---|---|---|---|
| 3×7 Gy | 0.5 cm depth | 74.0 | 66.4 |
| 4×6 Gy | 0.5 cm depth | 76.3 | 67.4 |
| 5×6 Gy | Vaginal surface | 84.3 | 73.4 |
| 4×7.0 Gy | Vaginal surface | 83.9 | 74.2 |

Adapted from guidelines from the American Brachytherapy Society (Nag et al. 2000)

**Table 8** Dose-fractionation schedules for high-dose-rate brachytherapy alone for inoperable primary endometrial cancer

| Fractionation | Dose-specification point (cm)[a] | Equivalent dose for tumor effects | Equiv. dose for late effects |
|---|---|---|---|
| 4×8.5 Gy | 2 | 52.4 | 42.6 |
| 5×7.3 Gy | 2 | 52.6 | 41.4 |
| 6×6.4 Gy | 2 | 52.5 | 40.3 |
| 7×5.7 Gy | 2 | 52.2 | 39.0 |

Adapted from guidelines from the American Brachytherapy Society
[a]HDR doses are prescribed to 2 cm from the midpoint of the intrauterine source (Nag et al. 2000)

– In the absence of CT/MRI-based treatment planning, the dose should be specified to a point 2 cm from the central axis of the intrauterine source.

# References

Creasman WT, Morrow CP, Bundy BN, Homesley HD, Graham JE, Heller PB (1987) Surgical pathologic spread patterns of endometrial cancer. A Gynecologic Oncology Group Study. Cancer 60(8 Suppl):2035–2041

Frei KA, Kinkel K, Bonel HM, Lu Y, Zaloudek C, Hricak H (2000) Prediction of deep myometrial invasion in patients with endometrial cancer: clinical utility of contrast-enhanced MR imaging-a meta-analysis and Bayesian analysis. Radiology 216(2):444–449

Heron DE, Gerszten K, Selvaraj RN, King GC, Sonnik D, Gallion H et al (2003) Conventional 3D conformal versus intensity-modulated radiotherapy for the adjuvant treatment of gynecologic malignancies: a comparative dosimetric study of dose-volume histograms. Gynecol Oncol 91(1):39–45

Keys HM, Roberts JA, Brunetto VL, Zaino RJ, Spirtos NM, Bloss JD et al (2004) A phase III trial of surgery with or without adjunctive external pelvic radiation therapy in intermediate risk endometrial adenocarcinoma: a Gynecologic Oncology Group study. Gynecol Oncol 92(3):744–751

Kitajima K, Murakami K, Kaji Y, Sakamoto S, Sugimura K (2011) Established, emerging and future applications of FDG-PET/CT in the uterine cancer. Clin Radiol 66(4):297–307

Mell LK, Mundt AJ (2008) Intensity-modulated radiation therapy in gynecologic cancers: growing support, growing acceptance. Cancer J 14(3):198–199

Mell LK, Roeske JC, Mundt AJ (2003) A survey of intensity-modulated radiation therapy use in the United States. Cancer 98(1):204–211

Nag S, Erickson B, Parikh S, Gupta N, Varia M, Glasgow G (2000) The American Brachytherapy Society recommendations for high-dose-rate brachytherapy for carcinoma of the endometrium. Int J Radiat Oncol Biol Phys 48(3):779–790

Naumann RW, Coleman RL (2007) The use of adjuvant radiation therapy in early endometrial cancer by members of the Society of Gynecologic Oncologists in 2005. Gynecol Oncol 105(1):7–12

Nout RA, Smit VT, Putter H, Jurgenliemk-Schulz IM, Jobsen JJ, Lutgens LC et al (2010) Vaginal brachytherapy versus pelvic external beam radiotherapy for patients with endometrial cancer of high-intermediate risk (PORTEC-2): an open-label, non-inferiority, randomised trial. Lancet 375(9717):816–823

Patel S, Liyanage SH, Sahdev A, Rockall AG, Reznek RH (2010) Imaging of endometrial and cervical cancer. Insights into imaging. Insights Imaging 1(5–6):309–328

Small W Jr, Mell LK, Anderson P, Creutzberg C, De Los Santos J, Gaffney D et al (2008) Consensus guidelines for delineation of clinical target volume for intensity-modulated pelvic radiotherapy in postoperative treatment of endometrial and cervical cancer. Int J Radiat Oncol Biol Phys 71(2):428–434

Smith-Bindman R, Kerlikowske K, Feldstein VA, Subak L, Scheidler J, Segal M et al (1998) Endovaginal ultrasound to exclude endometrial cancer and other endometrial abnormalities. JAMA 280(17):1510–1517

Toita T, Ohno T, Kaneyasu Y, Kato T, Uno T, Hatano K et al (2011) A consensus-based guideline defining clinical target volume for primary disease in external beam radiotherapy for intact uterine cervical cancer. Jpn J Clin Oncol 41(9):1119–1126

Yang R, Xu S, Jiang W, Wang J, Xie C (2010) Dosimetric comparison of postoperative whole pelvic radiotherapy for endometrial cancer using three-dimensional conformal radiotherapy, intensity-modulated radiotherapy, and helical tomotherapy. Acta Oncol 49(2):230–236

# Vulvar Cancer

John A. Vargo and Sushil Beriwal

## Contents

## 1  Anatomy and Patterns of Spread

- The vulva is a triangular-shaped structure composed of the labia and perineum immediately external to the vagina. Anatomically the urogenital diaphragm, clitoral hood, ischiopubic rami, and deep transverse perineal muscles bind the vulva.
- While as many as 5 % of vulvar cancers are multifocal, the most common site of involvement is the labia majora/minora (70–75 %).
- Extension to structures that maintain fecal/urinary continence or pelvic floor integrity such as anus/levator ani, urethra, vagina, obturator internus/piriformis muscles, and surrounding bone (pubis and ischium) define functional tumor resectability which is especially important for determining initial management strategies (see Fig. 1).
- For most vulvar cancers involving the labia and vestibule, the first echelon lymphatic drainage is to the superficial medial inguinal and deep femoral lymph nodes. The inguinal-femoral lymph nodes are an anatomically defined compartment laterally bound by the medial border of the iliopsoas, medially by the lateral border of the adductor longus, posteriorly by the iliopsoas muscle, and pectineus and anteriorly by the edge of the sartorius muscle and rectus femoris (Kim et al. 2012) (see Fig. 2).
- Vulvar lymphatic channels do not cross the labiocrural fold and generally do not cross the midline for well-lateralized lesions >1 cm from midline.
- Pelvic lymph nodes mainly represent second echelon lymphatics only affected when inguinal-femoral nodes are involved, the exception being small lymphatics of midline structures (clitoris or bulb of the vestibule) that drain directly to pelvic lymphatics via the internal pudendal and iliac lymphatics. As seen in GOG 37, 28 % of patients with inguinal node positivity had involvement of pelvic lymph nodes.
- A prior MRI study with injected iron oxide particles showed that 95 % of the common iliac, internal iliac,

J.A. Vargo, MD • S. Beriwal, MD (✉)
Department of Radiation Oncology, University of Pittsburgh
Cancer Institute, Pittsburgh, PA, USA
e-mail: beriwals@upmc.edu

N.Y. Lee et al. (eds.), *Target Volume Delineation for Conformal and Intensity-Modulated Radiation Therapy*,
Medical Radiology. Radiation Oncology, DOI: 10.1007/174_2014_981, © Springer International Publishing Switzerland 2014
Published Online: 12 November 2014

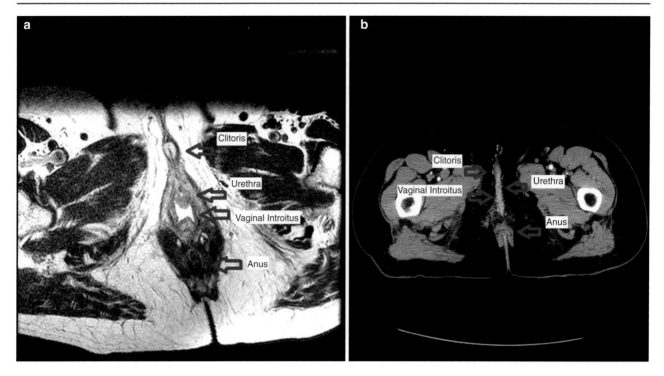

**Fig. 1** Functional pelvic anatomy determining vulvar cancer resectability: T2-weighted pelvic MRI with water-based endoluminal vaginal gel (**a**) and corresponding CT (**b**) imaging highlighting important pelvic structures integral in determining the functional resectability of vulvar cancers

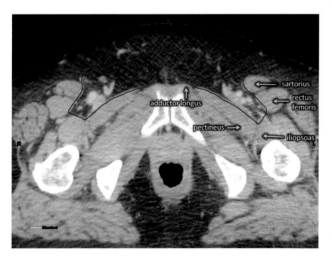

**Fig. 2** Inguinal-femoral lymph node compartment: anatomical compartment for the first echelon inguinal-femoral lymph nodes showing the muscles defining the compartment

medial and anterior external iliac, and obturator lymph nodes are located with 7 mm of the pelvic vasculature (Taylor et al. 2005). Conversely, for inguinal-femoral lymph nodes and the lateral external iliac region, variability of body habitus and prior lymph node dissection limits the applicability of the vessel surrogate plus 7 mm definition, where involved lymph nodes range from 0.9 to 3.5 cm from the vessel, and thus the anatomical compartment rather than fixed circumferential should be used in defining inguinal nodes (Kim et al. 2012).

## 2 Diagnostic Workup Relevant for Target Volume Delineation

- Initial physical examination should include a comprehensive gynecologic exam with specific attention paid to noting the local extent of the disease and inguinal nodal involvement. In GOG 37, 23.8 % of patients with clinically enlarged lymph nodes were found to have no evidence of disease on pathologic assessment, while 23.9 % of patients with a normal exam were found to have occult metastatic disease. Thus physical examination is neither sensitive nor specific in identifying the extent of nodal involvement. CT or PET-CT is therefore essential in workup and treatment planning.
- Extrapolating from other pelvic malignancies, most prominently anal cancer, where the role of PET-CT is well established, we recommend incorporating PET-CT-based planning for all vulvar patients to increase the sensitivity of identifying nodal disease that would otherwise be undetected by the combination of physical exam and CT imaging (Cotter et al. 2006).
- The use of gadolinium-enhanced pelvic MRI with and without water-based endoluminal vaginal gel is important in locally advanced disease to evaluate the relationship between tumor and functionally integral normal tissues such as the musculature of the anal sphincter and vagina that preclude surgical resection (see Fig. 3).
- When disease involves the vagina, a gold fiducial marker is placed during in-office speculum examination to identify the vaginal extent of disease aiding in GTV definition and daily setup.

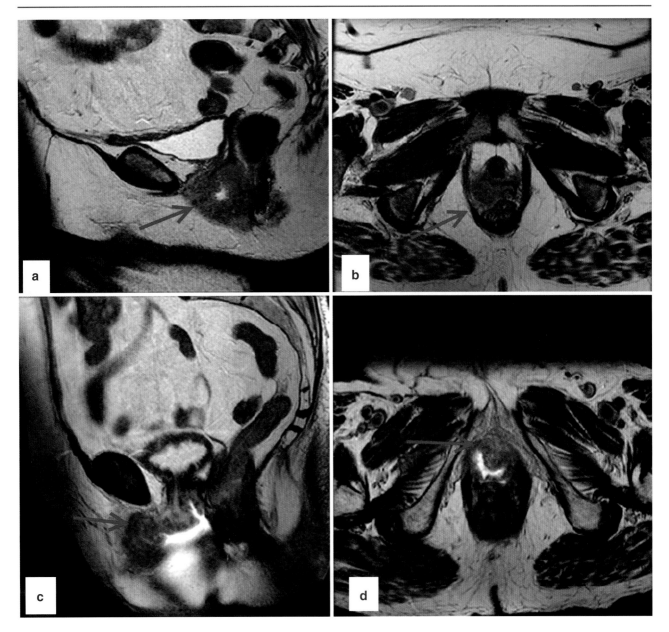

**Fig. 3** MR imaging of the locally advanced vulvar cancers. (**a**, **b**) Posterior vulvar lesion (highlighted by the *arrow*) extending to the anus and puborectalis muscle. (**c**, **d**) Anterior vulvar lesion with extensive urethral and preurethral involvement (highlighted by the *arrow*)

## 3    Simulation and Daily Localization

- CT or PET-CT simulation in the supine position with the lower extremities abducted ("frog-legged") and immobilized in a vacuum-evacuated device to assure reproducibility in setup. By abducting the lower extremities to the maximal extent allowable by the scanner, the dose to the medial thigh and groin folds is minimized.
- In order to assist in delineation of the tumor, radiopaque wire is used to identify areas of gross disease or the postoperative tumor bed (see Fig. 4).
- CT or PET-CT simulation using 3–5 mm thickness with IV and oral contrast. Oral contrast assists in the small bowel and rectum visualization, while the IV contrast aids

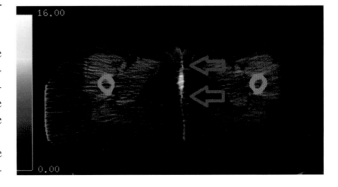

**Fig. 4** Radiopaque wire for simulation. PET-CT based simulation with gross disease outlined by a radiopaque wire placed at the time of simulation (highlighted by the *arrows*), corresponding to the PET avid disease seen on simulation imaging

in visualization of the vasculature structures for nodal contouring. We typically recommend a simulation scan from at least the L2 through the mid thigh. The isocenter is typically placed in the center of the pelvis if treating lymph nodes. In comparison, it is typically placed in the vulva at the level of pubic symphysis if targeting only the vulva.

- If the vagina is involved (and thus to be included in CTV1 as described below), we suggest performing the simulation with a full and empty bladder to create an ITV (internal target volume) for the vaginal region. It is recommended that all vulvar patients be treated with a full bladder and empty rectum irrespective of vaginal involvement. On the day prior to simulation, patients are instructed to take a fleet enema and are re-simulated if rectal distention is >3.0–3.5 cm since an empty rectum represents the most conservative posterior location for rectal filling effects on interfraction motion.

- We avoid the use of a vaginal obturator or marker as these devices distort anatomy and create non-reproducible anatomical deformation of the pliable vaginal mucosa. Additionally, the devices displace the vagina posteriorly, creating a situation prone to geographic miss.

- A customized bolus of 0.5–1 cm thickness is usually created for the vulvar region at the time of treatment planning and is used for daily treatments. Separate plans are generated with and without bolus at the time of initial IMRT planning, such that should the patient develop a brisk skin reaction, treatment can be continued without bolus and no attendant treatment interruption. Additionally a 1–2 cm thick bolus structure is extended in air for IMRT plan optimization only, which serves to extend the isodose line beyond the skin for flash to account for edema and swelling (see Fig. 5). The difference in monitor units with and without bolus should be minimal.

- Patients are typically set up with a combination of daily KV and CBCT imaging. Daily kV imaging is used to reduce interfraction motion based upon the bony anatomy or to fiducial markers placed at the vaginal extent of disease if present. For boost CBCT daily would be preferred for daily localization and matching with the soft tissue.

## 4 Target Volume Delineation and Treatment Planning

- The primary GTV includes all gross disease on physical examination and imaging. For pelvic and inguinal, GTV includes all lymph nodes ≥1 cm in the short axis, those with a necrotic center and/or PET avidity (see Table 1 and 2).

- CTV1 includes the GTV with at least a 1 cm margin including at minimum the entire vulvar region and excluding nearby uninvolved structures such as the muscles comprising the anal sphincter and bone (see Figs. 6 and 7). If uninvolved and posterior lesion, the mons pubis can be excluded from CTV1 to minimize the risk of long-term lymphedema (see Fig. 8a).

- For posterior vulvar lesions, the CTV1 also includes the perineum from the posterior fourchette to the anal verge. If the anal verge is involved, then CTV1 needs to include that with at least a 1–2 cm margin. If disease extends to the anal canal, then CTV1 also includes the entire meso-rectum from the anal verge to the rectosigmoid flexure to cover the perirectal lymph nodes (see Fig. 8a).

- For anterior vulvar lesions involving the urethra, CTV1 includes at least 2 cm proximal to the primary GTV or to the bladder neck (see Figs. 9a and 10a).

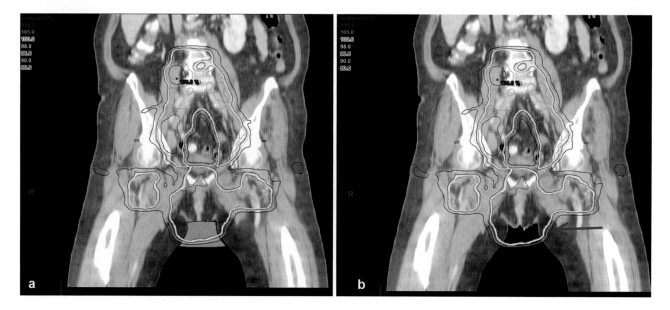

**Fig. 5** Customized bolus for IMRT optimization to generate flash. CT treatment planning images with and without a customized bolus structure generated for IMRT optimization to extend isodose lines beyond the vulva generating a flash of dose beyond the skin (highlighted by *arrow*)

**Table 1** Suggested IMRT dose fractionation schemes used for vulvar cancer

| Clinical situation | PTV1 (Gy) | PTV2 (Gy) | Dose per fraction |
|---|---|---|---|
| Preoperative GOG 205 (Moore et al. 2012) | 45–50.4 | 55.8–59.4 | 1.8 Gy daily |
| Definitive | 45–50.4 | 59.4–70.2 | 1.8 Gy daily |
| Adjuvant | 45–50.4 | 50.4–59.4 | 1.8 Gy daily |

- In the case of vaginal extension, the CTV1 includes the entire vagina from the apex to the vaginal introitus (see Fig. 9a).
- CTV1 for N0 patients encompasses the bilateral inguinal-femoral lymph nodes and the pelvic lymph nodes including the lower common iliac, bilateral external iliac, bilateral internal iliac, and bilateral obturator. Note the lower

**Table 2** Suggested target volumes at the high-risk subclinical region

| Target volumes | Definition and description |
|---|---|
| GTV | Primary: All gross disease on physical examination and imaging (see above regarding the importance of PET-CT and MRI) |
|  | Pelvic and inguinal nodes: All nodes ≥1 cm, or those with necrotic center, and/or PET avidity |
| CTV1 | GTV + 1 cm including the entire vulva (+/− perineum, vagina, or urethra if involved) with editing to exclude uninvolved bone, muscle, and adjacent organs |
|  | CTV1 includes the inguinal-femoral and pelvic lymph nodes (bilateral obturator and external and internal iliac) to the bifurcation of the external and internal iliac vessel |
|  | Include the entire common iliac chain to the aortic bifurcation if pelvic node positive |
|  | Include entire vagina if vaginal involvement and generate ITV for full and empty bladder if feasible |
|  | Include 2 cm of urethra proximal to primary GTV for anterior periurethral lesion or to the bladder neck if extensive urethral involvement |
|  | Include a 1–2 cm margin if anal verge is involved or the entire mesorectum if anal canal involvement |
| PTV1 | $CTV_1$ + 1 cm for the primary and 0.7–1 cm for lymph nodes |

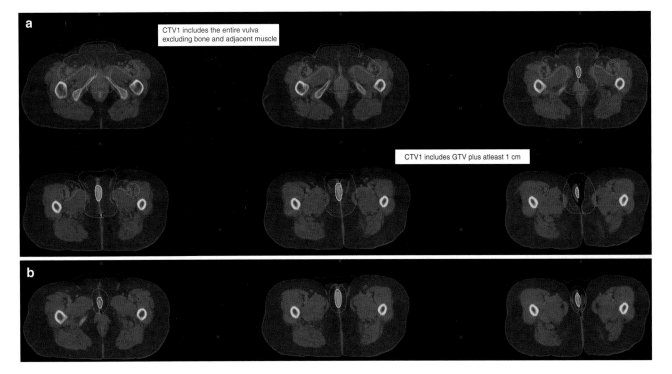

**Fig. 6** (**a**) **Preoperative vulvar cancer**. The patient had FIGO Stage IB squamous cell carcinoma of the vulva which approached but did not involve the urethra. However, the encochment on the urethra precluded initial margin negative resection; thus, she received preoperative chemoradiotherapy with weekly cisplatin 40 mg/m². The GTV for the primary lesion is noted in light green; note the midline lesion extended close to the urethral orifice. CTV1 (*red*) includes the entire vulva and the GTV plus at least 1 cm excluding adjacent bone/muscle as well as the inguinal-femoral lymph nodes (*red*) and pelvic lymph nodes (not shown). The PTV1 (*orange*) received 45 Gy in 25 fractions and a sequential IMRT photon boost of 12.6 Gy in seven fractions to a cumulative dose of 57.6 Gy in 32 fractions; she subsequently underwent successful partial vulvectomy with negative surgical margins and urethral preservation. (**b**) Preoperative vulvar cancer. GTV (*light green*) primary with corresponding boost PTV2 (*orange*) for the sequential IMRT photon boost of 12.6 Gy in seven fractions

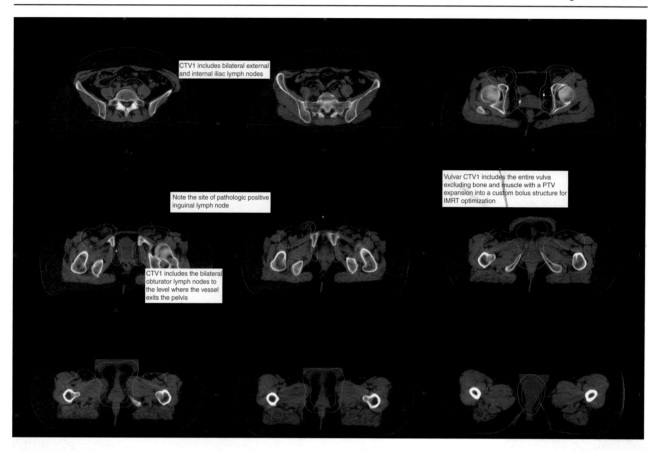

**Fig. 7** Postoperative vulvar cancer. The patient had FIGO Stage IIIA squamous cell carcinoma of the vulva. She underwent partial vulvectomy and bilateral sentinel lymph node biopsy. Final pathology showed a 1.7 cm lesion with lymphovascular space invasion, 0.3 mm depth of invasion, and 0.5 cm surgical margins. One of 2 right inguinal sentinel lymph nodes were involved measuring 0.5 cm, with involve-ment in 0 of 4 left sentinel lymph nodes. She completed adjuvant radiotherapy to 50.4 Gy in 28 fractions, for which the CTV1 (*red*) and PTV1 (*orange*) are shown above. The patient received an additional 9 Gy electron boost for a cumulative dose of 59.4 Gy for the close surgical margin

common iliac lymph node beds are not always treated with traditional fields; however, we believe inclusion is preferable with modern techniques.

- The pelvic nodal CTV1 contour begins superiorly with the lower common iliac lymph nodes and extends to the bifurcation of the external and internal iliac vessels. Inferiorly, the external iliac nodal contours are continued until the level of the femoral heads, marking the beginning of the obturator lymph nodes which extend to the level of the pelvic floor where the obturator vessels leave the pelvis.

- For patient with known disease in the pelvic lymph nodes, the superior border of CTV1 is extended to the take-off of the common iliac vessel from the descending aorta to include the entire common iliac nodes (see Figs. 9a and 10a).

- The inguinal-femoral compartment should extend caudally approximately 2 cm from the saphenous-femoral junction or to the level of the lesser trochanter with circumferential borders defined anatomically by musculature surrounding the compartment (see Fig. 2).

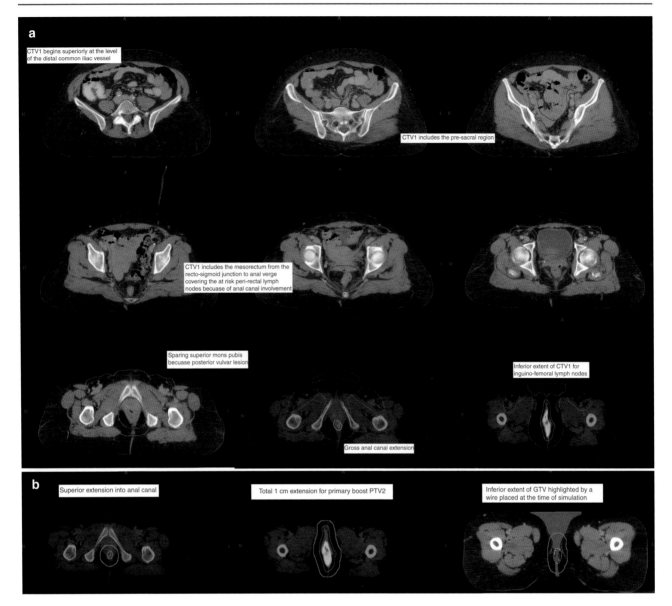

**Fig. 8** (**a**) **Locally advanced vulvar cancer** with anal canal extension. The patient had FIGO Stage IVA squamous cell carcinoma of the vulva with extension into the anal canal. She received preoperative chemoradiotherapy with concurrent weekly cisplatin 40 mg/m². The GTV (*green*) with extension into the anal canal, CTV1 (*red*) including the bilateral external iliac, internal iliac, obturator, presacral lymph nodes from S1–S4, inguinal-femoral lymph nodes, entire mesorectum from the anal verge to the rectosigmoid junction, and entire vulva. The corresponding PTV1 is shown in *orange*. Note for CTV1 the inclusion of the entire mesorectum and presacral region because of anal canal involvement, as well as the sparing of the superior mons pubis because of the posterior primary vulvar lesion. PTV1 was treated to 45 Gy in 25 fractions, with a sequential IMRT photon boost to the primary lesion for a cumulative dose of 59.4 Gy. (**b**) **Locally advanced vulvar cancer** with anal canal extension. GTV (*light green*) primary with corresponding boost PTV2 (*orange*) for the sequential IMRT photon boost of 14.4 Gy in eight fractions

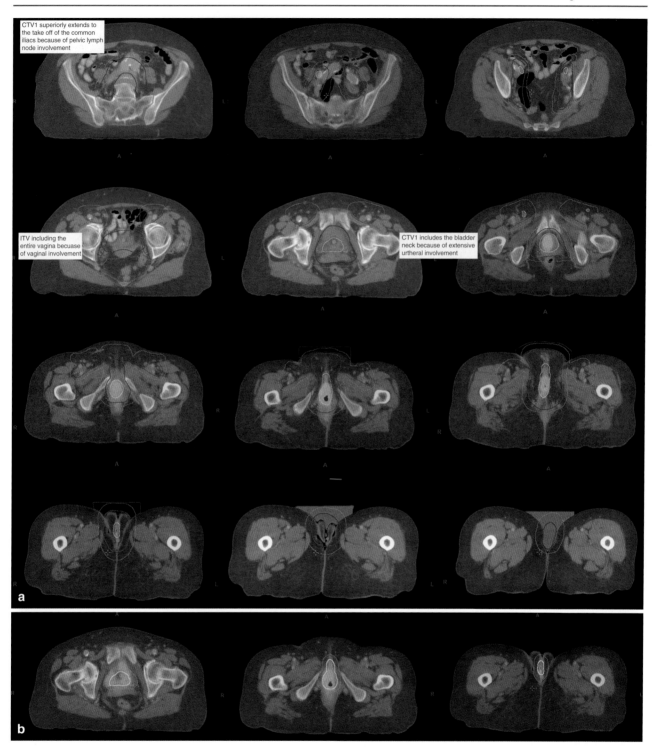

**Fig. 9** (a) **Locally advanced vulvar cancer** with extension to the vagina and bladder neck. The patient had FIGO stage IVB (based on pelvic node positive) squamous cell carcinoma of the vulva with vaginal extension and involvement of the urethra with extension superiorly to the bladder neck. She completed concurrent chemoradiotherapy with weekly cisplatin 40 mg/m². The GTV for the involved pelvic lymph nodes and primary is highlighted in green, and note the extensive involvement of urethra with extension to the bladder neck as well as vaginal involvement. CTV1 (*red*) and PTV1 (*orange*) including the entire urethra to the level of the bladder neck, and the entire vagina, contoured as an ITV to account for a full and empty bladder. PTV1 received a dose of 45 Gy in 25 fractions with an SIB to the involved lymph nodes to 55 Gy in 25 fractions and a sequential IMRT photon boost to a cumulative dose of 70.2 Gy to PTV2 in 39 fractions with complete metabolic and clinical response. Note the CTV1 and corresponding PTV1 extend into a custom bolus structure for IMRT optimization. (b) **Locally advanced vulvar cancer** with extension to the vagina and bladder neck. GTV (*light green*) primary with corresponding boost PTV2 (*blue green*) for the sequential IMRT photon boost of 25.2 Gy in 14 fractions

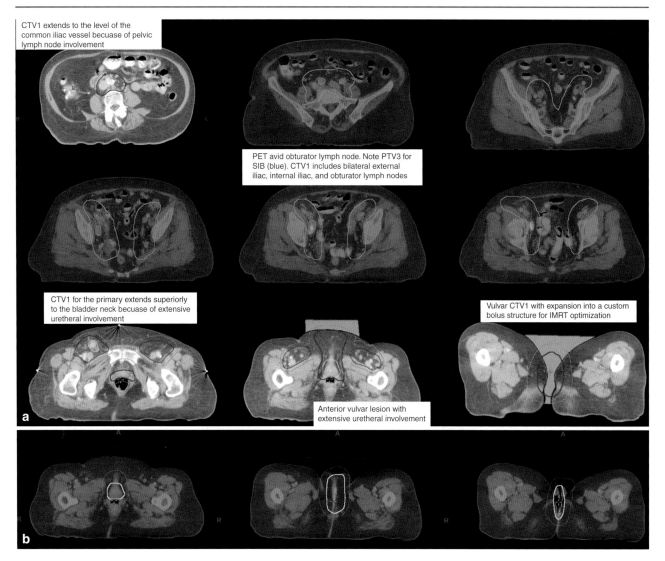

**Fig. 10** (**a**) **Locally advanced vulvar cancer** with bulky pelvic lymph node involvement. The patient had FIGO stage IVB (based on pelvic node positive) squamous cell carcinoma of the vulva with a bulky obturator lymph node and an anterior vulvar lesion with extensive periurethral involvement. GTV for involved pelvic and inguinal lymph nodes plus the primary is outlined in green. Note CTV1 (*red*), and corresponding PTV1 (*orange*) includes the common iliac lymph nodes to the level of the bifurcation of the descending aorta and includes the urethra to the level of the

bladder neck because of extensive periurethral involvement. She received concurrent cisplatin 40 mg/m$^2$ and radiotherapy to 45 Gy in 25 fractions followed by a 10.8 Gy IMRT photon boost to the primary. The involved lymph nodes received 55 Gy in 25 fractions using a SIB technique. The corresponding PTV3 for nodal SIB is shown in blue. (**b**) **Locally advanced vulvar cancer** with bulky pelvic lymph node involvement. GTV (*light green*) primary with corresponding boost PTV2 (*orange*) for the sequential IMRT photon boost to 10.8 Gy at 1.8 Gy per fraction

- For PTV1, CTV1 for the primary or tumor bed should be expanded by at least 0.7–1 cm to account for the previously mentioned uncertainties, whereas there is less variation in respect to the lymph nodes, and its CTV1 can be expanded by 0.5–0.7 cm for PTV based on frequency and type of imaging used for localization.
- When using a sequential boost for definitive dose, one should consider rescanning to account for response of exophytic tumor and subsequent adjustment of the targeted volume. For the primary, the GTV is expanded by a total of 1.0–2.0 cm for PTV2. For the involved lymph nodes, the GTV is expanded by a total of 0.7–1.0 cm to

create the final nodal boost volume, PTV3. The boost to the primary site can be delivered via IMRT, direct electron field, or interstitial brachytherapy depending on the response and location of remaining disease (see Table 1 and 3).

- An alternative in treating gross nodal disease is implementation of a simultaneous integrated boost (SIB) during the initial 45.0 Gy delivered to the pelvis, to a total of 55 Gy delivered at 2.2 Gy per fraction to the positive lymph node plus a total of 0.7–1.0 cm margin from GTV to PTV, which allows dose escalation without increasing the overall treatment time (see Fig. 10a).

**Table 3** Suggested target volumes for the boost

| Target volumes | Definition and description |
|---|---|
| GTV | Primary: All gross disease on physical examination and imaging (see above regarding the importance of PET-CT and MRI) |
| CTV2 | Primary: GTV+0.5–1 cm with editing to exclude uninvolved bone, muscle, and adjacent organs |
| PTV2 | Primary: $CTV_2$+0.5–1 cm depending on imaging used for localization |
| PTV3 | Involved Lymph Nodes: the entire GTV to PTV expansion is 0.7–1 cm depending on imaging used for localization |

**Table 4** Intensity-modulated radiation therapy normal tissue dose constraints

| Critical structures | University of Pittsburgh Cancer Institute[a] | RTOG[b] |
|---|---|---|
| Small bowel | Max<50 Gy, ≤35 % to receive ≥35 Gy | ≤ 30 % to receive ≥ 40 Gy |
| Anorectum | Max<50 Gy, ≤40–50 % to receive ≥40 Gy | ≤ 60 % to receive ≥ 40 Gy |
| Bladder | Max<50 Gy, ≤40–50 % to receive ≥40 Gy | ≤ 35 % to receive ≥ 45 Gy |
| Femoral heads | Max<50 Gy, ≤35 % to receive ≥35 Gy | ≤ 15 % to receive ≥ 35 Gy |
| Bone marrow | Max<50 Gy, ≤75–80 % to receive ≥20.0 Gy | ≤ 37 % to receive ≥ 40 Gy |

[a]Based on guidelines presently used at University of Pittsburgh Cancer Institute (Beriwal et al. 2006, 2008, 2013)
[b]Contemporary guidelines for pelvic radiotherapy as reflected in the ongoing RTOG 0921 and suggested on outcome analysis from RTOG 0418 (Klopp et al. 2013). Maximum doses can be increased depending on tumor location and potential PTV overlap

## 5　Plan Assessment

- The plan is considered acceptable if <5 % of the PTV receives <100 % of the prescribed dose and <10 % of the PTV receives >110 % of the prescribed dose. We attempt to avoid any hot spots in inguinal folds.
- At the time of the first treatment, a thermoluminescent dosimeter (TLD) should be placed under the bolus to confirm the delivered dose is within 7 % of the prescribed dose.
- For critical organs we advocate contouring the anorectum from the anal verge to rectosigmoid junction, the entire bladder with no overlap between the CTVs, small bowel including entire peritoneal cavity (instead of individual bowel loops) from the rectosigmoid junction to 1–2 cm above the final PTV, femoral heads caudally to level of the lesser trochanter, and in instances of concurrent chemotherapy the pelvic bone marrow including the lower lumbar spine, iliac, sacrum, and femoral heads (see Table 4).

## Suggested Reading

GOG 205 (Moore et al. 2012): Show feasibility of preoperative weekly cisplatin and dose-escalated radiotherapy to 57.6 Gy for locally advanced vulvar cancers.

Outcomes for Vulvar IMRT Beriwal et al. (2006, 2008, 2013): Reviews evolution, techniques, and outcomes for IMRT in vulvar cancer.

Australian Gastrointestinal Trials Group Contouring Atlas for Anal Cancer IMRT (Ng et al. 2012): Anatomical-based contouring guidelines for inguinal and pelvic lymph nodes, and for cases of anal involvement, delineate contouring for the entire mesorectum from the anal verge to rectosigmoid.

## References

Beriwal S, Heron DE, Kim H et al (2006) Intensity-modulated radiotherapy for the treatment of vulvar carcinoma: a comparative dosimetric study with early clinical outcome. Int J Radiat Oncol Biol Phys 64:1395–1400

Beriwal S, Coon D, Heron DE et al (2008) Preoperative intensity-modulated radiotherapy and chemotherapy for locally advanced vulvar carcinoma. Gynecol Oncol 109:291–295

Beriwal S, Shukla G, Shinde A et al (2013) Preoperative intensity modulated radiation therapy and chemotherapy for locally advances vulvar carcinoma: analysis of pattern of relapse. Int J Radiat Oncol Biol Phys 85:1269–1274

Cotter SE, Grigsby PW, Siegel BA et al (2006) FDG-PET/CT in the evaluation of anal carcinoma. Int J Radiat Oncol Biol Phys 65:720–725

Kim C, Olsen A, Kim H, Beriwal S (2012) Contouring inguinal and femoral nodes; how much margin is needed around the vessels. Pract Radiat Oncol 2:274–278

Klopp AH, Moughan J, Portelance L et al (2013) Hematologic toxicity in RTOG 0418: a phase 2 study of postoperative IMRT for gynecologic cancer. Int J Radiat Oncol Biol Phys 86:83–90

Moore DH, Ali S, Koh WJ et al (2012) A phase II trial of radiation therapy and weekly cisplatin chemotherapy for the treatment of locally advanced squamous cell carcinoma of the vulva: a gynecologic oncology group study. Gynecol Oncol 124:529–533

Ng M, Leong T, Chander S et al (2012) Australian Gastrointestinal Trials Group contouring atlas and planning guidelines for intensity modulated radiotherapy in anal cancer. Int J Radiat Oncol Biol Phys 83:1455–1462

Taylor A, Rockall AG, Reznek RH et al (2005) Mapping pelvic lymph nodes: guidelines for delineation in intensity-modulated radiotherapy. Int J Radiat Oncol Biol Phys 63:1604–1612

# Part VI

# Genitourinary System

# Prostate Adenocarcinoma

Neil B. Desai and Michael J. Zelefsky

## Contents

N.B. Desai • M.J. Zelefsky (✉)
Department of Radiation Oncology, Memorial Sloan Kettering
Cancer Center, New York, NY, USA
e-mail: zelefskm@mskcc.org

## 1   Introduction

- Advances in treatment delivery of external beam radiotherapy (EBRT) have facilitated improvement in treatment efficacy of radiotherapy (RT) for prostate cancer by enabling safe dose escalation. Intensity-modulated radiation therapy (IMRT) has become a standard current form of treatment delivery. Various protocols for fractionation exist, and EBRT is used in both the definitive and postoperative settings. However, all approaches rely on accurate target delineation, treatment planning, and patient setup. This chapter will describe the approach that is employed at Memorial Sloan Kettering Cancer Center (MSKCC).

## 2   Anatomy and Patterns of Spread

- The prostate is an approximately 25 cc gland that straddles the prostatic urethra in a craniocaudal axis between its broad base, where it abuts the bladder, and its narrow apex, where it terminates at the membranous urethra above the external urinary sphincter. This conical shape is framed laterally by the convergence of the obturator and levator ani muscles into the genitourinary diaphragm. The prostate is bounded anteriorly by a rich venous plexus and the pubis and posteriorly by the rectum. The neurovascular bundle, highlighted in nerve-sparing surgical approaches, is located within a cavernous plexus posterolateral to the prostate (Fig. 1).
- Four zones can be identified within the prostate of younger men (peripheral, central, transition, anterior fibromuscular). The peripheral zone lies adjacent to the rectum and is the site of the majority of tumors.
- Local tumor spread by extracapsular extension (ECE) is facilitated by defects in the prostatic capsule at the

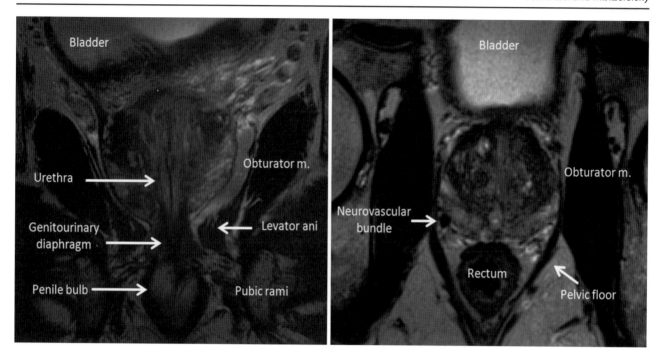

**Fig. 1** Relationship of prostate to surrounding anatomic landmarks on MRI T2-weighted sequences in a patient with clinically organ-confined disease. *Left*: Coronal view *Right*: Axial view

sites of entry of neurovascular structures (suggesting the importance of perineural invasion) or glandular ducts and at the prostatic apex, where the capsule is thin or absent. While involvement of the bladder neck and even trigone is more easily identified on workup, care must be taken not to underestimate the potential for spread into and beyond the anterior fibrostroma, where transrectal ultrasound (TRUS) and biopsy may undersample. Spread to the rectum is rare due to the reinforcement of the Denonvilliers fascia, formed by invagination of a peritoneal layer between the two structures.

- Regional spread is most common to the obturator lymph nodes and can also involve internal iliac, external iliac, and presacral nodes. Distant spread is overwhelmingly to bone, a predilection which is attributed to various hypotheses, including the anatomic ease of spread via the valveless Batson's venous plexus to the lumbar spine and biologic rationale. In particular, this causes concern for pathologic fracture from involvement of long bones and the pelvis, spinal cord compression or spinal instability from vertebral involvement, and cranial nerve palsies from skull base involvement.

## 3    Diagnostic Workup Relevant for Target Volume Delineation

- Initial case workup includes digital rectal examination, urinary and erectile function scores, and relevant labs. A history of prior transurethral resection of the prostate (TURP) or medication for benign prostatic hypertrophy is particularly important for optimizing treatment selection. In addition, knowledge of prior urethral surgery or visualization of the TURP defect is helpful so as to contour this area to insure that excessive doses are not given to this region.
- Standard imaging includes TRUS for initial assessment of gland size and biopsy guidance, with tumors appearing hypoechoic. The TRUS volume is also helpful for it provides prognostic data such as PSA density. Computed tomography (CT) of the pelvis provides limited information regarding evaluation for pelvic adenopathy. While the literature on its sensitivity is mixed, suspicious nodes may be noted for biopsy when carrying the potential to affect treatment.
- Magnetic resonance imaging (MRI) with 3T strength and with or without endorectal coil based on patient tolerance and level of detail needed (i.e. neurovascular bundle approximation relative to tumor prior to nerve sparing surgery is best seen with 3T + coil) is recommended at

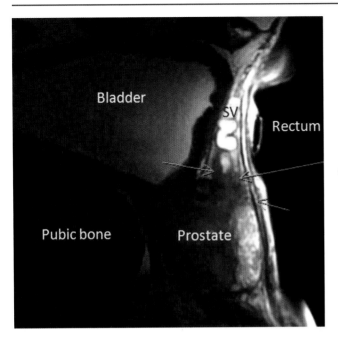

**Fig. 2** Seminal vesicle (SV) invasion by tumor (*green arrows*) is demonstrated on sagittal MRI T2-weighted sequence by irregular hypointense signal encroaching upon the hyperintense proximal SV

MSKCC for evaluation of intraprostatic anatomy and for ECE. This is performed at least 8 weeks following biopsy to allow for post-procedure changes to resolve. Tumors appear hypointense on T2 compared with normal gland, allowing assessment for dominant lesions and seminal vesicle invasion (Fig. 2). While blood products can also be hypointense on T2, they are hyperintense on T1, in contrast to tumor, allowing differentiation (Fig. 3). Disruption or irregularity of the well-defined capsule by tumor suggests ECE (Fig. 4). Sagittal view allows assessment of the extent of prior TURP defects and obstructive physiology, such as from a hypertrophied median lobe (Fig. 5). Finally, in the case of patients with MR-compatible prior hip arthroplasty, MRI fusion with CT-simulation images may facilitate basic visualization of target structures.

## 4 Simulation and Daily Localization

- CT simulation is performed with 2–3 mm slice thickness. Our approach at MSKCC includes:
  - Immobilization: Mold such as Aquaplast® in supine position with arms on chest and out of field.
  - Scan: Even if not treating pelvic nodes, scan cranial to prostate to allow full delineation of bladder, rectum to rectosigmoid junction, and the relevant areas of

small bowel that may fall adjacent to high-dose distributions.
  - Image guidance: Gold fiducials or Calypso™ beacons for daily inter-fraction or intra-fraction guidance, respectively, are placed at least 5 days prior to simulation.
  - Preparation: Bowel prep night prior, and oral contrast 90 min before simulation.
  - Special cases/regimens:
- Full bladder – 2 cups of water 45 min before scan.
  - This is required in postoperative therapy due to the tendency of small bowel to fall into the prostatectomy bed. If this is not achieved, a cone down may be required.
  - In definitive therapy, full bladder is useful when CT simulation scan demonstrates a) any small bowel within the high-dose region (rule of thumb 9mm separation from top slice of prostate/SV) or b) small overall bladder size that places a high percentage of bladder volume within the high dose region. If this is not achieved, a cone down may be required.
- Foley catheter for urethral delineation in treatment planning for stereotactic hypofractionation or combination therapy protocols.
  - We pretreat with ~5 cc of viscous lidocaine 2 % (i.e., Uro-Jet®) and employ a 12 or 14 French Coudé under sterile technique.
  - Isocenter is placed in the prostate.
- Daily setup: First, in room lasers are aligned to skin marks. Second, onboard kV orthogonal pair imaging is compared to the simulation-based digitally reconstructed radiograph (DRR) with projected fiducial contours. Our current image-guided RT (IGRT) protocol for daily inter-fraction adjustments requires a couch shift to align the kV verification film with a DRR fiducial-based match for deviations of >2 mm in any cardinal axis. Re-verification and readjustment as necessary is then performed before treatment is delivered.

## 5 Target Volume Delineation and Treatment Planning

- Target volume guidelines and delineation concepts are summarized in Table 1.
- Volume walkthroughs: See Figs. 6, 7, 8, 9, and 10 for examples of treatment of the prostate and seminal vesicles, pelvic nodes, and postoperative fossa. Special cases are highlighted in Figs. 11 and 12. General concepts of target delineation and quality assessment are highlighted:
  - Key anatomic boundaries and landmarks to guide interpretation
  - Quality assessment via 3-D projection

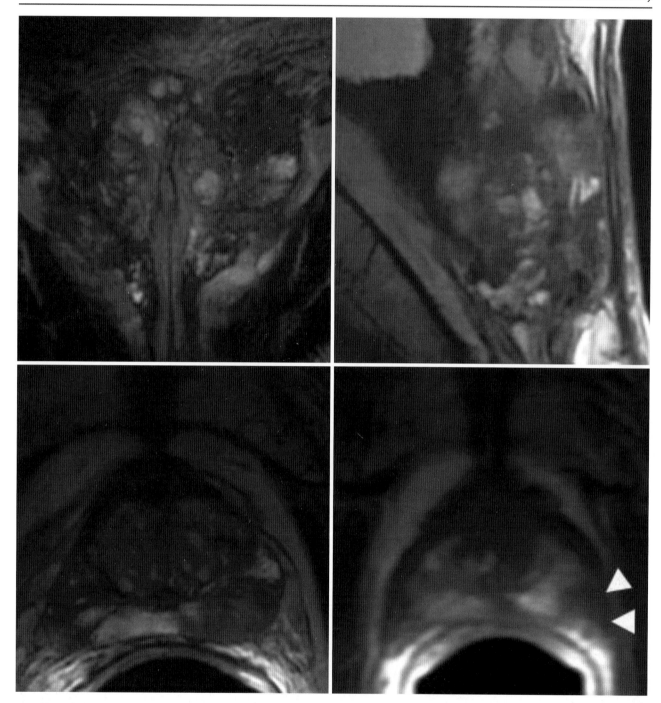

**Fig. 3** Demonstration of post-biopsy changes on MRI, which limits interpretation of disease extent. Diffuse signal irregularities are noted on T2-weighted sequences in the coronal (*top left*), sagittal (*top right*), and axial planes (*bottom left*), as well as on T1-weighted sequence in the axial plane (*bottom right*). Nonetheless, the distinct hypointensity in the left posterolateral gland on both T1- and T2-weighted sequences suggests a dominant peripheral zone tumor (*white arrowheads*)

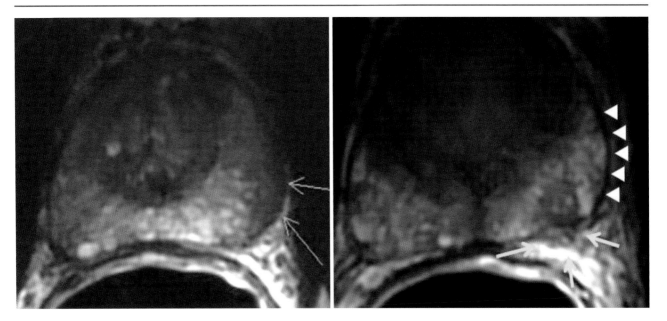

**Fig. 4** Extracapsular extension (ECE) detected by MRI T2-weighted axial sequences of the prostate. *Left*: Broad capsular contact is shown (*green arrows*) along the left posterolateral boundary without frank disruption. This would be called suspicious but not definite for ECE.

*Right*: In contrast, this image demonstrates a focal penetration (*yellow arrows*) of the capsule (*white arrowheads*) by a hypointense lesion, consistent with clear ECE

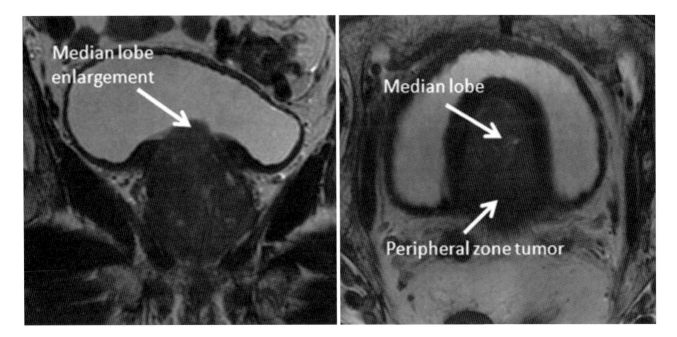

**Fig. 5** MRI T2-weighted sequences (*left* coronal, *right* axial) demonstrate enlargement of the median lobe of the prostate with invagination into the bladder due to both tumor and hypertrophy. Such features can be mistaken for bladder neck thickening on CT slices alone, leading to inadequate tumor coverage by PTV. In this case, this invagination of tissue into the bladder should be treated

**Table 1** Suggested target volumes for EBRT and contouring concepts

| Treatment setting | Protocol | Dose (cGy) | PTV margin | CTV description |
|---|---|---|---|---|
| Definitive | Conventional | 8,000–8,600 | 6 mm | • Prostate and seminal vesicles Fig. 6 |
| | Hypofractionated (full bladder, Foley) | 750 or higher × 5 | 5 mm except at the rectum (3 mm) | • Begin contours mid-gland where prostate borders are most easily identifiable<br>• Caudally, identify apex relative to GUD based on landmarks noted in the figure that identify the convergence of the levator ani (i.e., "slit" of McLaughlin et al. 2010)<br>• Lateral boundary = levator ani<br>• Anterior = anterior fibromuscular stroma (AFS)<br>• Posteriorly, rectum is opposed at mid-gland, but falls away caudally, so trace rectum from anal canal to avoid error<br>• Superiorly, incorporate SV but not the associated vasculature above into the final CTV. The SV can be contoured separately, but using one structure smoothens transition<br>• Check 3-D structure to assess for symmetry and interpretation errors. See Fig. 7 |
| Adjuvant/salvage | (Full bladder) | 7,200 ± dose painting boost to gross residual disease | 10 mm except at the rectum (6 mm) | Within RTOG guidelines Figs. 8 and 9<br>• Caudally begin just above GUD. Identify vesicourethral anastomosis (VUA) as slice below last with urine, and begin contouring 8–12 mm below. MRI fusion may aid.<br>• At superior border of pubic symphysis, pull back anterior border gradually over 3–4 slices to the 3 mm margin allowed on the bladder, forming a classic "dumbbell" shape noted in the figure<br>• Cranial border should extend approximately 2 cm above the pubic symphysis, but it is not necessary to encompass all hemostatic clips<br>• Laterally bound by obturator internus<br>• Dose paint gross residual disease on MRI Fig. 12b |
| Either | Pelvic nodes | 4,500 | 10 mm | Non-RTOG: See Fig. 10<br>• Target vessels: common iliac below the L5–S1 interspace, external iliac, internal iliac into pudendal and obturator vessels<br>• Posterior boundary of PTV (internal iliac branches) is most prone to over-contouring which would increase dose to the rectum<br>• Stopping points: end external iliac at the top of the femoral head, end inferior node contours (obturator/pudendal) at superior aspect of pubic symphysis |

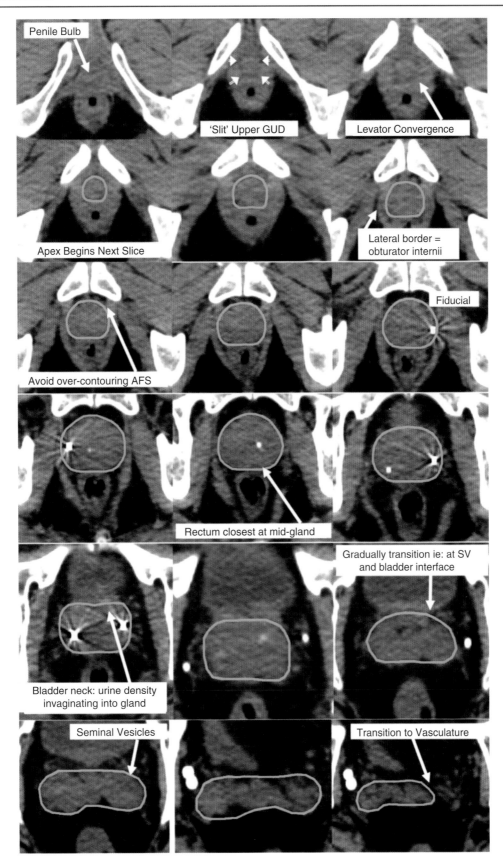

**Fig. 6** A patient with clinically organ-confined disease but with suggestion on MRI of possible seminal vesicle (SV) invasion treated to the prostate and SV. This series of representative images beginning at the apex from a 2 mm slice thickness CT simulation demonstrates general boundary discrimination and CTV delineation. Not all slices are shown. *AFS* anterior fibromuscular stroma, *GUD* genitourinary diaphragm

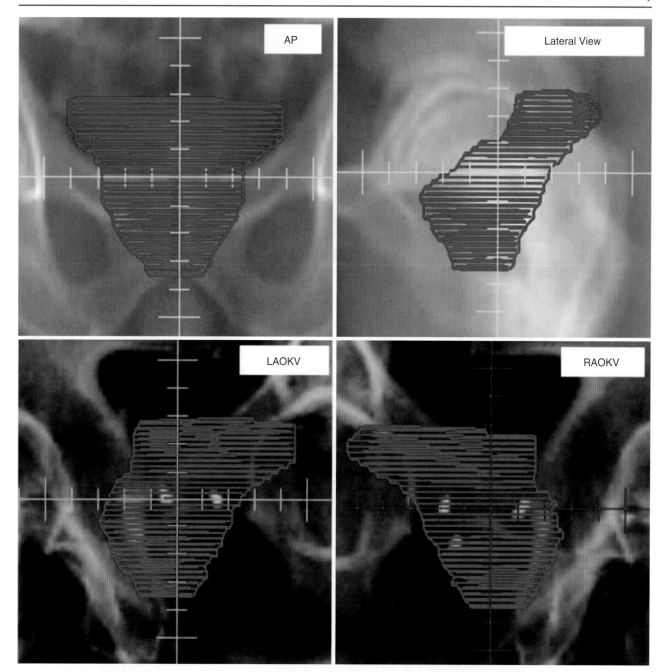

**Fig. 7** Three-dimensional projection of CTV in various views for quality assessment. Note the appearance of a relatively globular gland underneath a winged structure representing the seminal vesicles superiorly. Cross-referencing of these projections to axial contours allows for detection of common misinterpretations of anatomy (i.e., extending contours too far caudally into the genitourinary diaphragm will produce extension of a narrow pedestal-like structure inferiorly described by McLaughlin et al. 2010). Moreover, gross irregularities in the overall structure may reflect overcorrection from slice to slice that is not anatomically faithful, especially when averaging organ deformation and motion during treatment. *AP* anterior-posterior, *LAOKV* left anterior oblique kV, *RAOKV* right anterior oblique kV

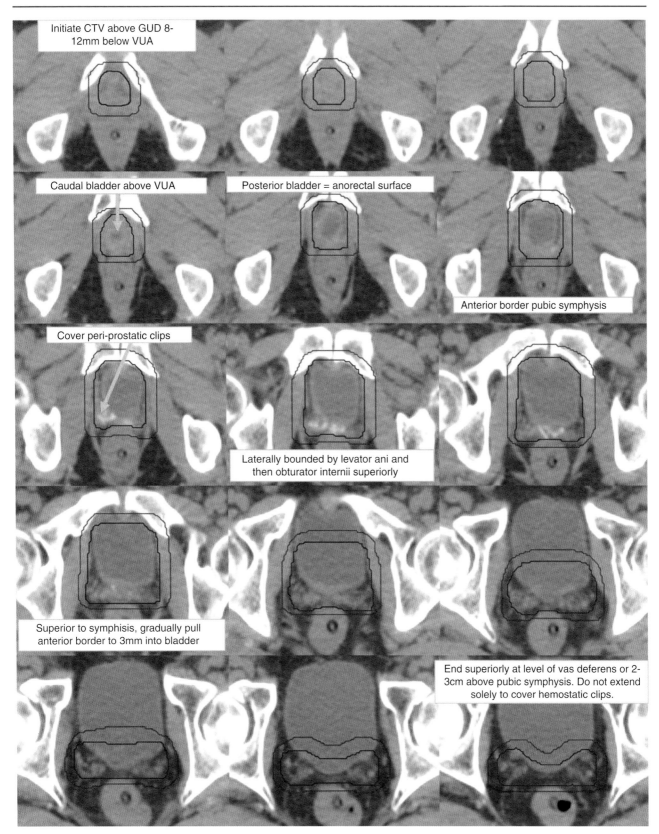

**Fig. 8** Post-robotic prostatectomy target delineation for salvage intent in a 60-year-old with high-risk pT3a, Gleason score 7, and PSA 6.8 adenocarcinoma with steadily rising PSA. Representative images from 2 mm slice thickness simulation CT with full bladder protocol begin caudally. Note that an iterative technique of contouring CTV, expansion to PTV, and modification of CTV before re-expansion is helpful in sensitive areas, such as cranially, where landmarks become subjective and critical structures sandwich the target volume. This helps avoid a "dumbbell" PTV shape from wrapping and overdosing the rectum, as suggested in the latter images. *GUD* genitourinary diaphragm, *VUA* vesicourethral anastomosis

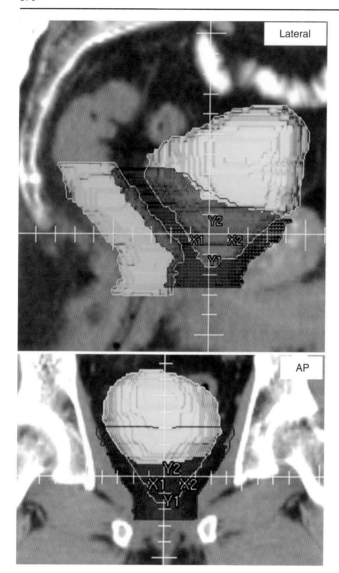

**Fig. 9** 3-D projection of PTV in orthogonal views for quality assessment. As opposed to an intact prostate treatment plan, the contours for a postoperative plan will necessarily approximate the bladder and rectum to cover areas of potential seeding. These areas include the anterior perirectal space, the vesicourethral anastomosis (VUA), and the new spaces created at the posterior bladder interface with the pelvic floor and VUA. The overlap of PTV margin with the rectum (*green*) and bladder (*yellow*) is highlighted here. In particular, a gradual tapering of the anterior PTV boundary superior to the pubic symphysis is ensured by inspection of the three-dimensional projection. Smoothing out this transition avoids abrupt changes in dose distribution that are susceptible to errant targeting based on day-to-day changes in bladder volume despite a full bladder protocol

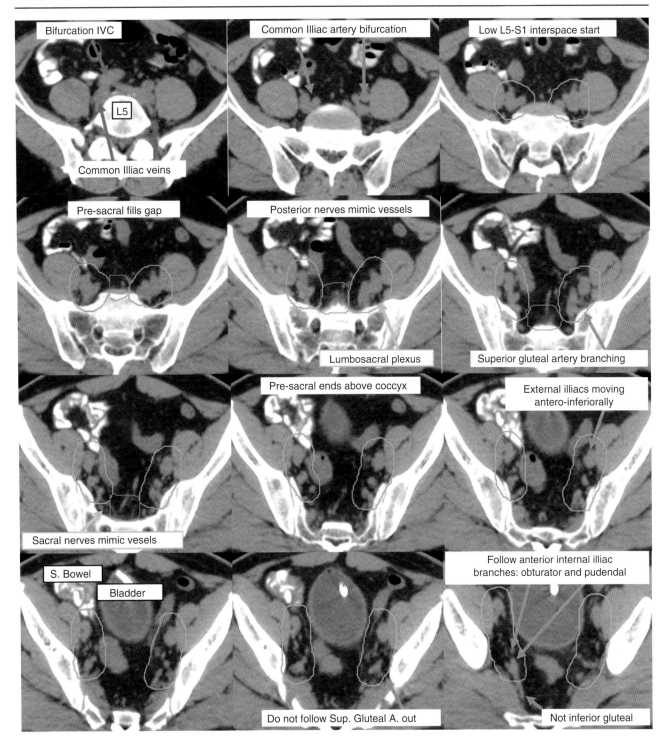

**Fig. 10** Pelvic lymph node target delineation. A 71-year-old man with National Comprehensive Cancer Network (NCCN) intermediate risk disease with MRI suggestion of seminal vesicle (SV) invasion undergoing combination high-dose rate (HDR) brachytherapy followed by external beam RT. Representative images from a 2 mm slice thickness CT simulation scan are provided beginning cranially and proceeding caudally. *IVC* inferior vena cava

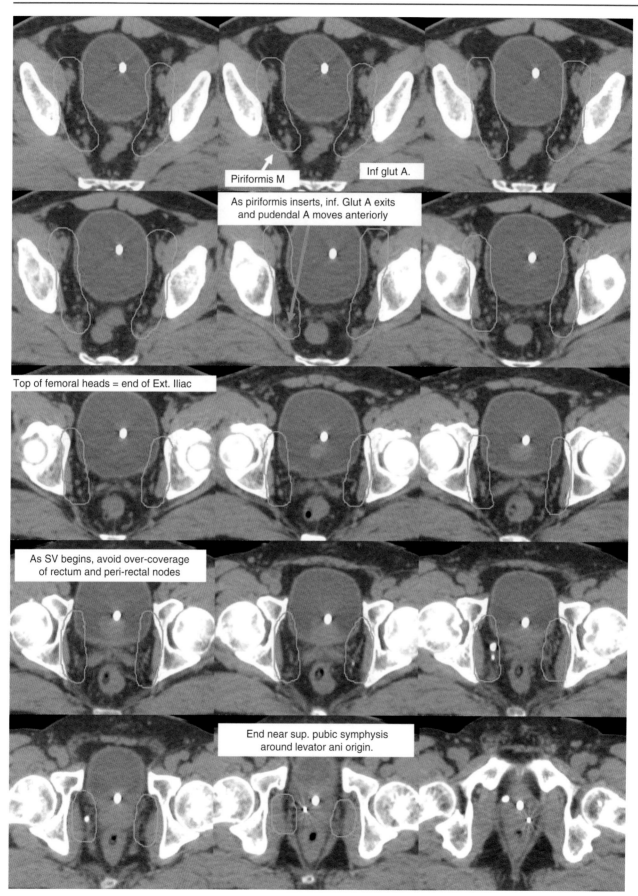

Piriformis M

Inf glut A.

As piriformis inserts, inf. Glut A exits and pudendal A moves anteriorly

Top of femoral heads = end of Ext. Iliac

As SV begins, avoid over-coverage of rectum and peri-rectal nodes

End near sup. pubic symphysis around levator ani origin.

**Fig. 10** (continued)

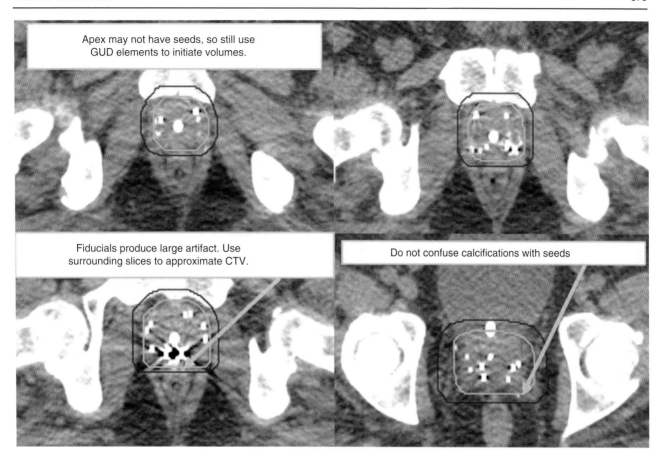

**Fig. 11** This case demonstrates special considerations in volume delineation of the prostate for combination therapy with external beam RT following brachytherapy. General concepts include seeds, do not assume that seed coverage peripherally delineates boundaries, interpolate to smoothen boundaries at areas of fiducial/seed scatter, and contour urethra via Foley for dosimetry. It is helpful to also have dosimetry from the implant to guide treatment planning of the external beam RT. *GUD* genitourinary diaphragm

a

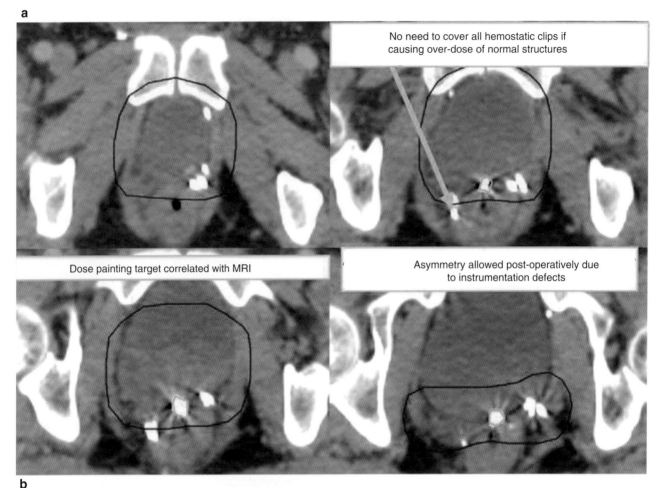

b

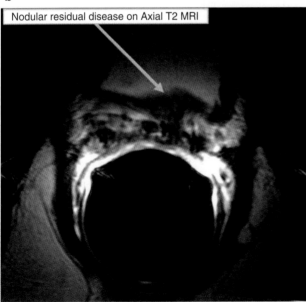

**Fig. 12** Dose painting in the post-prostatectomy setting with gross residual disease on CT (**a**) and MRI (**b**). Patient is a 49 year old with pT3aN0, Gleason score 8 disease who underwent retropubic prostatectomy with multifocal extracapsular extension, positive margins, and gross residual disease on follow-up MRI. The focus was marked for image-guided dose painting with ultrasound-guided placement of Calypso beacon (*blue*). A small margin (not shown) is applied, and boost dose is governed by what is achievable for an institution's given dose constraints for the bladder, rectum, and small bowel. Note that a degree of asymmetry is allowable in postoperative PTV (*red*) given the instrumentation. Also note that in contrast to the prior example of a post-robotic prostatectomy, a retropubic open approach usually leaves more hemostatic clips, which do not all need to be covered

## Suggested Reading and References

McLaughlin PW et al (2010) Radiographic and anatomic basis for prostate contouring errors and methods to improve prostate contouring accuracy. Int J Rad Onc Biol Phys 76(2):369–378

- Excellent demonstration of the anatomic features useful in determining boundaries to the clinical target volume and common errors in anatomic interpretation. Particularly useful are the comparisons of MRI to CT scan images.

RTOG 0534 Protocol Information: A phase III trial of short-term androgen deprivation with pelvic lymph node or prostate bed only radiotherapy (SPPORT) in prostate cancer patients with a rising PSA after radical prostatectomy. See Section 6.0 Radiation Therapy. Pollack A et al. 2010 Dec.

- Available online at RTOG website: http://www.rtog.org/ClinicalTrials/ProtocolTable/StudyDetails.aspx?action=openFile&FileID=4642
- General approach to both the postoperative fossa and pelvic lymph nodes are demonstrated in this protocol.
- These guidelines were formulated by consensus efforts coordinated by the RTOG study groups:
  - Lawton CA et al (2009) RTOG GU radiation oncology specialists reach consensus on pelvic lymph node volumes for high-risk prostate cancer. Int J Rad Onc Biol Phys 74(2):383–387
  - Michalski JM et al (2010) Development of RTOG consensus guidelines for the definition of the clinical target volume for postoperative conformal radiation therapy for prostate cancer. Int J Rad Onc Biol Phys 76(2):361–368

Boehmer D et al (2006) Guidelines for primary radiotherapy of patients with prostate cancer. Radiother Oncol 79(3):259–269

- EORTC guidelines for definitive therapy CTV delineation, which are not used in this manual.

Poortmans P et al (2007) Guidelines for target volume definition in post-operative radiotherapy for prostate cancer, on behalf of the EORTC Radiation Oncology Group. Radiother Oncol 84(2):121–127

- EORTC guidelines for postoperative target delineation. The EORTC volumes were formulated based on a pattern-of-failure study and appear to be somewhat smaller than the RTOG guidelines. Note that we more closely approximate RTOG guidelines for therapy.

# Bladder Carcinoma

Bret Adams, Dayssy A. Diaz, Alan Pollack,
and Matthew Abramowitz

## Contents

B. Adams • D.A. Diaz • A. Pollack • M. Abramowitz (✉)
Department of Radiation Oncology, University of Miami,
Miami, FL, USA
e-mail: mabramowitz@med.miami.edu

## 1    Anatomy and Patterns of Spread

- The bladder is a muscular reservoir that, when empty, is confined to the truc pelvis but fills anterosuperiorly entering the abdominal cavity and affects the position of the bowel. Anatomically it is divided into the base, apex, body, trigone, and neck. Tumors occur in all five of these regions and can often be multifocal.

- The apex extends anterior and superior reaching just above the pubic bone. The neck is located 3–4 cm behind the symphysis pubis and represents the most inferior portion of the bladder as well as the most anatomically fixed. In males, the neck approximates the prostate. The base of the bladder forms the posterior-inferior surface and is separated from the rectum by the vas deferens and seminal vesicles. In females, the bladder sits inferior to the uterus and anterior to the vagina. The trigone is a triangular area on the internal face of the posterior wall of the bladder containing the orifices of the ureters.

- Whereas many other cancers display monoclonality exhibited by a transformed cell that gives rise to many daughter cells, bladder cancer may display a field effect which indicates multifocality. New urothelial cancers can appear in the bladder or in the urothelial lining of the ureters or kidney and then may invade the basement membrane. As the cancer evolves into a more aggressive form, it is able to invade the extravesicular fat and finally into adjacent organs. Similarly, bladder carcinoma may dedifferentiate, invade, and spread along lymphatic channels.

- In patient series of cystectomy for bladder cancer pathologic subgroup, analysis shows that roughly 55 % of surgeries show organ-confined disease, 20 % show extravesicular extension, and 25 % show lymphatic spread (Stein et al. 2001; Madersbacher et al. 2003; Hautmann et al. 2006).

N.Y. Lee et al. (eds.), *Target Volume Delineation for Conformal and Intensity-Modulated Radiation Therapy*,
Medical Radiology. Radiation Oncology, DOI: 10.1007/174_2014_1003, © Springer International Publishing Switzerland 2014
Published Online: 31 October 2014

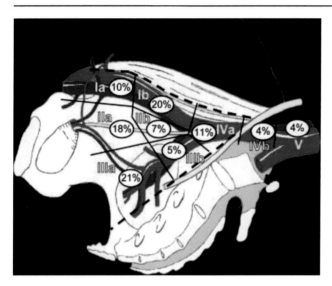

**Fig. 1** Primary lymphatic sites of bladder carcinoma: Distribution of positive nodes after cystectomy and PLND in 60 patients. The noted areas are the external iliac (*Ia*) distal and (*Ib*) proximal, obturator fossa (*IIa*) distal and (*IIb*) proximal, internal iliac (*IIIa*) distal and (*IIIb*) proximal, common iliac (*IVa*) distal and (*IVb*) proximal, (*V*) para-aortic/cava (Roth et al. 2010)

- The regional nodal levels are defined by primary and secondary drainage. The primary drainage levels include the hypogastric, obturator, iliac, perivesical, sacral, and presacral nodes. Common iliac nodes are defined as a secondary drainage region and not as metastatic disease. Figure 1 shows the location of noted positive nodes for bladder cancer in a series of surgically resected patients.

- In an analysis of the primary lymphatic sites of bladder carcinoma, it was discovered that 92 % of positive lymph nodes were distal and caudal to where the ureter crosses the common iliac arteries (Roth et al. 2010). All of those that were positive proximal to the crossing of the ureter over the common iliac arteries also showed endopelvic positive lymph nodes on extended pelvic lymph node dissection (PLND). Therefore, coverage superior to the ureters crossing the common iliac arteries would not aid in local control.

## 2 Diagnostic Workup Relevant for Target Volume Delineation

- Painless hematuria and voiding symptoms often initiate a workup which includes cystoscopy with cytology and urinalysis revealing carcinoma. Initial workup is recommended to include digital rectal and bimanual examinations as well as imaging of the upper tract. The presence of ureteral obstruction, hydronephrosis, or a nonfunctioning kidney predicts muscle-invasive disease in 90 % of cases (Messer et al. 2011; Hatch and Berry 1986). The importance of a proper workup cannot be overstated

for candidates for bladder preservation therapy since they are commonly understaged compared to those that undergo surgery.

- For patients who may be candidates for bladder preservation, a workup should include cystoscopy with a detailed description or illustrative mapping which provides direct visualization and enumeration of any biopsy-positive disease. Descriptors including size and location of any tumors are vital for target delineation.

- Patients with Ta or low-grade T1 tumors do not require an extensive metastatic workup. Those with muscle-invading tumors, however, have a risk of occult metastatic disease of up to 50 % and should undergo chest imaging and bone scanning if alkaline phosphatase is elevated.

- For patients with muscle-invasive disease, imaging of the upper tract is recommended and can include more common studies such as intravenous pyelogram or CT urography but may also include MRI urogram, ureteroscopy, or renal ultrasound with retrograde pyelogram. Locally advanced disease imaging with CT or MRI is imperative for proper staging, and MRI has shown improved specificity over CT scan due to its high soft tissue contrast and also has the advantage that contrast agents are non-nephrotoxic (Zhang et al. 2007). The contrast between fat and tissue is best defined on T1-weighted imaging or T1 subtraction sequences. Figure 2a shows how MRI can be used for staging as well as target delineation of the gross tumor volume (GTV) for a patient treated with IMRT. Notably, the contrast between the fat and tissue may be lost on the normal bladder wall several months after radiation treatment and limits the usefulness of follow-up MRI scans.

## 3 Simulation and Daily Localization

- CT simulation using 3 mm or less slice thickness should be performed prior to planning. For 3DCRT, set up the patient in supine position with the bladder emptied just prior to simulation for reproducibility. Similarly, patients are asked to void the contents of the rectum for daily reproducibility. When using 3DCRT technique, a sequential boost is added to the initial clinical target volume (CTV). A new simulation may be helpful with a partially distended bladder to limit dose to the entire bladder as well as the rectum depending on the location of the tumor. Many institutions continue the boost with the bladder empty since this provides reproducibility.

- If using IMRT with image guidance, the simulation is performed with the bladder partially full to allow for dose painting to the GTV daily. Bladder filling should be comfortable and reproducible by the patient. On board imaging capable of assessing bladder filling and volume is critical to treating with a full bladder. Simulation may include leg support for patient comfort which can aid in daily setup. Immobilization devices including Vak-Lok or Alpha Cradle may be used and vary by institution. Similarly, frog-leg positioning may be warranted to reduce skinfolds.

- IV contrast may be used to help guide the GTV target and vessels; however, renal function must be assessed and fusion of imaging from the patient's workup may be adequate. A simulation scan from the upper lumbar spine to mid-femur is recommended.

- Image registration and fusion applications with previously performed MRI and PET are recommended to help in the delineation of target volumes. However, the bladder mapping in conjunction with the surgeon is imperative for the CTV. Normal tissues should be outlined on all CT slices in which the structures exist. An example of how CT urography may aid in target delineation is provided in Fig. 3.

- Image-guided radiation therapy allows for adjustments to be made based on soft tissue anatomy prior to treatment delivery. Cone-beam CT can be performed in an effort to decrease uncertainty and therefore decrease treatment margins. It also allows for confirmation of bladder filling. While not the standard, IMRT is an option to reduce bowel dose as well as spare uninvolved bladder during a boost.

## 4 Target Volume Delineation and Treatment Planning

- Bladder preservation therapy is a multidisciplinary effort with concurrent chemotherapy and radiotherapy after maximal transurethral resection of bladder tumor (TURBT). Ideal candidates for bladder preservation include those with clinical T2-3a tumors that are unifocal, node negative, and with no evidence of ureteral obstruction or involvement with the ureteral orifice and good bladder function. Ideal candidates should have a complete resection by TURBT (Shipley et al. 1998; Tester et al. 1993).

- To properly plan the boost portion of therapy, bladder mapping from the pretreatment cystoscopy should be used as well as any findings on physical exam or imaging that display extravesicular extension.

- Suggested target volumes at the GTV and high-risk CTV are detailed in Table 1 for 3DCRT planning (Shipley et al. 1998).

- In 3DCRT a small pelvis field is followed by a boost to the bladder tumor. A boost to the bladder tumor with a margin as opposed to boosting the entire bladder has been determined to be safe in RTOG randomized trials. This involves close collaboration with the urologist with TURBT mapping. Once-daily fractionation is recommended at 1.8–2 Gy per fraction.

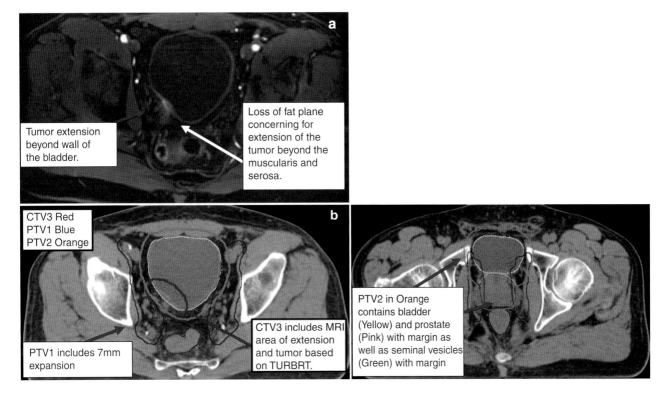

**Fig. 2** (**a**) MRI for patient showing axial T1-post-contrast subtraction sequence demonstrating invasion beyond the wall of bladder (*red arrow*) and loss of fat plane (*white arrow*). (**b**) CT contours for patient in Fig. 2a using IMRT. Target delineation CTV3$_{64.5\,Gy}$ (*red*), PTV1 $_{51\,Gy}$ (*blue*), and PTV2$_{54\,Gy}$ (*orange*) in a patient with muscle-invasive bladder cancer with focus at the primary site. GTV based on MRI and CT imaging. (**c**) CT contours for patient in Fig. X-X using IMRT. Target delineation CTV3$_{64.5\,Gy}$ (*red*), PTV1 $_{51\,Gy}$ (*blue*), and PTV2$_{54\,Gy}$ (*orange*) in a patient with muscle-invasive bladder cancer with focus at the primary site. Please note that these are representative slices and not all slices are included. Please note normal structure contours include bladder (*yellow*), seminal vesicles (*green*), and rectum (*brown*)

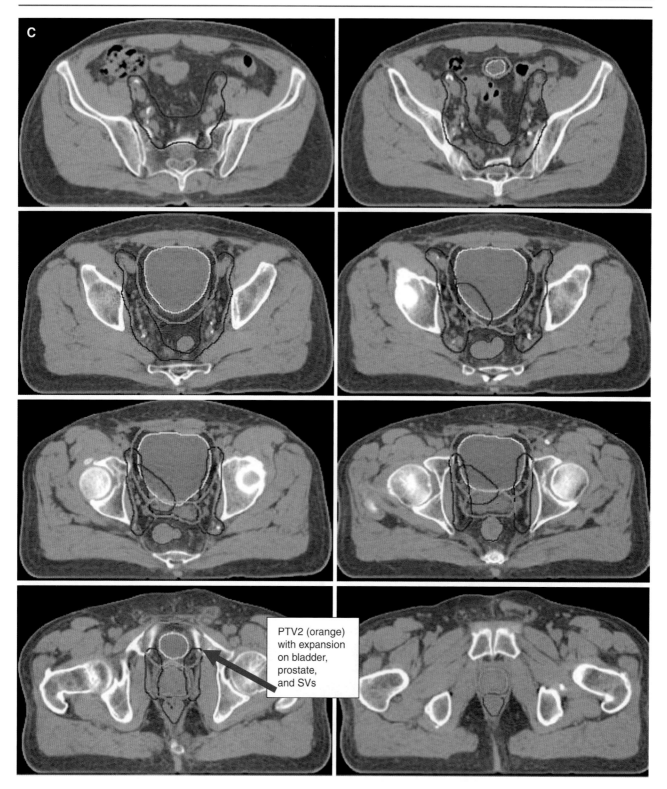

PTV2 (orange) with expansion on bladder, prostate, and SVs

**Fig. 2** (continued)

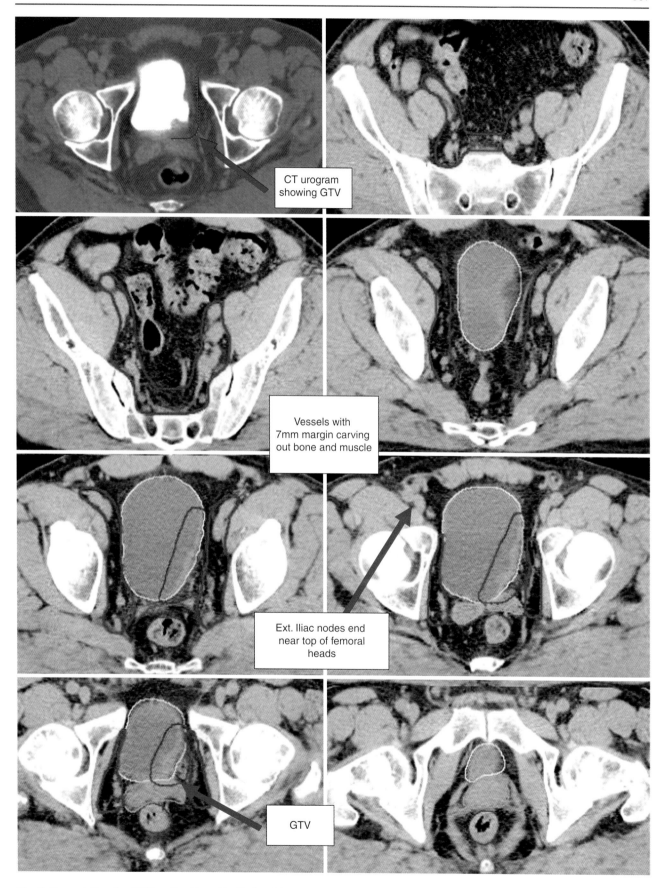

**Fig. 3** Target delineation GTV outlined in red is displayed in CT urogram. PTV$_1$ (*purple*) for lymph nodes is shown prior to expansion for planning. Please note that these are representative slices and not all slices are included. Please note normal structure contours include bladder (*yellow*), seminal vesicles (*green*), prostate (*pink*) and rectum (*brown*)

**Table 1** Suggested target volumes for bladder preservation (3DCRT)

| Target volumes | Field margins |
|---|---|
| Small pelvic fields (include CTV₁) (45 Gy) | *AP/PA*<br>*Superior-inferior field:* mid-sacro-iliac region (S2/S3) to just below the obturator foramen. Common iliac nodes will not be covered<br>*Anterior-posterior field:* 1.5–2.0 cm laterally beyond the medial aspect of the pelvic bone. Customized blocks should be used to reduce the exposure of the femoral heads |
| | *Lateral*<br>*Superior-inferior:* As AP/PA<br>*Anterior:* 1 cm anteriorly to the bladder boundary or 1 cm anterior to the tip of the symphysis<br>*Posterior:* 2.5 cm posteriorly to the bladder or any visible tumor. Customized block to protect bowel anterior to external iliac lymph nodes should be used since the bowel may be involved in future surgery as conduit or reservoir<br>Wedges must be considered depending on body contours |
| Whole bladder field (CTV₂) (54 Gy) | The field is constructed from the same simulation as the small pelvic field and contains the bladder volume as well as GTV. $PTV = CTV_2 + 2\ cm$ |
| Tumor boost field (CTV₃) (64 Gy) | $PTV = CTV_3 = GTV + 2\ cm$ |

- In 3DCRT planning a dose of 40–45 Gy is delivered to the pelvic lymph nodes and areas at risk defined by CTV1. The whole bladder field will receive 54 Gy and boost field receives 60–65 Gy. The Nodal XRT fields are conservative to reduce small bowel toxicity so that diversions can later be accomplished without complications. The tumor boost field only treats partial bladder and incorporates all information for the location of GTV prior to TURBT. An example of digitally reconstructed radiographs for treatment is provided in Fig. 4a, b revealing established borders.

- Hypofractionation has been investigated and shown to have similar disease outcome status with recent reports showing acceptable toxicities with once-daily fractionation utilizing IMRT (Turgeon et al. 2013).

- IMRT planning requires more detailed knowledge of anatomical structures for accurate dose delivery. The benefits of IMRT can be negated by patient and organ motion; therefore, setup and reproducibility are imperative. For this reason, rigid immobilization and cone-beam CT (CBCT) are often used to aid in reduction of uncertainty. As mentioned previously, when utilizing IMRT, the target volumes may be simulated with a comfortably full bladder. This difference in simulation may displace the bowel as well as provide more accurate delineation of the target since TURBT with tumor resection is performed with a full bladder. Furthermore, this may promote long-term bladder function by sparing a larger percentage of the bladder receiving the highest doses of radiation.

- Delineated target volumes for bladder preservation therapy include a GTV and multiple clinical target volumes: CTV1, CTV2, and CTV3. See Table 2 for more details regarding CTV.

- Planning target volumes (PTVs) are created for each CTV. The separate PTVs are based on uncertainty regarding internal organ motion and they are combined for a final PTV. For IMRT planning, the GTV is defined as all

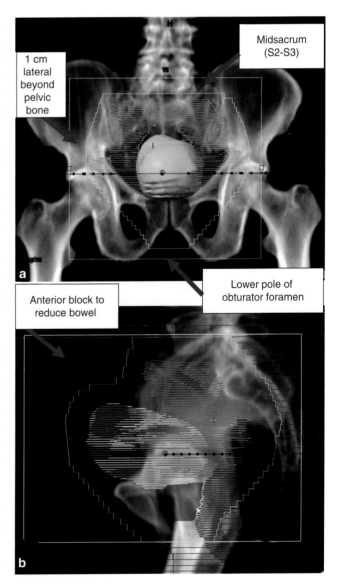

**Fig. 4** Digitally reconstructed radiographs for (**a**) AP portal image and (**b**) lateral portal image of small pelvic field for 3D

**Table 2** Suggested target volumes for IMRT planning

| IMRT | |
|---|---|
| Target volumes | Structures |
| Small pelvic fields (include CTV$_1$) (51 Gy/30 fractions @ 1.7 Gy/Fx) | The CTV1 is defined as regions at high risk for microscopic disease. Lymph node volumes extend anteriorly to include the lateral external iliac nodes with CTV extending laterally to the pelvic side wall. This volume joins the internal iliac vessels to form a single volume on each side of the pelvis and should include an expansion of 7 mm from the vessels where lymph nodes may reside. Also included are the presacral and the obturator nodes. The presacral CTV extends superiorly to S2/S3 |
| Whole bladder field (CTV$_2$) (54 Gy/30 fractions @ 1.8 Gy/Fx) | The entire bladder, prostate, and prostatic urethra are included due to the multifocal nature of bladder cancer |
| Tumor boost field (CTV$_3$) (64.5 Gy/30 fractions @ 2.15 Gy/fx) | This volume is defined by the GTV and includes the area of bladder involved with tumor based on TURBRT, imaging, or palpable disease plus 7 mm. The CTV3 encompasses the GTV for the boost portion of the plan |
| PTV$_1$ | *CTV$_1$ + 7 mm* |
| PTV$_2$ | *CTV$_2$ + 10 mm* |
| PTV$_3$ | *CTV$_3$ + 7 mm* |

*The final PTV is then generated by combination of* PTV$_1$, PTV$_2$, *and* PTV$_3$

known gross disease determined from CT, MRI, clinical information, and cystoscopy.

- Figure 2a–c shows MRI and utilization of T1 post-contrast subtraction sequence for GTV definition. The CTV$_3$ is shown for delineation prior to PTV expansion. Bowel is not contoured but is defined by potential space. The ano-rectum is shown contoured in brown and begins inferiorly at the ischial tuberosity and continues superiorly until it projects anteriorly connecting to the sigmoid colon.

- Figure 3a, b displays patient treated with IMRT with lymph nodes contoured prior to PTV expansion. Patient did not receive staging MRI and CT urogram was utilized for GTV delineation. Lymph node volumes include 7 mm circumscribing the internal and external iliac vessels prior to 7 mm expansion. MRI was unavailable for staging, and a slightly more generous GTV was created due to

increased uncertainty of target volume based on imaging modality characteristics.

- Figure 5a, b shows T1 axial MRI and comparable CT scan to reveal invasion into vagina in a post-hysterectomy female patient. The vagina is not a target of interest or organ at risk but contoured for educational purposes.

## 5  Plan Assessment

- At least 95 % of the volume of each PTV should receive 100 % of prescribed dose. Generally, a minimum dose of 95 % and a max dose of 115 % is set for PTV$_3$.

- Several critical normal structures surround the bladder and therefore need to be outlined for dose constraints including the anorectum, femoral heads, and bowel (Table 3).

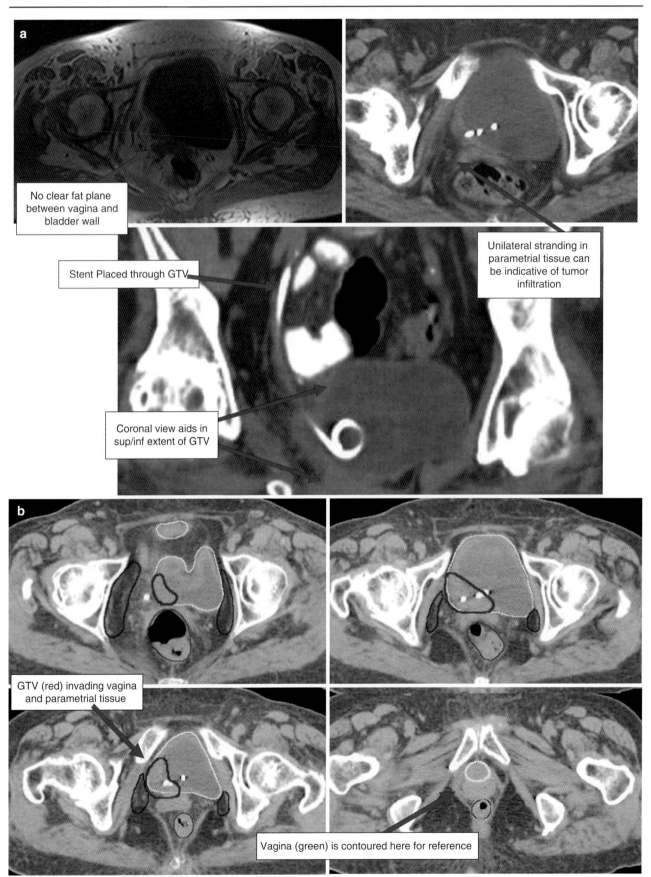

**Fig. 5** (**a**) Target delineation is aided by T1 axial MRI. Contrast was unable to be used increasing uncertainty relating to GTV. There is eccentric wall thickening of the right posterolateral bladder wall at the ureterovesical junction and questionable extension posteriorly to the vagina. MRI in conjunction with coronal and axial CT scans defines GTV. (**b**) CT contours for patient in Fig. 5a. Target delineation for the GTV/CTV$3_{64.5\,Gy}$ (*red*), PTV1 $_{51\,Gy}$ (*blue*), as well as the bladder and vaginal cuff in post-hysterectomy patient with muscle-invasive bladder cancer. Please note that these are representative slices and not all slices are included. Please note normal structure contours include bladder (*yellow*), vagina (*green*), and rectum (*brown*)

**Table 3** Intensity-modulated radiation therapy: normal tissue dose constraints

| Critical structures | Constraints |
|---|---|
| Femoral heads | Max <45 Gy |
| Spinal cord | Max <45 Gy or 1 cc of the PTV cannot exceed 50 Gy |
| Rectum | 50 % of the volume should receive less than 55 Gy |
| Bowel | <300 ccs receiving a dose greater than 45 Gy |

A DVH for the femoral heads, rectum, and bladder is advised and an example of an acceptable plan is displayed in Fig. 6a. This figure shows that a high volume of the bladder is receiving the highest dose of radiation (red arrow), and for comparison, a patient simulated (Fig. 6b) with the bladder full is also depicted (white arrow)

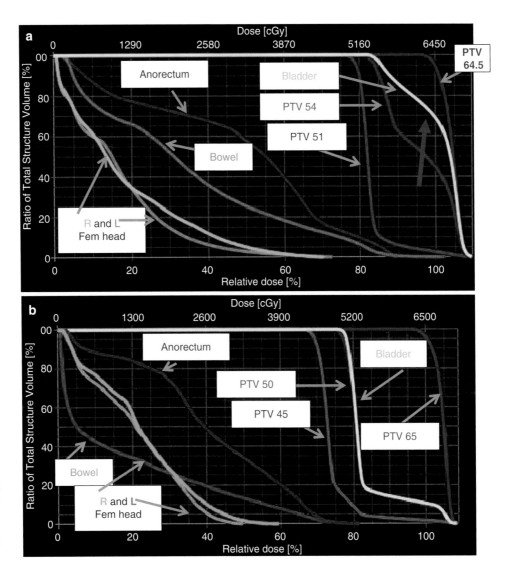

**Fig. 6** Plan evaluation PTVs and OARs in a patient with muscle-invasive bladder cancer. Below are two DVHs. A patient who underwent simulation with bladder empty (**a**) is shown compared to the DVH of a patient who was simulated with bladder full (**b**)

## Suggested Reading

RTOG 8903 and RTOG 0233: Describes RTOG recommended treatment guidelines for bladder cancer

Male and female RTOG normal pelvic contouring atlases

Kaufman D, Shipley W, Feldman A (2009) Review of current treatment paradigms and trial results. Lancet 374(9685):239–249

## References

Hatch T, Berry J (1986) The value of excretory radiography in staging bladder cancer. J Urol 135:49

Hautmann RE, Gschwend JE, de Petriconi RC et al (2006) Cystectomy for transitional cell carcinoma of the bladder: results of a surgery only series in the neobladder era. J Urol 176(2):486–492

Madersbacher S, Hochreiter W, Burkhard F et al (2003) Radical cystectomy for bladder cancer today–a homogeneous series without neoadjuvant therapy. J Clin Oncol 21(4):690–696

Messer JC, Terrell JD, Herman MP et al (2011) Multi-institutional validation of the ability of preoperative hydronephrosis to predict advanced pathologic tumor stage in upper-tract urothelial carcinoma. Urol Oncol 31(6):904–908

Roth B, Wissmeyer MP, Zehnder P et al (2010) A new multimodality technique accurately maps the primary lymphatic landing sites of the bladder. Eur Urol 57(2):205–211

Shipley WU, Winter KA, Kaufman DS et al (1998) Phase III trial of neoadjuvant chemotherapy in patients with invasive bladder cancer treated with selective bladder preservation by combined radiation therapy and chemotherapy: initial results of Radiation Therapy Oncology Group 89–03. J Clin Oncol 16:3576–3583

Stein JP, Lieskovsky G, Cote R et al (2001) Radical cystectomy in the treatment of invasive bladder cancer: long-term results in 1,054 patients. J Clin Oncol 19(3):666–675

Tester W, Porter A, Asbell S et al (1993) Combined modality program with possible organ preservation for invasive bladder carcinoma: results of RTOG protocol 85–12. Int J Radiat Oncol Biol Phys 25:783–790

Turgeon G-A, Souhami L, Cury FL, Faria SL et al (2013) Hypofractionated intensity modulated radiation therapy in combined modality treatment for bladder preservation in elderly patients with invasive bladder cancer. Int J Radiat Oncol Biol Phys 88(2):326–331

Zhang J, Gerst S, Lefkowitz RA, Bach A (2007) Imaging of bladder cancer. Radiol Clin North Am 45(1):183–205

# Testicular Seminoma

Sean M. McBride

## Contents

S.M. McBride, MD, MPH
Department of Radiation Oncology,
Memorial Sloan-Kettering Cancer Center,
New York, NY, USA
e-mail: mcbrides@mskcc.org

N.Y. Lee et al. (eds.), *Target Volume Delineation for Conformal and Intensity-Modulated Radiation Therapy*,
Medical Radiology. Radiation Oncology, DOI: 10.1007/174_2014_982, © Springer International Publishing Switzerland 2014
Published Online: 22 October 2014

# 1 Anatomy and Patterns of Spread

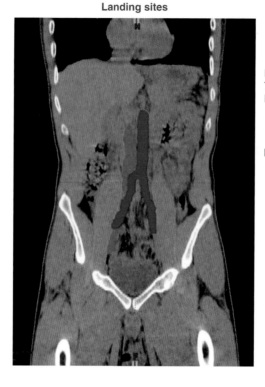

**Right:**
Testicular vein →
vena cava

**Aortocaval nodes**

Inguinal nodes if prior
ing/pevic surgery

**Left**:
Testicular vein →
L renal vein

**Para-aortic nodes**

- R testicular seminoma tends to drain to the vena cava and aortocaval nodes.
- L testicular seminoma tends to drain to the L renal vein and para-aortic nodes.

## 2 Diagnostic Workup Relevant for Target Volume Delineation

- A suspicious testicular mass should prompt a complete history and physical exam, serum tumor markers (α-fetoprotein, β-human chorionic gonadotropin, and LDH), chemistry panel, and CXR. Always *REMEMBER SPERM BANKING*.
- After orchiectomy, patients should complete staging with a CT of the abdomen and pelvis (and include CT chest if suspicious nodes on CT A/P) and have repeat of beta-hCG, LDH, and AFP.

- At some institutions, a PET/CT will be part of initial workup. This could conceivably help with target delineation.

## 3 Simulation and Daily Localization

- Simulation in the supine position with arms in wing-board and wedge under knees.
- One could consider using alpha-cradle to help to enhance immobilization.
- A clamshell shield must be added to decrease dose to the remnant testicle.
- Move the penis out of the field with mesh.
- Tattoos must be placed at the level of the isocenter anteriorly and laterally.
- IV contrast can be used to help better identify both the vessels and any gross disease.
- If available, a PET/CT simulation may be helpful in stage II cases for delineation of gross nodal disease.

## 4    Target Volume Delineation and Treatment Planning

- Stage I: It is the strong recommendation of the National Comprehensive Cancer Network Treatment (NCCN) that all patients with stage I seminoma undergo post-orchiectomy surveillance. Treatment of these patients risks late morbidity, most notably secondary malignancies. However, if a patient refuses active imaging surveillance, based on results from MRC TE 10 and TE 18, patients with stage I seminoma can receive adjuvant radiotherapy confined to para-aortic lymph nodes to a dose of 20 Gy unless there is prior inguinal or scrotal violation (lymphatic alteration) (Fossa et al. 1999; Jones et al. 2005). Fields for stage I disease are outlined below. Besides radiotherapy, carboplatinum ×1 cycle is also an option for stage I patients who refuse surveillance (National Comprehensive Cancer Network 2014).
- Stage II: Radiotherapy to a traditional "dog-leg" field is the typical standard of care for stage IIa patients as outlined below; for stage IIb patients, options include radiotherapy as outlined or chemotherapy (etoposide + cisplatinum ×4 cycles or bleomycin, etoposide, cisplatinum ×3 cycles); stage IIc patients should be treated with chemotherapy (same) (National Comprehensive Cancer Network 2014).
- Volume recommendations were derived from Wilder et al. Excellent reference (Wilder et al. 2012) (Tables 1 and 2; Figs. 1 and 2).

## 5    Plan Assessment

- IMRT offers a dosimetric disadvantage in terms of mean and D50 % to the liver, bowel, and kidneys compared to 3DRT (Zilli et al. 2011); proton therapy may offer significant sparing of normal tissues (Efstathiou et al. 2012); this is under investigation in early phase clinical trials.
- For AP-PA beams, one can consider equally weighted fields; however, to improve target coverage, unequal weighting may be necessary.
- V100 % should be 95 % for PTVs.
- D50 % $\leq$8 Gy for each kidney for PTV initial (or PTV for stage I).

**Table 1** Suggested target volumes for stage IA, IB, or IS

| Target volumes | Definition and description |
| --- | --- |
| CTV | *Based on CT imaging (preferred)*: contour out the inferior vena cava and aorta from 2 cm below the top of the kidney superiorly to bifurcations inferiorly → provide a 1.2 cm expansion on IVC and 1.9 cm expansion on the aorta → contour out the bone, muscle, and bowel → merge two expanded volumes<br>*Based on bony landmarks*: superior border at T11, inferior border at L5, lateral borders at transverse processes |
| PTV | Dependent on institution but can expand by 0.5 cm. Additional 0.7 cm to block edge for penumbral effect |

PTV receives 20 Gy in AP/PA prescribed to midplane

**Table 2** Suggested target volumes for stage IIA and IIB

| Target volumes | Definition and description |
| --- | --- |
| CTV initial | Based on CT anatomy:<br>The same instructions as stage I re: aorta + IVC → contour out common iliacs, proximal internal iliac vessels (until takeoff of superior gluteal), and external iliac vessels down to the upper border of the acetabulum → place aortic and IVC expansions as per stage I and place 1.2 cm expansions around common, internal, and external iliac volumes → merge to create CTV vessels and contour out the bone, muscle, and bowel<br>Contour gross nodal disease (GTV) → expand GTV nodes by 0.8 cm to create CTV nodes (exclude bones, muscle, bowel)<br>Merge CTV vessels and CTV nodes to create CTV initial |
| PTV initial | Expansion by 0.5 cm on CTV initial; 0.7 cm to block edge for penumbral effect |
| PTV conedown | Expansion by 0.5 cm on CTV nodes; 0.7 cm to block edge for penumbral effect |

PTV initial treated to 25.5 Gy in 1.7 Gy fractions in an attempt to reduce toxicity to late responding normal tissues
PTV conedown gets a boost to approximately 30 Gy in 2 Gy fractions for stage IIA disease and approximately 36 Gy in 2 Gy fractions for stage IIB disease

- For PTV initial in stage II, mean dose for combined kidney volume should be $\leq$9 Gy.
- For the boost volumes, D50 % should be $\leq$2 Gy for each kidney. Mean dose to combined volume should be $\leq$ 3 Gy.

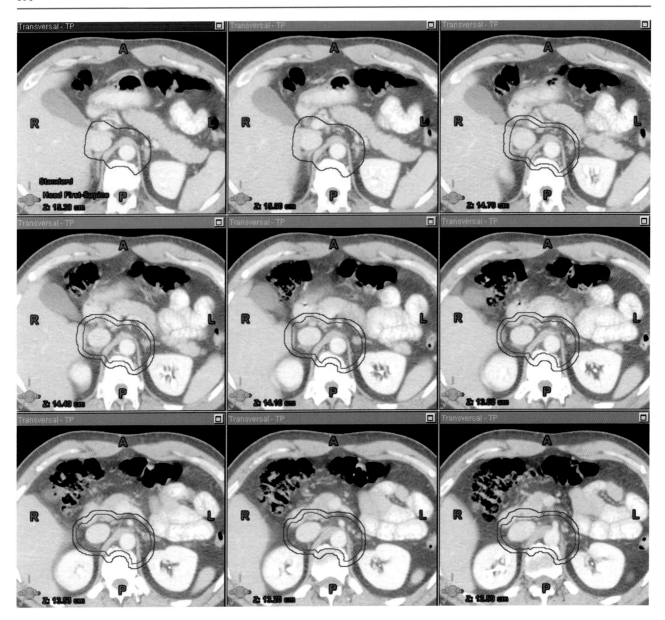

**Fig. 1** Volumes for clinical stages IA, IB, and IS (CTV = *red*, PTV = *blue*); slices are superior to inferior

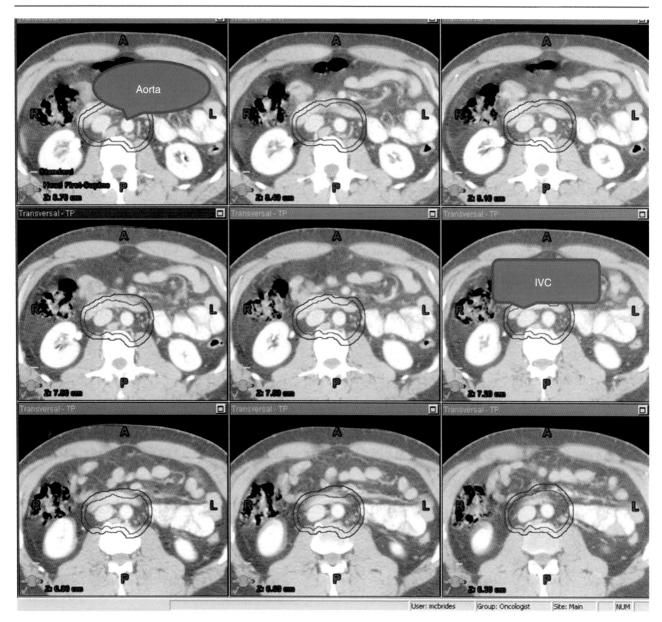

**Fig. 1** (continued)

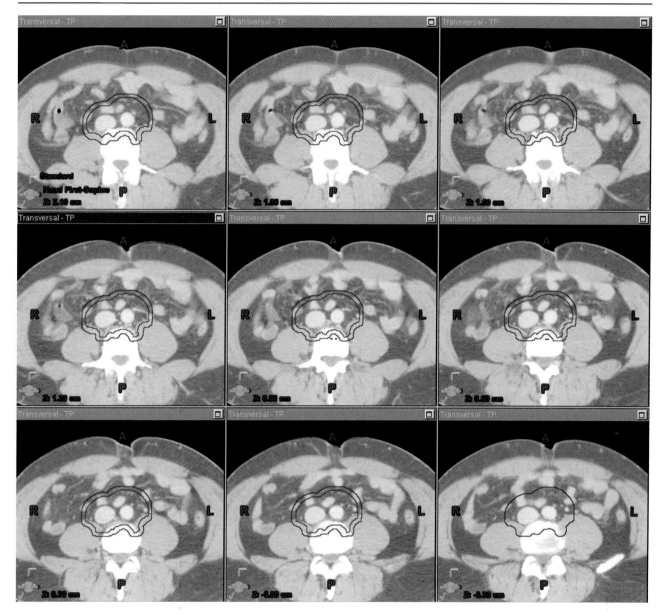

**Fig. 1** (continued)

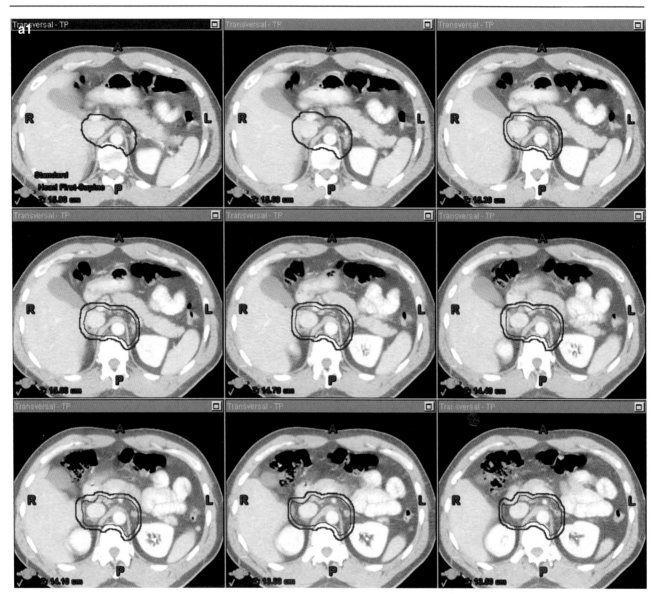

**Fig. 2** (**a**) Initial volumes for stage IIA or IIB (CTV = *red*, PTV = *blue*) with BEV; slices are superior to inferior. (**b**) Boost volumes for stage IIA case (GTV = *yellow*, CTV = *red*, PTV = *blue*); slices are superior to inferior

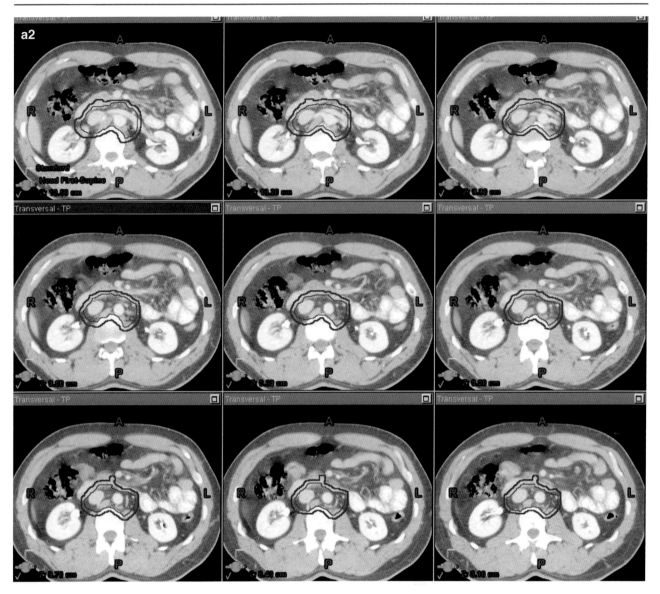

**Fig. 2** (continued)

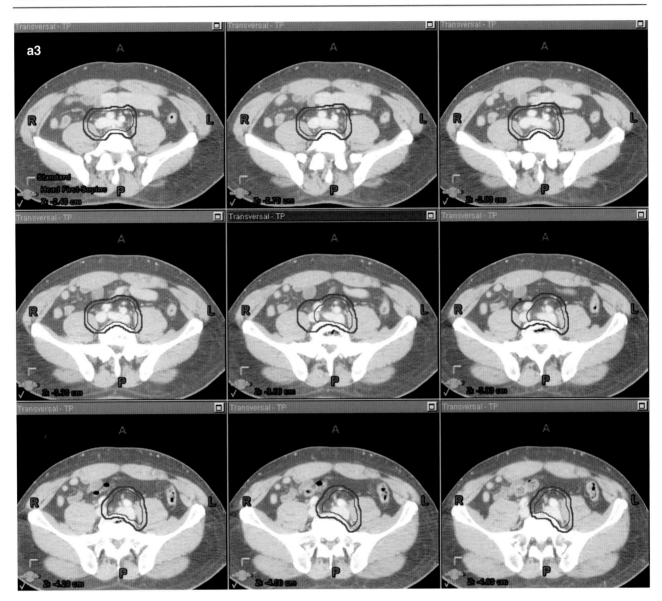

**Fig. 2** (continued)

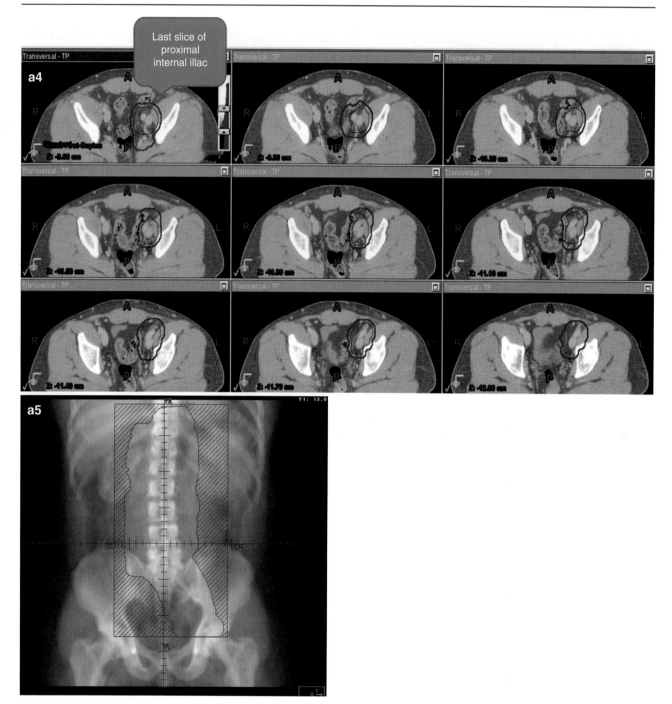

Last slice of proximal internal iliac

**Fig. 2** (continued)

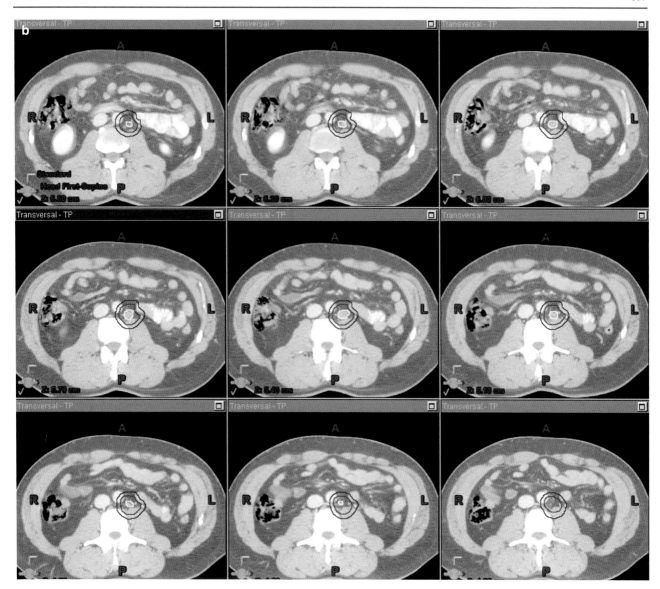

**Fig. 2** (continued)

## References

Efstathiou JA et al (2012) Adjuvant radiation therapy for early stage seminoma: proton versus photon planning comparison and modeling of second cancer risk. Radiother Oncol 103(1):12–17

Fossa SD et al (1999) Optimal planning target volume for stage I testicular seminoma: A Medical Research Council randomized trial. Medical Research Council Testicular Tumor Working Group. J Clin Oncol 17(4):1146

Jones WG et al (2005) Randomized trial of 30 versus 20 Gy in the adjuvant treatment of stage I Testicular Seminoma: a report on Medical Research Council Trial TE18, European Organisation for the Research and Treatment of Cancer Trial 30942 (ISRCTN18525328). J Clin Oncol 23(6):1200–1208

National Comprehensive Cancer Network. Testicular Cancer (Version 1.2014). http://www.nccn.org/professionals/physician_gls/pdf/testicular.pdf. Accessed 7 Feb 2014

Wilder RB et al (2012) Radiotherapy treatment planning for testicular seminoma. Int J Radiat Oncol Biol Phys 83(4):e445–e452

Zilli T et al (2011) Bone marrow-sparing intensity-modulated radiation therapy for stage I seminoma. Acta Oncol 50(4): 555–562

# Benign Intracranial Disease: Benign Tumors of the Central Nervous System, Arteriovenous Malformations, and Trigeminal Neuralgia

Rupesh Kotecha, Samuel T. Chao, Erin S. Murphy, and John H. Suh

## Contents

R. Kotecha
Department of Radiation Oncology,
Cleveland Clinic Foundation, Cleveland, OH, USA
e-mail: kotechr2@ccf.org

S.T. Chao • E.S. Murphy • J.H. Suh (✉)
Department of Radiation Oncology,
Cleveland Clinic Foundation, Cleveland, OH, USA

Taussig Cancer Institute,
Cleveland Clinic Foundation, Cleveland, OH, USA

Burkhardt Brain Tumor and Neuro-Oncology Center,
Cleveland Clinic Foundation, Cleveland, OH, USA
e-mail: suhj@ccf.org

# 1    Anatomy and Patterns of Spread

## 1.1    Meningioma

- The meninges are the membranes that envelop the brain and spinal cord and consist of three separate layers. The dura mater is the outer connective tissue layer, itself composed of an outer endosteal layer and an inner meningeal layer. The dura mater forms a double fold to create the falx cerebri (separates the cerebral hemispheres), tentorium cerebelli (separates the occipital lobes of the cerebrum from the cerebellum), falx cerebelli (separates the cerebellar hemispheres), and the diaphragma sellae (covers the pituitary gland). The middle layer, the arachnoid membrane, and the inner layer, the pia mater, together are referred to as the leptomeninges. Cerebrospinal fluid flows through the space between the arachnoid membrane and the pia matter (Schünke et al. 2007).

- Meningiomas can develop in many locations including the parasagittal/falcine (25 %), convexity (19 %), sphenoid ridge (17 %), suprasellar (9 %), posterior fossa (8 %), olfactory groove (8 %), middle fossa/Meckel's cave (4 %), tentorial (3 %), peri-torcular (3 %), lateral ventricle (1–2 %), foramen magnum (1–2 %), and orbit/optic nerve sheath (1–2 %) (Lee 2008).

- A majority of the parasagittal meningiomas occur over the anterior one-third of the falx cerebri (49 %), while 29 % occur in the middle third and 22 % occur in the posterior third (Rohringer et al. 1989) (Fig. 1a, b).

- Multiple meningiomas, also known as meningiomatosis, occur in only 2.5 % of cases (Lee 2008).

## 1.2    Pituitary

- The pituitary gland, located in the sella turcica, is typically 8 mm in males and 10 mm in females in the superior-inferior dimension. Pituitary tumors that are smaller than 10 mm are referred to as microadenomas, while tumors

N.Y. Lee et al. (eds.), *Target Volume Delineation for Conformal and Intensity-Modulated Radiation Therapy*,
Medical Radiology. Radiation Oncology, DOI: 10.1007/174_2014_983, © Springer International Publishing Switzerland 2014
Published Online: 20 September 2014

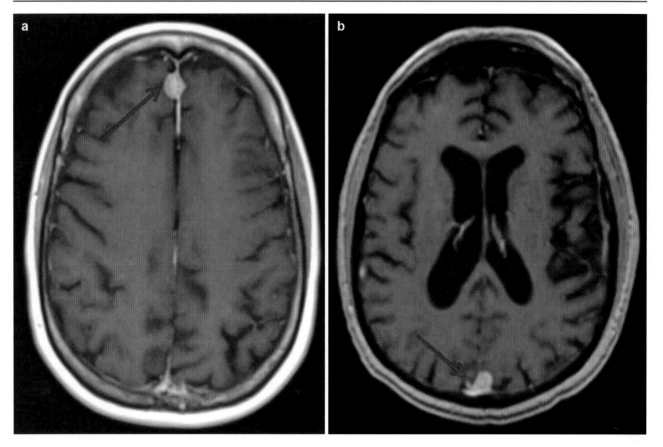

**Fig. 1** (**a**) Axial T1-weighted post-contrast MRI demonstrates a homogeneously enhancing meningioma in the frontal falx cerebri causing mild mass effect on the adjacent frontal gyri (*arrow*). (**b**) Axial T1-weighted post-contrast MRI demonstrates a small homogeneously enhancing dural-based lesion along the left aspect of the posterior falx cerebri adjacent to the parieto-occipital sulcus with mild extension into the patent adjacent superior sagittal sinus (*arrow*)

larger than this are referred to as macroadenomas. Pituitary adenomas are also subdivided into functioning (secreting) and nonfunctioning (non-secreting) types.

- The pituitary gland and paired cavernous sinuses are located in the sellar and parasellar region of the middle cranial base. The boundaries of the sella turcica include the tuberculum sellae and anterior clinoid processes anteriorly and the dorsum sellae and posterior clinoid processes posteriorly. The sella is defined inferiorly by the portion of the sphenoid bone that also marks the superior margin of the sphenoid sinus. The superior border of the sella is covered by the diaphragma sellae. The lateral border is bounded by the cavernous sinuses which bridge the superior orbital fissure to the apex of the petrous bone (Swearingen and Biller 2008).

- The cavernous sinus contains a segment of the carotid artery and is the location where multiple veins from the cerebrum and cerebellum connect with draining venous sinuses. From superior to inferior, the oculomotor (CN III), trochlear (CN IV), and ophthalmic nerves (CN V1) are located in the lateral segment of the cavernous sinus; the abducens nerve (CN VI) is located in the medial segment (Swearingen and Biller 2008; Dolenc and Rogers 2009) (Fig. 2).

- To estimate the likelihood of cavernous sinus invasion by a pituitary adenoma, it is helpful to evaluate the extent of encasement of the carotid artery. In general, if there is a plane of normal-appearing pituitary tissue between the adenoma and the cavernous sinus, there is little to no risk of cavernous sinus invasion. On the other hand, complete encasement of the carotid artery is indicative of cavernous sinus invasion. In between, if there is less than 25 % encasement of the carotid artery, there is a small chance of cavernous sinus invasion, but if there is at least 67 % encasement of the carotid artery, the probability is quite high (Swearingen and Biller 2008) (Fig. 3).

## 1.3    Vestibular Schwannoma

- Vestibular schwannomas are divided into four stages based on location and size: intracanalicular, cisternal, brainstem compressive, and hydrocephalic.

**Fig. 2** Coronal section through the cavernous sinus depicting the location of the cranial nerves, carotid artery, and pituitary gland

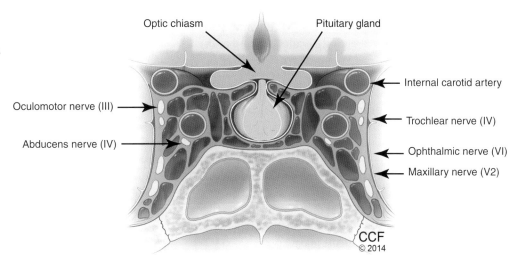

Optic chiasm

Pituitary gland

Internal carotid artery

Oculomotor nerve (III)

Trochlear nerve (IV)

Abducens nerve (IV)

Ophthalmic nerve (VI)

Maxillary nerve (V2)

CCF
© 2014

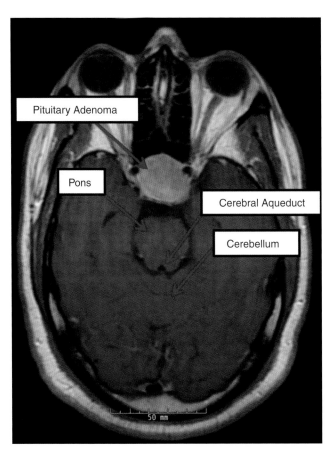

Pituitary Adenoma

Pons

Cerebral Aqueduct

Cerebellum

50 mm

**Fig. 3** Axial T1-weighted post-contrast MRI demonstrates a bulky intrasellar pituitary adenoma with suprasellar extension and extension into the bilateral cavernous sinuses, sphenoid sinus, clivus, and basisphenoid sinus. The bony sella is expanded, remodeled, extensively invaded, and demineralized. Retroclival extension is also present

- Vestibular schwannomas that are contained within the internal auditory meatus, known as intracanalicular schwannomas, are usually round or oval in shape. If the

tumor contains an extrameatal component, that portion is typically spherical and tapers towards the internal auditory meatus (Sriskandan and Connor 2011).

- The boundaries of the cerebellopontine angle (CPA) are the brainstem medially, the cerebellum superiorly and posteriorly, and the temporal bone laterally. The inferior extent of the CPA is bounded by the glossopharyngeal (CN IX), vagus (CN X), and spinal accessory nerves (CN XI) (Kutz et al. 2012).

- The vestibular nerve root arises from the vestibular apparatus, and the cochlear nerve root arises from the auditory apparatus to form the vestibulocochlear nerve which courses through the internal auditory meatus to the cerebellopontine angle (CPA) (Schünke et al. 2007).

- Vestibular schwannomas often arise from the superior or inferior branches of the vestibular nerve.

- Additional important structures traversing the CPA include the anterior inferior cerebellar artery and the facial nerve (CN VII).

## 1.4    Arteriovenous Malformations (AVMs)

- AVMs occur more commonly in the cerebral hemispheres (85 %) than in the posterior cranial fossa (15 %) (Kornienko and Pronin 2009).

- The arterial blood supply to an AVM may arise either directly from the feeding artery or indirectly from supplementary arteries transmitting blood from the supply region of a single artery. Additionally, the afferent arterial vessels can form various vascular channels, aneurysms, or pseudoaneurysms. In 27–32 % of AVMs, the arterial supply arises from a combination of intracranial arteries, dural arteries, and extracranial arteries (Kornienko and Pronin 2009).

- Venous drainage of an AVM may be directed through a single large or numerous small veins. The draining veins of an AVM are visualized during the arterial phase of the angiogram (Kornienko and Pronin 2009).

## 1.5    Trigeminal Nerve (CN V)

- The trigeminal nerve contains sensory afferent fibers and visceral efferent fibers. The somatic afferent fibers are responsible for sensation from the face, nasopharyngeal mucosa, and anterior two-thirds of the tongue (Schünke et al. 2007).
- The three major divisions of the trigeminal nerve are the ophthalmic division (V1) which travels through the superior orbital fissure to the orbit, the maxillary division (V2) which travels through the foramen rotundum to the pterygopalatine fossa, and the mandibular division (V3) which travels through the foramen ovale to the base of the skull (Schünke et al. 2007).
- The individual divisions of the trigeminal nerves converge at the anterior aspect of the trigeminal ganglion. The trigeminal ganglion is enveloped by dura mater and located in Meckel's cave, a depression in the petrous part of the temporal bone lateral to the cavernous sinus.

## 2    Diagnostic Workup Relevant for Target Volume Delineation

### 2.1    General Principles

- A thorough history should be obtained, and an appropriate physical examination with a specific emphasis on the neurologic exam should be performed.
- A patient's performance status should be evaluated using a validated scale such as the Karnofsky performance scale (KPS), ECOG performance status, neurologic function status (NFS), or mini mental status exam (MMSE).
- All patients should have an MRI of the brain performed for diagnostic and treatment planning purposes. MRI sequences should include precontrast T1-weighted, precontrast T2-weighted, and fluid-attenuated inversion recovery (FLAIR) images. Multiplanar (axial, sagittal, and coronal) post-contrast gadolinium-enhanced T1-weighted images should also be obtained. For enhancing tumors, high-resolution modes such as magnetization-prepared rapid gradient echo (MP-RAGE) are utilized for accurate delineation of the disease of interest. A constructive interference in steady state (CISS) or 3D fast imaging with steady state acquisition (3D FIESTA) may be useful for identifying the cranial nerves. Fat suppression MRI scans are also useful in determining target volumes for some tumors such as optic nerve sheath meningiomas.

## 2.2    Meningiomas

- On diagnostic CT scans, meningiomas appear as well-circumscribed, extra-axial masses that displace adjacent parenchymal tissue. They are isodense or hyperdense when compared to the normal brain tissue and demonstrate strong homogeneous contrast enhancement. Calcifications may be visualized in 20–30 % of meningiomas, and approximately half of cranial base meningiomas are associated with adjacent bone changes such as hyperostosis and osteolysis (Pieper et al. 1999).
- Typically, meningiomas are isointense or hypointense to gray matter on T1-weighted MR images and isointense, hypointense, or hyperintense on T2-weighted images. On the FLAIR sequence, meningiomas are typically hyperintense to gray matter (Tsuchiya et al. 1996).
- Approximately 90 % of meningiomas demonstrate strong homogenous enhancement with gadolinium; 10 % demonstrate mild enhancement (Pamir et al. 2010) (Fig. 4a, b).
- Approximately two-thirds of meningiomas exhibit a characteristic dural thickening, classically known as a "dural tail," which extends 0.5–3.0 cm from the meningioma mass. Imaging criteria for defining the dural tail include (Rokni-Yazdi and Sotoudeh 2006; Goldsher et al. 1990):
  – Presence on at least two consecutive slices in more than one imaging plane
  – Tapering of the tail from the meningioma mass
  – More enhancing than the meningioma mass
- Approximately 60 % of meningiomas are accompanied by peritumoral edema, seen most frequently with meningiomas of the olfactory groove, parasagittal region, and convexity (Pamir et al. 2010).

## 2.3    Pituitary Adenomas

- On diagnostic CT scans, pituitary microadenomas appear hypodense and exhibit less contrast enhancement than a normal pituitary gland (Swearingen and Biller 2008).
- Typically, pituitary microadenomas are hypointense to the normal pituitary gland on T1-weighted MR images, but can be isointense in 25 % of cases (Bonneville et al. 2005). The isointensity of pituitary adenomas on T2-weighted images can be quite variable; for example, approximately 80 % of prolactinomas and 67 % of GH-secreting microadenomas are isointense or hypointense (Swearingen and Biller 2008; Bonneville et al. 2005).
- Macroadenomas exhibit variable MRI features, but are typically hypointense on T1-weighted MR images and hyperintense to the normal pituitary gland on T2-weighted MR images (Swearingen and Biller 2008).

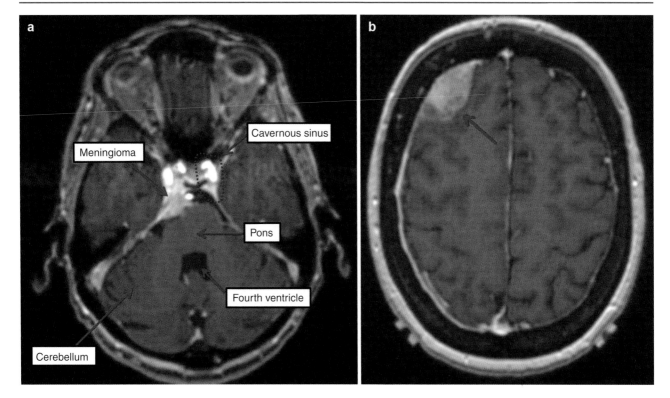

**Fig. 4** (**a**) Axial T1-weighted post-contrast MRI demonstrates a homogeneously enhancing meningioma centered along the anterior right tentorium with extension in the right cavernous sinus. There is also posterior extension along the right aspect of the clivus and mild mass effect on the adjacent undersurface of the right cerebral peduncle and the ventral aspect of the pons. There is partial encasement of a segment of the right posterior cerebellar artery. (**b**) Axial T1-weighted post-contrast MRI shows an enhancing extra-axial soft tissue mass overlying the lateral aspect of the right frontal pole with heterogeneous enhancement medially and moderate compression of the underlying parenchyma consistent with a convexity meningioma (*arrow*)

- Pituitary adenomas that are partially cystic may be hypointense on T1-weighted MR images. If there is a significant protein or lipid concentration in the pituitary cysts or if there is intralesional hemorrhage, there may be areas of hyperintensity observed on T1-weighted MR images.
- Pituitary adenomas demonstrate heterogeneous, partial, or incomplete enhancement with gadolinium (in contrast to the strong homogeneous enhancement visualized with sellar or parasellar meningiomas) (Taylor et al. 1992) (Fig. 5a, b).
- In pituitary adenomas with suprasellar extension, it is important to measure the extent of disease through the diaphragm sellae, including the closest distance between the tumor and the optic chiasm and optic nerves (Fig. 6a, b).
- A complete hormonal evaluation should be performed including measurement of the serum prolactin concentration, serum insulin-like growth factor (IGF)-1, serum growth hormone levels after a glucose load, 24-h urine cortisol, ACTH, LH, FSH, free T4, T3, and serum TSH.
- Visual field and visual acuity testing should be performed to determine any pattern of vision loss.

## 2.4    Vestibular Schwannoma

- On diagnostic CT scans, vestibular schwannomas appear as well-demarcated isodense masses that demonstrate enhancement with IV contrast. The absence of calcifications helps to differentiate these tumors from meningiomas radiographically.
- Typically, vestibular schwannomas are isointense or hypointense to the pons on T1-weighted MR images and heterogeneously hyperintense on T2-weighted images (Fig. 7).
- Vestibular schwannomas demonstrate strong homogeneous enhancement with gadolinium.
- For diagnostic evaluation of vestibular schwannomas, a thin-slice T1-weighted gadolinium-enhanced MRI of the cerebellopontine angle is helpful.
- A constructive interference in steady state (CISS) or 3D fast imaging with steady state acquisition (3D FIESTA) sequence can produce high-resolution images of the tumor and vestibulocochlear nerve by outlining the structures surrounded by CSF.

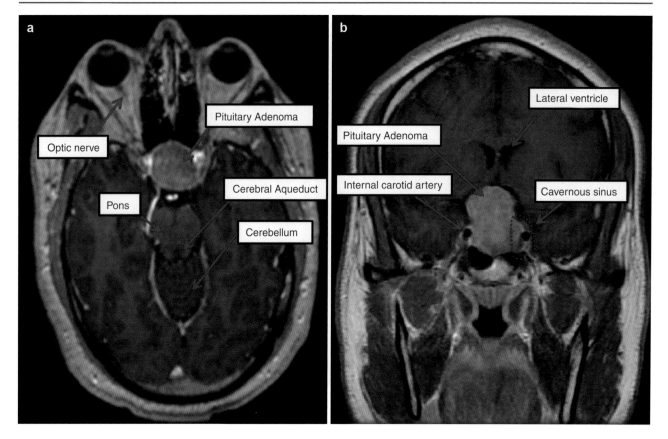

**Fig. 5** (**a**, **b**) Axial T1-weighted MRI demonstrates a well-circumscribed heterogeneous sellar/suprasellar mass with remodeling and expansion of the sella turcica. This mass also extends into the left cavernous sinus region, and the suprasellar portion of the mass abuts the medial aspect of the supraclinoid internal carotid arteries with uplifting of the optic chiasm and floor of the third ventricle

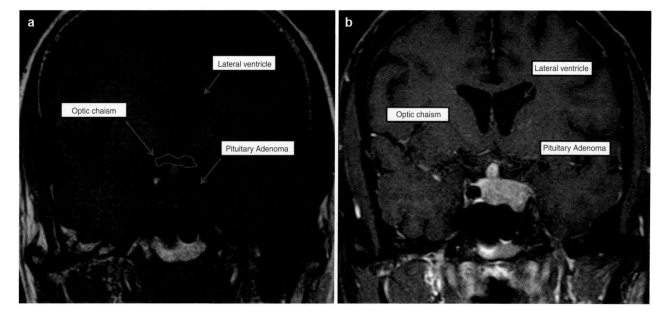

**Fig. 6** (**a**, **b**) Coronal T1-weighted non-contrast and post-contrast MRIs show the heterogeneously enhancing pituitary macroadenoma in the sella that is expanding the infundibulum. The mass extends into the cavernous sinus on the left with mild displacement and elevation of the optic chiasm. The optic chiasm is outlined in red

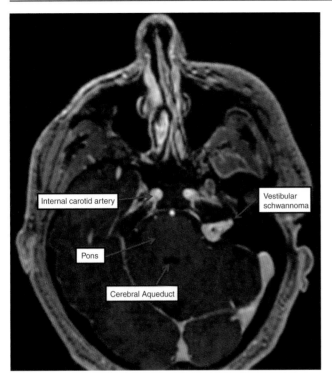

**Fig. 7** T1-weighted post-contrast MRI demonstrates an enhancing vestibular schwannoma with internal cystic changes in the left internal auditory canal extending into the cerebellopontine angle

- Ancillary testing performed at diagnosis includes pure tone and speech audiometry, brainstem-evoked response audiometry, and vestibular testing.

## 2.5 Arteriovenous Malformations (AVMs)

- On CT scans, AVMs appear as tortuous vessels that are isodense or hyperdense. Calcifications may be present in the vessels or the surrounding brain. AVMs demonstrate strong enhancement with IV contrast. Hemorrhages may be visualized around the nidus and the adjacent brain.
- On CTA, the feeding arteries and draining veins demonstrate enhancement.
- Typically, AVMs appear as hypointense flow voids on both T1-weighted and T2-weighted MR images.
- The nidus of the AVM demonstrates strong gadolinium enhancement, and the draining veins are also visualized on contrast-enhanced MR images (Fig. 8a, b).
- Invasive angiography is the best imaging modality to clearly delineate the feeding arteries, nidus, and venous drainage pattern.
- AVMs are graded from 1 to 5 by adding the points from the Spetzler-Martin classification system; see Table 1.

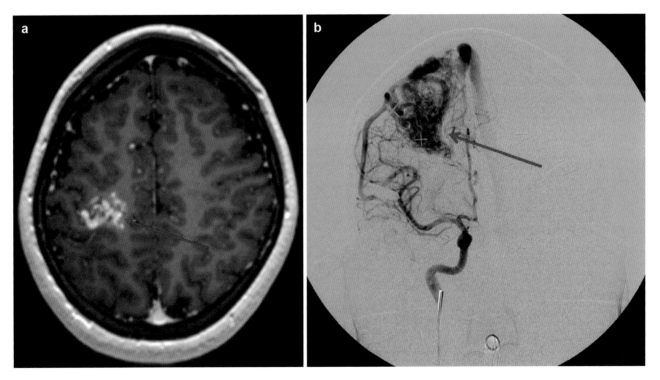

**Fig. 8** (a) Axial T1-weighted post-contrast MRI demonstrates a vascular malformation in the right frontoparietal lobe, right MCA territory, with draining veins without edema or hemorrhage (*arrow*). (b) Right frontoparietal AVM, elongated vertically, and located in the precentral-central region. Feeders originate from a large right MCA branch and a large right ACA branch (*arrow*)

**Table 1** Spetzler-Martin classification system (Olesen and Steiner 2004)

| | Points assigned |
|---|---|
| *Size* | |
| Small (0–3.0 cm) | 1 |
| Medium (3.1–6 cm) | 2 |
| Large (>6.0 cm) | 3 |
| *Location* | |
| Noneloquent brain area (frontal lobe, temporal lobe, or cerebellar hemisphere) | 0 |
| Eloquent brain area (sensorimotor, language, visual cortex, hypothalamus, thalamus, brainstem, cerebellar nuclei, or regions directly adjacent to these structures) | 1 |
| *Pattern of venous drainage* | |
| Superficial only | 0 |
| Deep | 1 |

**Table 2** Classic trigeminal neuralgia diagnostic criteria (Olesen and Steiner 2004)

| |
|---|
| Paroxysmal attacks of pain lasting from a fraction of a second to 2 min, affecting one or more divisions of the trigeminal nerve |
| Pain has at least one of the following characteristics: |
|    Intense, sharp, superficial, or stabbing |
| Precipitated from trigger areas or by trigger factors |
| Attacks are stereotyped in the individual patient |
| There is no clinically evident neurologic deficit |
| Not attributed to another disorder |

## 2.6 Trigeminal Neuralgia

- The International Headache Society provides diagnostic criteria for classic trigeminal neuralgia; see Table 2.
- On T1-weighted and T2-weighted MRI images, the trigeminal nerve can be visualized as it exits laterally from the pons and becomes the trigeminal ganglion.
- A CISS sequence or 3D FIESTA can produce high-resolution images of the trigeminal nerve by outlining the structures surrounded by the CSF.
- Ancillary trigeminal nerve testing includes a blink reflex and masseter inhibitory reflex.

## 3 Simulation and Daily Localization

- For simulation, the patient should be set up in the supine position, arms at the sides, with the head and neck in a neutral position parallel to the treatment table.
- A noninvasive stereotactic immobilization system should be used during simulation and treatment. Commonly utilized examples include a 3-point thermoplastic fixation mask and a modified stereotactic frame.
- A spiral CT simulation using 2.0–3.0 mm slice thickness with IV contrast should be performed from the vertex of the head to the mid-cervical spine to delineate the target volume. The isocenter should be placed in the center of the visualized tumor volume at least 1.5 cm deep to the surface.

- Image co-registration and fusion of the planning CT scans with diagnostic MRI scans helps to accurately delineate the extent of the tumor volume and is useful in identifying critical structures, including the brainstem and the optic chiasm. The target structures and organs at risk should be contoured on the corresponding simulation CT scans.
- For benign CNS tumors, the GTV should be delineated by the outer edge of gadolinium enhancement as seen on the T1-weighted post-contrast sequences. The GTV and normal structures should be outlined on all CT slices in which the structures exist.
- General planning strategies include 3D-CRT, IMRT, and VMAT depending on the orientation, location, and size of the tumor. The typical energy used is 6 MV photons or higher.
- IGRT examples commonly integrated into treatment units and utilized when treating CNS tumors include orthogonal KV X-rays and volume-based cone-beam CTs.

## 4 Target Volume Delineation and Treatment Planning

- Suggested target volumes and selected dose fractionation schemes for meningiomas, pituitary adenomas, and vestibular schwannomas are detailed in Tables 3, 4, and 5, respectively (Figs. 9, 10, 11, 12, 13, 14, 15, 16, 17, and 18).

**Table 3** Suggested target volumes for a benign meningioma

| Target volumes | Definition and description |
|---|---|
| $GTV_{54}^{a}$ (The subscript 54 denotes the radiation dose delivered) | The tumor bed as defined as the enhancing mass on the post-contrast T1-weighted MRI. For postsurgical cases, the GTV should be defined by the tumor bed and any residual nodular enhancement |
| | [a]Do not enlarge the contoured volume to cover the surrounding cerebral edema, if any |
| | The "dural tail" is defined as the linearly enhancing dura immediately adjacent to the primary meningioma mass (see above). This is thought to represent hypervascular dura; however, microscopic meningioma cells have been found in this region. If there is nodularity in the enhancing dura, it should be included in the GTV. If there is no nodularity, the proximal millimeters of dura can be included in the GTV electively; however, more extensive coverage of the distal portion is not recommended. In most planning cases, the adjacent portion of the dural tail is usually covered in the PTV expansion |
| $CTV_{54}$ | For benign meningiomas, the CTV=GTV, although a small margin of 0.5–1 cm may be added, especially if the dural tail is not covered or if there is uncertainty based on the MRI |
| $PTV_{54}$ | $CTV_{54}+3.0$–5.0 mm, depending on setup error and the reproducibility of patient positioning |
| SRS dosing | 12–15 Gy in a single fraction prescribed to the 50 % isodose line to the GTV |

- The recommended PTV margin expanded from CTV is 3.0–5.0 mm, depending on the accuracy of the daily patient positioning. A PTV expansion of 3.0 mm can be used if daily IGRT is utilized. If the tumor PTV margins overlap with a defined organ at risk (OAR), do not modify the PTV to exclude these structures. Instead, define a planning risk volume (PRV) for each OAR using a 3.0 mm margin on the contoured structure of interest. The dose to the OAR PRV should be as close to the recommend prescription dose while not exceeding the acceptable dose tolerance of the OAR (Table 6).

## 4.1    Trigeminal Neuralgia

- The target volume is the entry of the trigeminal nerve root at the level of the pons or the trigeminal ganglion.
- A single 4 mm collimator is used and is placed in the center of the trigeminal nerve (Kondziolka 2006).
- The recommended dose is 80–90 Gy to the 100 % isodose line. The exact prescription dose varies with the dose to the brainstem and the age of the patient (Lunsford and Sheehan 2009) (Fig. 19).

## 4.2    AVMs

- The target volume is the nidus of the AVM as demonstrated on angiography with image co-registration to an MRI and CT.
- Single or multiple isocenter dose plans may be used to create a radiosurgical volume that conforms to the area of mixed signal intensity (Niranjan et al. 2012).
- The recommended dose is 16–27 Gy to the peripheral margin (50 % or greater isodose line). The exact prescription dose may vary with the size of the AVM and its location (Niranjan et al. 2012).
- For AVMs that are large in size (>15 cc), a staged radiosurgery approach is recommended with two treatments performed approximately 6 months apart (Figs. 20 and 21a, b).

**Table 4** Suggested target volumes for a pituitary adenoma

| Target volumes | Definition and description |
| --- | --- |
| GTV$_{45-54}$[a] | The tumor bed as defined as the enhancing mass on the post-contrast T1-weighted MRI |
| | Nonfunctional tumors: 45 Gy in 25 fractions |
| | Functional tumors: 50.4–54 Gy in 28–30 fractions |
| CTV$_{45-54}$ | For pituitary adenomas, the CTV = GTV |
| PTV$_{45-54}$ | GTV$_{45-54}$ + 3.0–5.0 mm, depending on setup error and the reproducibility of patient positioning |
| SRS dosing[a] | Nonfunctional tumors: 14–16 Gy in a single fraction prescribed to at least the 50 % isodose line |
| | Functional tumors: 16–25 Gy in a single fraction prescribed to at least the 50 % isodose line. Higher doses are preferred |
| | [a]Fractionated radiation therapy is recommended for tumors in close proximity to the optic chiasm (3 mm) or with marked extension into the cavernous sinus (Fig. 12) |
| | Consideration is given to a temporary discontinuation of medical therapy for patients with functional pituitary adenomas to increase the radiation therapy response (Pollock et al. 2007) |

**Table 5** Suggested target volumes for a vestibular schwannoma

| Target volumes | Definition and description |
| --- | --- |
| GTV$_{45-54}$ | The tumor bed as defined as the enhancing mass on post-contrast T1-weighted MRI |
| CTV$_{45-54}$ | For vestibular schwannomas, the CTV = GTV |
| PTV$_{45-54}$ | GTV$_{45-54}$ + 3.0–5.0 mm, depending on setup error and the reproducibility of patient positioning |
| SRS dosing | 12–13 Gy in a single fraction prescribed to at least the 50 % isodose line |

## 5    Plan Assessment

There are many critical structures that need to be outlined for dose constraint analysis in CNS cases including the lens, globes, optic nerves, optic chiasm, pituitary, hypothalamus, cochlea, brainstem, and spinal cord.

**Table 6** Intensity-modulated radiation therapy and radiosurgery normal tissue dose constraints

| Critical structures | Recommend constraints[a,b] | Maximum allowed constraint[a,b] |
| --- | --- | --- |
| Lens | Max < 5 Gy | Max < 7 Gy |
| Retinae | Max < 45 Gy | Max < 50 Gy |
| Optic nerves | Max < 50 Gy | Max < 55 Gy |
| Optic chiasm | Max < 54 Gy | Max < 56 Gy |
| | For SRS dosing: 8 Gy (Leber et al. 1998) | For SRS dosing: 10 Gy (Leber et al. 1998) |
| Spinal cord | Max < 45 Gy | Max < 56 Gy |
| Brainstem | Max < 55 Gy | Max < 60 Gy |
| | For SRS dosing: < 12.5 Gy | |
| Cochlea mean cochlea < 35 Gy | | Mean cochlea < 45 Gy |
| For SRS dosing < 4 Gy (Kano et al. 2009) | | For SRS dosing: 12–14 Gy |

[a]Maximum point dose defined as a volume greater than 0.03 cc
[b]Constraints partially based on RTOG 0539

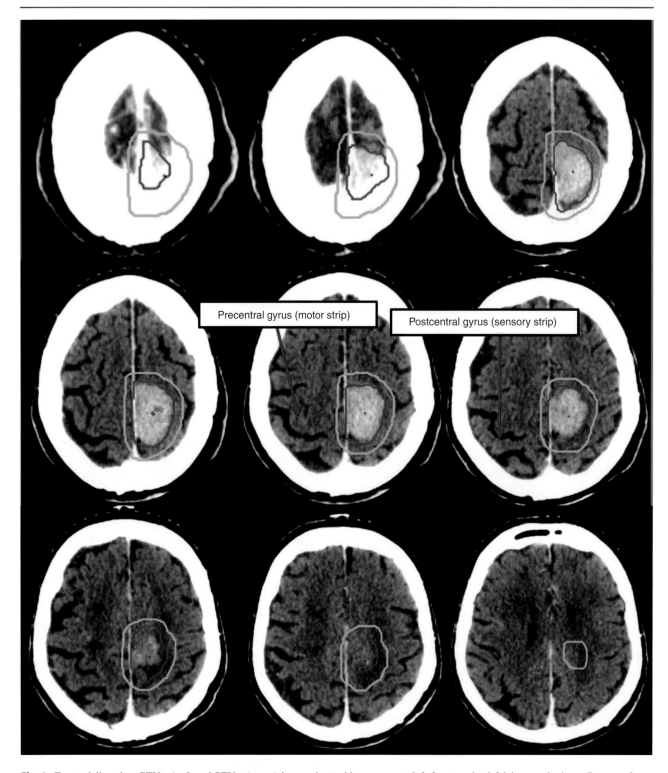

**Fig. 9** Target delineation $GTV_{54}$ (*red*) and $PTV_{54}$ (*green*) in a patient with a recurrent left frontoparietal falcine meningioma 7 years after a Simpson grade 2 resection. Please note that these are representative slices and not all slices are included

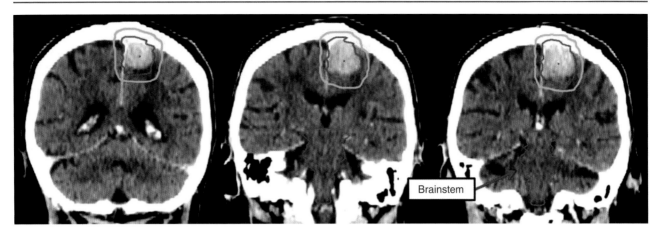

**Fig. 10** Representative coronal sections of the GTV$_{54}$ (*red*) and PTV$_{54}$ (*green*) in a patient with a recurrent left frontoparietal falcine meningioma 7 years after a Simpson grade 2 resection. Please note that these are representative slices and not all slices are included

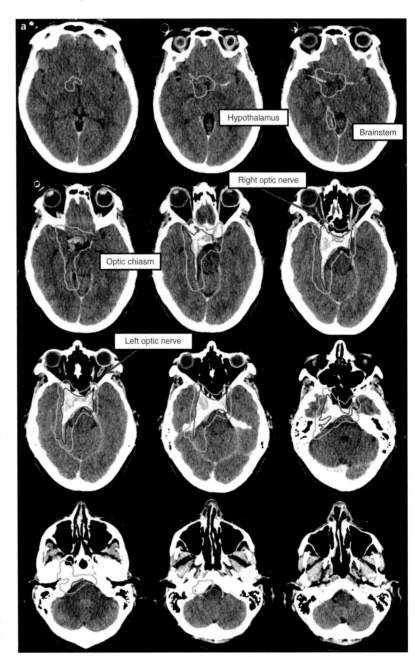

**Fig. 11** (**a**) Target delineation GTV (*red*) and CTV (*green*) in a patient with a right cavernous sinus meningioma encompassing the internal carotid artery. Please note that these are representative slices and not all slices are included. Note the dural tail is included in this case as the GTV. Areas determined to be thicker than the representative contralateral dura were felt to represent the dural tail. (**b**) Target delineation in a patient with a right cavernous sinus meningioma encompassing the internal carotid artery. To determine the extent of the dural tail as contoured above, use the T1-weighted post-contrast MRI to outline the area of enhancement and exclude the bone on the corresponding CT axial slices. Areas determined to be thicker than the representative contralateral dura were felt to represent the dural tail

**Fig. 11** (continued)

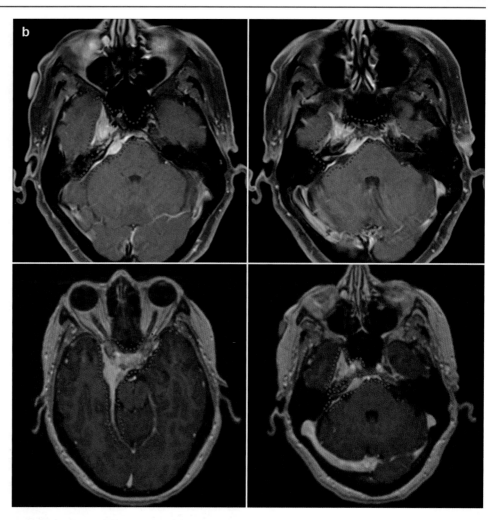

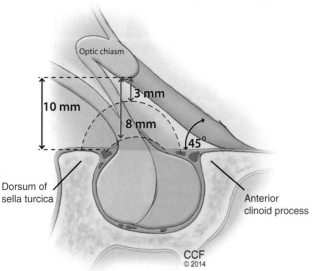

**Fig. 12** Illustration of the anatomic relationship between the pituitary gland and the optic chiasm. When considering different radiation therapy techniques for treatment of pituitary adenomas, it is important to measure the distance between the superior edge of the tumor and the optic chiasm. For example, a tumor 8 mm from the optic chiasm (*green shade*) is amenable to treatment with stereotactic radiosurgery or fractionated radiation therapy. On the other hand, for tumors extending within 3 mm of the optic chiasm (*yellow shade*), fractionated radiation therapy is recommended

## 5.1 Meningiomas

Ideally, at least 95 % of the volume of $PTV_{54}$ should receive 54 Gy. In addition, the minimum dose within $PTV_{54}$ should be 51 Gy. The maximum dose received by 0.03 cc of the $PTV_{54}$ should be less than or equal to 62 Gy. At least 98 % of the volume of the GTV should receive the prescription dose.

## 5.2 Pituitary Adenomas

Ideally, at least 95 % of the volume of $PTV_{54}$ should receive the prescription dose (based on functional/nonfunctional subtype). At least 98 % of the volume of the GTV should receive the prescription dose.

## 5.3 Vestibular Schwannomas

Ideally, at least 95 % of the volume of $PTV_{54}$ should receive the prescription dose (45–54) Gy. At least 98 % of the volume of the GTV should receive the prescription dose.

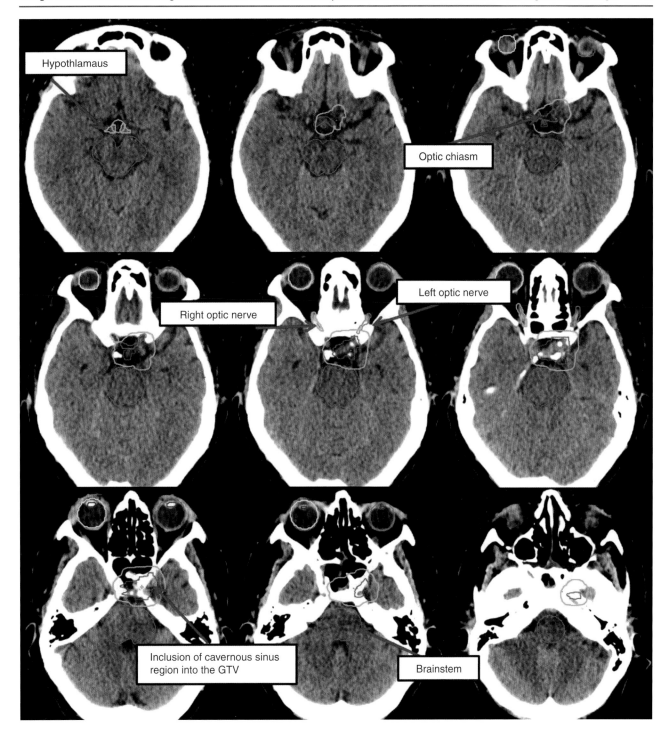

**Fig. 13** Target delineation GTV (*red*) and PTV (*green*) in a patient with residual pituitary adenoma in the left sella extending into the left cavernous sinus and adjacent clivus after a transnasal transsphenoidal resection and sellar reconstruction. Please note that these are representative slices and not all slices are included

For radiosurgery cases, three planning calculations to perform are (Balagamwala et al. 2012):

- Conformality Index: Prescription isodose volume/tumor volume ≤2
- Heterogeneity Index: Maximum dose to the tumor volume/ prescribed dose ≤2
- Gradient Index: Ratio of the volume receiving half the prescription isodose to the volume receiving the full prescription isodose ≥3

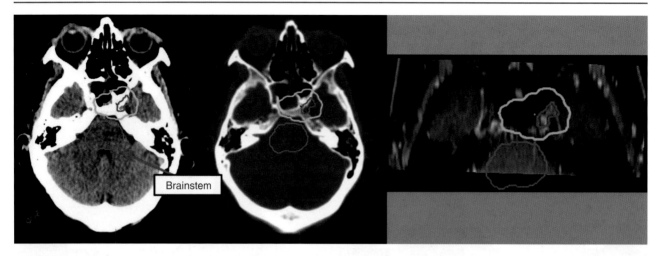

**Fig. 14** Soft tissue and bone window views of the GTV (*red*) and PTV (*green*) in a patient with residual pituitary adenoma in the left sella extending into the left cavernous sinus and adjacent clivus after a transnasal transsphenoidal resection and sellar reconstruction. MRI can be used for delineation of the tumor volume, and reconstructed bone windows can be useful for determining the extent of coverage of the adjacent bony structures

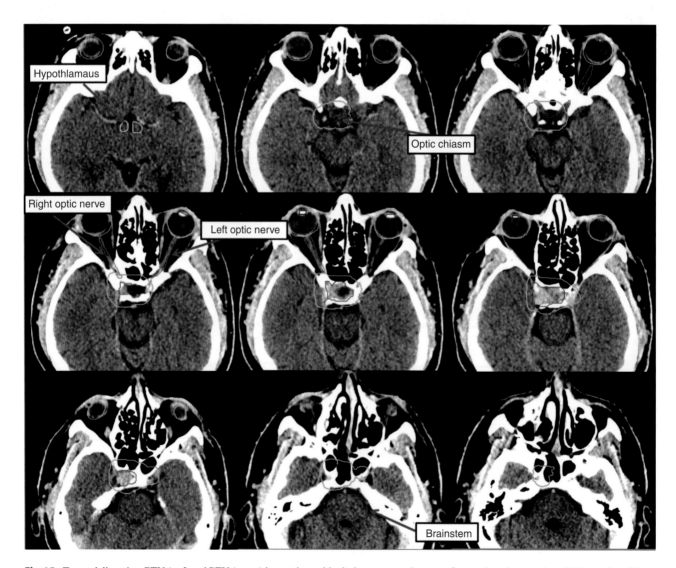

**Fig. 15** Target delineation GTV (*red*) and PTV (*green*) in a patient with pituitary macroadenoma after a subtotal transsphenoidal resection. Please note that these are representative slices and not all slices are included

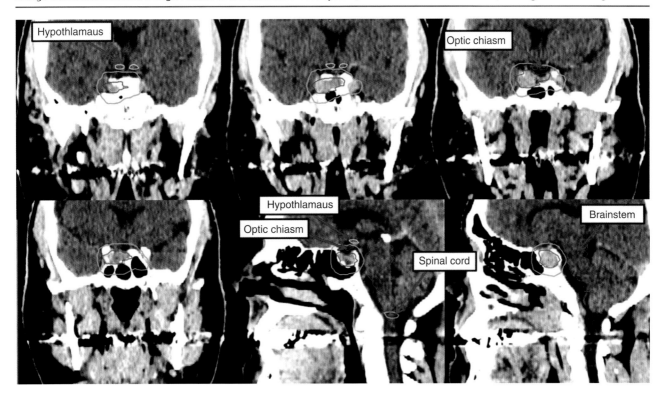

**Fig. 16**  Coronal and sagittal views of the GTV (*red*) and PTV (*green*) in a patient with pituitary macroadenoma after a subtotal transsphenoidal resection. Please note that these are representative slices and not all slices are included

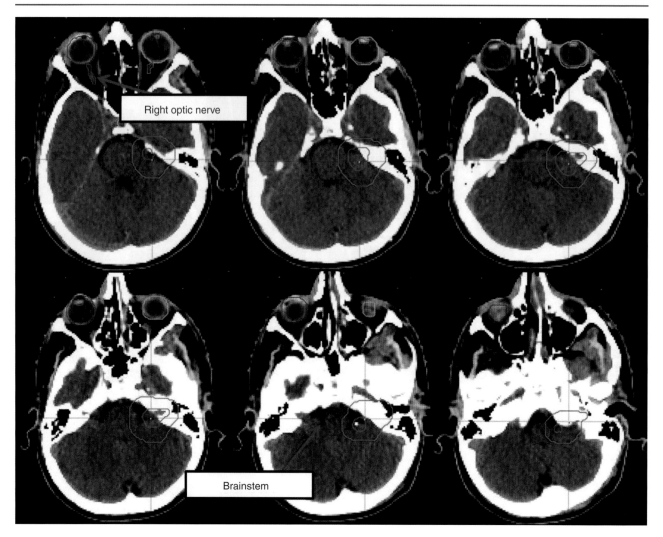

**Fig. 17** Target delineation GTV (*green*) and PTV (*light purple*) in a patient with a left-sided vestibular schwannoma. Please note that these are representative slices and not all slices are included

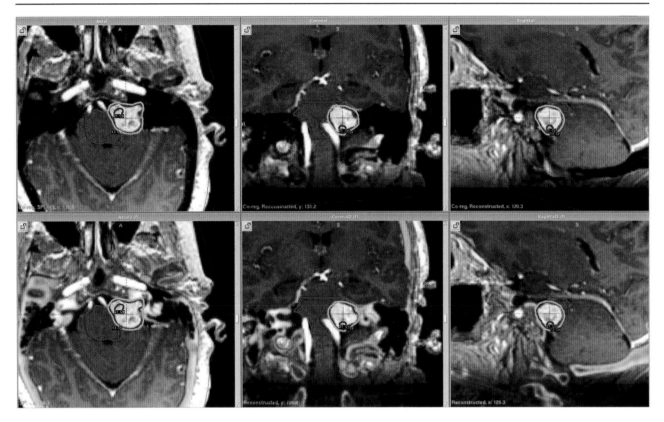

**Fig. 18** Gamma Knife radiosurgery treatment plan for a patient with a left-sided vestibular schwannoma. Note that the tumor causes moderate effacement of the left brachium pontis, but the cerebral aqueduct is pat- ent. The brainstem is *outlined in pink*; the tumor volume is *outlined in red*. The *green outline* represents the 13 Gy isodose line, and the *blue outline* represents the 21 Gy isodose line

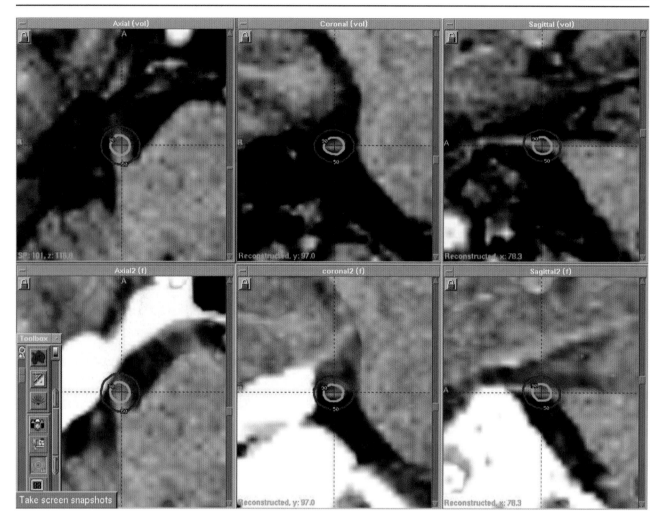

**Fig. 19** Gamma Knife radiosurgery treatment for trigeminal neuralgia refractory to medication. The root entry zone of the right trigeminal nerve is receiving a dose of 8,000 cGy prescribed to the 100 % isodose line using a 4 mm collimator. The *green outline* represents the 90 % isodose line, and the *red outline* represents the 50 % isodose line

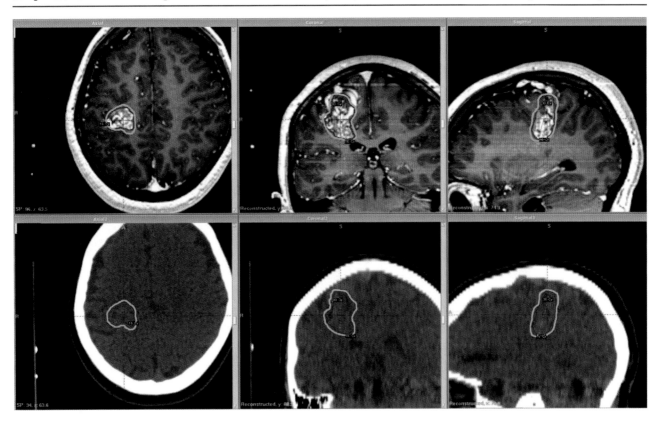

**Fig. 20**  Gamma Knife radiosurgery treatment for a right motor strip AVM. The *red outline* defines the target volume. The *green outline* represents the 16 Gy isodose line, and the *blue outline* represents the 30 Gy isodose line

**Fig. 21** (**a**, **b**). Staged Gamma Knife radiosurgery treatment for a 25×35×55 mm right mesial temporal Spetzler-Martin grade III AVM. (**a**) The part of the AVM *outlined in blue* represents the target volume as part of staged procedure. The *red outline* represents the 11 Gy isodose line, and the *green outline* represents the 19 Gy isodose line. (**b**) The part of the AVM *outlined in light blue* represents the previously treated region. The *dark blue outline* represents the target treatment region

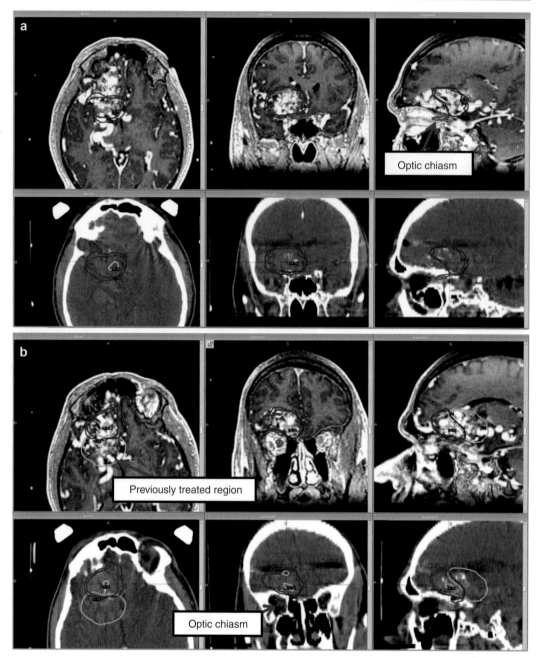

## Suggested Reading

Gaffney DK (2013) Radiation oncology: imaging and treatment. Amirsys, Altona

RTOG 0539 protocol. Phase II trial of observation for low-risk meningiomas and of radiotherapy for intermediate- and high-risk meningiomas. Online: http://www.rtog.org/ClinicalTrials/ProtocolTable/StudyDetails.aspx?study=0539

## References

Balagamwala EH, Suh JH, Barnett GH et al (2012) The importance of the conformality, heterogeneity, and gradient indices in evaluating gamma knife radiosurgery treatment plans for intracranial meningiomas. Int J Radiat Oncol Biol Phys 83(5):1406–1413

Bonneville J-F, Bonneville F, Cattin F (2005) Magnetic resonance imaging of pituitary adenomas. Eur Radiol 15(3):543–548

Dolenc VV, Rogers LA (2009) Cavernous sinus: developments and future perspectives. Springer, Wien/New York

Goldsher D, Litt A, Pinto R, Bannon K, Kricheff I (1990) Dural "tail" associated with meningiomas on Gd-DTPA-enhanced MR images: characteristics, differential diagnostic value, and possible implications for treatment. Radiology 176(2):447–450

Kano H, Kondziolka D, Khan A, Flickinger JC, Lunsford LD (2009) Predictors of hearing preservation after stereotactic radiosurgery for acoustic neuroma: clinical article. J Neurosurg 111(4):863–873

Kondziolka D (2006) Radiosurgery: 7th International Stereotactic Radiosurgery Society Meeting, Brussels, September 2005. Basel, Switzerland

Kornienko V, Pronin I (2009) Diagnostic neuroradiology. Springer, Berlin

Kutz JWJ, Roland PS, Isaacson B (2012) Acoustic neuroma. Accessed 12 March 2013

Leber KA, Berglöff J, Pendl G (1998) Dose–response tolerance of the visual pathways and cranial nerves of the cavernous sinus to stereotactic radiosurgery. J Neurosurg 88(1):43–50

Lee JH (2008) Meningiomas: diagnosis, treatment, and outcome. Springer, London

Lunsford LD, Sheehan JP (2009) Intracranial stereotactic radiosurgery. Thieme, New York

Niranjan A, Kano H, Lunsford LD (2012) Gamma knife radiosurgery for brain vascular malformations. Basel, Switzerland

Olesen J, Steiner T (2004) The International classification of headache disorders, 2nd edn (ICDH-II). J Neurol Neurosurg Psychiatry 75(6):808–811

Pamir MN, Black PM, Fahlbusch R (2010) Saunders Elsevier Philadelphia, Pennsylvania

Pieper DR, Al-Mefty O, Hanada Y, Buechner D (1999) Hyperostosis associated with meningioma of the cranial base: secondary changes or tumor invasion. Neurosurgery 44(4):742–746

Pollock BE, Jacob JT, Brown PD, Nippoldt TB (2007) Radiosurgery of growth hormone-producing pituitary adenomas: factors associated with biochemical remission. J Neurosurg 106(5):833–838

Rohringer M, Sutherland GR, Louw DF, Sima AA (1989) Incidence and clinicopathological features of meningioma. J Neurosurg 71(5):665–672

Rokni-Yazdi H, Sotoudeh H (2006) Prevalence of "dural tail sign" in patients with different intracranial pathologies. Eur J Radiol 60(1):42–45

Schünke M, Schulte E, Schumacher U, Rude J (2007) Thieme atlas of anatomy: head and neuroanatomy, vol 3. Thieme, Stuttgart/New York

Sriskandan N, Connor S (2011) The role of radiology in the diagnosis and management of vestibular schwannoma. Clin Radiol 66(4):357–365

Swearingen B, Biller BM (2008) Diagnosis and management of pituitary disorders. Springer; Totowa, NJ

Taylor SL, Barakos JA, Harsh GR IV, Wilson CB (1992) Magnetic resonance imaging of tuberculum sellae meningiomas: preventing preoperative misdiagnosis as pituitary macroadenoma. Neurosurgery 31(4):621–627

Tsuchiya K, Mizutani Y, Hachiya J (1996) Preliminary evaluation of fluid-attenuated inversion-recovery MR in the diagnosis of intracranial tumors. AJNR Am J Neuroradiol 17(6):1081–1086

# Glioma

Kruti Patel and Minesh P. Mehta

## Contents

K. Patel, MD
Department of Radiation Oncology,
University of Maryland Medical Center,
Baltimore, MD, USA
e-mail: kpatel3@umm.edu

M.P. Mehta, MD (✉)
Department of Radiation Oncology,
University of Maryland School of Medicine,
Baltimore, MD, USA
e-mail: mmehta@umm.edu

## 1   Anatomy and Patterns of Spread

- Gliomas can arise in any part of the brain. The origins of these tumors are unknown, but at least one hypothesis supports a localized stem cell compartmental derivation with the spread of clonogenic tumor cells along cortical pathways and localization to regions of high growth factor activity. Brainstem gliomas account for 15 % of pediatric cases but are uncommon in adults (Gondi et al. 2013).
- High-grade glial (HGG) neoplasms can grow rapidly within the parenchyma, but extracranial metastasis through hematogenous or lymphatic spread is exquisitely rare. In contrast, lower-grade tumors can remain indolent for years. The incidence of leptomeningeal spread is quite low in either case (Gondi et al. 2013).
- These tumors are generally highly infiltrative through adjacent brain matter, although exceptions (such as pilocytic astrocytoma and pleomorphic xanthoastrocytoma) do exist. The infiltrative capacity allows for spread to more "distant" brain regions: for example, a mass in close proximity to the corpus callosum can cross midline through direct invasion (as seen in Fig. 1), and separate compartments of enhancement create the somewhat inaccurate concept of "multifocality."
- Low-grade gliomas (LGGs) demonstrate a propensity for progression to a higher grade over time, possibly through accumulation of additional genetic events. Malignant transformation can occur in as many as 80 % of low-grade diffuse astrocytomas (Gondi et al. 2013).
- An adequate understanding of intracranial anatomy is essential when approaching these tumors. Accurate assessment of location of gliomas and proximity to critical structures is crucial in determining the appropriate degree of surgical intervention. These factors must also be taken into account when designing a target for radiation therapy.

N.Y. Lee et al. (eds.), *Target Volume Delineation for Conformal and Intensity-Modulated Radiation Therapy*,
Medical Radiology. Radiation Oncology, DOI: 10.1007/174_2014_989, © Springer International Publishing Switzerland 2014
Published Online: 22 October 2014

- Pertinent anatomic structures to delineate in a patient with a glioma include (Fig. 2):
- Lenses
- Eyes (retina)
- Lacrimal glands
- Optic nerves
- Optic chiasm
- Hippocampus (not routinely done)
- Pituitary gland
- Cochleae

- Brainstem and upper cervical spinal cord (as appropriate)
- Specific cranial nerves (in select circumstances)

## 2 Diagnostic Workup Relevant for Target Volume Delineation

- Prior to surgery, it can be helpful to obtain functional MR imaging to determine potential injury that could result from aggressive tumor resection, based on location.

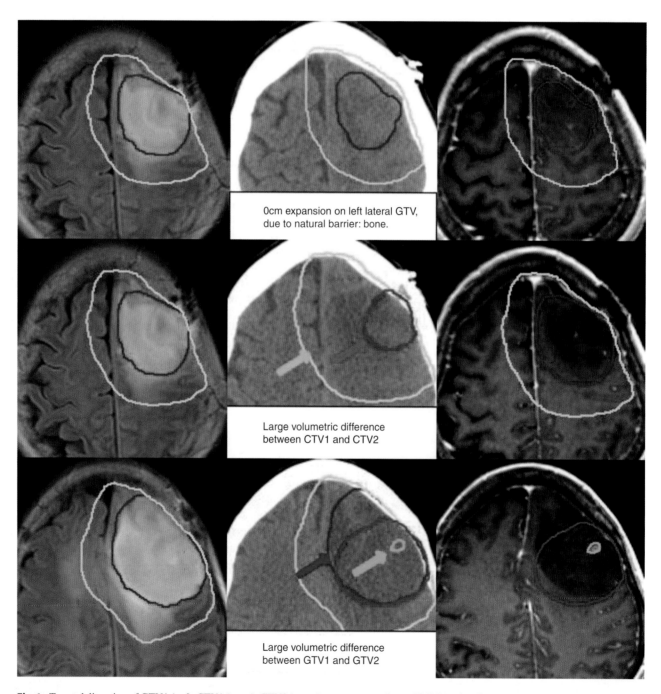

**Fig. 1** Target delineation of GTV1 (*red*), CTV1 (*aqua*), GTV2 (*green*), and CTV2 (*purple*) in a patient with a left frontotemporal GBM (post-biopsy only) on axial MRI FLAIR sequence (*left*), CT (*middle*), and T1 contrast-enhanced MRI (*right*) slices. In this case, there was significant edema, resulting in a dramatic difference in volumes between GTV1 and GTV2, as well as CTV1 and CTV2

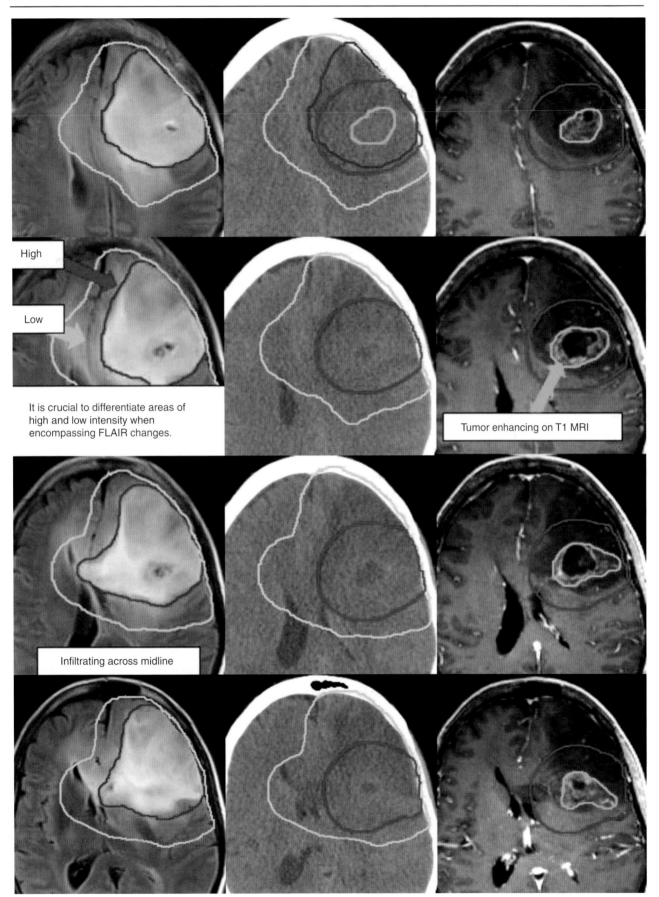

High

Low

It is crucial to differentiate areas of
high and low intensity when
encompassing FLAIR changes.

Tumor enhancing on T1 MRI

Infiltrating across midline

**Fig. 1** (continued)

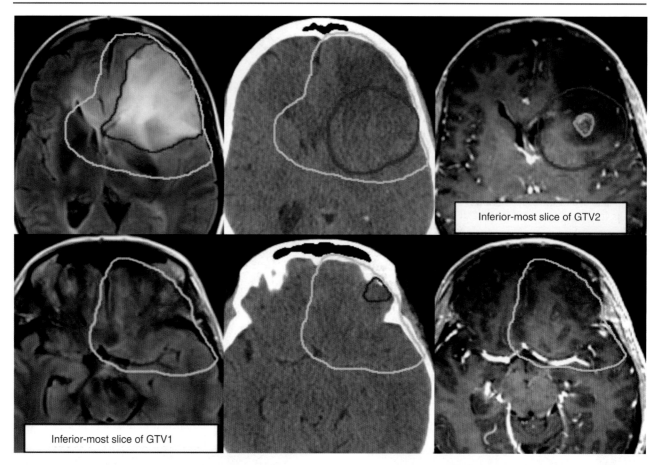

**Fig. 1** (continued)

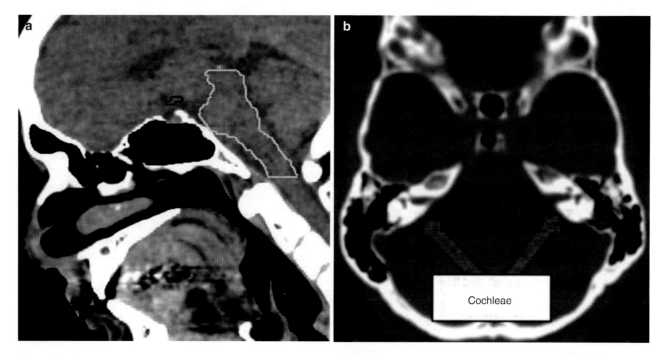

**Fig. 2** (**a**) Sagittal CT showing the chiasm (*purple*) and brainstem (*light orange*) contours. (**b**) CT scan on bone windows facilitates identification of the cochleae. (**c**) Bilateral lenses (*yellow* & *pink*), eyes (*teal* & *lavender*), lacrimal glands (*orange* & *green*), and brainstem (*light orange*) outlined on axial CT. (**d**) Axial CT of pituitary gland (*green*). (**e**) Sagittal CT of the pituitary gland (*green*). (**f**) Axial CT of hippocampus (*orange*). (**g**) Sagittal of hippocampus (*orange*). Hippocampi are best contoured on MRI and transposed to the CT images

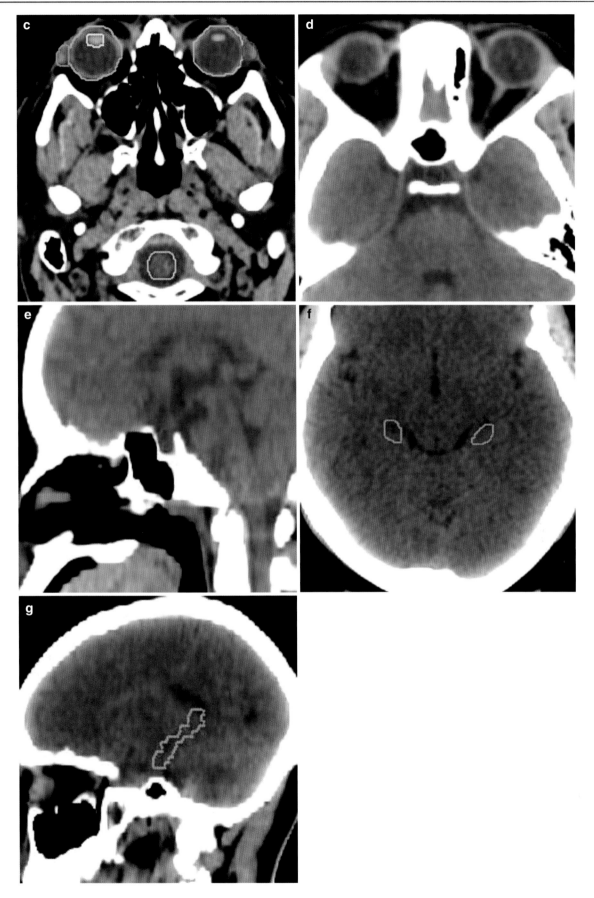

**Fig. 2** (continued)

Intraoperative monitoring is often employed to further decrease the risk of adversely affecting function.

- Following surgical intervention, immediate (within 48 h) postoperative MR imaging with contrast is strongly recommended. Thin slices (e.g., 1–2 mm) are preferred for enhanced image resolution and more accurate fusion with the planning CT images, which should ideally match the slice thickness of the MR images.
- Radiographic imaging is helpful in treatment planning but almost universally underestimates the true extent of disease.
  – In 35 glioblastoma multiforme (GBM) patients, 78 % of recurrences were found to be within 2 cm of the tumor as visualized on CT at autopsy in a study by Hochberg and Pruitt (1980). This pattern was validated by Wallner et al. (1989). These data are the basis for the definition of the boost gross tumor volume (GTV), treated to higher doses (e.g., 60 Gy).
  – In a study by Kelly et al. (1987), isolated tumor cells were noted to extend to cover T2 changes and beyond

on MR imaging. This was confirmed with serial stereotactic biopsies. These data are the foundation for the definition of the initial GTV, treated to lower doses (e.g., 46 Gy).

- For patients with extensive edema and only a small volume of enhancing tumor, a diagnostic MR image at mid-treatment is recommended. In such cases, emergence of further areas of enhancement can be seen, requiring expansion of the boost (GTV2) volume to cover these areas. Figures 3, 4, and 5 include images that show multifocal edema and a small unifocal enhancing tumor. It is possible that enhancing disease may develop in other areas of edema over a span of weeks.
- MR fluid-attenuated inversion recovery (FLAIR), T1, and T2 (if significantly different from FLAIR) sequences should be fused with the simulation CT scan for contouring guidance.
- In situations in which cranial nerve abutment is a concern, a 3D fast imaging employing steady-state acquisition

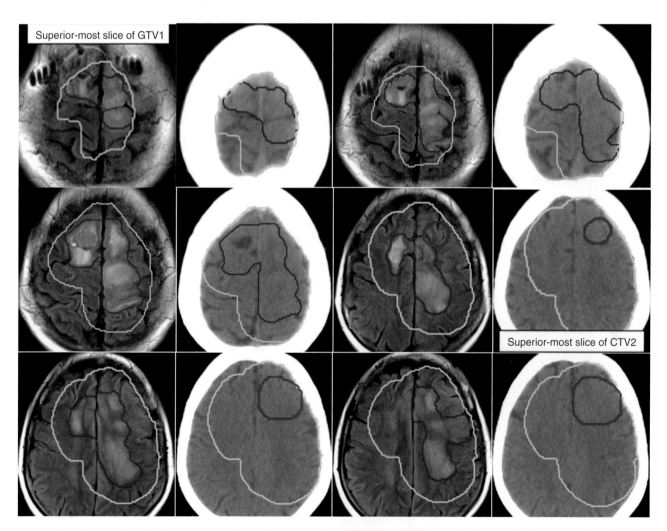

**Fig. 3** (**a**) Axial FLAIR and CT images of a patient with multifocal GBM demonstrating superior sections of GTV1 (*red*), CTV1 (*aqua*) and CTV2 (*purple*). A 1.5 cm expansion, rather than 2 cm, was used to create both CTVs given the expansive FLAIR changes and concern for volume of normal brain being irradiated. (**b**) Axial FLAIR, CT and TI contrast-enhanced images of the same patient with a multifocal GBM. Contoured structures include GTV1 (*red*), CTV1 (*aqua*), GTV2 (*green*) and CTV2 (purple)

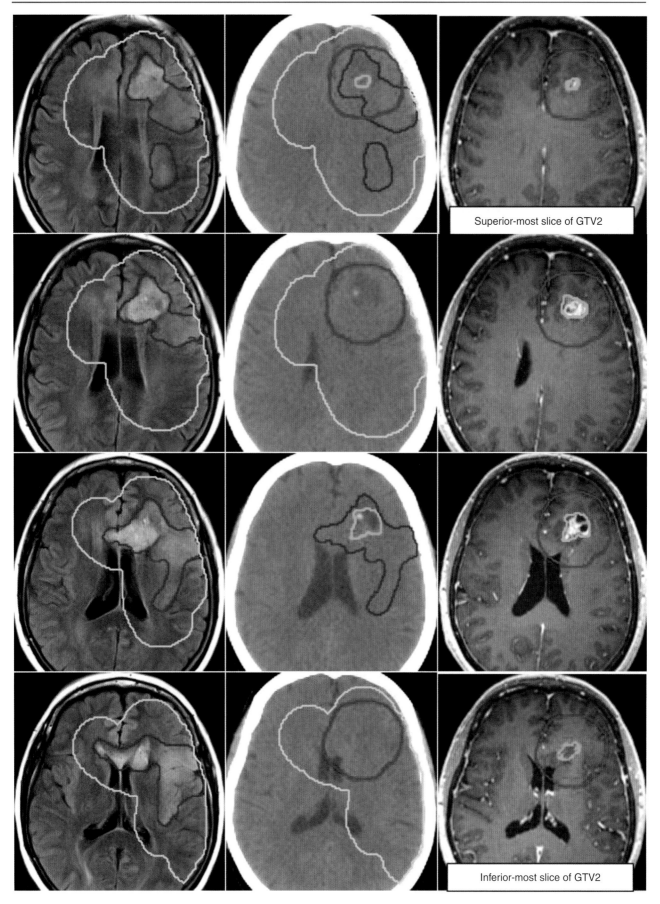

Superior-most slice of GTV2

Inferior-most slice of GTV2

**Fig. 3** (continued)

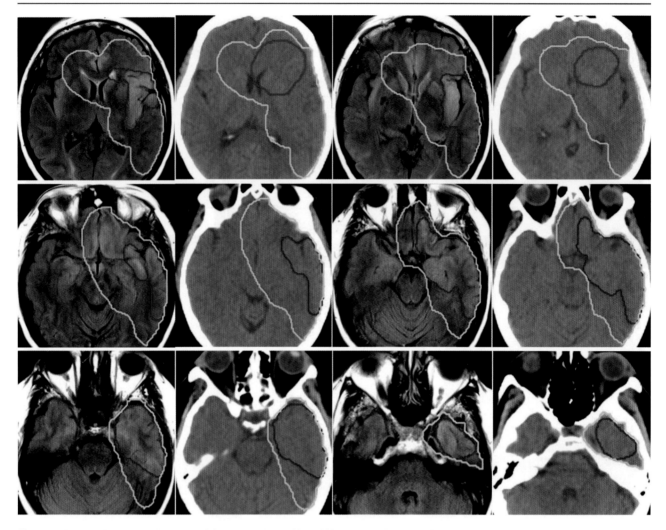

**Fig. 4** Axial MRI FLAIR and CT views of the same patient with multifocal GBM demonstrating inferior portion of GTV1 (*red*), CTV1 (*aqua*), and CTV2 (*purple*)

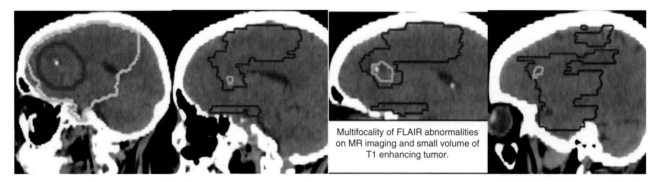

Multifocality of FLAIR abnormalities on MR imaging and small volume of T1 enhancing tumor.

**Fig. 5** Sagittal CT views of the same patient with multifocal GBM demonstrating GTV1 (*red*), CTV1 (*aqua*), GTV2 (*green*), and CTV2 (*purple*)

(FIESTA) MR series can be helpful in visualizing and sparing the nerves. A 3D spoiled gradient recalled (SPGR) MR image can facilitate contouring of the hippocampus.

- For patients with recurrent GBM, the addition of PET/CT imaging should be considered. Because it is difficult to distinguish between postradiation changes and disease recurrence on MR imaging, PET occasionally can be helpful. In these instances, PET/CT should be fused to the tumor on simulation CT and to MR imaging. Amino acid PET imaging for this purpose is frequently used in Europe but is not approved for this use in the United States.

# 3 Simulation and Daily Localization

- In the majority of situations, patients should undergo CT simulation supine with the head in a neutral position. Intravenous contrast is not recommended.
- The head and neck must be immobilized, preferably up to the shoulders, using a custom mold or mask to increase setup accuracy. Bite blocks can be useful in those situations in which angular rotations are a problem (in our practice, these are used infrequently). One specific advantage of a bite block is the possibility of incorporating into it markers that can be tracked by cameras, so that intrafraction motion can be monitored. This would be useful in fractionated stereotactic approaches.
- Thin-slice CT imaging is recommended (at 1–2 mm intervals) and, for ease of fusion, ideally should match the MR image slice thickness.
- Multimodal MR fusion, using at least the contrast-enhanced T1 and FLAIR sequences, should be fused to the planning CT. Although the entire anatomic volume should be matched, the primary matching focus is the tumor. PET/CT fusion can be helpful in select situations, as mentioned above.

# 4 Target Volume Delineation and Treatment Planning

- Standards for treatment of HGGs are directed by data from three seminal studies from the 1980s that highlighted the extent of microscopic disease well beyond enhancing tumors or radiographic changes (Hochberg and Pruitt 1980; Wallner et al. 1989; Kelly et al. 1987). This finding drives the principles of contour generation in these cases.
- Because the infiltrative nature of HGGs results in large fields, the GTV is divided into two components: one that incorporates all (or almost all) *possible* malignancy and one that focuses on a region of known or gross disease or the region at highest risk of developing recurrence.
- MR imaging should be used for the creation of most of the regions of interest (both target and avoidance structures).

- CT can be helpful for target volume contouring if the tumor has questionable bone involvement or if it contains calcifications, as frequently seen in oligodendrogliomas. CT should be used to contour the lenses, eyes, and cochleae. See Fig. 2b, c.
- From the postoperative MR imaging dataset, the FLAIR sequence is preferred for delineation of the initial volume (GTV1) for HGGs (Figs. 1, 3, and 6). The T2 sequence is appropriate to use as well; however, FLAIR is somewhat superior for this purpose. The rationale for utilizing the FLAIR images is to include microscopic disease that is known to extend beyond enhancing tumor. This area is difficult to evaluate, especially in the context of significant vasogenic edema, which has MR characteristics similar to that of infiltrative tumor. In cases with substantial FLAIR changes, low-intensity changes should be distinguished from high-intensity changes (Fig. 1).
- In cases with marked improvement of edema with use of steroids, it is not necessary to include all FLAIR changes in GTV1 (Fig. 7). Steroid responsiveness usually implies vasogenic edema, as opposed to infiltrative tumor.
- A contrast-enhanced T1 postoperative MR image should be used for delineation of GTV2, which entails gross residual disease and/or the surgical bed as demonstrated in Figs. 1 and 3.
- GTVs are expanded by 1.5–2.5 cm to generate clinical target volumes (CTVs) for HGGs, with the recognition that expansions must be tailored and individualized to respect natural barriers and organs at risk (Figs. 8 and 9).
- For LGGs, FLAIR abnormalities are used to designate a single GTV (Fig. 10). These tumors are typically non-enhancing, thereby obviating the need for T1 MR image fusion. An exception is unresected pilocytic astrocytoma, in which T1 enhancement should be the basis for contour generation. The patient in Figs. 11 and 12 underwent multiple resections for recurrent pilocytic astrocytoma. At the time of treatment, minimal T1 enhancement remained. For this reason, FLAIR changes were the basis for the GTV.
- GTV-to-CTV expansion for LGGs also ranges from 1.5 to 2.5 cm because of their equally diffuse and infiltrative nature. Exceptions include very well-circumscribed glial neoplasms, such as pilocytic astrocytomas; in such cases, the CTV margin should be smaller.
- A summary of the suggested target volumes is listed in Table 1.
- Expansion from CTV to PTV in all cases requires consideration of factors specific to the patient and treating facility, including but not limited to immobilization, reproducibility, planning technique (3D CRT vs. intensity-modulated radiation therapy [IMRT] vs. proton therapy),

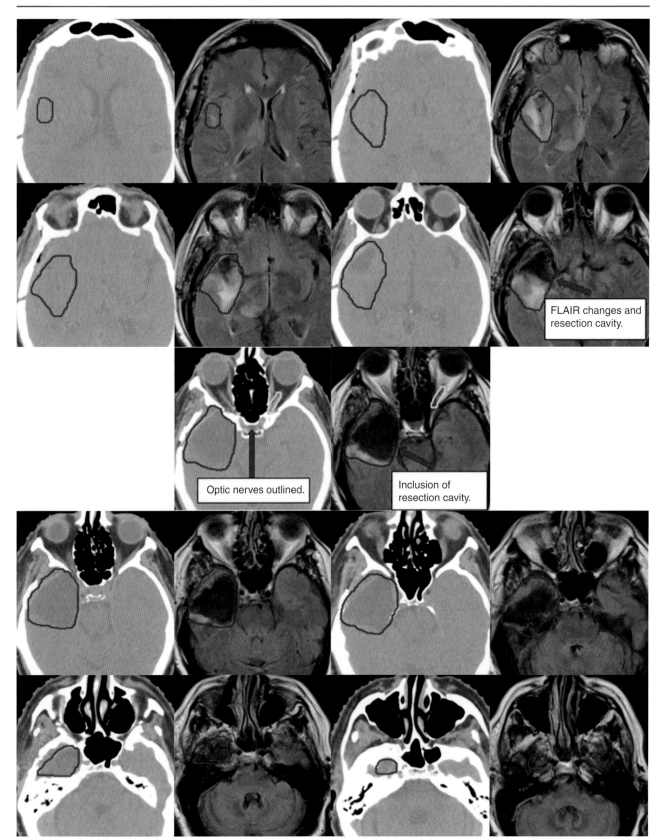

**Fig. 6** Target delineation of GTV1 (*red*) in a patient with a right temporal GBM (post gross total resection) on CT and fused corresponding MRI FLAIR sequence

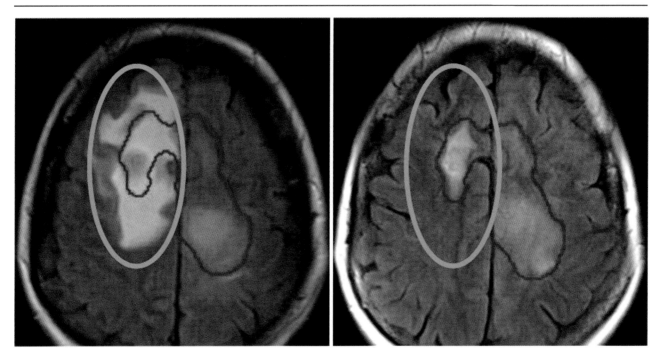

**Fig. 7** Reduction in FLAIR changes in 3 weeks in a patient with multifocal GBM. The entirety of the initial FLAIR abnormalities (*blue*) was not covered in the GTV1 (*red*) because they improved with steroid therapy alone

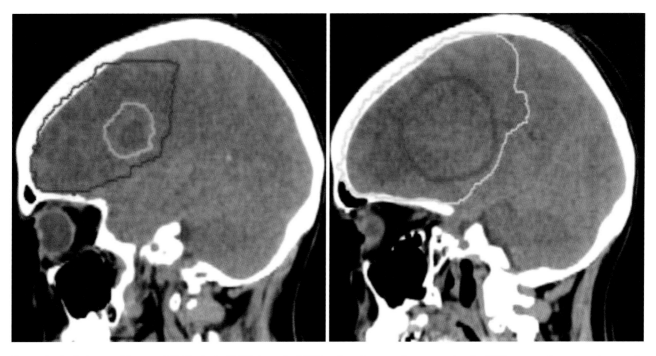

**Fig. 8** Sagittal view on CT scan of GTV1 (*red*), GTV2 (*green*), CTV1 (*aqua*), and CTV2 (*purple*) in a patient with a left frontotemporal GBM (post-biopsy only). The marked difference in volume is apparent in these images when comparing the CTV generated to cover microscopic extent of disease (CTV1) vs. visible disease (CTV2)

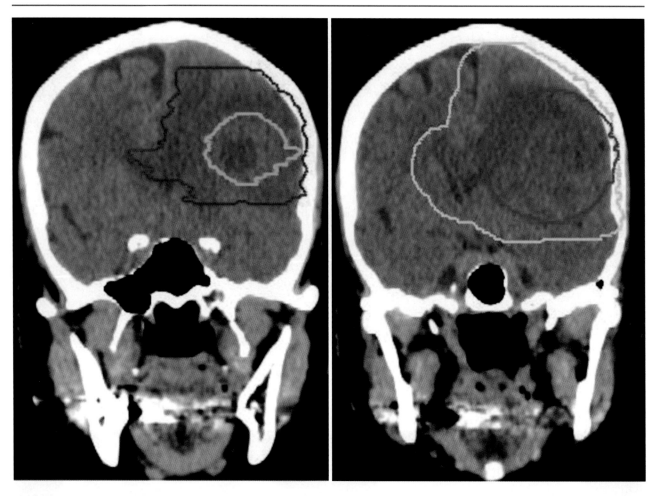

**Fig. 9** Coronal view on CT scan of GTV1 (*red*), GTV2 (*green*), CTV1 (*aqua*), and CTV2 (*purple*) in a patient with a left frontotemporal GBM (post-biopsy only)

quality of CT and MR image fusion, and institutional measurements relative to setup accuracy.

• Accepted alternative approaches to volume generation and expansion deviate from the above method, which is similar to the Radiation Therapy Oncology Group (RTOG) standards.

  – The European Organisation for Research and Treatment of Cancer (EORTC) uses one GTV instead of two, with a 2–3 cm margin to form a CTV.

  – Other institutions have also adopted similar contouring guidelines, which result in smaller fields.

• The University of Texas MD Anderson Cancer Center (MDACC) has reported on a cohort of patients treated with a single GTV technique who experienced recurrence and underwent hypothetical replanning using RTOG guidelines (Chang et al. 2007).

  – This analysis showed that all out-of-field recurrences would have remained outside the target had the larger volumes been treated.

• Kumar et al. (2012) presented results from a small, relatively underpowered randomized trial in GBM patients not stratified by MGMT methylation status to treatment with the RTOG volumes or to the MDACC approach.

  – Data revealed a statistically smaller treatment volume using the MDACC method than with RTOG volumes (246 and 436 cc, respectively), as well as improved mean overall survival (18.4 and 14.8 mo, respectively).

• For CTV coverage, 3D conformal radiation therapy techniques produce acceptable plans in most patients. However, for sparing of critical normal structures, IMRT may be required.

• Setup verification should be a function of technique employed and margins applied.

  – If the CTV-to-PTV margin is ≥5 mm, orthogonal imaging should suffice. In such cases, the bony anatomy on both image sets should be matched.

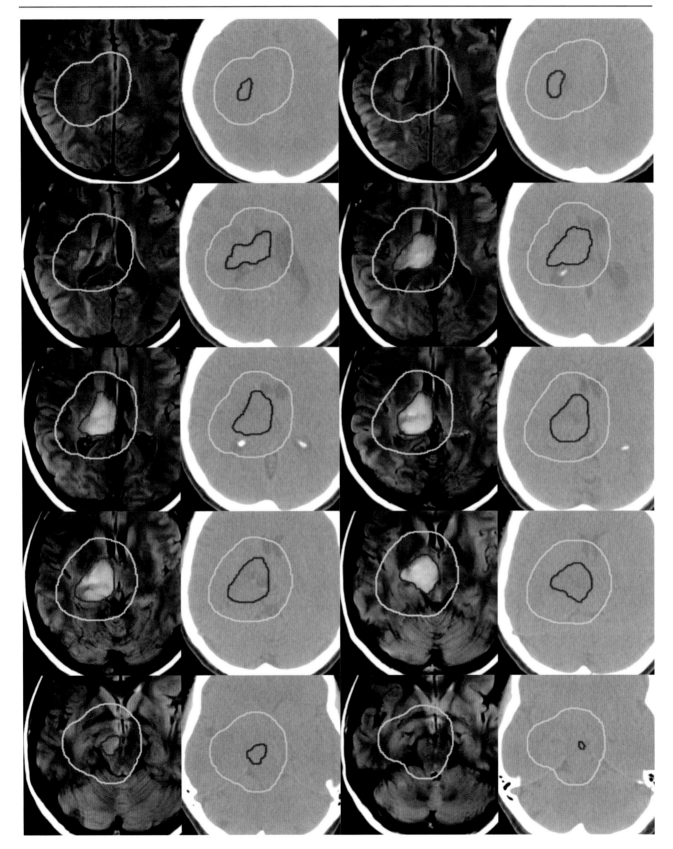

**Fig. 10** Target delineation of GTV (*red*) and CTV (*aqua*, using a 1.5 cm margin) using a FLAIR MR sequence in a patient with a grade 2 astrocytoma of the right thalamus who underwent biopsy only (as a result of the eloquent location of tumor)

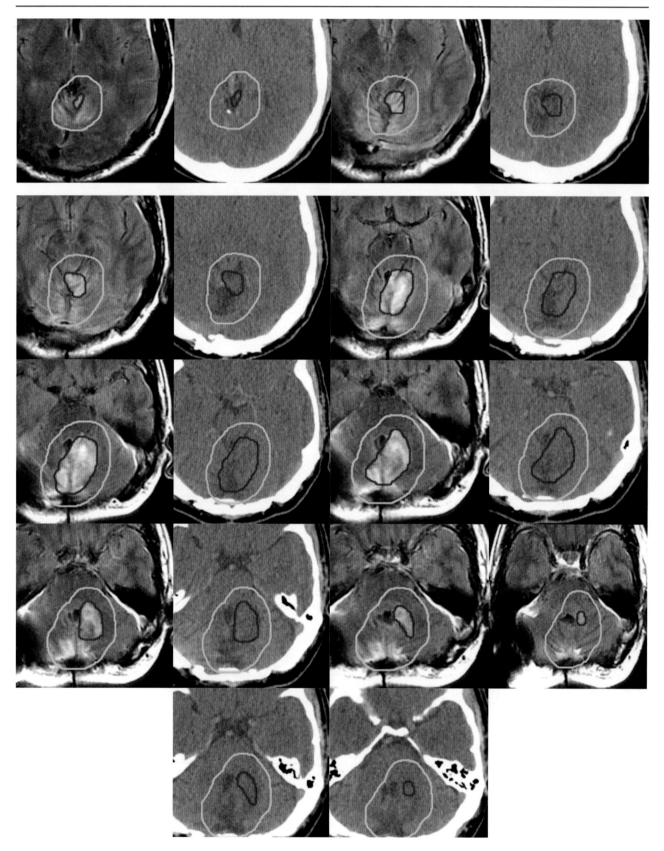

**Fig. 11** Axial CT and FLAIR MRI views of a patient with multiply recurrent pilocytic astrocytoma treated with surgical resection and no adjuvant radiation therapy in the past. GTV (*red*) was drawn using the FLAIR sequence, to which a 1 cm margin was added to create the CTV (*aqua*)

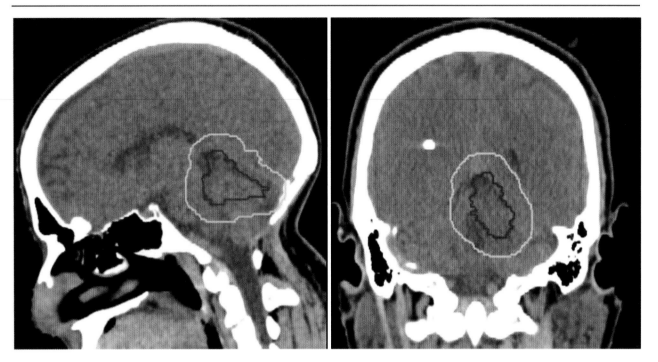

**Fig. 12** Sagittal and coronal views of CT images reflecting GTV (*red*) and CTV (*aqua*) in a patient with a recurrent pilocytic astrocytoma

**Table 1** Suggested target volumes

| Target | Volume |
|---|---|
| HGG GTV1 | FLAIR abnormalities to encompass microscopic disease |
| HGG GTV2 | Contrast-enhanced T1 changes to cover resection cavity and/or residual tumor |
| HGG CTV | GTV + 1.5–2.5 cm except at natural barriers |
| LGG GTV | FLAIR abnormalities to include resection cavity and/or residual tumor |
| LGG CTV | GTV + 1.5–2.5 cm except at natural barriers or in well-circumscribed tumors |

- If margins are tighter (≤3 mm) or if the plan consists of IMRT fields with multiple small segments, daily verification is highly recommended with a volumetric technique, such as megavoltage or cone-beam CT.
- Recommended doses are summarized in Table 2.

---

## 5    Plan Assessment

- Balancing ideal target coverage and appropriate sparing of organs at risk can be challenging. In these instances, consideration of the patient's overall prognosis must be factored into plan evaluation.

**Table 2** Suggested dose

| Target | Dose |
|---|---|
| HGG PTV1 | 45 Gy in 25 fractions or 46 Gy in 23 fractions |
| HGG PTV2 | 59.4 Gy in 33 fractions or 60 Gy in 30 fractions |
| LGG PTV | Controversial, 45–54 Gy acceptable in 1.8 Gy or 2 Gy per fraction[a] |

[a]The preferred dose at the University of Maryland Medical Center is 54Gy

- For example, superseding the optic nerve dose may be less acceptable in a patient with a low-grade 1p/19q co-deleted oligodendroglioma than in a patient with a GBM, because the former patient would be more likely to survive for a long period of time and therefore be at greater risk for late toxicities. On the other hand, he/she would also be more likely to live to have a recurrence, so that compromising on CTV coverage should not be taken lightly.
- Generally, ≥95 % of the PTV should receive 100 % of the prescribed dose. 100 % of the GTV should be covered by 100 % of the dose. The maximum dose to any point should be limited to 105 % of the prescription dose and ideally should be located in the GTV.
- Commonly used dose limitations to organs at risk are summarized in Table 3.

**Table 3** Normal tissue dose constraints

| Critical structures | Constraints |
|---|---|
| Lenses | Max <7 Gy |
| Retina | Max <50 Gy |
| Lacrimal glands | Max <35 Gy[a] |
| Optic nerves | Max <54 Gy or 1 % of PTV cannot exceed 60 Gy |
| Optic chiasm | Max <54 Gy or 1 % of PTV cannot exceed 60 Gy |
| Hippocampus | Max ≤16 Gy and no more than 9 Gy to 100 % volume |
| Pituitary gland | Max <45 Gy |
| Cochleae | Max <45 Gy |
| Brainstem | Max <54 Gy or 1 % of PTV cannot exceed 60 Gy |

Based on the University of Maryland treatment planning guidelines
[a]This may change to include V20<25 % as new data emerges (Batth et al. 2013)

## Suggested Reading

Chao ST, Suh JH (2011) Radiation for glioblastoma. In: Mehta MP (ed) Principles and practices of neuro-oncology. A multidisciplinary approach. Demos Medical Publishing, New York, pp 744–751

Fischer I, Sulman E, Aldape K (2011) Molecular pathogenesis of glioma: overview and therapeutic implications. In: Mehta MP (ed) Principles and practices of neuro-oncology. A multidisciplinary approach. Demos Medical Publishing, New York, p 88–99

For delineation of normal structures: www.imaios.com

Laack NN, Brown PD (2011) Low-grade glioma radiation therapy. In: Mehta MP (ed) Principles and practices of neuro-oncology. A multidisciplinary approach. Demos Medical Publishing, New York, pp 760–768

Pacholke HD, Amdur RJ, Schmalfuss IM, Louis D, Mendenhall WM (2005) Contouring the middle and inner ear on radiotherapy planning scans. Am J Clin Oncol 28:143–147

Radiation Therapy Oncology Group. RTOG 0933 Hippocampal atlas. Available at: http://www.rtog.org/corelab/contouringatlases/hippocampalsparing.aspx. Accessed 20 Feb 2014

RTOG 0424. A phase II study of a temozolomide-based chemoradiotherapy regimen for high risk low-grade gliomas. Updated December 26, 2013. Protocol information available at: http://www.rtog.org/ClinicalTrials/ProtocolTable/StudyDetails.aspx?study=0424. Accessed 20 Feb 2014

RTOG 0837. Randomized, phase II, double-blind, placebo-controlled trial of conventional chemoradiation and adjuvant temozolomide plus cediranib versus conventional chemoradiation and adjuvant temozolomide plus placebo in patients with newly diagnosed glioblastoma. Updated 2/14/12. Protocol information available at: http://www.rtog.org/ClinicalTrials/ProtocolTable/StudyDetails.aspx?study=0837. Accessed 27 Feb 2014

Siker ML, Mehta MP (2011) Anaplastic glioma. In: Mehta MP (ed) Principles and Practices of neuro-oncology. A multidisciplinary approach. Demos Medical Publishing, New York, pp 752–759

## References

Batth SS, Sreeraman R, Dienes E et al (2013) Clinical-dosimetric relationship between lacrimal gland dose and ocular toxicity after intensity-modulated radiotherapy for sinonasal tumours. Br J Radiol 86:20130459

Chang EL, Akyurek S, Avalos T et al (2007) Evaluation of peritumoral edema in the delineation of radiotherapy clinical target volumes for glioblastoma. Int J Radiat Oncol Biol Phys 68:144–150

Gondi V, Vogelbaum MA, Grimm S, Mehta MP (2013) Primary intracranial neoplasms. In: Halperin EC, Wazer DE, Perez CA, Brady LW (eds) Perez & Brady's principles and practice of radiation oncology, 6th edn. Wolters Kluwer, Philadelphia, pp 652–653

Hochberg FH, Pruitt A (1980) Assumptions in the radiotherapy of glioblastoma. Neurology 30:907–911

Kelly PJ, Daumas-Duport C, Scheithauer BW, Kall BA, Kispert DB (1987) Stereotactic histologic correlations of computed tomography and magnetic resonance imaging-defined abnormalities in patients with glial neoplasms. Mayo Clinic Proc 62:450–459

Kumar N, Kumar R, Sharma S et al To compare the treatment outcomes of two different target delineation guidelines (RTOG vs. MD Anderson) in glioblastoma multiforme patients: a prospective randomized study. Presented at the 17th annual scientific meeting of the society for neuro-oncology, Washington, DC, 16 Nov 2012

Wallner KE, Gallcich JH, Krol G, Arbit E, Malkin MG (1989) Patterns of failure following treatment for glioblastoma multiforme and anaplastic astrocytoma. Int J Radiat Oncol Biol Phys 16: 1405–1409

# Palliative Radiation for Brain Metastases

Nicholas S. Boehling, David C. Weksberg, Jiade J. Lu, and Eric L. Chang

## Contents

N.S. Boehling • D.C. Weksberg
Department of Radiation Oncology,
M.D. Anderson Cancer Center, Houston, TX, USA
e-mail: nboehling@gmail.com

J.J. Lu
Shanghai Proton and Heavy Ion Center,
Shanghai, China
e-mail: jiade.lu@sphic.org.cn

E.L. Chang (✉)
Department of Radiation Oncology,
USC Keck School of Medicine, Los Angeles, CA, USA
e-mail: eric.chang@health.usc.edu

## 1     Anatomy and Patterns of Spread

- The brain is one of the most common sites of cancer metastasis. Approximately half of the patients who develop brain metastases will be diagnosed with a single metastatic lesion. Spread is through hematogenous dissemination commonly to the watershed area at the gray/white matter junction. Metastases follow blood supply with the most occurring in the supratentorial brain. Some histologies, notably small cell lung cancer, prostate and gastrointestinal cancers are commonly found in the cerebellum.

- Tumors break the blood-brain barrier and often grow spherically with resultant cerebral edema. Metastases from melanoma, renal cell carcinoma, and choriocarcinoma have a higher rate of hemorrhage.

- Leptomeningeal carcinomatosis is a rare diagnosis but carries a grim prognosis in which metastases spread to the meninges surrounding the brain and the spinal cord. Findings may be detected on MRI with enhancement of sulci, cerebellar folia, or cranial nerve enhancement and confirmed by CSF cytology.

- In the setting of leptomeningeal disease or lymphoreticular metastases, involvement of the ocular structures and cribriform plate requires special consideration.

## 2     Diagnostic Imaging for Target Volume Delineation

- MRI with gadolinium contrast is the best diagnostic tool. MRI is more effective at detecting small lesions and leptomeningeal involvement as compared to CT imaging. Sagittal and coronal images should be obtained.
  - If hippocampal avoidance (HA-WBRT) is planned, 1.25 mm slice thickness spoiled-gradient MRI is preferred for image fusion.

N.Y. Lee et al. (eds.), *Target Volume Delineation for Conformal and Intensity-Modulated Radiation Therapy*,
Medical Radiology. Radiation Oncology, DOI: 10.1007/174_2014_984, © Springer International Publishing Switzerland 2014
Published Online: 14 October 2014

- It is important to consider other diagnoses including abscess, radiation necrosis, or second primary if history and imaging are incongruous. If MRI cannot be obtained due to a pacemaker, contrast-enhanced CT imaging can be obtained as an alternative.
- MR series can assist in target identification.
  - T1 non-contrast series can assess for hemorrhage.
  - T2/FLAIR series best demonstrates cerebral edema.
  - T1 post-contrast can best identify metastases.
  - For the purposes of radiosurgery, a volumetric, thin-slice (1 mm) T1 fast spoiled-gradient sequence with contrast is obtained.

# 3  Simulation and Daily Localization

- For WBRT simulation, the patient should be imaged in the supine position, using a head holder and an immobilizing thermoplastic mask. Non-contrast CT imaging with 3–5 mm slice thickness is preferred for treatment planning; however, clinical patient setup can be performed in the emergent setting. Axial images from the vertex through the upper cervical spine should be obtained. Daily kV imaging is commonly utilized for IMRT-based whole-brain treatment.
- For frame-based SRS, a stereotactic head frame should be placed by a neurosurgeon. Optimally, a volumetric (1 mm slices, up to 2 mm), contrast-enhanced MRI is used for target delineation and treatment planning. In multi-isocenter, cobalt-based SRS systems (Gamma Knife), this MRI can be directly used for treatment planning. However, for linear accelerator (LINAC)-based SRS, a thin-slice CT must be acquired for dose calculation and additional scans (i.e., volumetric MRI) can be co-registered for treatment planning.

# 4  Target Volume Delineation and Treatment Planning

## 4.1  WBRT

- Whole-brain radiation therapy (WBRT) using conventional external beam radiation is most commonly employed (Fig. 1). Stereotactic radiosurgery (SRS) can be used in the adjuvant or upfront settings for patients with limited number of intracranial metastatic foci, sufficient extracranial disease control, and appropriate performance status.
- The typical treatment technique consists of opposed lateral photon beams. Field design is demonstrated in Fig. 1 and should take care to provide adequate coverage of the cribriform plate and temporal lobes. Figure 2 illustrates variations of the standard WBRT fields to account for differing clinical situations.
- A wide variety of dose and fractionation schemes are used for WBRT, with 30 Gy in 10 fractions being the most common. For patients with a relatively long life expectancy (and greater concern for neurocognitive sequelae), more protracted fractionation schemes (30 Gy in 12 fractions, 37.5 in 15 fractions) can be considered. The most commonly recommended dose for PCI in SCLC is 25 Gy in 10 daily fractions. For CNS leukemia, a total dose of 18–24 Gy is given at 1.8 Gy per fraction.
- For lymphoreticular involvement, radiation fields should include the posterior 1/3 of the orbit and cribriform plate (Fig. 2).
- IMRT can be used for HA-WBRT (Fig. 3). The standard dose scheme is 30 Gy in 10 fractions with a maximal hippocampal dose of 10 Gy. The CTV is defined as the entire brain parenchyma. The PTV is defined as the CTV minus the hippocampus + 3–5 mm volumetric expansion. Hippocampus contouring is best seen on T1 series MRI to identify the gray matter in the medial temporal horn. The RTOG atlas (see suggested reading) is available for further guidance.
- Reirradiation is done on a selective basis with a lowered total dose of 20–25 Gy in 10 fractions and a time interval of at least 4–6 months between the initial and repeat course. Blocking radiosensitive organ at risk (OAR) structures, including the optic nerve and chiasm, is accomplished by creating a block with a 3 mm expansion on the OAR, as demonstrated in Fig. 4.

## 4.2  SRS

- The optimal use of SRS in conjunction with WBRT or as stand-alone treatment remains controversial. Randomized data supports the addition of SRS before or after WBRT for patients with 1–3 metastases (Andrews et al. 2004). SRS alone may also be offered to patients with 1–3 lesions (Chang et al. 2009; Aoyama et al. 2006), provided that close imaging follow-up can be obtained to monitor for additional disease.
- SRS is generally appropriate for lesions less than 4 cm in largest diameter. Independent of size, neurosurgical management may be preferred for lesions causing symptoms and mass effect. Fractionated stereotactic radiotherapy in 3–5 fractions is preferred for larger lesions.
- For frame-based SRS, the gross tumor volume (GTV) is contoured as the visualized lesion on contrast-enhanced MRI (Fig. 5). No CTV or PTV expansions are used (in frameless systems, a 1–2 mm PTV expansion should be

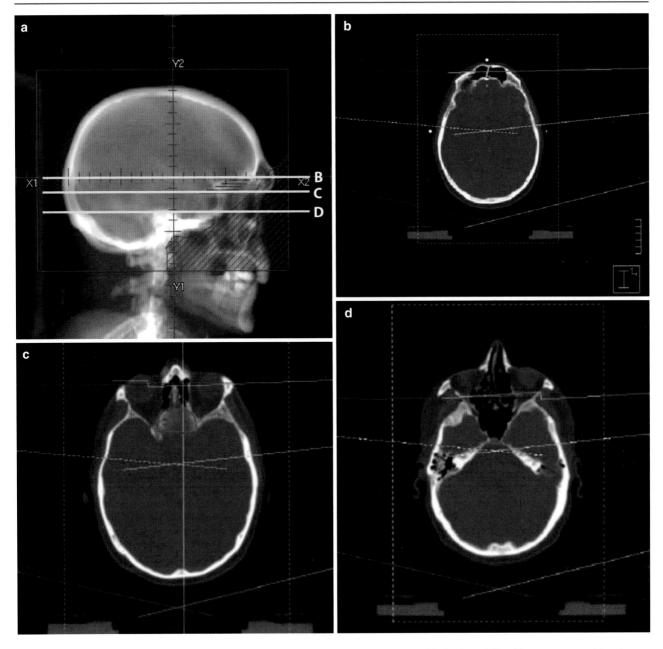

**Fig. 1** Standard WBRT fields. Conventional opposed lateral fields are rotated slightly off-axis (RAO/LAO) (*red/green*) to create coplanar anterior field edges which do not diverge into the lenses. (**a**) Beam's eye view (RAO) and blocking (diagonal red lines) as defined by graticule measurments X and Y. The inferior field edge is set at C1 with at least 2 cm of flash posteriorly and superiorly. The block begins at the anterior aspect of the C1 vertebral body and is designed to spare nontarget tissues (e.g., parotid glands), while taking care to provide adequate margin on the temporal lobes and cribriform plate (*blue*). (**b**) Central axis view showing coplanar anterior field edges. (**c**) Axial slices demonstrating adequate margin on the cribriform plate (*blue*) and avoidance of divergent dose through the lenses. (**d**) Axial slice demonstrating adequate margin on the temporal lobes

created depending on the setup accuracy). Dose is typically prescribed to the 50 % isodose line for Gamma Knife and 75–95 % for LINAC-based SRS, with the choice of prescription dose determined by lesion size (Table 1). SRS can create a highly conformal dose distribution, allowing for treatment of lesions in close proximity to critical OAR structures (Fig. 6); however, care must be paid to normal tissue tolerance (Table 2).

- Postoperative cavity SRS in lieu of WBRT as a routine adjuvant treatment remains controversial. When indicated, any residual disease is contoured as the GTV to be included within a CTV that encompasses the surgical cavity (Fig. 7). A small margin of 2 mm to create a PTV is recommended (Choi et al. 2012). Dose in a single fraction setting is decreased for microscopic disease levels at 15–20 Gy based on volume according to NCCTG N107C protocol.

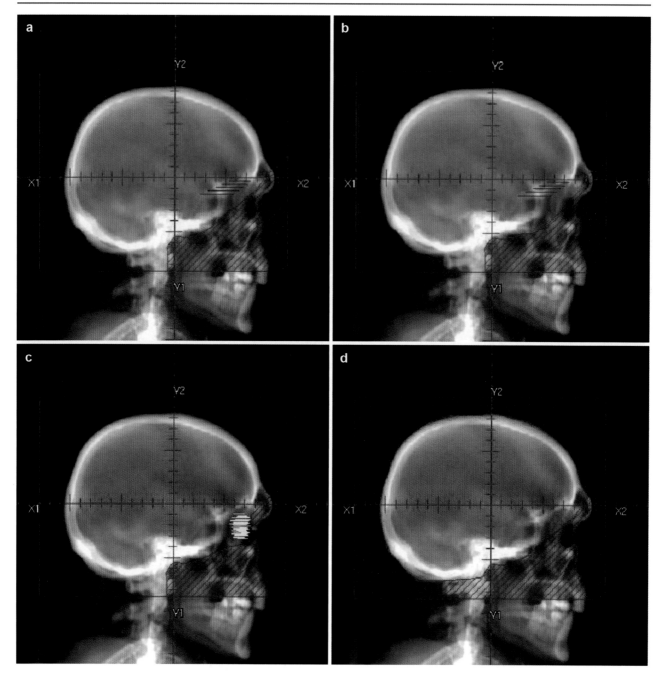

**Fig. 2** Variations on WBRT fields. (**a**) Conventional fields (RAO/LAO) as described in Fig. 1. (**b**) More generous WBRT fields used in the setting of leptomeningeal disease – these fields provide additional margin on the cribriform plate (*blue*). (**c**) Conventional fields (RAO/LAO) covering the traditional WBRT target with the addition of coverage of the bilateral retinas (*yellow*) in the setting of proven retinal involvement (e.g., CNS lymphoma, CNS prophylaxis for leukemia, leukemic infiltrate to the retina) with blocking of the lens (*green*) and anterior chamber. (**d**) Scalp-sparing WBRT fields – the block edge is set at the outer table of the calvarium to minimize alopecia in patients for whom cosmesis is of particular concern. The blocked field is represented by the diagonal red lines

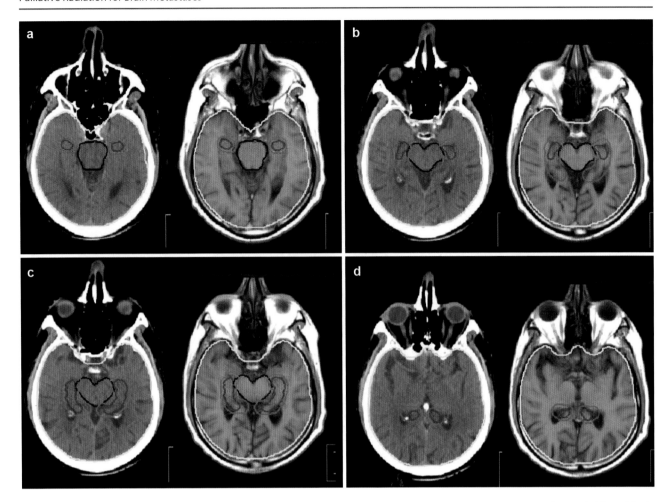

**Fig. 3** Hippocampal avoidance WBRT. Axial slices are presented from caudal (**a**) to cranial (**d**) extent with CT and matched T1 series MRI. Structures highlighted include the hippocampal formation of interest (*red*), expansion (*blue*), normal brain tissue (khaki), and brain stem (*black*). The CTV contains all normal brain tissue with the hippocampal formation expansion removed from the target

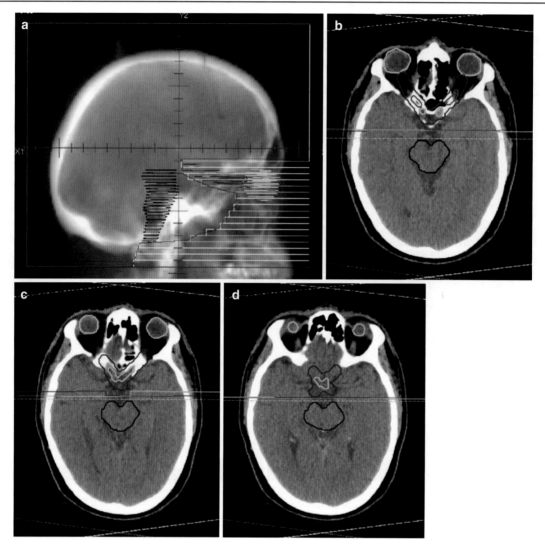

**Fig. 4** Reirradiation using a peninsula block. (**a**) Optic nerves (*pink*) and chiasm (*green*) are blocked with a 3 mm OAR PTV (*purple*). A standard WBRT is modified to include a block covering the PTV as well as the spinal cord caudal to the brain stem (*black*). Axial slices from caudal (**b**) to cranial (**d**) are shown with MLC blocks from the RAO beam (*red*) and LAO beam (*green*)

Lesion 1        Lesion 2        Lesion 3

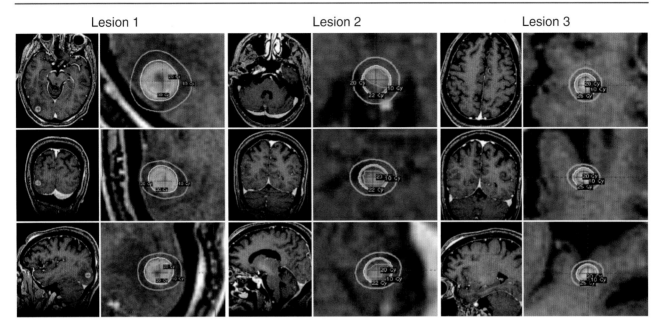

**Fig. 5** SRS treatment of 3 metastatic lesions. A Leksell Gamma Knife was used for the treatment of a patient with 3 metastatic lesions from non-small cell lung cancer. Contrast-enhanced volumetric MRI (1 mm cuts) demonstrated three enhancing lesions in the right parietal lobe (*lesion 1*), right cerebellar hemisphere (*lesion 2*), and right occipital lobe (*lesion 3*). All three lesions were prescribed 20 Gy based on size criteria (Table 1). Axial, coronal, and sagittal images from the planning MRI are depicted, as well as representative slices from the treatment plan showing the prescription isodose line in *yellow*, with additional isodose lines shown in *green*

**Table 1** SRS dose prescriptions by lesion size (Shaw et al. 2000)

| Tumor size (cm) | Prescription dose (Gy) |
|---|---|
| <2 | 20–24 |
| 2–3 | 18 |
| 3–4 | 15 |

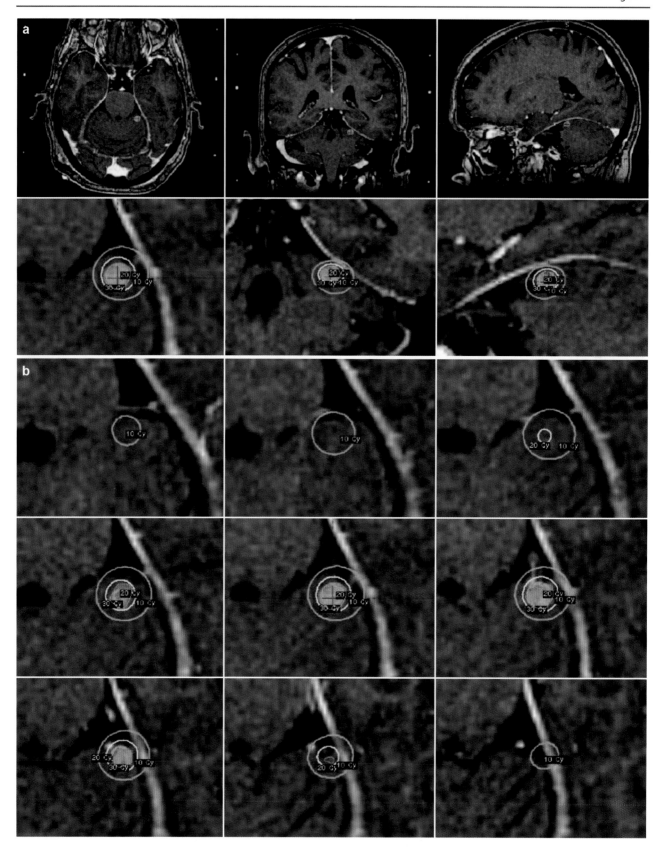

**Fig. 6** SRS treatment of a cerebellar lesion in close proximity to the brain stem. (**a**) Axial, coronal, and sagittal slices from a volumetric (1 mm) contrast-enhanced MRI through the center of the metastatic lesion, contoured in orange. The 20 Gy prescription isodose line is shown in *yellow*, with 30 Gy and 10 Gy lines in *green*. (**b**) Serial axial images delineating the entire volume receiving 10 Gy. The sharp dose falloff allows treatment of this lesion adjacent to the brain stem (see Table 2 for dose constraints)

**Table 2** Critical structure dose constraints

| Organ at risk | Dose constraint ($D_{max}$) (Gy) |
| --- | --- |
| Brain stem | 12 |
| Optic structures | 8 |

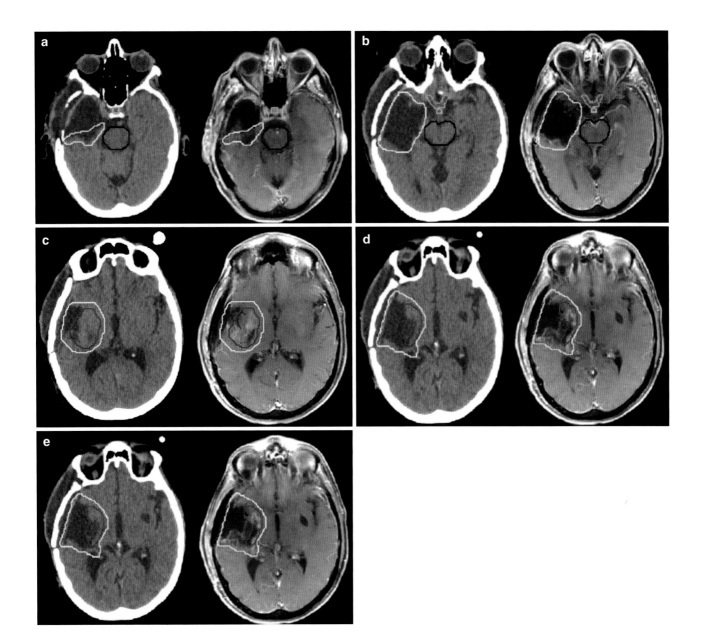

**Fig. 7** SRS treatment of a postoperative resection cavity. Axial slices are presented from caudal (**a**) to cranial (**e**) with matched T1 post-contrast MRI slices. The surgical cavity (khaki) is outlined with an area of gross residual disease (*red*). The pituitary (*light blue*), brain stem (*black*), and optic chiasm (*green*) are outlined due to proximity. A long thermoplastic mask was utilized for immobilization. Cone beam CT and ExacTrac imaging was utilized for image guidance. The patient was treated with a simultaneous integrated boost technique with 21 Gy to the cavity and 24 Gy to the residual disease in three fractions

## Suggested Reading

RTOG Hippocampal Sparing Atlas (http://www.rtog.org/
    CoreLab/ContouringAtlases/HippocampalSparing.aspx)
Additional references for further reading are provided below
    (Patchell et al. 1990, 1998; Kocher et al. 2011; Sperduto
    et al. 2012; Boehling et al. 2012; Gaspar et al. 1997, 2010;
    Kalkanis et al. 2010; Linskey et al. 2010; Tsao et al.
    2012).

## References

Andrews DW et al (2004) Whole brain radiation therapy with or with-
    out stereotactic radiosurgery boost for patients with one to three
    brain metastases: phase III results of the RTOG 9508 randomised
    trial. Lancet 363(9422):1665–1672
Aoyama H et al (2006) Stereotactic radiosurgery plus whole-brain radi-
    ation therapy vs stereotactic radiosurgery alone for treatment of
    brain metastases: a randomized controlled trial. JAMA 295(21):
    2483–2491
Boehling N et al (2012) Stereotactic radiosurgery for brain metastases:
    current status and future directions. J Radiat Oncol 1(3):245–253
Chang EL et al (2009) Neurocognition in patients with brain metastases
    treated with radiosurgery or radiosurgery plus whole-brain irradia-
    tion: a randomised controlled trial. Lancet Oncol 10(11):1037–1044
Choi CY et al (2012) Stereotactic radiosurgery of the postoperative resec-
    tion cavity for brain metastases: prospective evaluation of target mar-
    gin on tumor control. Int J Radiat Oncol Biol Phys 84(2):336–342
Gaspar L et al (1997) Recursive partitioning analysis (RPA) of prognos-
    tic factors in three Radiation Therapy Oncology Group (RTOG)

brain metastases trials. Int J Radiat Oncol Biol Phys 37(4):
    745–751
Gaspar LE et al (2010) The role of whole brain radiation therapy in the
    management of newly diagnosed brain metastases: a systematic
    review and evidence-based clinical practice guideline. J Neurooncol
    96(1):17–32
Kalkanis SN et al (2010) The role of surgical resection in the manage-
    ment of newly diagnosed brain metastases: a systematic review and
    evidence-based clinical practice guideline. J Neurooncol 96(1):
    33–43
Kocher M et al (2011) Adjuvant whole-brain radiotherapy versus obser-
    vation after radiosurgery or surgical resection of one to three cere-
    bral metastases: results of the EORTC 22952–26001 study. J Clin
    Oncol 29(2):134–141
Linskey ME et al (2010) The role of stereotactic radiosurgery in the
    management of patients with newly diagnosed brain metastases: a
    systematic review and evidence-based clinical practice guideline.
    J Neurooncol 96(1):45–68
Patchell RA et al (1990) A randomized trial of surgery in the treatment
    of single metastases to the brain. N Engl J Med 322(8):494–500
Patchell RA et al (1998) Postoperative radiotherapy in the treatment of
    single metastases to the brain: a randomized trial. JAMA 280(17):
    1485–1489
Shaw E et al (2000) Single dose radiosurgical treatment of recurrent
    previously irradiated primary brain tumors and brain metastases:
    final report of RTOG protocol 90–05. Int J Radiat Oncol Biol Phys
    47(2):291–298
Sperduto PW et al (2012) Summary report on the graded prognostic
    assessment: an accurate and facile diagnosis-specific tool to esti-
    mate survival for patients with brain metastases. J Clin Oncol 30(4):
    419–425
Tsao MN et al (2012) Radiotherapeutic and surgical management for
    newly diagnosed brain metastasis(es): an American Society for
    Radiation Oncology evidence-based guideline. Pract Radiat Oncol
    2(3):210–225

# Hodgkin Lymphoma

Bradford S. Hoppe and Richard T. Hoppe

## Contents

B.S. Hoppe, MD, MPH (✉)
Department of Radiation Oncology,
University of Florida, Jacksonville, FL 32206, USA
e-mail: bhoppe@floridaproton.org

R.T. Hoppe, MD
Department of Radiation Oncology,
Stanford University, Palo Alto, Stanford, CA 94304, USA

N.Y. Lee et al. (eds.), *Target Volume Delineation for Conformal and Intensity-Modulated Radiation Therapy*,
Medical Radiology. Radiation Oncology, DOI: 10.1007/174_2014_985, © Springer International Publishing Switzerland 2014
Published Online: 31 October 2014

# 1    Introduction

**Table 1** ILROG planning definitions for ISRT in lymphoma (Specht et al. 2013; Illidge 2014)

| Volume | | Description |
|---|---|---|
| Gross tumor volume (GTV) | Pre-chemotherapy/surgery GTV (GTVp) | Contains gross tumor volume as identified on diagnostic imaging prior to chemotherapy and/or surgery |
| | Post-chemotherapy/surgery GTV (GTVr) | Contains gross tumor volume as identified on diagnostic and/or planning imaging after management with chemotherapy and/or surgery |
| | No prior treatment GTV (GTV) | Contains gross tumor volume identified on diagnostic and/or planning imaging in the absence of prior chemotherapy or surgery (e.g., in the case of primary or salvage RT) |
| Clinical target volume (CTV) | | Contains entire post-chemotherapy/surgery or "no prior treatment" GTV |
| | | Generally contains pre-chemotherapy/surgery GTV (unless volume is unable to be safely treating in its entirety) |
| | | Excludes extent of pre-chemotherapy/surgery GTV that displaced normal, uninvolved tissue (bone, organs, muscles, etc.) prior to chemotherapy or surgery |
| | | Includes consideration of the following: |
| | |    Image accuracy and quality. CTV should be increased in size to account for uncertainties such as suboptimal fusion of pre- and post-chemotherapy/surgery images to planning images or in the absence of pre-chemotherapy/surgery images |
| | |    Changes in volume since the time of imaging |
| | |    Pattern of disease spread |
| | |    Potential subclinical involvement. Consider including nodes of unknown status near the site of disease, particularly if the questionable nodes belong to a nodal chain or group already partially encompassed by the CTV |
| | |    Adjacent organ dose constraints |
| | | Can contain separate nodal volumes if ≤5 cm apart. Lesions >5 cm apart are treated with separate CTVs |
| Internal target volume (ITV) | | Contains the CTV plus an internal margin that accounts for variation in CTV shape, size, and position (e.g., target movement with respiration) |
| | | Most relevant for targets within the chest and abdomen; may be unnecessary for other sites |
| Planning target volume (PTV) | | Contains CTV or ITV plus a margin to account for setup uncertainties associated with patient position and beam alignment |
| | | *Note that CTV to PTV expansions are patient- and institution-specific; any recommendations in this chapter or elsewhere must be adjusted to reflect factors unique to the patient and institution* |
| Organs at risk (OAR) | | Includes uninvolved normal structures at risk of RT-related toxicity for which RT planning or dose may be altered |

# 2    Anatomy and Patterns of Spread

- Hodgkin lymphoma is a malignancy of the lymphatic system. Consequently, the pattern of spread generally follows that of the lymphatic system in a predictable manner. The most common sites of disease are the mediastinum and cervical/supraclavicular regions.
- Although pretreatment imaging may occasionally show non-contiguity, subclinical disease is likely to be harbored in the lymphatic region lying between two regions shown to be involved on CT or PET/CT scan.
- Splenic involvement almost always accompanies para-aortic involvement. Splenic disease is always present if there is bone marrow or liver involvement.

- Bone marrow involvement occurs more commonly in patients with B symptoms and more advanced disease. PET/CT scan is sufficient for diagnosing bone marrow involvement, allowing patients to forgo bone marrow biopsies.

# 3    Diagnostic Workup Relevant for Target Volume Delineation

- All patients should undergo a contrast-enhanced CT of the neck, chest, abdomen, and pelvis along with a PET/CT scan prior to starting any systemic therapy (including steroids). Nodes that are palpable on exam, enlarged on

CT, or positive on FDG-PET are considered to be positive. Unusual or non-contiguous sites of disease should be biopsied to confirm involvement.

(i) When possible, PET/CT scan and contrast CT scan should be performed in the treatment position to assist in fusion with the CT simulation scan following chemotherapy. This may require careful coordination with radiology and medical oncology and developing a special "lymphoma" imaging protocol to be used when a patient is undergoing staging for lymphoma or when lymphoma is high on the differential diagnosis list.

    1. Arms slightly akimbo or at the side allow for more reproducible setup and fusion with CT scan, when axillary nodes are involved. However, arms above the head may provide better access to the mediastinum if IMRT or rapid arc is contemplated.

    2. Neutral or slightly extended neck, which allows for potentially less mandible to be included in the treatment field. Hyperextended neck may drop the brain further into the field when the high cervical nodes are involved. Diagnostic scans are often done in a head-neutral or head-flexed position.

    3. Performing the initial staging scans with deep inspiration breath-hold technique may allow for further reduction in radiation dose to the heart and lung.

- Chest X-ray still is the preferred way to characterize mediastinal bulk, due to its use in prior clinical trials. Masses greater than one-third of the maximum intrathoracic diameter or greater than 10 cm are considered to be unfavorable.

- MRI and MRI/PET scans may also be used, especially in pediatric Hodgkin lymphoma. Although these modalities will reduce the radiation dose compared with a PET/CT scan, they may not fuse as well with CT simulation and may, in fact, lead to larger radiation targets, due to the uncertainties with the fusion. FDG-PET remains the most effective way to define initial sites of disease.

- One should familiarize themselves with the Deauville criteria for evaluating treatment response in Hodgkin lymphoma (1, no uptake; 2, uptake <= mediastinum; 3, uptake > mediastinum but <= liver; 4, uptake > liver at any site; 5, uptake > liver and new sites of disease).

## 4  Simulation and Daily Localization

- The vast majority of patients with Hodgkin lymphoma will undergo radiotherapy as consolidation following chemotherapy. Since target delineation is based on pre-chemotherapy sites of involvement and since disease is expected to regress following chemotherapy, improved image registration with the pre-chemotherapy staging scans will allow for reduced size in target volume (due to less margin for fusion uncertainty). However, repositioning the patient may be required to avoid the OARs, despite requiring more margin for fusion uncertainties. For example, if the pretreatment PET/CT scan is performed with the head flexed, maintaining the same position for treatment would lead to unnecessary irradiation of the salivary glands and oral cavity in the presence of high cervical nodal disease. Planning treatment with the neck in a different position than the pretreatment PET/CT will require increasing the size of the CTV because of the uncertainty in image registration.

- When the supraclavicular or cervical region is involved, a face mask is used to help stabilize the patient in a reproducible manner and keep the chin from falling into the treatment field.

(i) When a face mask is used, it is advisable to avoid putting arms above the head, as this can cause significant pain and discomfort for some patients during their treatment.

- When axillary nodes require treatment, it is important to try and reproduce the initial staging scan patient setup. Although axillary nodes that were initially involved might be quite small, the axilla is a large nodal station, and the nodes can move considerably depending on patient arm position. Since these nodes may be difficult to identify at the time of simulation, larger margins will need to be used when discrepancies in arm setup are present between the staging scan and CT simulation. In this situation, it may be preferable to have the arms at the patient's side with a Vac-Lok bag and arm pulls to prevent the patient's arms from drifting during treatment.

- CT simulation should be performed with at a minimum 3 mm slices, starting at least 5 cm above the most superior level of disease from the staging scans and end at least 5 cm below the most inferior level of disease from the staging scans. Make sure to include adjacent OAR in their entirety to ensure an accurate DVH (i.e., include the entire lungs, even if the entire mediastinum is not included).

- IV contrast can help differentiate between residual Hodgkin lymphoma and the OARs and major vessels. It may also be helpful for contouring cardiac structures, including coronary vessels and valves.

- Wire scars from biopsies to define prior lymph node involvement, especially when the staging scans were done after the patient had an excisional biopsy.

- When the mediastinum, lung, para-aortics, and/or spleen are to be irradiated, one should consider respiratory motion management strategies. These may include:

   (i) 4D CT simulation to assess respiratory motion and either develop the GTV and CTV based on all 10 phases of the respiratory cycle or consider adding a uniform superior-inferior margin to the GTV and CTV drawn on the average scan to account for motion throughout the breathing cycle

   (ii) Deep inspiration breath-hold technique

   (iii) Abdominal compression (may increase lung dose when mediastinum or lung undergoing treatment, due to smaller lung volumes)

- Deep inspiration breath hold might be considered for patients with mediastinal involvement to help pull the heart away from the disease involvement and to increase lung volume, which may help reduce overall dose to the heart and lungs. This must be done with care, and it is important to have the staging CT scan performed with a breath-hold technique, to reduce uncertainties in image registration.

(i) Image guidance can be done with orthogonal kV imaging, CT on rails, or cone-beam CT scan.

   (i) The advantage of CT on rails or cone-beam CT is that the patient can undergo soft tissue alignment. However, patients are exposed to higher doses of radiation with this type of IGRT. Some consider subtracting this additional daily dose from the planned daily treatment (i.e., .05 Gy from IGRT/day and 1.75 Gy/day for RT treatment).

   (ii) The advantage to orthogonal kV imaging is that there is less radiation dose compared with a cone-beam CT scan or CT on rails. However, bony alignment or fiducial alignment is generally used, since the soft tissue cannot be seen well. Special attention to the alignment of clavicles can be helpful when axilla, infraclavicular, or supraclavicular regions are being treated.

## 5    Radiation Dose

- Pediatric patients are generally treated per specific pediatric protocols. In general, these protocols generally omit radiation in patients with rapid early response midway through chemotherapy and a complete response following chemotherapy, while patients with slow response or bulky mediastinal mass generally receive radiation doses of 21 Gy. Radiation oncologists should review the specific protocol the patient was treated to clarify the radiation dose and field design appropriate for the patient's care.

- Patients with early stage (I–IIA) non-bulky disease and with a complete response (by CT scan criteria) after 2 cycles of ABVD may do well with an additional 2 cycles of ABVD without any radiation (Meyer et al. 2012).

- Patients treated with favorable risk early stage disease that meets the entry criteria for the German Hodgkin Study Group protocol can receive 20 Gy (2 Gy/fraction × 10 fractions) as consolidation following 2 cycles of ABVD (Engert et al. 2010).

- Patients who do not meet the entry criteria for GHSG protocol should receive 30–36 Gy (1.8–2 Gy/fraction) as consolidation following chemotherapy (Hoppe et al. 2012a).

- Patients with residual PET avid disease > background level of the liver (Deauville criteria 4 or 5) should receive higher doses of radiation to 39.6–45 Gy (Hoppe et al. 2012a).

- Patients receiving definitive treatment for lymphocyte-predominant Hodgkin lymphoma without chemotherapy should receive doses of 30–36 Gy (Hoppe et al. 2012a).

## 6    Target Volume Delineation and Treatment Planning

- Treatment fields that have been used for Hodgkin lymphoma (in decreasing size) are total lymphoid (TL), subtotal lymphoid (STL), extended field (EF), involved field (IF), involved site (IS), and involved node (IN) irradiation.

- The larger fields (TL, STL, and EF irradiation) are infrequently used, due to common management with combined modality therapy. Clinical trials have shown an equivalence between IF and larger fields in this setting.

- IF irradiation is poorly defined. It is meant to be a field that includes the Ann Arbor lymph node groups involved with lymphoma at the time of diagnosis, but variations in the definition were employed by different investigators or clinical trial groups. The field borders were developed at the time of 2D simulation techniques, when field borders were generally determined based on bony landmarks and the concepts of GTV, CTV, and PTV were not utilized (Yahalom and Mauch 2002).

- IS and IN irradiation are intended to replace IF (Specht et al. 2013; Girinsky et al. 2006). These treatment fields incorporate modern ICRU definitions for GTV, CTV, ITV, and PTV and encourage the use of highly conformal treatment planning to help reduce radiation exposure to the OARs. In some treatment protocols, such as after 12 weeks of Stanford V or in patients with Stage III/IV disease, the radiation field is the IS to just the areas of bulky disease or slow-responding disease, excluding all other areas Table 1.

(i) The gross tumor volume (GTVr) is the residual disease seen at the time of CT simulation and can be visualized best with IV contrast.

(ii) The clinical target volume (CTV) includes all of the disease prior to chemotherapy. This includes the most superior and inferior extension of disease at presentation (GTVp), even if it has significantly regressed. However, normal structures that were clearly uninvolved should be excluded from the CTV. For example, a large bulky mediastinal mass, should not have the CTV extend into the lung on the CT simulation. Rather the post-chemotherapy lateral extension of the mediastinal disease should be used. This is best delineated after registering the CT simulation with the pre-chemotherapy PET/CT scan. When a perfect fusion exists between the CT simulation and the pretreatment PET/CT scan, the CTV delineated is consistent with IN irradiation. In most cases the fusion between the pretreatment PET/CT and CT simulation is not perfect. In that case, a margin needs to be considered to address the uncertainty of the fusion, and the CTV delineated is defined as IS irradiation.

(iii) When involving a structure that moves with the respiration, an ITV margin can be added based on the 4D CT scan. When no respiratory motion occurs, the ITV is the same as the CTV.

(iv) The planning target volume (PTV) includes the ITV with a margin to account for setup uncertainties. When using a face mask for immobilization with daily IGRT, then a 5 mm margin could be used. If the thorax is targeted, then a larger PTV margin should be considered of 5–8 mm. The larger the field, the more likely there will be setup uncertainty, and consideration of even larger margins is warranted. When IGRT is not being used, larger margins should be used of 10–15 mm depending on the region of interest.

(v) Patients with nodular lymphocyte-predominant Hodgkin lymphoma NOT receiving chemotherapy represent a unique group. Involved lymph nodes should still be present and contoured as GTV. The lymph node chain where the involved nodes are located should be contoured on the axial image as the CTV (to include the GTV) and should be extended to include interruptions between the involved nodes and extended superiorly and inferiorly 2–4 cm. In a recent poll of radiation oncology lymphoma experts, the majority (>60 %) felt the extension should be 4 cm.

- Effective treatment plans may include 3D CRT, IMRT, VMAT, or proton therapy. Although more conformal techniques reduce the high dose region, one must be mindful of the increased volume of low dose radiation exposure that may occur (especially with IMRT and VMAT). Doses as low as 5 Gy have been associated with increased risk of radiation-induced breast cancer, lung cancer, and cardiac mortality in long-term survivors of Hodgkin lymphoma (Travis et al. 2002; Travis et al. 2003; Tukenova et al. 2010).

(i) 3D CRT is generally done with AP/PA field arrangement; however, alternative field arrangement can be used to reduce the dose to the OARs.

(ii) When treating mediastinal fields with IMRT, consider avoiding lateral fields, which may increase lung dose unnecessarily.

(iii) When proton therapy is being used, try to use fewer fields to reduce integral dose. When anterior mediastinal disease is present, try to just use anterior fields to reduce the dose to the heart (Hoppe et al. 2012b).

- DVH analysis

(i) CTV and PTV coverage should be the highest priority. In general, the CTV D99%=100 %, 95 % of the PTV should receive 100 % of the dose, and 100 % of the PTV should receive 95 % of the dose. In some cases, target coverage must be compromised to reduced dose to the OAR. In that case, the authors try and get 95 % of the PTV covered by 95 % of the dose.

(ii) OAR constraints include mean lung dose <14–17 Gy, mean heart dose <15–20 Gy, mean total parotid dose <20–26 Gy, and maximum spinal cord dose <45 Gy.

(iii) Occasionally, one must increase the dose to one OAR to reduce the dose to another OAR. Based on causes of death in long-term survivors, the OAR most responsible for death is the heart. On the other hand, the most frequently encountered radiation-induced cancers are the lung (men) and breast (women). Consequently, the authors consider dose to the heart, lung, breast, stomach, and thyroid especially given that doses as low as 5 Gy or higher have been associated with increased risk of cardiac mortality and secondary cancers.

## 7 Cases

- A 75-year-old woman with stage IA favorable non-bulky nodular sclerosing Hodgkin lymphoma involving left-sided periparotid and upper cervical lymph nodes, who received 2 cycles of ABVD and consented to consolidative ISRT to 20 Gy (2 Gy/fraction × 10 fractions).

(i) Figure 1a reveals the sagittal view of the image fusion between the pretreatment PET/CT scan and the CT simulation. Notice poor fusion due to PET/CT scan

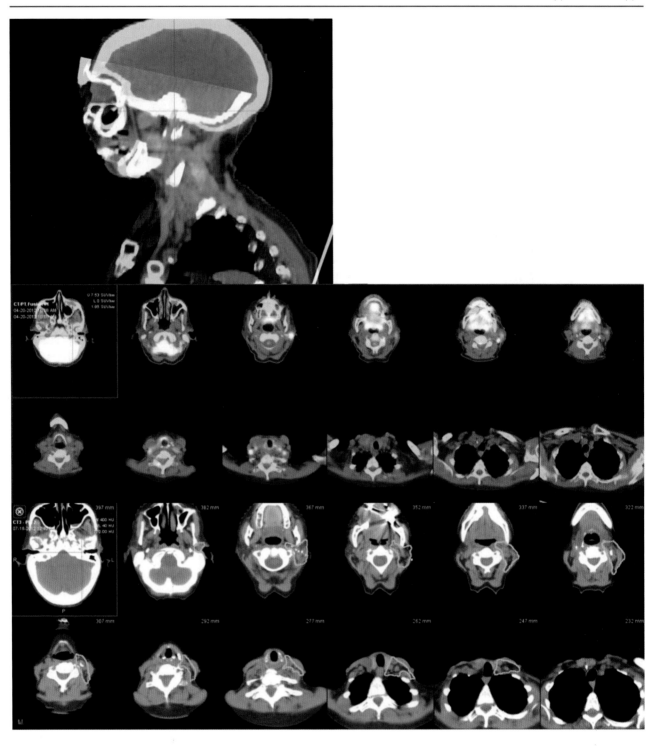

**Fig. 1**

being done with a flexed neck on a pillow and the CT sim with neck positioned neutral in a head rest.

(ii) Figure 1b reveals the pretreatment PET/CT scan. What is not seen is the excised periparotid lymph node that was performed prior to the PET/CT scan as part of the excisional biopsy. Normal uptake is seen in the brain, base of tongue, floor of mouth, and salivary glands. Additionally, uptake is seen bilater- ally on images in the 2nd row, 2nd and 3rd from the left and was attributed to muscle activity and not involved lymph nodes. PET activity correlating with disease includes the surgical bed around the parotid (row 1, image 3–6 from the left), the cervical lymph node (row 1, image 5). An additional cervical node is located between the 3rd and 4th image in row 2, but cannot be seen on these wide cuts.

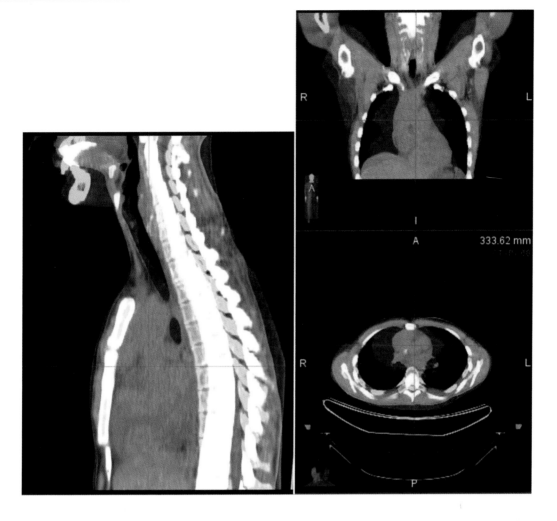

**Fig. 2**

(iii) Figure 1c reveals the CT simulation with the CTV outlined in green. Note the wire outlining the cervical scar in the 1st row, 4th image from the left. Extra margin was included on the CTV, due to the poor fusion between the two scans.

- A 21-year-old male with stage IIA bulky (17 cm in greatest transverse dimension) nodular sclerosing Hodgkin lymphoma involving the following regions: right supraclavicular and anterior mediastinal ending onto the diaphragm. The patient was treated with 6 cycles of ABVD chemotherapy with a complete response by PET scan, but a PR by CT scan. The patient received 30.6 Gy at 1.8 Gy/fraction as consolidation.

  (i) Figure 2a demonstrates a reasonably good fusion between the pre-chemotherapy PET/CT scan in red and the CT simulation in gray from a standpoint of the normal anatomy. On the coronal and axial images, one can appreciate the considerable regression in tumor size, which can lead to changes in normal anatomy positioning, especially with regard to the lung and heart.

  (ii) Figure 2b represents the fused axial images from the pretreatment PET/CT scan (bottom) and CT simulation (top). GTV is contoured in pink, and CTV is contoured in blue. Due to extension of the initial mass along the anterior pericardium, the initial extension along the pericardium is used as the lateral border. Some disagreement exists among radiation oncology lymphoma experts whether to include the pretreatment pericardial extension in a recent poll. However, the majority (>70 %), including these authors, used the pre-chemotherapy extension along the pericardium as depicted in this case in blue. A 32-year-old female with stage IIB bulky (15 cm greatest transverse dimension) nodular sclerosing Hodgkin lymphoma involving the following lymph node groups: bilateral cervical, bilateral supraclavicular, left axilla, left infraclavicular/subpectoral, mediastinal, left internal mammary, and left diaphragmatic. The patient received 4 cycles of ABVD complicated by bleomycin toxicity with a complete response by PET/CT scan.

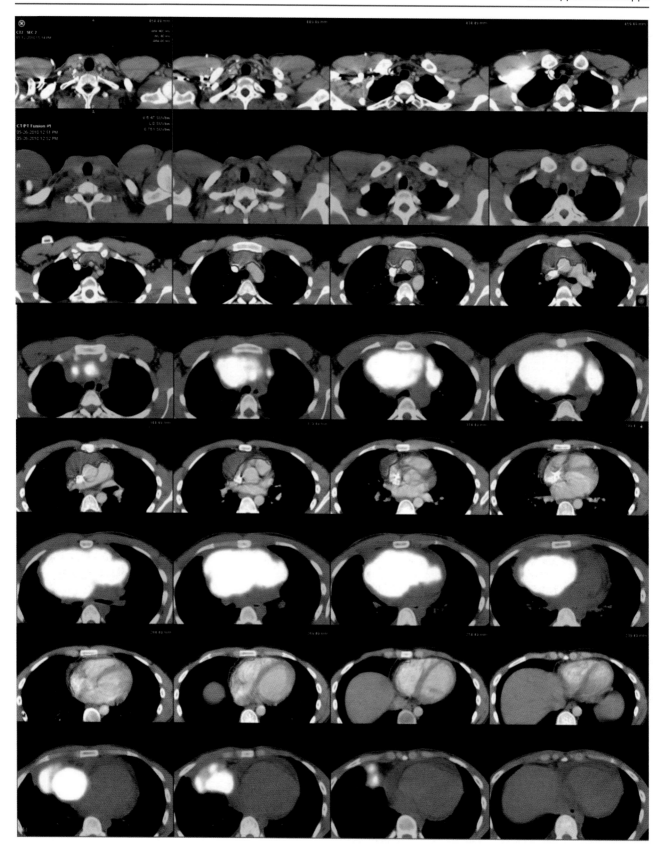

**Fig. 2** (continued)

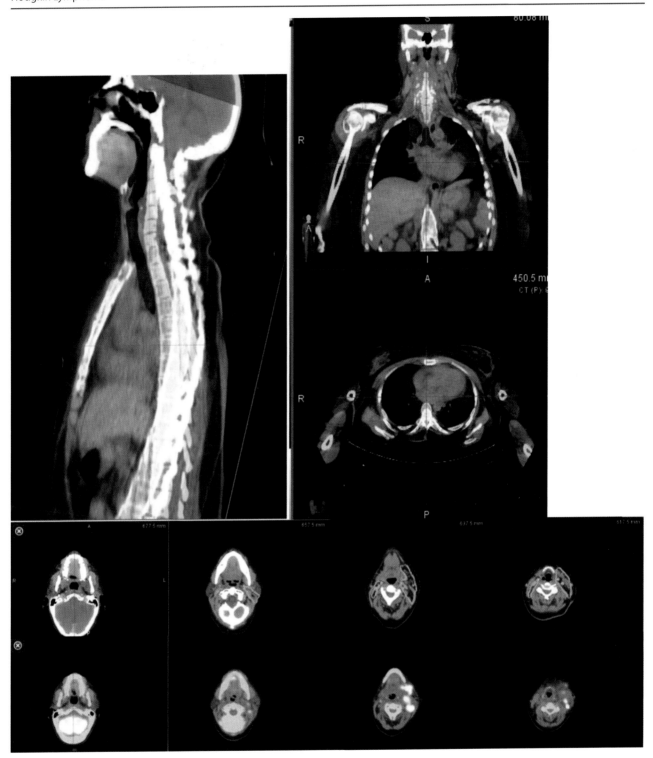

**Fig. 3**

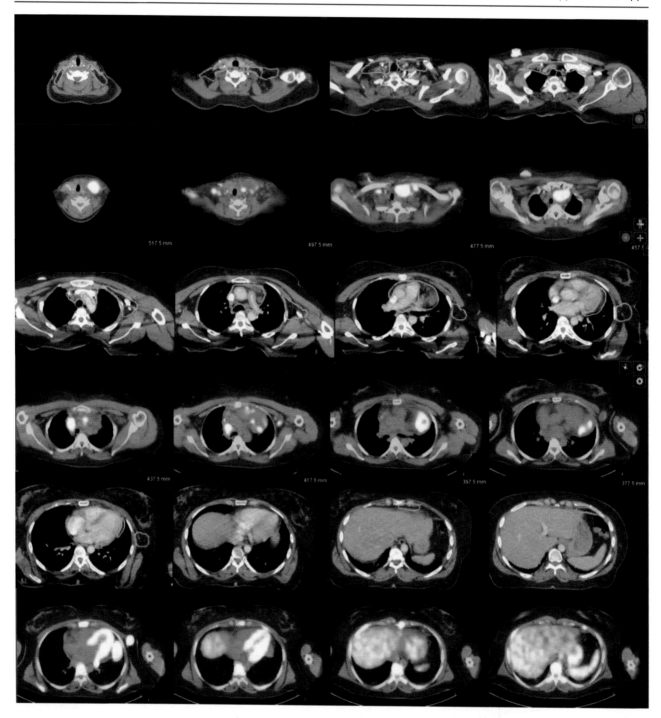

**Fig. 3** (continued)

(i) Figure 3a demonstrates the registration between the pre-chemotherapy PET/CT scan in red and the CT simulation in gray. Notice poor alignment of the spine and neck on sagittal view, due to a flexed neck at time of PET/CT scan and slightly extended neck at simulation. On axial image, one can appreciate the difference in arm position (despite both being by the patient's side), due to the need to lower arms to allow for fields

to treat the axillary region. In patients with large fields, sometimes the registration between the two scans must be performed multiple times throughout the planning process to ensure the most accurate contouring.

(ii) Figure 3b demonstrates the fused axial images from the pre-chemotherapy PET/CT scan (bottom) and the CT simulation (top). The CTV is depicted in green. Larger volumes are located in the axilla, due

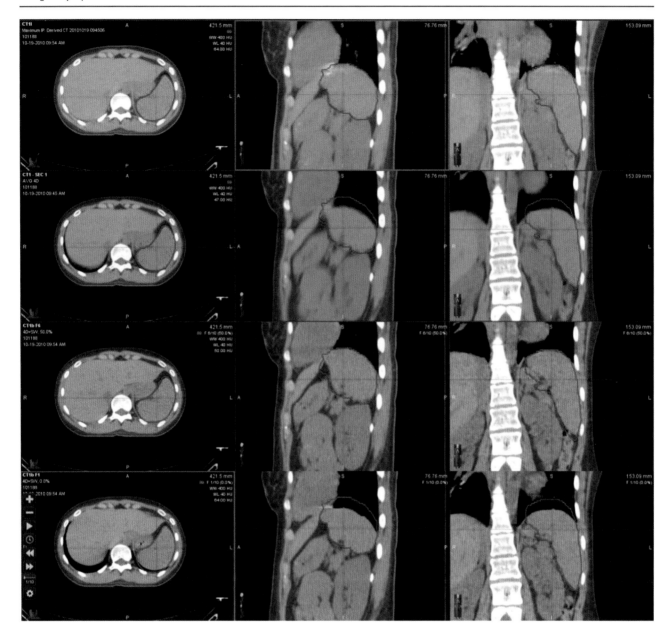

**Fig. 4**

to larger uncertainties regarding the location of the axillary node because of different arm position. The last two slices demonstrate the CTV to cover the diaphragmatic nodes. In a recent survey, most (>70 %) radiation oncology lymphoma experts would include the prior involved diaphragmatic nodes in the CTV as depicted in these slices.

• A 20-year-old female with stage IV mixed cellularity Hodgkin lymphoma was initially treated with BEACOPP × 8 cycles, then relapsed 1 year later in the bilateral neck, mediastinum, para-aortics, and spleen. She received 2nd-line chemotherapy with ICE × 3 with a complete response except within the spleen. The patient went on to receive high-dose chemotherapy with BEAM followed by autologous stem cell rescue (ASCR). Recommendations were made for consolidative radiotherapy to the spleen following recovery from her ASCR to 30.6 Gy at 1.8 Gy/fraction.

(i) Figure 4a demonstrates the spleen movement with respiration and demonstrates the MIP(maximum intensity projection), AVG (average scan), 50 % phase of the respiratory cycle, and the 0 % phase of the respiratory cycle. The spleen from the MIP image is contoured in pink and superimposed on the other scans to demonstrate the movement of the spleen with respiration.

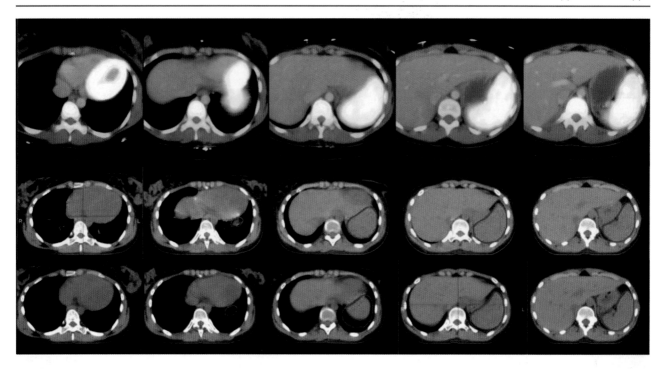

**Fig. 4** (continued)

(ii) Figure 4b represents the axial images from the pre-ASCR PET/CT scan with the PET avid spleen (top), MIP axial images (middle), and average images from the 4D CT simulation (bottom). The spleen as contoured on the MIP is the CTV in pink.

• A 40-year-old male with stage IIA nodular lymphocyte-predominant Hodgkin lymphoma involving the bilateral iliacs and bilateral inguinal regions. The patient was treated to 30.6 Gy at 1.8 Gy/fraction without chemotherapy.

(i) Figure 5 shows a PET/CT simulation scan with the involved nodes contoured in yellow and the CTV contoured in blue. Normal PET activity is seen in the bowel, bladder, and testis.

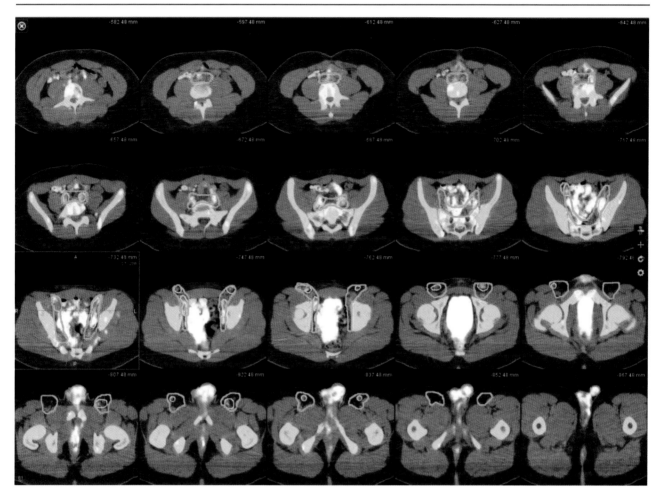

**Fig. 5**

## References

Engert A, Plutschow A, Eich HT et al (2010) Reduced treatment intensity in patients with early-stage Hodgkin's lymphoma. N Engl J Med 363(7):640–652

Girinsky T, van der Maazen R, Specht L et al (2006) Involved-node radiotherapy (INRT) in patients with early Hodgkin lymphoma: concepts and guidelines. Radiother Oncol 79(3):270–277

Hoppe RT, Advani RH, Ai WZ et al (2012a) Hodgkin lymphoma, version 2.2012 featured updates to the NCCN guidelines. J Natl Compr Canc Netw 10(5):589–597

Hoppe BS, Flampouri S, Su Z et al (2012b) Consolidative involved-node proton therapy for Stage IA-IIIB mediastinal Hodgkin lymphoma: preliminary dosimetric outcomes from a Phase II study. Int J Radiat Oncol Biol Phys 83(1):260–267

Illidge T, Specht L, Yahalom J (2014) Modern Radiation Therapy for Nodal Non-Hodgkin Lymphoma—Target Definition and Dose Guidelines From the International Lymphoma Radiation Oncology Group. IJROBP 89 (1):49–58

Meyer RM, Gospodarowicz MK, Connors JM et al (2012) ABVD alone versus radiation-based therapy in limited-stage Hodgkin's lymphoma. N Engl J Med 366(5):399–408

Specht L, Yahalom J, Illidge T et al (2013) Modern radiation therapy for Hodgkin lymphoma: field and dose guidelines from the International Lymphoma Radiation Oncology Group (ILROG). Int J Radiat Oncol Biol Phys

Travis LB, Gospodarowicz M et al (2002) Lung cancer following chemotherapy and radiotherapy for Hodgkin's disease. J Natl Cancer Inst 94:182–92

Travis LB, Hill DA et al (2003) Breast cancer following radiotherapy and chemotherapy among young women with Hodgkin disease. JAMA 290:465–75

Tukenova M, Guibout C et al (2010) Role of cancer treatment in long-term overall and cardiovascular mortality after childhood cancer. J Clin Oncol 28:1308–15.

Yahalom J, Mauch P (2002) The involved field is back: issues in delineating the radiation field in Hodgkin's disease. Ann Oncol 13(Suppl 1):79–83

# Non-Hodgkin Lymphoma

Sara Alcorn, Harold Agbahiwe, and Stephanie Terezakis

## Contents

S. Alcorn • S. Terezakis (✉)
Department of Radiation Oncology and Molecular Radiation
Sciences, The Johns Hopkins Hospital, Baltimore, MD, USA
e-mail: sterezak@jhmi.edu

H. Agbahiwe
Department of Radiation Oncology, Sibley Memorial Hospital,
Johns Hopkins Medicine, Washington, DC, USA

N.Y. Lee et al. (eds.), *Target Volume Delineation for Conformal and Intensity-Modulated Radiation Therapy*,
Medical Radiology. Radiation Oncology, DOI: 10.1007/174_2014_997, © Springer International Publishing Switzerland 2014
Published Online: 1 November 2014

# 1    Introduction

**Table 1**  ILROG planning definitions for ISRT in lymphoma (Specht et al. 2013; Illidge 2014)

| Volume | | Description |
|---|---|---|
| Gross tumor volume (GTV) | Pre-chemotherapy/surgery GTV (GTVp) | Contains gross tumor volume as identified on diagnostic imaging prior to chemotherapy and/or surgery |
| | Post-chemotherapy/surgery GTV (GTVr) | Contains gross tumor volume as identified on diagnostic and/or planning imaging after management with chemotherapy and/or surgery |
| | No prior treatment GTV (GTV) | Contains gross tumor volume identified on diagnostic and/or planning imaging in the absence of prior chemotherapy or surgery (e.g., in the case of primary or salvage RT) |
| Clinical target volume (CTV) | | Contains entire post-chemotherapy/surgery or "no prior treatment" GTV |
| | | Generally contains pre-chemotherapy/surgery GTV (unless volume is unable to be safely treating in its entirety) |
| | | Excludes extent of pre-chemotherapy/surgery GTV that displaced normal, uninvolved tissue (bone, organs, muscles, etc.) prior to chemotherapy or surgery |
| | | Includes consideration of the following:<br><br>Image accuracy and quality. CTV should be increased in size to account for uncertainties such as suboptimal fusion of pre- and post-chemotherapy/surgery images to planning images or in the absence of pre-chemotherapy/surgery images<br><br>Changes in volume since the time of imaging<br><br>Pattern of disease spread<br><br>Potential subclinical involvement. Consider including nodes of unknown status near the site of disease, particularly if the questionable nodes belong to a nodal chain or group already partially encompassed by the CTV<br><br>Adjacent organ dose constraints |
| | | Can contain separate nodal volumes if ≤5 cm apart. Lesions >5 cm apart are treated with separate CTVs |
| Internal target volume (ITV) | | Contains the CTV plus an internal margin that accounts for variation in CTV shape, size, and position (e.g., target movement with respiration) |
| | | Most relevant for targets within the chest and abdomen; may be unnecessary for other sites |
| Planning target volume (PTV) | | Contains CTV or ITV plus a margin to account for setup uncertainties associated with patient position and beam alignment |
| | | *Note that CTV to PTV expansions are patient- and institution-specific; any recommendations in this chapter or elsewhere must be adjusted to reflect factors unique to the patient and institution* |
| Organs at risk (OAR) | | Includes uninvolved normal structures at risk of RT-related toxicity for which RT planning or dose may be altered |

# 2    Background

- Non-Hodgkin lymphoma (NHL) is a heterogeneous group of B-cell, T-cell, and natural killer (NK)-cell neoplasms that lack the pathologic characteristics seen in Hodgkin disease (HD).
- The World Health Organization (WHO) has classified approximately 80 unique forms of NHL (Swerdlow et al. 2008). These are traditionally grouped by tumor aggres-siveness into indolent, aggressive, and highly aggressive NHL categories, as described in Table 2.
- NHL can be further divided into nodal versus extra-nodal lymphomas. Although treatment of both nodal and extra-nodal NHL depends on tumor aggressiveness, extent of disease, and response to systemic therapies, management of extra-nodal lymphoma with radiother-apy (RT) is more clearly driven by site-specific considerations.

## 2.1 Evolution of Radiation Fields for Lymphoma

- Historically, HD and NHL were managed with RT alone using extended fields such as mantle and inverted Y configurations, with higher rates of late toxicity associated with larger field size (Fig. 1a, b).
- By the 1990s, combined modality therapy became a mainstay of lymphoma management. With the addition of increasingly successful chemotherapies and advancements in target localization such as 3D simulation, RT fields have become progressively smaller (Fig. 1).
- Until recently, the standard of care for RT in both HD and NHL was involved field radiotherapy (IFRT). This began to change in 2006, when EORTC-GELA Lymphoma Group published guidelines for involved nodal radiotherapy (INRT) for HD (Girinsky et al. 2006) (Fig. 1c).
- Unlike traditional IFRT fields that treat adjacent uninvolved lymph nodes, INRT limits treatment to only pre- and post-chemotherapy involved nodal volumes plus margin. Whereas IFRT traditionally uses bony landmarks to identify field borders, INRT volumes are delineated using definitions of gross tumor volume (GTV), clinical target volume (CTV), and planning target volume (PTV) per the International Commission on Radiation Units and Measurements (ICRU) Report 83 (Hodapp 2012).
- However, INRT requires precisely fused pre- and post-chemotherapy imaging performed in the treatment position, which is often unattainable in clinical practice. To address this limitation, the International Lymphoma Radiation Oncology Group (ILROG) published consensus guidelines for the use of involved site radiotherapy (ISRT) for HD (Specht et al. 2013). ISRT targets the sites of pre- and post-chemotherapy disease involvement but also offers less stringent treatment volume definitions than ISRT to allow for uncertainties associated with less than optimal imaging.
- ILROG has recently published consensus guidelines for the use of ISRT for nodal NHL(reference below), with similar guidelines pending for extra-nodal NHL (Illidge 2014). Although ISRT for NHL has not yet been validated through randomized trials, single-arm and retrospective data suggest comparable control with such reduced field sizes (Campbell et al. 2010; Zhang et al. 2012; Yu et al. 2010).
- As ISRT is evolving to be the standard of care for RT in NHL, this chapter will focus on ISRT for both nodal and extra-nodal lymphomas. For recommendations regarding involved fields, reference should be made to Yahalom and Mauch's guidelines for IFRT in HD (Yahalom and Mauch 2002).

**Table 2** Select non-Hodgkin lymphoma histologies arranged by tumor aggressiveness (Swerdlow et al. 2008; Pileri et al. 1998; National Cancer Institute 2014)

| Indolent | Aggressive | Highly aggressive |
|---|---|---|
| Follicular lymphoma (grades I and II) | Follicular lymphoma (grade III) | Burkitt's lymphoma |
| Marginal zone B-cell lymphoma: extra-nodal (MALT lymphoma), nodal (monocytoid), splenic | Diffuse large B-cell lymphoma (DLBCL) | Precursor B-cell or T-cell lymphoblastic lymphoma/ leukemia |
| Small lymphocytic lymphoma | Mantle cell lymphoma | |
| T-cell granular lymphocytic lymphoma | Anaplastic large cell lymphoma | |
| | Peripheral T-cell lymphoma | |
| | Angiocentric T-cell lymphoma | |
| | Angioimmunoblastic T-cell lymphoma | |

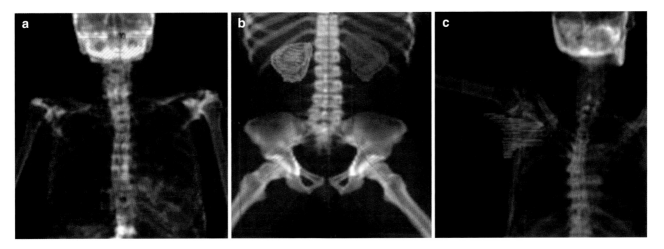

**Fig. 1** Historical RT fields. Digitally reconstructed radiographs (DRR) of (**a**) mantle and (**b**) inverted Y extended fields and (**c**) axilla involved field RT

**Table 3** Management of nodal B-cell NHL

| Aggressiveness | Stage[a] or clinical status | Treatment modality | RT dose (1.8–2 Gy fraction) | Target delineation considerations |
|---|---|---|---|---|
| Indolent B cell | Stages I–II | RT alone | 24–30 Gy | CTV should generously cover adjacent nodes when RT is used as definitive therapy (e.g., CTV of at least 1–2 cm depending on the clinical scenario) |
| | Stages III–IV | Rituximab, palliative RT, or observation | 4–30 Gy | – |
| Aggressive B cell | Stages I–II and favorable | R-CHOP×3–4 cycles+RT; R-CHOP×6–8 cycles | 30–36 Gy | For planned combined chemoRT, CTV includes entire pre-chemotherapy GTV (minus uninvolved displaced tissues) For RT to sites of residual disease, the treatment volume can be limited to sites with residual PET-avidity on post-chemotherapy imaging |
| | Stages I–II and unfavorable | R-CHOP×6–8 cycles +/− RT for sites of bulky disease or partial response | 30–40 Gy | |
| | Stages III–IV | R-CHOP×6–8 cycles +/− RT for sites of bulky disease or partial response | 30–40 Gy | |
| Highly aggressive | – | Chemotherapy alone, with palliative RT to symptomatic sites | 4–30 Gy | – |

*R-CHOP* rituximab, cyclophosphamide, doxorubicin, vincristine, and prednisone/prednisolone
[a]Traditionally by Ann Arbor staging system (Rosenberg 1977)

## 2.2 General Principles of Involved Site Radiotherapy

- ISRT requires 3D simulation with CT, PET-CT, or MRI. Pre-chemotherapy or pre-surgery diagnostic imaging is strongly recommended, particularly PET-CT with IV contrast as well as PO contrast for abdominopelvic sites. Post-chemotherapy PET-CT is also useful for identifying areas of residual FDG avidity.
- These studies should be fused to simulation imaging when feasible. Although not a requirement for ISRT, diagnostic imaging should be performed in the treatment position whenever possible to optimize fusion.
- The ILROG volume definitions for ISRT are summarized in Table 1 (Specht et al. 2013; Illidge 2014).
- Simulation and immobilization will be discussed by treatment site.

## 3 Nodal NHL

### 3.1 Principles of Management

- In nodal NHL, RT may be indicated as primary therapy; consolidation following chemotherapy for bulky, residual, or unfavorable disease; or salvage for chemotherapy-refractory or recurrent disease.

- RT dose varies by tumor aggressive, extent of disease and chemotherapy response.
- See Table 3 for management strategies of nodal B-cell NHL (Illidge 2014).

### 3.2 General Considerations for Cervical/Supraclavicular Nodal ISRT

- The patient should be simulated in the supine position with hyperextension of the neck and the use of a long thermoplastic mask extending to the shoulder region for immobilization.
- 3D simulation should be performed with IV contrast.
- GTV to CTV margin should be at least 1 cm. If applicable, the final CTV should also encompass the pre-chemotherapy/surgery GTV extent, excluding normal, uninvolved tissue that was displaced by the tumor prior to chemotherapy or surgery.
- Relevant OARs include the cervical spinal cord, brachial plexus, and salivary glands.
- For treatment with AP/PA technique:
  - A posterior cervical cord block can be placed if cord dose exceeds 36 Gy.
  - A posterior mouth block is recommended to inhibit divergence through the mouth.
  - A laryngeal block can be added after 18 Gy or a 50% partial transmission laryngeal block can be used for

the full duration of treatment unless prohibited by the presence of medial cervical lymph nodes (Fig. 2).

## 3.3 General Considerations for Axillary Nodal ISRT

- The patient should be simulated in the supine position with a custom mold for immobilization. In adults, treatment with arms above the head shifts axillary nodes away from the chest wall and improves the ability to block the lungs. In children, treatment with arms akimbo allows for improved blocking of the humeral heads, which protects sensitive epiphyseal growth plates.
- 3D simulation should be performed with IV contrast.

- GTV to CTV margin should be at least 1 cm. If applicable, the final CTV should also encompass the pre-chemotherapy/surgery GTV extent, excluding normal, uninvolved tissue that was displaced by the tumor prior to chemotherapy or surgery.
- Relevant OARs include the cervical and thoracic spinal cord, brachial plexus, and lungs (Fig. 3).

## 3.4 General Considerations for Mediastinal Nodal ISRT

- The patient should be simulated in the supine position with a custom mold for immobilization. Arms may be placed at the sides, akimbo, or above the head.

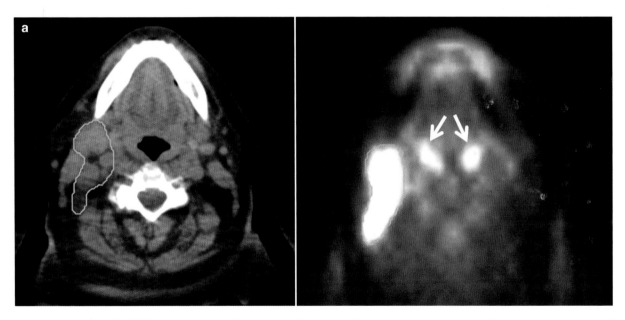

**Fig. 2** (**a–c**) Cervical nodal ISRT planning images for a patient with stage IA diffuse large B-cell lymphoma with near-complete response after three cycles of R-CHOP. (**a**) The pre-chemotherapy FDG-avid GTV is delineated in purple. Also noted is benign physiologic pharyngeal uptake (*white arrows*). There were no other areas of FDG-avid disease. (**b**) Axial CT slices from the post-chemotherapy planning CT (*left column*) and the pre-chemotherapy PET-CT (*right column*) are fused to create a pre-chemotherapy GTV (*orange*), post-chemotherapy GTV (*red*), and CTV (*green*). Fusion of the two image sets is limited by differences in neck extension and arm position; this is particularly noticeable when locating the region of the pre-chemotherapy right level IV lymph node on the post-chemotherapy planning CT (*red arrows*). To account for greater uncertainty in target localization, the CTV in the corresponding regions is larger than the typical 1 cm CTV expansion. (**c**) post-chemotherapy GTV (*red*), CTV (*green*), and PTV (*blue*) are shown in on (*1*) coronal, (*2*) sagittal, and (*3*) axial slices. In this case, the GTV to CTV expansion is at least 1 cm, and the CTV to PTV expansion is 0.5 cm. Note that CTV to PTV margins depend on patient- and institution-specific factors, and therefore, universal recommendations for appropriate expansions cannot be provided

Post-chemotheragy          Pre-chemotheragy

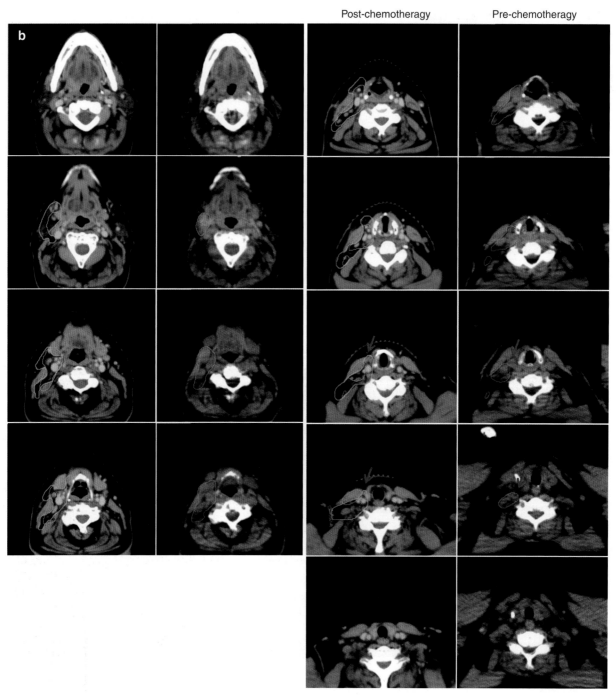

**Fig. 2** (continued)

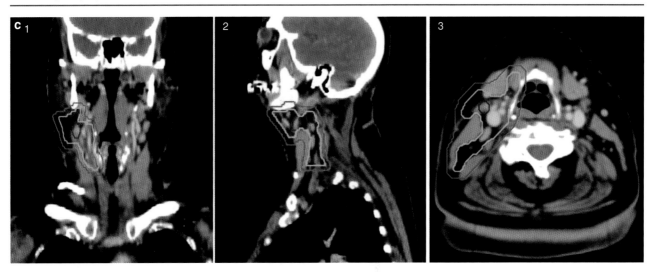

**Fig. 2** (continued)

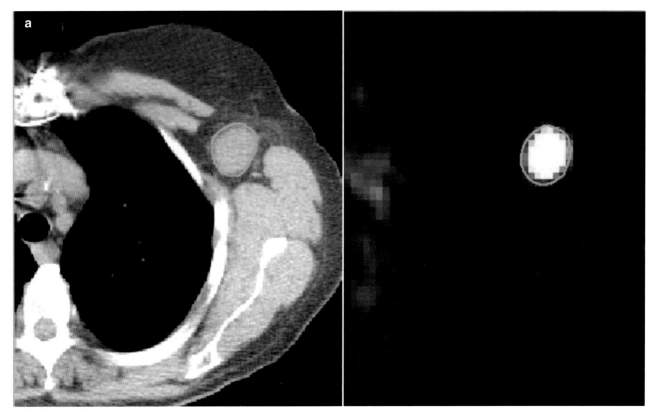

**Fig. 3** (**a–c**) Axillary nodal ISRT planning images for a patient with a history of stage IIIA diffuse large B-cell lymphoma with initial complete response following six cycles of R-CHOP. Within 18 months, the patient was found to have a single site of FDG-avid recurrence in the left axilla and elected ISRT as a first step in salvage therapy. (**a**) A single area of recurrent FDG-avid disease (*purple*) is seen in the left axilla on PET-CT. (**b**) Axial slices from the planning CT demonstrate the FDG-avid GTV (*red*) and CTV (*green*). Small lymph nodes of unknown status that were not FDG avid were included in the treatment volume, as they were felt to be suspicious for lymphomatous involvement. Note the GTV of interest in this case is the "no prior treatment" GTV, which should generally be used if there has been considerable time between last chemotherapy and current RT. (**c**) GTV (*red*), CTV (*green*), and PTV (*blue*) are shown in on (*1*) coronal, (*2*) sagittal, and (*3*) axial slices. In this case, the GTV to CTV expansion is at least 1 cm, and the CTV to PTV expansion is 0.5 cm. Note that CTV to PTV margins depend on patient- and institution-specific factors, and therefore, universal recommendations for appropriate expansions cannot be provided

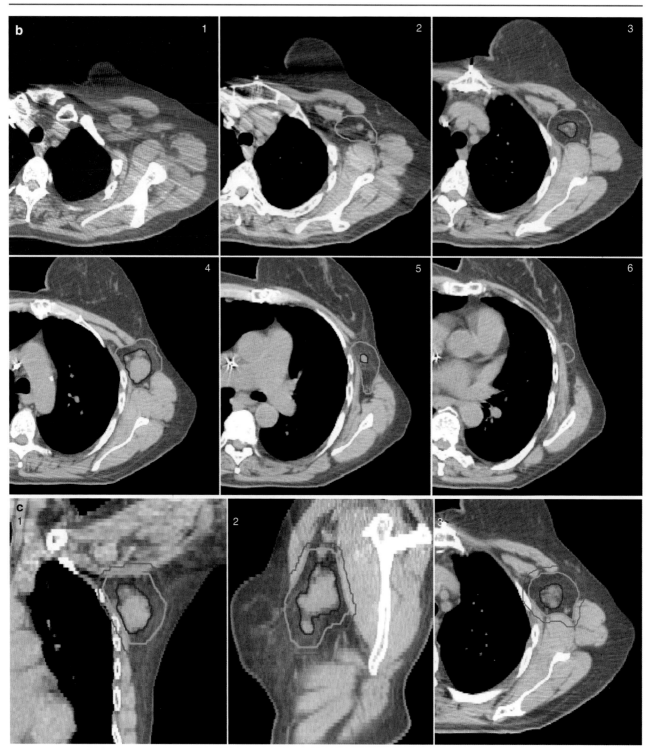

**Fig. 3** (continued)

- 3D simulation should be performed with IV contrast. As target movement with respiration may be seen, 4DCT or fluoroscopy, with consideration for deep inspiration breath hold, is recommended to allow for creation of an ITV.
- GTV to CTV/ITV margin should be at least 1 cm. If applicable, the final CTV/ITV should also encompass the pre-chemotherapy/surgery GTV extent, excluding normal, uninvolved tissue that was displaced by the tumor prior to chemotherapy or surgery.
- Relevant OARs include the thoracic spinal cord, lungs, and esophagus. The RTOG breast contouring atlas (White et al.) may be used to estimate and avoid excessive radiation dose, particularly in young females (Fig. 4).

## 3.5 General Considerations for Para-aortic Nodal ISRT

- The patient should be simulated in the supine position with a custom mold for immobilization. Arms may be placed on the chest or at the sides.
- 3D simulation should be performed with IV and PO contrast. As target movement with respiration may be seen, a 4DCT or fluoroscopy should be considered to allow for creation of an ITV.
- GTV to CTV/ITV margin should be at least 1 cm. If applicable, the final CTV/ITV should also encompass the pre-chemotherapy/surgery GTV extent, excluding nor-

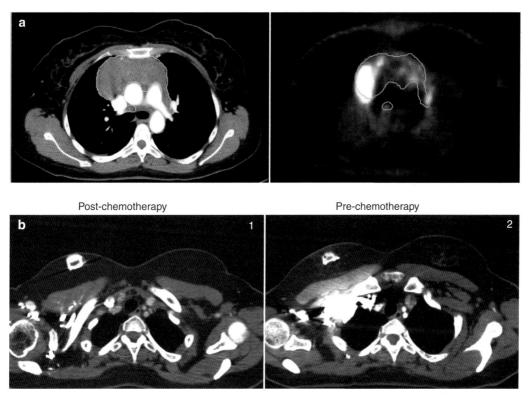

**Fig. 4** (**a–d**) Mediastinal nodal ISRT planning images for a patient with stage IIA diffuse large B-cell lymphoma with bulky mediastinal adenopathy, demonstrating response to six cycles of RCHOP. Post-chemotherapy imaging demonstrates response to six cycles of R-CHOP. (**a**) The initial FDG-avid volume is delineated in purple on pre-chemotherapy PET-CT. Note that planning accuracy can be limited by misregistration between the PET and CT components. Post-chemotherapy imaging demonstrated resolution of FDG avidity on PET and decreased size of the mediastinal soft tissue mass on CT. (**b**) Axial CT slices from post-chemotherapy planning CT (*left column*) and the pre-chemotherapy PET-CT (*right column*) are fused to create a pre-chemotherapy GTV (*orange*), post-chemotherapy GTV (*red*), and CTV (*green*). Fusion of the two image sets is limited by differences in arm positioning, which is particularly noticeable when locating the region of the pre-chemotherapy right subpectoral lymph node on the post-chemotherapy planning CT (*red arrow*). To account for greater uncer-

tainty in target localization, the CTV in the corresponding regions is larger than the typical 1 cm CTV expansion. Note that the CTV excludes normal, uninvolved tissue that was displaced by the tumor prior to chemotherapy. (**c**) The patient was simulated with a 4DCT to account for respiratory motion, and axial images from the free-breathing planning CT (*1*) were fused with images from two phases associated with maximum target excursion (*2, 3*). CTV was contoured on each phase independently. Image *4* shows all three CTVs overlaid on the free-breathing CT, and image *5* shows the ITV (*yellow*), determined by combining these volumes. (**d**) The post-chemotherapy GTV (*red*), ITV (*yellow*), and PTV (*blue*) are shown in on (*1*) coronal, (*2*) sagittal, and (*3*) axial slices. In this case, the GTV to CTV/ITV and the CTV/ITV to PTV expansion were both at least 1 cm. Note that CTV/ITV to PTV margins depend on patient- and institution-specific factors, and therefore, universal recommendations for appropriate expansions cannot be provided

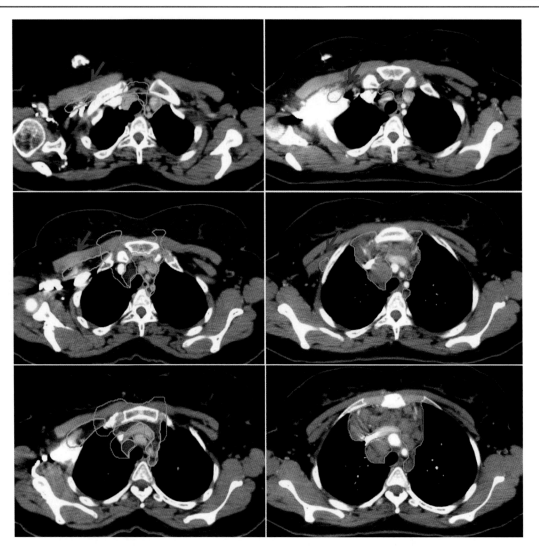

**Fig. 4** (continued)

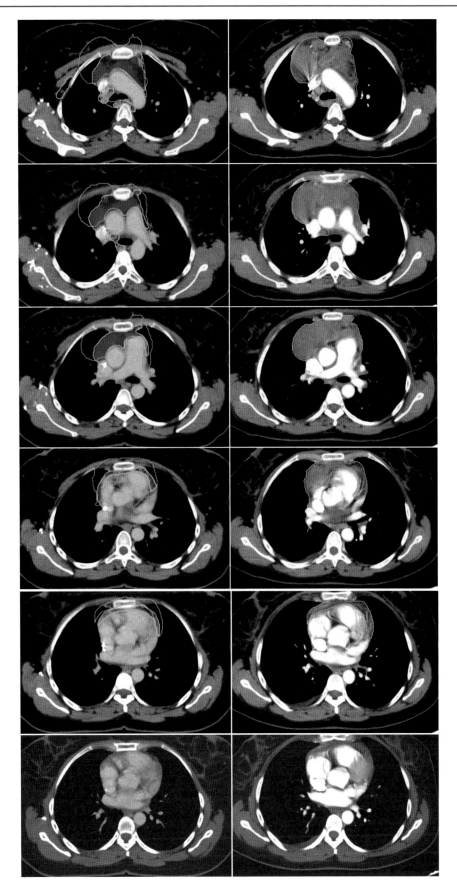

**Fig. 4** (continued)

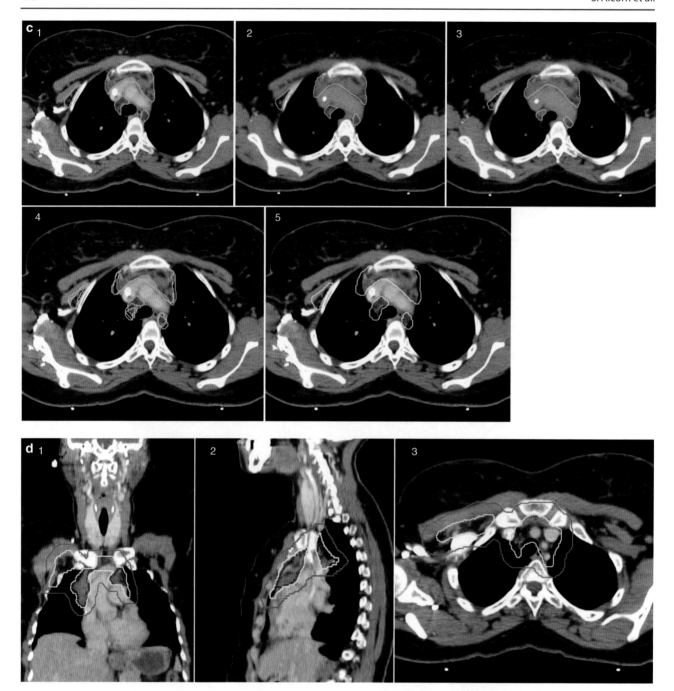

**Fig. 4** (continued)

mal, uninvolved tissue that was displaced by the tumor prior to chemotherapy or surgery.

- Relevant OARs include the thoracic and lumbar spinal cord, bowel, and kidneys.
- Consider testicular shielding, fertility counseling, egg or sperm banking, and/or repositioning of the ovaries if the reproductive organs are at risk (Fig. 5).

## 3.6 General Considerations for Pelvic and Inguinal ISRT

- The patient should be simulated in the supine position with a custom mold for immobilization. Arms may be placed on the chest or at the sides. If the inguinal nodes are treated, position the patient in the "frog-leg" position

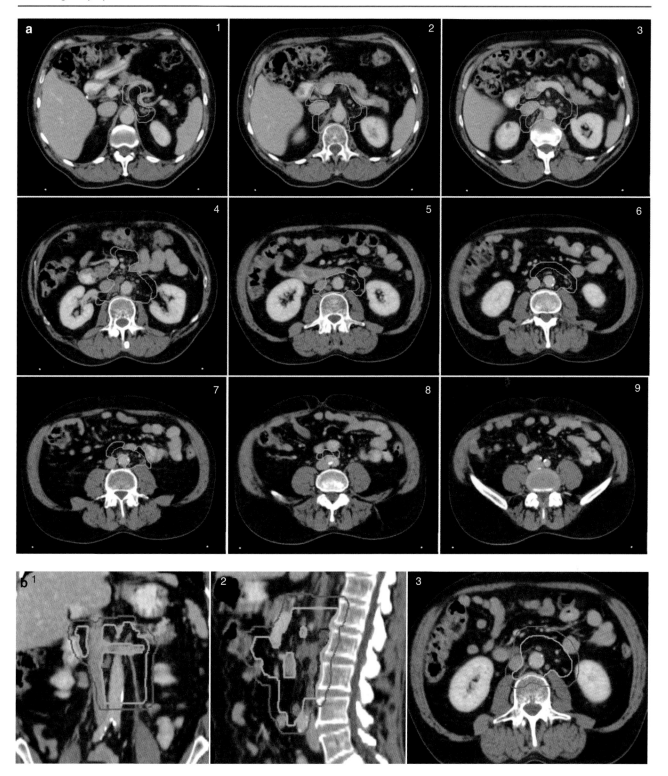

**Fig. 5** (**a, b**) Para-aortic nodal ISRT planning images for a patient with stage IVB diffuse large B-cell lymphoma with bulky para-aortic disease, showing response after six cycles of R-CHOP and four cycles of prophylactic intrathecal chemotherapy with cytarabine. PET-CT revealed residual FDG avidity in several small para-aortic lymph nodes. (**a**) Axial slices from the post-chemotherapy planning CT are shown. Pre-chemotherapy GTV (*orange*), post-chemotherapy GTV (*red*), and CTV (*green*) are delineated. Although both pre- and post-chemotherapy PET-CTs were performed, these could not be fused with the planning study. While this does not preclude management with ISRT, estimations of pre-chemotherapy GTV as well as CTV were generous to account for imaging uncertainties. Also note that the patient had several small involved lymph nodes ≤5 cm apart, which were able to be treated with the same CTV. (**b**) The post-chemotherapy GTV (*red*), CTV (*green*), and PTV (*blue*) are shown in (*1*) coronal, (*2*) sagittal, and (*3*) axial slices. In this case, the GTV to CTV and CTV to PTV expansions were both at least 1 cm. Note that CTV to PTV margins depend on patient- and institution-specific factors, and therefore, universal recommendations for appropriate expansions cannot be provided

Post-chemotherapy          Pre-chemotherapy

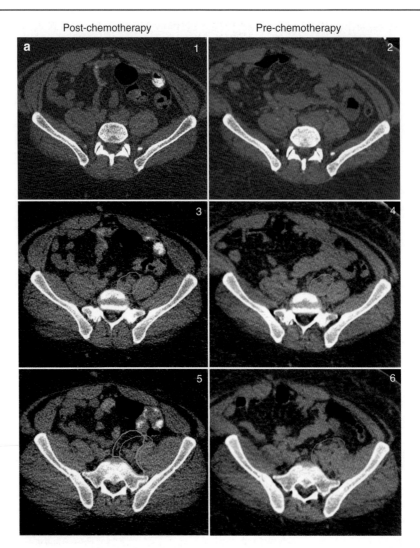

**Fig. 6** (**a**, **b**) Pelvic nodal ISRT planning images for a patient with stage IIIA diffuse large B-cell lymphoma with bulky pelvic adenopathy. The patient showed partial response after eight cycles of R-CHOP, with a residual pelvic mass. (**a**) Axial slices from post-chemotherapy planning CT (*left column*) and the pre-chemotherapy CT (*right column*) are fused to create a pre-chemotherapy GTV (*orange*), post-chemotherapy GTV (*red*), and CTV (*green*). The patient declined pre- and post-chemotherapy PET-CT and had renal insufficiency prohibiting IV contrast administration. Although these factors do not eliminate the option to treat with ISRT, they support the use of a generous CTV. Simulation was performed with PO contrast. Note that the CTV excludes normal, uninvolved tissue that was displaced by the tumor prior to chemotherapy. (**b**) The post-chemotherapy GTV (*red*), CTV (*green*), and PTV (*blue*) are shown in (*1*) coronal, (*2*) sagittal, and (*3*) axial slices. In this case, the GTV to CTV expansion is at least 1 cm, and the CTV to PTV expansion is 0.5 cm. Note that CTV to PTV margins depend on patient- and institution-specific factors, and therefore, universal recommendations for appropriate expansions cannot be provided

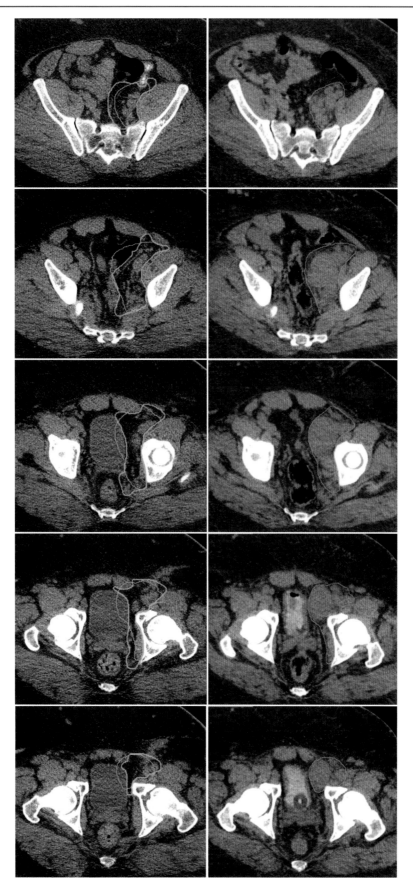

**Fig. 6** (continued)

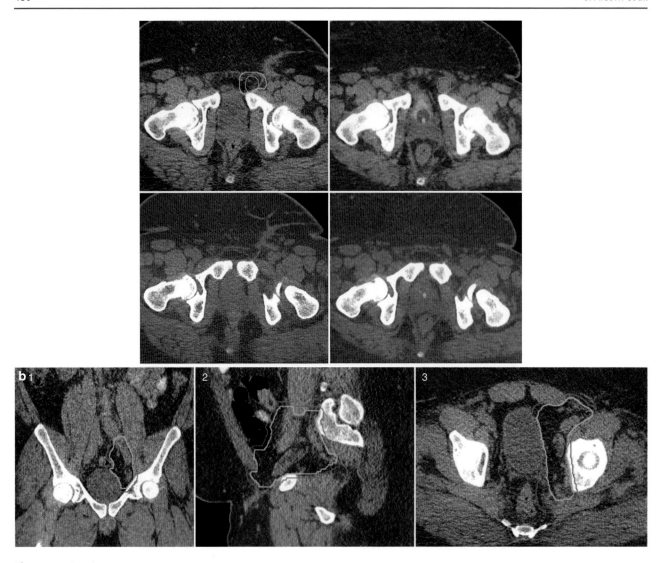

**Fig. 6** (continued)

to minimize skin reaction at the groin fold. Testicular shielding with a clamshell should be placed.

- 3D simulation should be performed with IV and PO contrast.
- GTV to CTV margin should be at least 1 cm. If applicable, the final CTV should also encompass the pre-chemotherapy/surgery GTV extent, excluding normal, uninvolved tissue that was displaced by the tumor prior to chemotherapy or surgery.
- Relevant OARs include the lumbar spinal cord, bowel, and reproductive organs.
- Consider fertility counseling, egg or sperm banking, and/or repositioning of the ovaries (Fig. 6).

# 4 Extra-nodal NHL

## 4.1 Principles of Management

- As in nodal NHL, RT may be indicated as primary therapy; consolidation following chemotherapy for bulky, residual, or unfavorable disease; or salvage for chemotherapy-refractory or recurrent disease.
- For extra-nodal NHL, ISRT generally treats the entire involved organ, although RT targeting select involved tissues can also be performed. Table 4 describes management of several sites of extra-nodal NHL.

## 4.2 General Considerations for RT in Primary CNS Lymphoma (PCNSL)

- PCNSL is characterized by multifocal involvement, generally by DLBCL. Relapse can occur within the eyes due to continuity with the CNS via the optic nerves. As such, the RT is delivered to a whole-brain field with coverage of at least the posterior portion of the orbits.
- Pre- and post-chemotherapy imaging with brain MRI is recommended. Ophthalmologic exams should be performed at baseline, and the RT field should be extended to cover entire orbit if there is evidence of ocular involvement.

**Table 4** Management of select sites of extra-nodal NHL

| Site | Tumor aggressiveness | Treatment modality | RT dose | Target delineation considerations |
|---|---|---|---|---|
| Primary CNS | – | High-dose methotrexate + RT | 24 Gy for complete response; 36–45 Gy for partial response; 40–50 Gy if chemotherapy is contraindicated | CTV = whole-brain fields + posterior orbits. CTV should include the whole orbit if there is baseline ocular involvement |
| Nasal type NK/T cell | – | RT +/− chemotherapy (e.g., SMILE) | 50 Gy with 5–10 Gy boost for RT alone; 45–54 Gy (depending on response) after chemotherapy | *For RT alone* |
| | | | | Confined to unilateral nasal cavity: CTV = bilateral nasal cavities + bilateral anterior ethmoid sinuses + part or all of the ipsilateral maxillary sinus + GTV (inclusion of the hard palate can be considered) |
| | | | | Bilateral nasal cavity: CTV may also include part or all of the bilateral maxillary sinuses |
| | | | | Posterior nasal cavity or nasopharyngeal extension: CTV should also include nasopharynx |
| | | | | Anterior ethmoid sinus extension: CTV should also include bilateral posterior ethmoid sinuses |
| | | | | Lymph node positive: CTV should also include involved lymph nodes |
| | | | | *After complete response to chemotherapy* |
| | | | | CTV = at least pre-chemotherapy GTV with appropriate margins |
| Orbital | Indolent | RT alone | 24–30 Gy (1.5-2 Gy/fraction) | For conjunctival NHL, CTV = whole conjunctiva + GTV |
| | Aggressive | R-CHOP or appropriate chemotherapy +/- RT | 30 Gy for complete response; 30–36 Gy + boost to 40–45 Gy for partial response, relapse, or RT alone | For non-conjunctival sites, whole orbital fields are generally used, where CTV = whole bony orbit + GTV |
| | | | | If treatment is targeting less than the whole orbit, CTV = organ of involvement + GTV |
| Gastric | Indolent | *H. pylori* positive: antibiotics + PPI | 30 Gy (1.5 Gy/fraction) | CTV = stomach from GE junction to duodenal bulb + visible perigastric nodes + GTV |
| | | *H. pylori* negative: RT | | |
| | Aggressive | R-CHOP or appropriate chemotherapy + RT | 30–36 Gy depending on response | |

*SMILE* steroid (dexamethasone), methotrexate, ifosfamide, L-asparaginase, and etoposide

- The patient should be simulated in the supine position with a thermoplastic mask for immobilization.
- 3D simulation may be performed without IV contrast.
- Relevant OARs include the cervical cord, brain stem, and optic apparatus.
- Typical whole-brain field borders:
  - Flash anteriorly, posteriorly, and superiorly.
  - The inferior border typically extends to below C2.
  - A margin of approximately 2 cm from the brain with coverage of the posterior aspect orbits should be applied. Coverage should be extended to the entire orbit if there is evidence of ocular involvement.
- Beam arrangement is typically opposed laterals.

## 4.3 General Considerations for RT in Orbital NHL

- Orbital lymphoma is most commonly characterized by indolent disease involving the uvea, conjunctiva, lacrimal structure, eyelid, and retrobulbar areas. The site of disease directs management, as described in Table 4.
- Pretreatment MRI and CT of the orbits as well as ophthalmologic examination are recommended.
- The patient should be simulated in the supine position with a short thermoplastic mask for immobilization. Apply bolus for superficial lesions including the conjunctiva.
- 3D simulation may be performed without IV contrast.
- For whole-orbit irradiation, treat with superior-inferior wedge pairs, 3DCRT, or IMRT. Localized, indolent conjunctival NHL may be treated with en face electrons or electron/photon mixed energy.
- Relevant OARs include the optic apparatus, lens, and lacrimal glands.
- For lesions at the periphery of the conjunctiva, consider a lens shield if possible without compromising margin coverage.
- The CTV should cover the whole orbit, with at least a 1 cm expansion of the GTV if gross disease extends outside the confines of the orbit.

## 4.4 General Considerations for RT in Nasal-Type NK-/T-Cell NHL

- Nasal-type NK-/T-cell lymphoma can be locally invasive, with microscopic submucosal infiltration common; as such, they it requires RT to the whole involved sinus or nasal cavity, as well as with consideration of RT to proximate structures as well.
- Pre-chemotherapy MRI and PET-CT are recommended but may be limited by inflammatory changes of the sino-nasal mucosa.
- The patient should be simulated in the supine position with a thermoplastic mask for immobilization.
- 3D simulation with IV contrast is recommended. MRI simulation may be useful in delineated head and neck anatomy.
- Relevant OARs include the brain stem, optic apparatus, and salivary glands.
- Planning with 3DCRT or IMRT may be required to avoid excess toxicity to nearby critical structures.
- Table 4 outlines CTV considerations.

## 4.5 General Considerations for RT in Gastric NHL

- Gastric lymphoma often presents with multifocal disease requiring whole-stomach irradiation.
- Endoscopic ultrasound and gastric mapping should be performed to identify areas of involvement.
- The patient should be simulated in the supine position with arms up and a custom mold for immobilization. Two to four hours prior to simulation and treatments, the patient should abstain from oral intake.
- 3D simulation with IV and PO contrast is recommended. As target movement with respiration may be seen, a 4DCT or fluoroscopy is recommended to allow for creation of an ITV.
- GTV to CTV/ITV margin should be at least 1–2 cm.

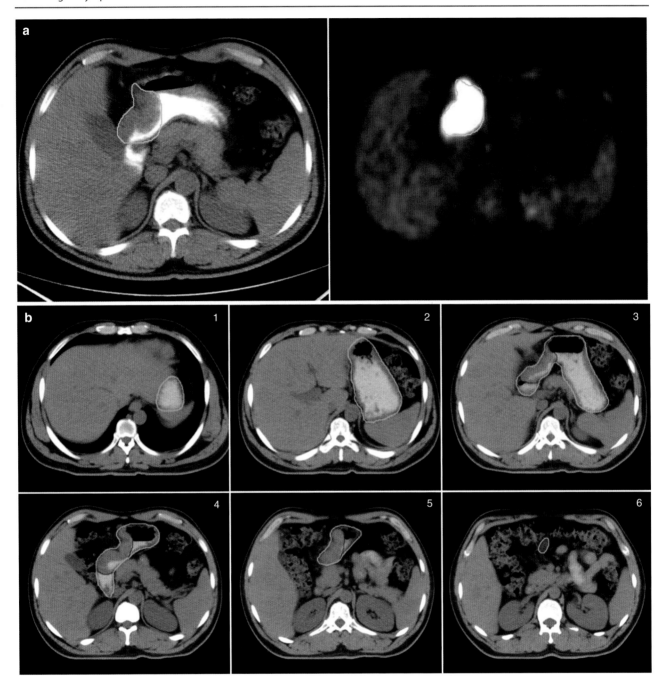

**Fig. 7** (**a–c**) Gastric RT planning images for a patient with a diffuse large B-cell lymphoma of the stomach with residual FDG-avid disease following four cycles of R-EPOCH and two cycles of RICE chemotherapy. (**a**) Residual FDG-avid volume is delineated in purple on PET-CT. There were no other areas of FDG-avid disease. (**b**) The patient was simulated with PO contrast; a 4DCT was performed. Axial slices show the PET-avid GTV (*red*) as well as the CTV (*green*). For gastric lymphomas, the CTV encompasses the GTV as well as the entire stomach including the stomach wall from the gastroesophageal junction to the duodenal bulb as well as any perigastric lymph nodes visible. (**c**) The GTV (*red*), CTV (*green*), and ITV (*yellow*) based on 4DCT, and PTV (*blue*) are shown in (*1*) coronal, (*2*) sagittal, and (*3*) axial slices. In this case, there is at least 1 cm expansion both from GTV to ITV and from ITV to PTV. Note that CTV/ITV to PTV margins depend on patient- and institution-specific factors, and therefore, universal recommendations for appropriate expansions cannot be provided

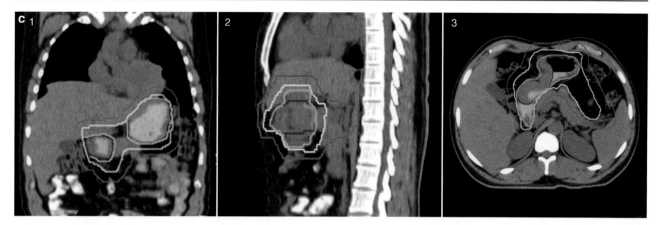

**Fig. 7** (continued)

- Relevant OARs include the thoracic spinal cord, kidneys, liver, bowel, and esophagus.
- Planning with 3DCRT or IMRT may be required to avoid excess toxicity to nearby critical structures (Fig. 7).

## 5 Plan Assessment

- For ISRT, the decision to treat with conventional versus conformal techniques is guided by considerations including the size of the treatment field, treatment dose, and proximity to critical structures.
- In general, treatment to nodal NHL of the abdomen and pelvis as well as extra-nodal NHL at gastric and sinonasal sites require conformal techniques due to location near dose-limiting structures.
- It may be necessary to plan by both conventional and conformal techniques in order to choose the optimal DVH on a case-by-case basis.
- OAR should be delineated in a site-dependent manner. Normal tissue dose constraints can be found by references such as QUANTEC (Marks et al. 2010) or RTOG protocols (RTOG 2014).

## Suggested Reading

IFRT guidelines: Yahalom J, Mauch P (2002) The involved field is back: issues in delineating the radiation field in Hodgkin's disease. Ann Oncol 13 Suppl 1:79–83

EORTC-GELA's INRT guidelines for Hodgkin lymphoma: Girinsky T et al (2006) Involved-node radiotherapy (INRT) in patients with early Hodgkin lymphoma: concepts and guidelines. Radiother Oncol 79:270–277

ILROG's ISRT guidelines for Hodgkin lymphoma: Specht L et al (2013) Modern radiation therapy for Hodgkin lymphoma: field and dose guidelines from the International Lymphoma Radiation Oncology Group (ILROG). Int J Radiat Oncol Biol Phys

## References

Campbell BA et al (2010) Long-term outcomes for patients with limited stage follicular lymphoma: involved regional radiotherapy versus involved node radiotherapy. Cancer 116:3797–3806

Girinsky T et al (2006) Involved-node radiotherapy (INRT) in patients with early Hodgkin lymphoma: concepts and guidelines. Radiother Oncol 79:270–277

Hodapp N (2012) The ICRU Report 83: prescribing, recording and reporting photon-beam intensity-modulated radiation therapy (IMRT). Strahlenther Onkol 188:97–99

Illidge T, Specht L, Yahalom J (2014) Modern Radiation Therapy for Nodal Non-Hodgkin Lymphoma—Target Definition and Dose Guidelines From the International Lymphoma Radiation Oncology Group. IJROBP 89 (1):49–58

Marks LB et al (2010) Use of normal tissue complication probability models in the clinic. Int J Radiat Oncol Biol Phys 76:S10–S19

National Cancer Institute (2014) Adult non-Hodgkin lymphoma treatment (PDQ): cellular classification of adult NHL. Available at http://www.cancer.gov/cancertopics/pdq/treatment/adult-non-hodgkins/HealthProfessional/page3#Reference3.9

Pileri SA, Milani M, Fraternali-Orcioni G, Sabattini E (1998) From the R.E.A.L. Classification to the upcoming WHO scheme: a step toward universal categorization of lymphoma entities? Ann Oncol 9:607–612

Rosenberg SA (1977) Validity of the Ann Arbor staging classification for the non-Hodgkin's lymphomas. Cancer Treat Rep 61: -1023–1027

RTOG (2014) RTOG clinical trials listed by subject number. Available at http://www.rtog.org/clinicaltrials/protocoltable.aspx

Specht L et al (2013) Modern radiation therapy for Hodgkin lymphoma: field and dose guidelines from the International Lymphoma Radiation Oncology Group (ILROG). Int J Radiat Oncol Biol Phys. doi:10.1016/j.ijrobp.2013.05.005

Swerdlow S et al (2008) WHO classification of tumours of haematopoietic and lymphoid tissues, 4th edn. IARC

White J et al. Breast cancer atlas for radiation therapy planning: consensus definitions. Available at http://www.rtog.org/CoreLab/ContouringAtlases/BreastCancerAtlas.aspx

Yahalom J, Mauch P (2002) The involved field is back: issues in delineating the radiation field in Hodgkin's disease. Ann Oncol 13(Suppl 1).79–83

Yu J, Nam H et al (2010) Involved-lesion radiation therapy after chemotherapy in limited-stage head-and-neck diffuse large B cell lymphoma. Int J Radiat Oncol Biol Phys 78:507–512

Zhang Y, et al (2012) Personalized assessment of kV cone beam computed tomography doses in image-guided radiotherapy of pediatric cancer patients. Int J Radiat Oncol Biol Phys 83:1649–1654

# Pediatric Sarcoma

Arthur K. Liu and Arnold C. Paulino

## Contents

A.K. Liu, MD, PhD (✉)
Department of Radiation Oncology,
University of Colorado Denver, Aurora, CO, USA

A.C. Paulino, MD
Department of Radiation Oncology,
MD Anderson Cancer Center, Houston, TX, USA
e-mail: apaulino@mdanderson.org

- Pediatric sarcomas are a diverse group of diagnoses. The three most common types that involve radiation therapy for local control are Ewing sarcoma (EWS), rhabdomyosarcoma (RMS), and non-rhabdomyosarcoma soft tissue sarcoma (NRSTS). In this chapter, we will discuss the treatment of EWS and RMS which are predominantly seen in the pediatric and young adult population.

## 1   Anatomy and Patterns of Spread

- EWS and RMS can occur in essentially any location of the body. EWS is most commonly located in the extremity followed by the pelvis, while RMS is most commonly seen in the head and neck region followed by the extremity and genitourinary sites. As such, a general description of relevant normal anatomy is beyond the scope of this chapter.
- There are some general guidelines regarding patterns of spread for these two tumors. Uninvolved bone and intraosseous membranes typically provide boundaries for microscopic spread. Also, the margin to create the clinical target volume (CTV) is less compared to the typical adult NRSTS, secondary to the inherent sensitivity of most of these tumors to the combination of chemotherapy and radiotherapy.
- Volume reduction is performed for "pushing" rather than invasive such as tumors that displace the lung, intestine, or bladder that show clear return to a more normal anatomic position after chemotherapy.
- Nodal regions are not electively treated for EWS or RMS. While the nodal metastasis is uncommon in EWS, it is seen in approximately 15–50 % of RMS arising in the extremity and genitourinary sites. It is believed that

N.Y. Lee et al. (eds.), *Target Volume Delineation for Conformal and Intensity-Modulated Radiation Therapy*,
Medical Radiology. Radiation Oncology, DOI: 10.1007/174_2014_986, © Springer International Publishing Switzerland 2014
Published Online: 4 November 2014

**Table 1** Ewing sarcoma volume definitions

| Initial target volumes | Definition and description |
|---|---|
| GTV1 | Gross disease (including unresected enlarged lymph nodes) at presentation, prior to chemotherapy or surgery. GTV1 can be modified for tumors that extend into body cavities, such as the pelvis or thorax that regress with chemotherapy. In these cases, the edge of GTV1 can be defined as the post-chemotherapy volume |
| CTV1 | GTV1 + 1 cm. CTV1 includes involved (pathologically or clinically) nodal regions |
| PTV 1 | CTV1 + institutional setup margin |
| Volume reduction | |
| GTV2 | Residual tumor after induction chemotherapy. For definitive radiation therapy, include all initial areas of bony involvement |
| CTV2 | GTV2 + 1 cm |
| PTV2 | CTV2 + institutional setup margin |

*GTV* gross tumor volume, *CTV* clinical target volume, *PTV* planning target volume

**Table 2** Ewing sarcoma doses in 1.8 Gy per fraction

| | PTV1 (Gy) | PTV2 (Gy) |
|---|---|---|
| Definitive radiotherapy (all sites except vertebra) | 45 | 10.8 |
| Definitive radiotherapy (vertebra) | 45 | 5.4 |
| Extraosseous with complete response (CR) to chemotherapy | 50.4 | 0 |
| Postoperative with microscopic residual with >90 % necrosis | 0 | 50.4 |
| Postoperative with microscopic residual with <90 % necrosis | 50.4 | 0 |
| Postoperative with gross residual | 45 | 10.8 |

*PTV* planning target volume

**Table 3** Rhabdomyosarcoma target volume definitions

| Initial target volumes | Definition and description |
|---|---|
| GTV | Gross disease (including unresected enlarged lymph nodes) at presentation, prior to chemotherapy or surgery. GTV can be modified for tumors that extend into body cavities, such as the pelvis or thorax, that regress with chemotherapy. In these cases, the edge of GTV can be defined as the post-chemotherapy volume |
| CTV | GTV + 1 cm. CTV includes involved (pathologically or clinically) nodal regions |
| PTV | CTV + institutional setup margin |

*GTV* gross tumor volume, *CTV* clinical target volume, *PTV* planning target volume

subclinical involvement of nodal regions is appropriately addressed by chemotherapy, and only gross or microscopic nodal disease receives additional treatment in the form of radiotherapy.

## 2 Diagnostic Imaging for Target Volume Definition

- Both CT scans and MRI scans are helpful for definition of the gross tumor volume (GTV) and the CTV.
- CT scan provides better definition of bony involvement, while MRI provides better definition of soft tissue involvement.
- The role of positron emission tomography (PET) scans in pediatric sarcomas is still unclear, but increasingly is used to help delineate the gross tumor volume.

## 3 Target Volume Delineation and Treatment Planning

- For EWS, target volumes include an initial target volume defined at presentation prior to chemotherapy or surgery (GTV1, CTV1) and a volume reduction defined after chemotherapy and surgery (GTV2, CTV2). An additional margin is added to the CTV to account for treatment setup uncertainty to create the PTV (PTV1 for the initial volume and PTV2 for the boost volume). See Table 1 for additional target definitions. Suggested doses (based on the Children's Oncology Group protocol AEWS1031) are given in Table 2.
- In comparison to EWS, RMS typically uses only a single course of treatment with a single set of target volumes. Table 3 shows the target volume definitions for RMS, while Table 4 shows the recommended dose according to histologic subtype and group.

**Table 4** Rhabdomyosarcoma doses in 1.8 Gy per fraction

| Group | Histology | Dose (Gy) |
|---|---|---|
| I | Embryonal | 0 |
| I | Alveolar | 36 |
| II, node negative | Embryonal or alveolar | 36 |
| II, node positive | Embryonal or alveolar | 41.4 |
| III | Embryonal or alveolar | 50.4 (except orbit 45) |

**Table 5** Normal tissue constraints

| Organ | Volume (%) | Dose (Gy) |
|---|---|---|
| Heart | 100 | 30 |
| Lung (bilateral) | 20 | 20 |
|  | 100 | 15 |
| Liver | 100 | 23.4 |
|  | 50 | 30 |
| Kidney (bilateral) | 50 | 24 |
|  | 100 | 14.4 |
| Bladder | 100 | 45 |
| Rectum | 100 | 45 |
| Small bowel | 50 | 45 |
| Optic chiasm/optic nerve | 100 | 54 |
| Spinal cord | Point max | 45 |
| Lens | 100 | 6 |
| Lacrimal gland/cornea | 100 | 41.4 |
| Cochlea | 100 | 40 |

These suggested normal tissue constraints are based on the most recent Children's Oncology Group EWS and RMS protocols. For organs where there was a discrepancy between the two diseases, the most conservative constraint is given

- Three examples of target volume delineation for pediatric sarcomas are given below.

# 4 Simulation, Daily Localization, and Treatment Devices

- Immobilization during CT simulation will depend on the sites to be treated. For pelvic primaries, a custom Alpha Cradle or VacLok bag should be used to immobilize the pelvis and upper legs. For thoracic primaries, the arms are often positioned up, and a custom Alpha Cradle/VacLok

bag or wingboard are used. For head and neck primaries, both the head and shoulders should be immobilized using an aquaplast mask. For extremities, immobilization usually involves the use of a custom Alpha Cradle or VacLok bag and needs to also account for the potential treatment angles.

- The type and frequency of image guidance usually defines the PTV expansion. For example, with daily image guidance, many institutions use 3 mm for PTV expansion. The smaller PTV is especially helpful when normal tissues will receive near- or above-tolerance doses, which commonly occurs with head and neck primaries.
- In the treatment of boys with pelvic and proximal lower extremity sarcomas, the patient may need to be in a frog leg position to accommodate a testicular shield.

# 5 Plan Assessment

Acceptable plans typically have 95 % of the prescription dose covering the PTV, with no more than 10 % of the PTV receiving greater than 110 % of the prescription dose. Dose to surrounding organs is kept within tolerance doses. Table 5 shows the normal tissue dose constraints in the Children's Oncology Group studies on EWS and RMS.

## Suggested Reading

Donaldson SS (2004) Ewing sarcoma: radiation dose and target volume. Pediatr Blood Cancer 42:471–476

Donaldson SS, Torrey M, Link MP et al (1998) A multidisciplinary study investigating radiotherapy in Ewing's sarcoma: end results of POG #8346. Pediatric Oncology Group. Int J Radiat Oncol Biol Phys 42:125–135

Lin C, Donaldson SS, Meza JL et al (2012) Effect of radiotherapy techniques (IMRT vs. 3DCRT) on outcome in patients with intermediate-risk rhabdomyosarcoma enrolled in COG D9803 – a report from the Children's Oncology Group. Int J Radiat Oncol Biol Phys 82:1764–1770

Million L, Anderson J, Breneman J et al (2011) Influence of noncompliance with radiation therapy protocol guidelines and operative bed recurrences for children with rhabdomyosarcoma and microscopic residual disease: a report from the Children's Oncology Group. Int J Radiat Oncol Biol Phys 80:333–338

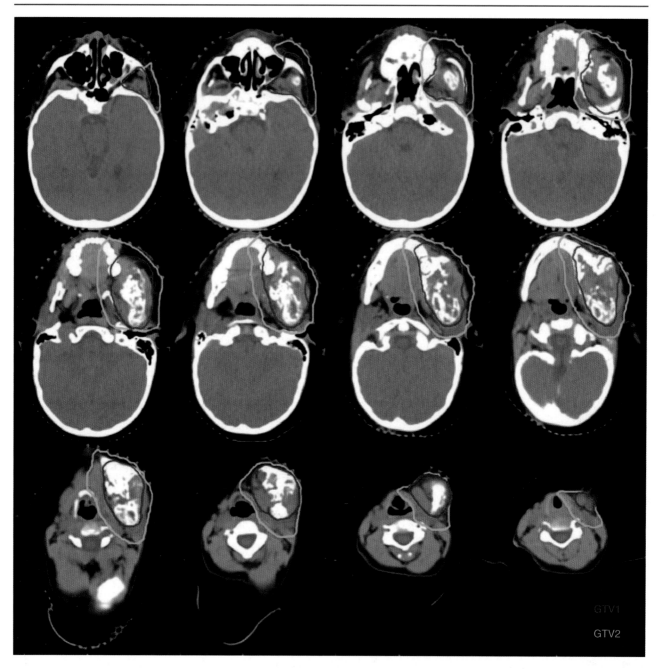

**Fig. 1** Ewing Sarcoma of the left mandible. There was no involvement of the skull, so the CTV was limited to be outside of the skull. *GTV* gross tumor volume, *CTV* clinical target volume

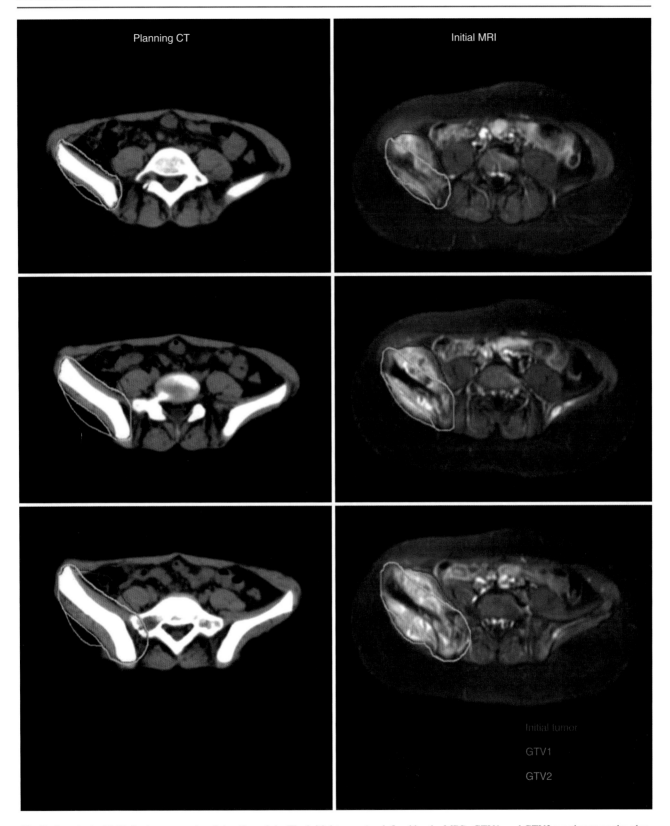

**Fig. 2** A patient with Ewing's sarcoma involving the pelvis. The initial tumor (as defined by the MRI), GTV1, and GTV2 are shown on the planning CT and initial MRI. For clarity, CTVs are not shown but are GTV + 1 cm

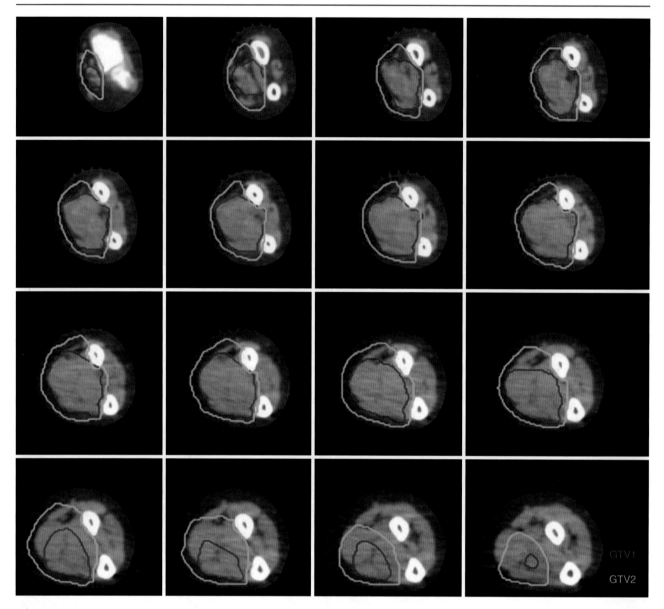

**Fig. 3** Rhabdomyosarcoma of the forearm. The clinical target volume (CTV) was limited by the interosseous membrane. *GTV* gross tumor volume

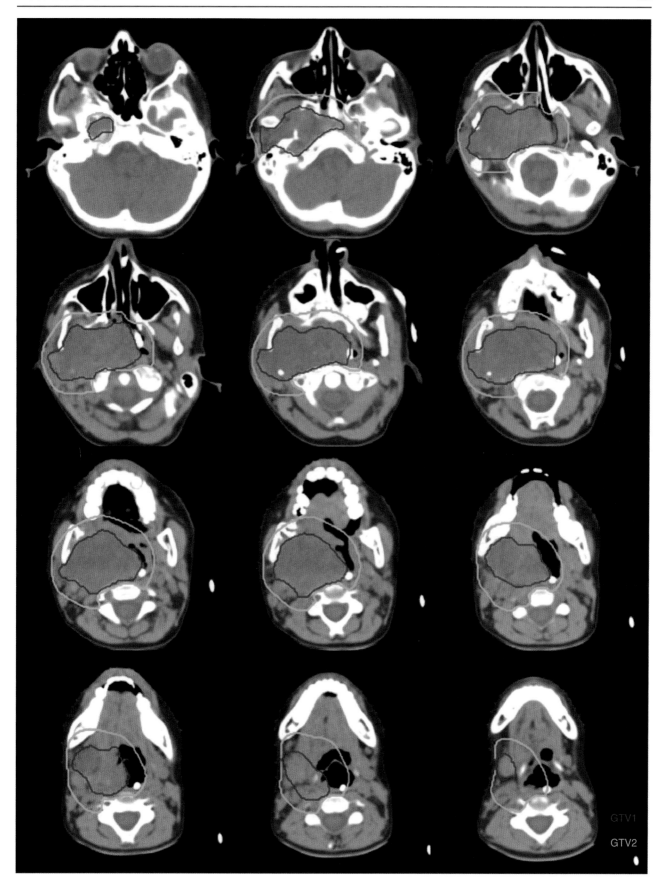

**Fig. 4** Rhabdomyosarcoma of the parapharyngeal region. The clinical target volume (CTV) is limited posteriorly by the vertebra. The CTV is not limited by the right mandible as there was mandibular involvement of tumor. *GTV* gross tumor volume

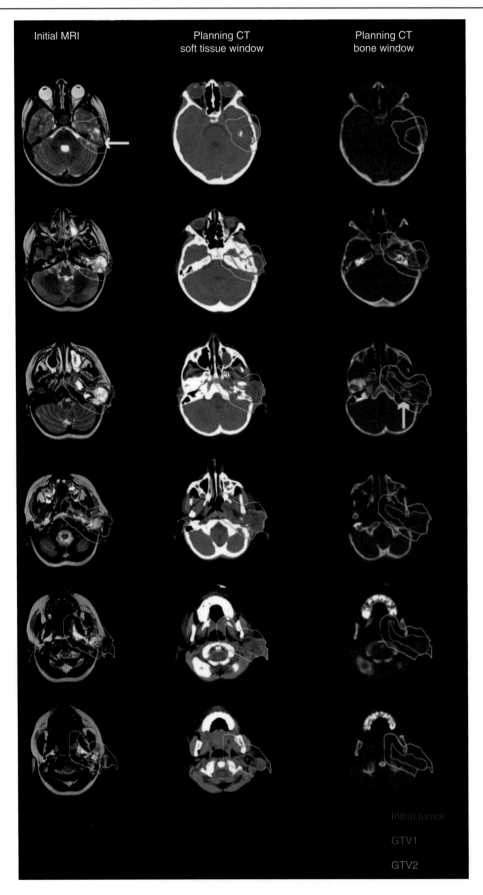

**Fig. 5** A patient with rhabdomyosarcoma involving the middle ear. The initial tumor (as defined by the MRI), GTV, and CTV are shown on the initial MRI and planning CT (both bone and soft tissue windows). The patient has intracranial extension (*white arrow*) and significant bony destruction of the middle ear (*yellow arrow*)

# Pediatric Brain Tumors

Jeffrey Buchsbaum and Arnold C. Paulino

## Contents

J. Buchsbaum, MD, PhD
Department of Radiation Oncology,
Indiana University, Bloomington, IN, USA
e-mail: leen2@mskcc.org

A.C. Paulino, MD (✉)
Department of Radiation Oncology,
MD Anderson Cancer Center, Houston, TX, USA
e-mail: apaulino@mdanderson.org

## 1 Medulloblastoma

### 1.1 General Principles of Planning and Target Delineation

- Volumetric planning is the standard method for definitive craniospinal and boost radiation therapy for medulloblastoma. Treatment can be delivered using a number of techniques such as proton therapy, intensity-modulated radiation therapy (IMRT), and 3D conformal therapy; however, accurate delineation of target volumes is universally required.

- In addition to a thorough physical examination, adequate imaging studies should be obtained for diagnosis, staging, and planning. Unless contraindicated, all patients should undergo contrast-enhanced MRI scans of the brain (preoperative and postoperative), preferably with 1–3 mm thickness. In addition, MRI of the spine and cerebrospinal fluid cytology from a lumbar tap are part of staging to rule out tumor dissemination. Children who are M0 and <1.5 $cm^2$ residual on postoperative MRI are classified as having standard-risk disease, while those with M1–M4 disease and/or ≥1.5 $cm^2$ residual have high-risk disease.

- CT simulation without contrast should be performed in order to have a data set for target delineation. Because digitally reconstructed radiographs tend to be of higher quality with thinner slices, one should use a slice thickness setting that both optimizes planning and treatment delivery image guidance. Planning system slice capacity is often the limiting factor. DRR quality for use in image guidance generally improves with thinner slices at simulation. Thinner slices in the CSI portion of data collection allow for superior image resolution for fusion and for digitally reconstructed radiograph (DRR) formation to be used in imaged guidance. The range of the CT scan must include all immobilization devices and generally includes an image data set beyond the top of the head to below the gonads.

N.Y. Lee et al. (eds.), *Target Volume Delineation for Conformal and Intensity-Modulated Radiation Therapy*,
Medical Radiology. Radiation Oncology, DOI: 10.1007/174_2014_992, © Springer International Publishing Switzerland 2014
Published Online: 20 September 2014

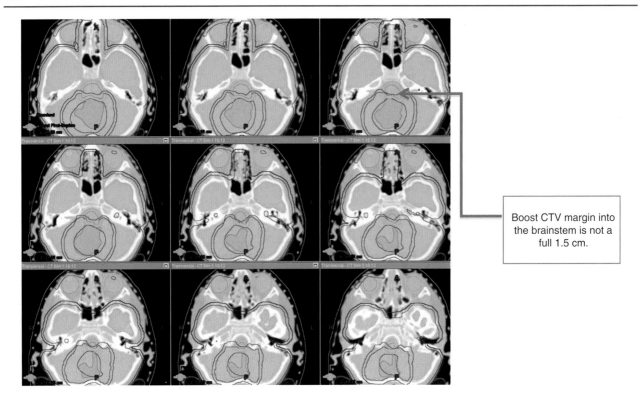

Boost CTV margin into the brainstem is not a full 1.5 cm.

**Fig. 1** A patient with standard-risk medulloblastoma. This patient was simulated using a 1.5 mm CT slice thickness. Note the coverage of the cribriform plate as part of the target volume (the *dark blue line* is the PTV$_{CSI}$, while the inner *red line* is the CTV$_{CSI}$). Also note the PTV$_{tbboost}$ (*purple line*), CTV$_{tbboost}$ (*orange line*), and GTV (*shaded purple*) contours. Note that the CTV margin anteriorly in the brainstem is less compared to the posterior and lateral margins

- Immobilization for setup reproducibility involves the construction of a body immobilization device and a mask, regardless of whether the patient is set up in the prone or supine position. Both prone and supine patients need body immobilization device (i.e., Vac-Lok bag, Alpha Cradle) and a mask. If the patient is positioned prone, a customized forehead and chin rest is used and the head is immobilized with a mask. If general anesthesia is used, prone patients often require an endotracheal (ET) tube. Supine patients may sometimes be treated with a nasal cannula or a laryngeal mask airway (LMA). The LMA offers better airway control than the nasal cannula as secretions during extended sedation time can be significant. For this reason, it is the authors' preference to use the LMA in the supine position.
- Target volumes need to be delineated on every slice of the planning CT (Figs. 1 and 2). The recommended target volumes for the craniospinal axis, tumor bed boost, and posterior fossa boost are detailed in Tables 1, 2, and 3.
- In the case of a growing child, the entire vertebral body must be contoured and included in the CTV when treating the craniospinal axis. An example is shown in Fig. 3. In a full-grown child or adult, the entire vertebral does

- not need to be included in the CTV. An example is shown in Fig. 4.
- Fusion of MR to CT is not perfect, so each slice of MR-based contours should ultimately be reviewed on the CT scan to make sure it is reasonable.
- The standard recommendation for determining the caudal extent for the CTV$_{CSI}$ is to use the MRI scan to find the termination of the thecal sac. In the past the caudal margin has been set to the bottom of the S2 vertebral level; however, we now know that in one-third of cases, the termination will be higher or lower than S2. Going more inferiorly than necessary may deliver more exit dose into the gonads. When proton therapy is used for the craniospinal axis, the exit dose to the gonads is not of concern.
- The current recommended dose to the craniospinal axis for standard-risk disease is 23.4 Gy in 13 fractions while for high-risk disease is 36 Gy in 20 fractions. In both cases, the recommended total dose to the CTV boost volume is 54 Gy. An ongoing Children's Oncology Group study is looking at reducing the CSI dose from 23.4 to 18 Gy in children <7 years of age with standard-risk disease.
- For the boost field, an ongoing COG study is examining the question of the appropriate boost volume for

medulloblastoma. In this study, the two types of boost volumes include the entire posterior fossa ($CTV_{pf}$) versus the tumor bed with a margin ($CTV_{tbboost}$). Several single institutional studies have been published that support the safety and efficacy of the tumor bed boost. Normal anatomic constraints may limit the CTV boost volume in such a way that a uniform margin around the GTV is not necessary. The tentorium cerebelli (separates the posterior fossa and the supratentorial brain) and bony skull are considered as barriers of spread; therefore, the CTV should be limited not to extend beyond these barriers. Invasion into the brainstem is possible so expansion into the brainstem may be needed. In cases where the tumor is touching the brainstem, a limited margin of 2–3 mm has

often been used for the anterior expansion of the CTV boost volume. In cases where tumor is not in contact with the brainstem such as in a case of a well-lateralized medulloblastoma, the brainstem is an anatomic barrier to spread and hence need not be included in the CTV boost volume (Figs. 5, 6, and 7).

• When treating the entire posterior fossa as the boost volume, the anterior border includes the posterior clinoids and the entire contents of the posterior fossa. The brainstem in its entirety is included in the CTV. One can see this outlined in graphical format via the website dedicated to the COG trial comparing the two different boost methods at www.qarc.org/ACNS0031Atlas.pdf (Figs. 5, 6, and 7).

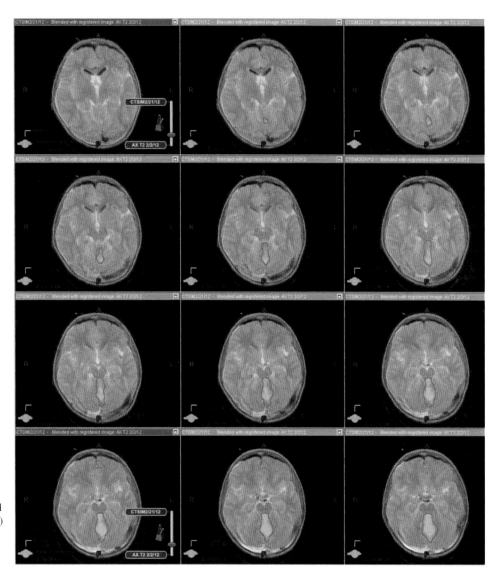

**Fig. 2** MRI slices fused to CT simulation images from a similar patient who had a gross total resection of a medulloblastoma. This is an example of a tumor bed boost. The GTV (resection cavity) is shown in *blue*, $CTV_{tbboost}$ in *light orange*, and $PTV_{tbboost}$ in *purple*

**Fig. 2** (continued)

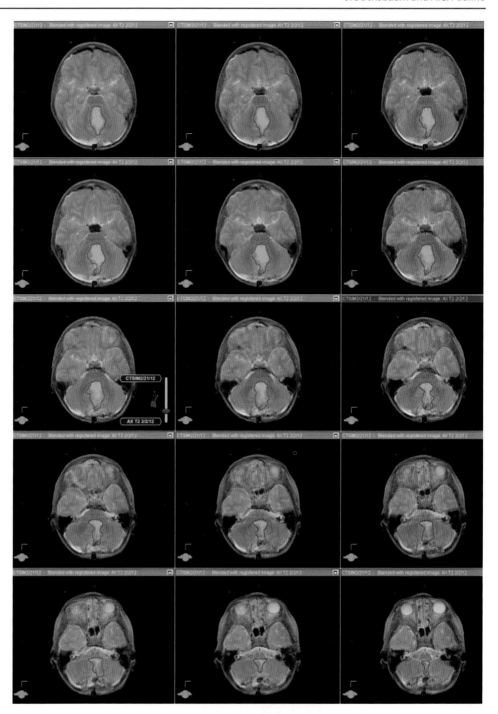

**Table 1** Recommended target volumes for the craniospinal (CSI) portion of the treatment

| Target volumes | Definition and description |
| --- | --- |
| GTV | Tumor bed includes all gross disease and the walls of the resection cavity as noted on the MRI. Surgical defects caused by the procedure (the route to and from the tumor bed) are not considered part of the cavity |
| CTV$_{CSI}$ | The entire volume contained by the dura matter and in contact with the cerebrospinal fluid is the CTV. The cribriform plate should be included in the CTV. Because the spinal cord can in theory move in the canal, the CTV is defined as limits of the spinal canal down to the thecal sac termination as defined by the spinal MRI |
| | For the CSI portion, the entire vertebral body may need to be treated in a growing child so that growth is symmetric (Fig. 3). Such is not the case in a grown child or adult (Fig. 4) |
| PTV$_{CSI}$ | CTV + 3–10 mm, depending on comfort level of daily patient positioning and institutional experience |

**Table 2** Recommended target volumes of the tumor bed boost within the posterior fossa

| Target volumes | Definition and description |
|---|---|
| GTV | Tumor bed includes all gross disease and the walls of the resection cavity as noted on the MRI. Surgical defects caused by the procedure (the route to and from the tumor bed) are not considered part of the cavity |
| CTV$_{tbboost}$ | CTV$_{tbboost}$ should include the entire GTV with a 1–1.5 cm margin |
| | Clinical limits to CTV expansion include the normal anatomic barriers to tumor spread such as the brainstem, the bone, and the tentorium. If there is brainstem invasion, then a portion of the brainstem in included in the CTV |
| PTV$_{tbboost}$ | CTV$_{tbboost}$+3–5 mm, depending on institutional experience |

**Table 3** Recommended target volumes for the entire posterior fossa boost

| Target volumes | Definition and description |
|---|---|
| GTV | Tumor bed includes all gross disease and the walls of the resection cavity as noted on the MRI. Surgical defects caused by the procedure (the route to and from the tumor bed) are not considered part of the cavity |
| CTV$_{pf}$ | CTV$_{pf}$ should include the posterior fossa. The brainstem is included in the posterior fossa compartment |
| | Clinical limits to CTV expansion include the normal anatomic barriers to tumor spread such as the bone and the tentorium |
| PTV$_{pf}$ | CTV$_{pf}$+3–5 mm, depending on institutional experience |

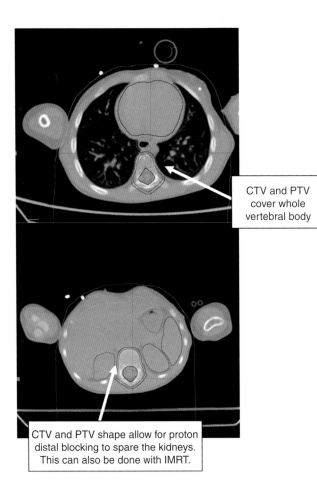

CTV and PTV cover whole vertebral body

CTV and PTV shape allow for proton distal blocking to spare the kidneys. This can also be done with IMRT.

**Fig. 3** Example of CTVs displayed on bone windows of the spine in a growing child. The CTV could cut across the vertebral body in a fully grown child or an adult

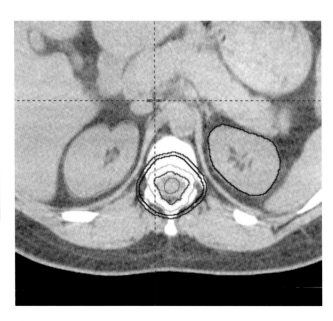

**Fig. 4** This shows how the spine field changes for a fully grown patient. Note how the CTV (*blue*) and PTV (*purple*) lines are not outside of the bone anteriorly

## 2 Ependymoma

### 2.1 General Principles of Planning and Target Delineation

- Volumetric planning is the standard method for radiation therapy planning for intracranial ependymoma. Treatment can be delivered using a number of techniques such as

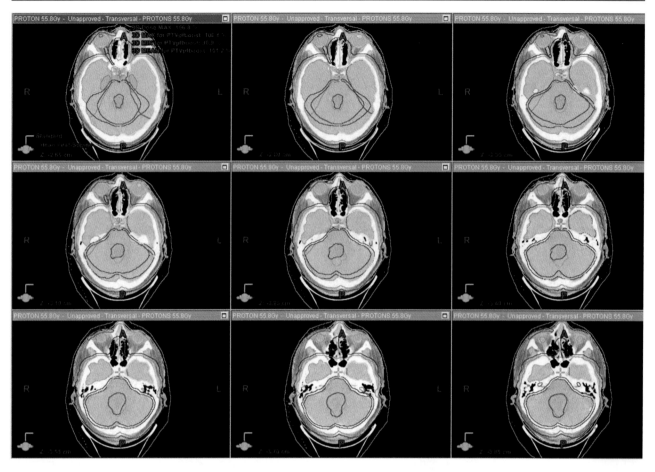

**Fig. 5** The posterior fossa contours in a series of CT slices

proton therapy, intensity-modulated radiation therapy (IMRT), and 3D conformal therapy; however, accurate delineation of target volumes is universally required.

- In addition to a thorough physical examination, adequate imaging studies should be obtained for diagnosis, staging, and planning. Unless contraindicated, all patients should undergo contrast-enhanced MRI scans of the brain (preoperative and postoperative), preferably 1–3 mm slice thickness.
- In addition, MRI of the spine and cerebrospinal fluid cytology from a lumbar tap are part of staging to rule out tumor dissemination. Tumor dissemination is usually seen in <10 % of intracranial ependymoma cases at initial diagnosis.
- CT simulation without contrast should be performed in order to have a data set for target delineation. Because digitally reconstructed radiographs tend to be of higher quality with thinner slices, one should use a slice thickness setting that both optimizes planning and treatment delivery image guidance. DRR quality for use in image guidance generally improves with thinner slices at

simulation. The range of the CT scan must include all the surrounding organs that need a dose volume histogram; therefore, the inferior border should be inferior to C7 vertebral level so that the normal cervical spinal cord can be outlined in its entirety.

- Immobilization for setup reproducibility involves the construction of a mask in the supine position. A mask that extends to cover the shoulders may be needed if the tumor extends down to the cervical spinal cord. Given the young age of many of these patients, general anesthesia may need to be used. In making the mask, the anesthesiologist should be involved to ensure a secure airway.
- The GTV includes any residual tumor and the postoperative resection cavity. The CTV is usually the GTV with a 1 cm margin. The PTV is the CTV with a 3–5 mm margin, depending on institutional experience. In cases where image-guided radiotherapy is used, a 3 mm margin is usually adequate. All target volumes are contoured on each CT slice (Table 1) (Figs. 8, 9, 10, and 11).
- In cases where there is residual tumor remaining, reresection should be entertained if the risk of complications is

**Fig. 6** The posterior fossa contours can be seen in this series of MRI slices fused to the simulation CT. These are from the above patient. MRI fusion is critical for these cases. The CTV is bounded by the tentorium in these images

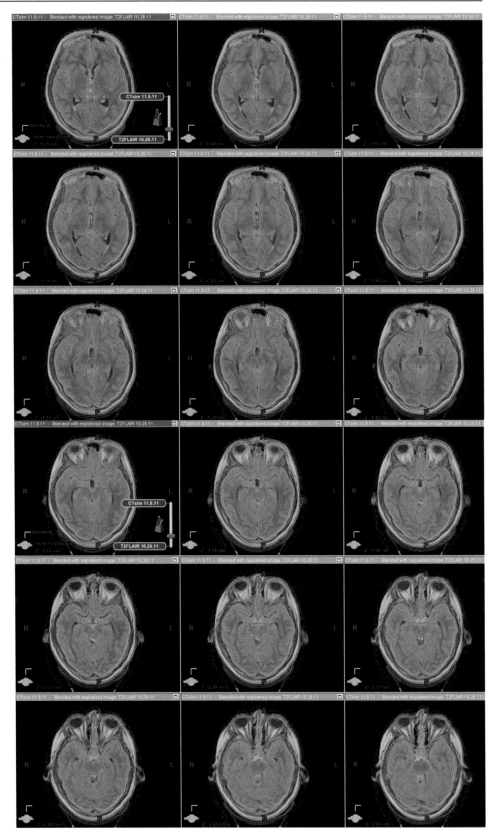

**Fig. 6** (continued)

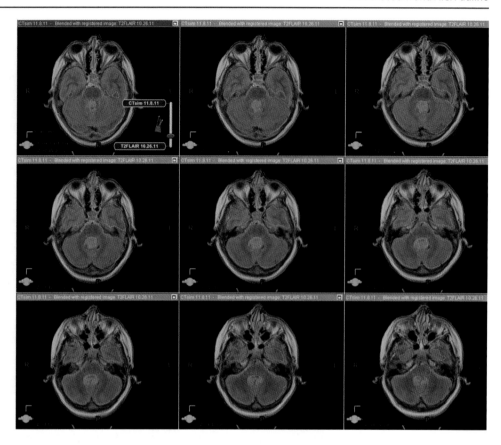

low. The degree of tumor resection is the most important prognostic factor in intracranial ependymoma.

## 3 Pure Germinoma

### 3.1 General Principles of Planning and Target Delineation

- Volumetric planning is the standard method for radiation therapy planning for intracranial ependymoma. Treatment can be delivered using a number of techniques such as proton therapy, intensity-modulated radiation therapy (IMRT), and 3D conformal therapy; however, accurate delineation of target volumes is universally required.
- In addition to a thorough physical examination, adequate imaging studies should be obtained for diagnosis, staging, and planning. Unless contraindicated, all patients should undergo contrast-enhanced MRI scans of the brain (preoperative and postoperative), preferably 1–3 mm slice thickness.
- In addition, MRI of the spine and cerebrospinal fluid cytology from a lumbar tap are part of staging to rule out tumor dissemination. Tumor dissemination is usually seen in <10 % of intracranial germinoma cases at initial diagnosis.

- Serum and CSF beta-human chorionic gonadotropin (b-HCG) and alpha-fetoprotein (AFP) are drawn to rule out a non-germinomatous germ cell tumor (NCCCT) component. NGGCT is treated differently compared to pure germinoma. Patients with elevated AFP and/or b-HCG ≥50 IU/L are treated as NGGCT.
- Immobilization for setup reproducibility involves the construction of a mask in the supine position. In cases where there is evidence of tumor dissemination, CSI is used, and the immobilization will be similar to the CSI component for the medulloblastoma patient.
- For localized disease and classic bifocal germinoma (suprasellar and pineal involvement), the standard radiotherapy field includes treatment of the whole ventricular volume followed by a boost to the primary tumor. Target volumes include gross tumor volume pre-chemotherapy and post-chemotherapy, the ventricles, and the normal structures of elegant brain that are nearby (hearing, hormonal systems, visual pathways, memory and learning pathways, and the brainstem).
- It is unclear how often or if one should repeat an MR scan for the possibility that the ventricular shape will change when the primary tumor shrinks.
- For localized disease and classic bifocal germinoma (suprasellar and pineal component), the current recommendation when treating with RT alone is to treat the full

ventricular volume plus the initial tumor volume with a CTV margin of 1–1.5 cm. A cone-done boost after about 21 Gy at 1.5 Gy per fraction is then employed to treat the pre-chemotherapy volume plus a 1–1.5 cm. The PTV used is typically 3–5 mm and depends on institutional experience. The boost dose is typically 24 Gy at 1.5 Gy per fraction. The total dose to the primary tumor is 45 Gy (Table 5) (Figs. 12, 13, and 14).

- In cases when neoadjuvant chemotherapy is used and the primary tumor achieves a complete response, a whole ventricular RT dose of 21 Gy followed by a 9 Gy boost may be used, such that the total dose to the primary tumor is 30 Gy. The pre-chemotherapy GTV is used for target delineation. A 1 cm margin is added to create the CTV. Another 3–5 mm is added to the CTV to create the PTV (Fig. 14).

**Fig. 7** Details of the posterior fossa boost contours at the level of the cochleae. Note the craniospinal PTV in *purple* is covering the full bones of the base of skull and still is coving some areas of the cribriform plate to make sure it is covered by at least 5 mm

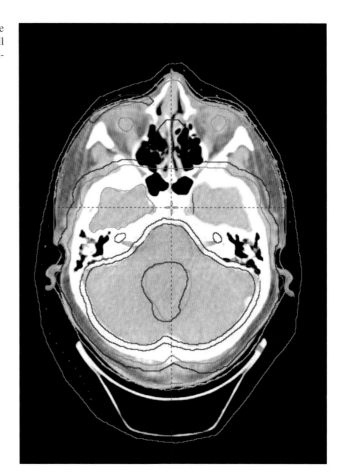

**Table 4** Recommended target volumes for ependymoma

| Target volumes | Definition and description |
| --- | --- |
| GTV | The GTV is generally defined by the postoperative cavity and any residual tumor. While the postoperative MRI is crucial for the determination of the surgical cavity and residual tumor, the preoperative MRI will be useful to help determine where the tumor was previously located to help better delineate the operative bed |
| $CTV_{54}$ and $CTV_{59.4}$ | CTV expansion is usually 10 mm. One has to take bone and tentorial constraints into consideration. In the most recent Children's Oncology Group study ACNS0121, the prescribed dose was 59.4 Gy. For the $CTV_{54}$, the entire tumor bed is treated. For $CTV_{59.4}$, the volume of CTV inferior to the foramen magnum is not included to respect the tolerance of the cervical spinal cord |
| $PTV_{54}$ and $PTV_{59.4}$ | The $PTV_{54}$ is the $CTV_{54}$ with a 3–5 mm margin for setup uncertainty. The $PTV_{59.4}$ has the same border inferiorly as the $CTV_{59.4}$. The PTV is purposely underdosed to respect the tolerance of the cervical spinal cord (Fig. 12) |

**Fig. 8** Target volume contours for an 18-month-old boy with an infratentorial ependymoma. Note that the brainstem was in contact with the tumor but was not formally invaded, so the CTV was taken into the brainstem by 3 mm. The CTV does not include regions outside of the skull. CTV (*orange*), PTV (*purple*)

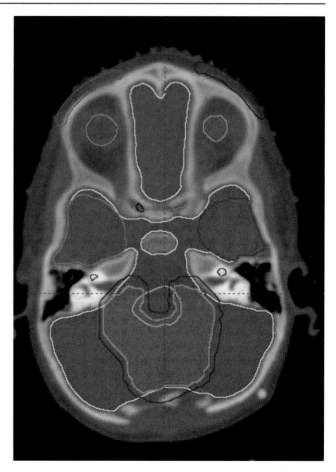

**Fig. 9** Contours of a patient with infratentorial ependymoma. GTV (*red*), CTV (*purple*), and PTV (*pink*). The bilateral cochlea are also contoured in *purple* and *green*

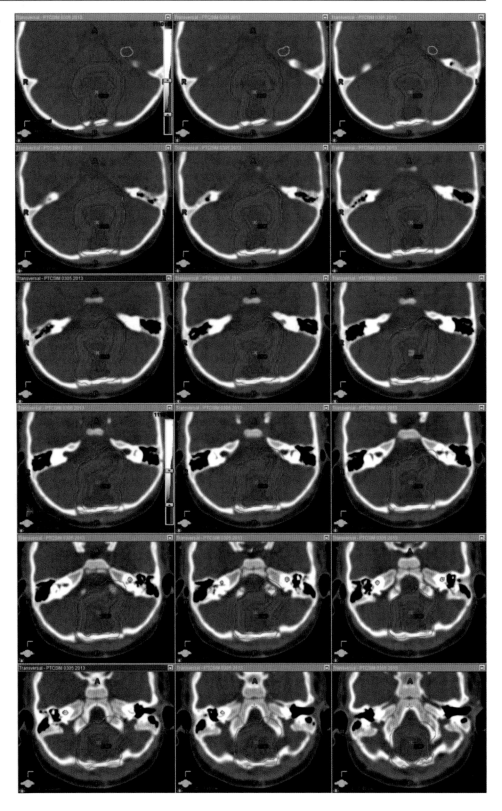

**Fig. 10** MRI slices fused to the CT scan in a child with infratentorial ependymoma. GTV (*blue*), CTV (*orange*), PTV (*purple*), brainstem (*aquamarine*)

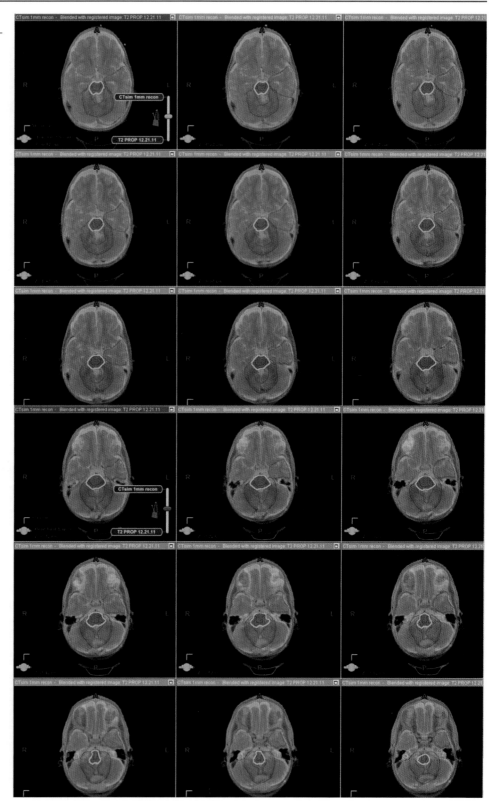

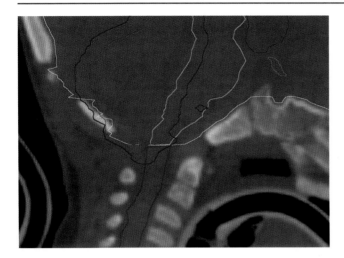

**Fig. 11** Sagittal view of the same ependymoma infant showing the use of a PTV$_{54}$ (*purple*) and a PTV$_{59.4}$ (*pink*). The spinal cord is in *brown* and the brainstem is in *light blue*

**Table 5** Recommended target volumes for whole ventricular and boost for pure germinoma

| Target volumes | Definition and description |
| --- | --- |
| GTV | GTV is the pre-chemotherapy volume of tumor. The GTV is incorporated in both the CTV$_{ventricles}$ and the CTV$_{boost}$ |
| CTV$_{ventricles}$ | CTV expansion is usually 10–15 mm from the ventricles and primary tumor. One has to take the bone and tentorium as anatomic barriers to spread. For the whole ventricular portion of treatment, there is variability nationally on what is defined as this volume; in particular the inclusion of the CSF-bearing space anterior to the brainstem is a subject of debate (Figs. 12, 13, and 14) |
| CTV$_{boost}$ | GTV with a 10–15 mm margin (Fig. 14) |
| PTV$_{ventricles}$ and PTV$_{boost}$ | PTVs are expanded by 3–5 mm beyond the CTV listed according to institutional experience (Figs. 12 and 13) |

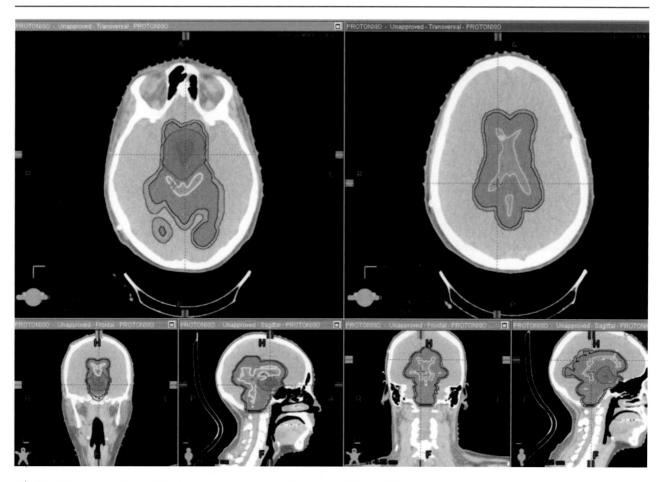

**Fig. 12** Whole ventricular used for treatment of a pure germinoma. The same plan on the same patient is shown with two sets of orthogonal slices. Note the initial hypothalamic CTV pushing out the ventricle-based CTV. In this case, the area anterior to the brainstem is considered part of the target and one can see coverage of this region. Every patient will have different ventricles, so it is not possible to generalize the approach too much. Critical is noting patients that have ventricles that are changing in volume or that might and addressing these patients with on treatment simulations (weekly simulations are not unreasonable). Frequent physical examination of these patients is a must

**Fig. 13** Detailed view of the contours used in whole ventricular therapy in orthogonal views. The ventricles at simulation are in *red*. The preoperative tumor volume is in *green*. Other structures include the CTV (*blue*), PTV (*purple*), brain (*yellow*), and brainstem (*aquamarine*)

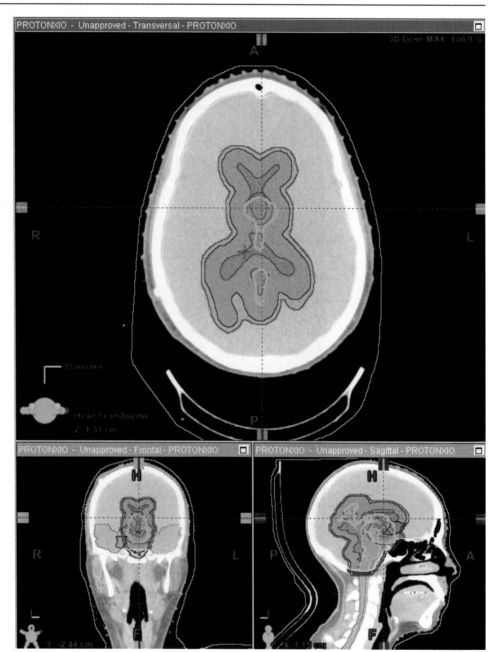

**Fig. 14** MRI slices of a whole ventricular case for a different patient. Shown are the ventricles (*orange*), the gross tumor volume (*red*), whole ventricular clinical target volume (*aquamarine*), boost clinical target volume (*blue*), and boost planning target volume (*purple*)

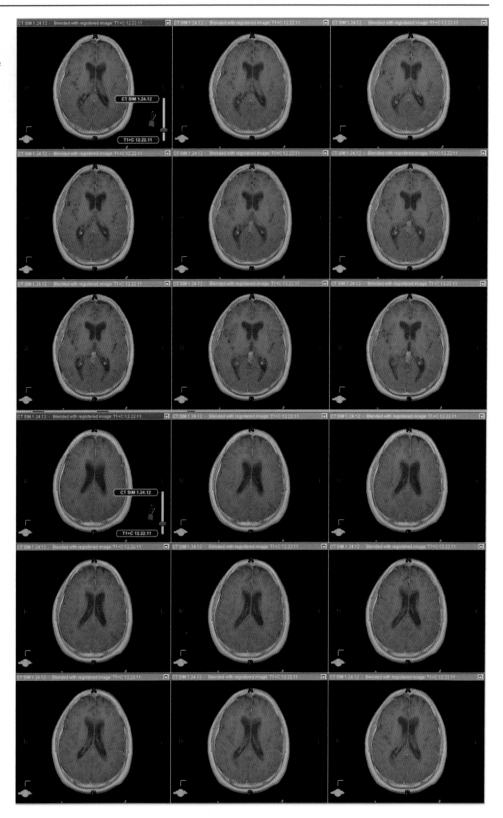

**Fig. 14** (continued)

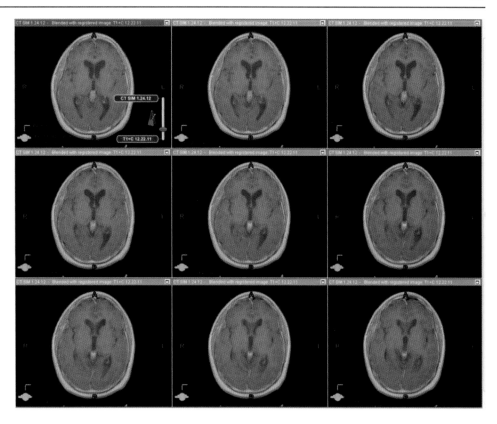

## Suggested Reading

Merchant TE, Li C, Xiong X et al (2009) Conformal radiotherapy after surgery for paediatric ependymoma: a prospective study. Lancet Oncol 10:258–266

Paulino AC, Mazloom A, Teh BS et al (2011) Local control after craniospinal irradiation, intensity-modulated radiotherapy boost, and chemotherapy in childhood medulloblastoma. Cancer 117: 635–641

Raggi E, Mosleh-Shirazi MA, Saran FH (2008) An evaluation of conformal and intensity- modulated radiotherapy in whole ventricular radiotherapy for localized primary intracranial germinomas. Clin Oncol (R Coll Radiol) 20:253–260

Roberge D, Kun LE, Freeman CR (2005) Intracranial germinoma: on whole-ventricular irradiation. Pediatr Blood Cancer 44:358–362

Wolden SL, Dunkel IJ, Souweidane MM et al (2003) Patterns of failure using a conformal radiation therapy tumor bed boost for medulloblastoma. J Clin Oncol 21:3079–3083

# Soft Tissue Sarcoma

Colleen Dickie and Brian O'Sullivan

## Contents

C. Dickie, MSc, MRT(T)(MR)
Radiation Medicine Department, Princess Margaret Hospital,
University of Toronto, Toronto, ON, USA
e-mail: colleen.dickie@rmp.uhn.on.ca

B. O'Sullivan, MD, FRCPC (✉)
Department of Radiation Oncology, Princess Margaret Hospital,
University of Toronto,
610 University Avenue, Toronto, ON M5G 2M9, USA
e-mail: brian.osullivan@rmp.uhn.on.ca

## 1 Anatomy and Patterns of Spread

- Anatomic location, size, depth (with respect to the superficial fascia separating subcutaneous tissue from the muscle groups), and pathological features dictate the management of soft tissue sarcoma (STS).

- Invasion is typically in the longitudinal direction within or along muscle and confined to the compartment of origin. Suspicious peritumoral changes, henceforth referred to as *edema*, may harbor microscopic disease. Edema is most often pronounced in the craniocaudal dimension and should ordinarily be encompassed in the radiotherapy target volume.

- STS generally respect barriers to tumor spread such as bone, interosseous membrane, and major fascial planes. This characteristic should be exploited in tissue/function preserving radiotherapy planning, especially in extremity lesions.

- Some tumors may exceptionally demonstrate multifocal or others patterns of spread that must be considered in surgical and radiotherapy planning.

- Retroperitoneal tumors commonly grow to a large size and initially displace but can eventually invade adjacent organs and tissues. They are by definition classified as deep tumors.

- In the event of an "unplanned" surgical resection with positive margins (surgical error), the RT target volume needs to generously include the disturbed muscles and other structures in addition to any other tissues considered to be directly involved. This may require treatment of most of a compartment where this may not have been needed at the clinical presentation initially.

- In general, lymph node metastasis is uncommon

- The most common distant metastatic site is the lung, generally determined by a profile predicted by the size, depth, and grade of the tumor.

## 2 Diagnostic Workup Relevant for Target Volume Delineation

- Pre-biopsy, adequate cross-sectional imaging (CT +/− MRI) is necessary of the primary tumor. A plain radiograph is optional.
- Biopsy and pathology assessment should be carefully planned along the future resection axis to establish grade and histologic subtype.
- Biopsy should comprise a core needle or incisional biopsy. Fine needle aspiration may be acceptable in institutions where pathologists have proven experience in its interpretation.
- Biopsy intrusions need to be addressed by inclusion either in the RT treatment volume or in the surgical resection.
- Chest CT should be used to assess for distant metastases.
- Chest CT or chest x-ray is recommended for low-grade T1 lesions for metastatic assessment.
- CT abdomen/pelvis should be planned for abdominal/retroperitoneal lesions. It is usual to perform intravenous pyelogram at baseline CT scan or a differential renal isotope scan to appreciate the function of the kidney contralateral to the side involved by the disease for abdominal/retroperitoneal lesions.
- A creatinine clearance test should be performed for abdominal/retroperitoneal lesions.
- Consider MRI of the total spine for myxoid/round cell liposarcoma.
- Consider CNS imaging for alveolar soft part sarcoma.
- Consider bone marrow examination and bone scintigraphy in cases of non-pleomorphic rhabdomyosarcoma and CSF examination if originating in parameningeal sites with lymph node involvement.

## 3 Simulation and Daily Localization

- Diagnostic imaging must be reviewed and discussed among the multidisciplinary team to confirm location/extent of disease and muscle compartment involvement prior to positioning/immobilizing the patient for RT simulation.

- Image-guided RT techniques require neutral patient positioning and the least cumbersome immobilization devices possible. This is to achieve imaging during treatment and mechanical clearance of the treatment unit from the patient's anatomy.
- For all extremity tumors, appropriate attention to limb rotational position is important to effectively isolate the affected muscle compartments (see Fig. 1a, b). This is needed to:
  - Achieve optimal normal tissue avoidance in RT planning
  - Facilitate the most straightforward RT beam arrangement
- A reproducible marking on the patient should be defined for daily setup points of reference (i.e., permanent tattoos).
- A six-point patient setup system is ideal, with three setup points chosen along the central axis plane and three along the sagittal plane.
- Preferably, these points should be placed above and below a joint to assess and maintain the joint angle throughout RT and should also be placed beyond any anticipated tumor volume changes as shown in Fig. 1c–f.
- For highly conformal RT techniques, reinforcement of limb stability is important to ensure fixed rotation is maintained throughout the treatment. This can be accomplished with a thermoplastic sheet molded, as in head and neck immobilization for radiotherapy, over the top of the limb and secured to the treatment couch.
- Any chosen immobilization device should attach to the RT treatment couch securely to reinforce stability in all dimensions and maximize setup reproducibility. Various immobilization devices appropriate to different anatomic sites are available.
- Pelvic, abdominal, and retroperitoneal patients require positional support for their arms, which must be spatially separated from the treatment volume (e.g., optimally supported above their head). This can be accomplished with a large polystyrene vacuum cushion or other commercial device that supports the desired arm position (see Fig. 1f).
- Daily image guidance is preferred. For example, 2D KV/2D MV for orthogonal localization or 3D image guidance (i.e., cone beam CT) for target volume/soft tissue localization.

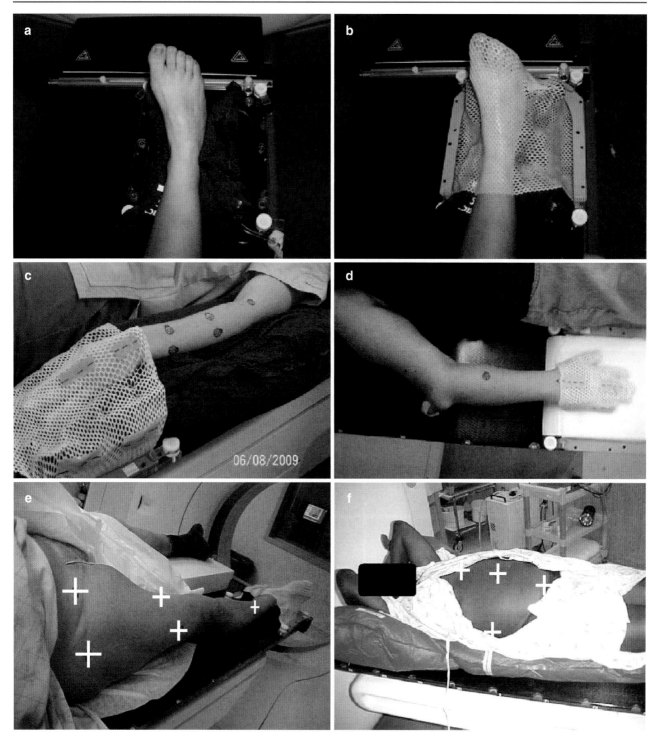

**Fig. 1** Example of soft tissue sarcoma radiotherapy immobilization. (**a**) A right foot immobilized for a radical course of radiotherapy to the right thigh. Rotation is secured by the mini vacuum cushion placed underneath the limb which also provides patient comfort for the longer RT treatment delivery times typical of IMRT/IGRT/Tomotherapy/3D CRT. (**b**) A thermoplastic shell is molded over the limb to reduce patient setup uncertainty in all dimensions. This immobilization system attaches to the radiotherapy treatment couch. It can be used for upper and lower extremity immobilization. (**c**) Upper extremity immobilization for an STS sarcoma of the elbow. A larger mini vacuum cushion is utilized to support the contour change from the shoulder to the wrist typical of this anatomic area. (**d**) Another STS sarcoma of the elbow using a modified version of the device shown in (**a**). Styrofoam is used instead of the vacuum cushion for superior hand

definition in the thermoplastic mold. Both systems attach to the radiotherapy treatment couch. (**e**) Medial upper thigh sarcoma immobilized with a device placed on the foot to secure rotation and reduce setup uncertainty. Five permanent tattoos are used to enhance patient setup consistency; the tattoos are artificially depicted by the *white crosses* in this image. The tattoos were used for daily patient positional reproducibility and alignment, in addition to other marks placed on the immobilization device. The scrotum is retracted from the treatment volume. (**f**) A retroperitoneal sarcoma setup using a large polystyrene vacuum cushion to support the arms away from the treatment volume with 5 setup tattoos. One is placed on each side of the patient for rotational reproducibility and 3 along the central axis for patient alignment (see 4 *white crosses* depicting the 3 *central axis tattoo* points with the right lateral visible tattoo point)

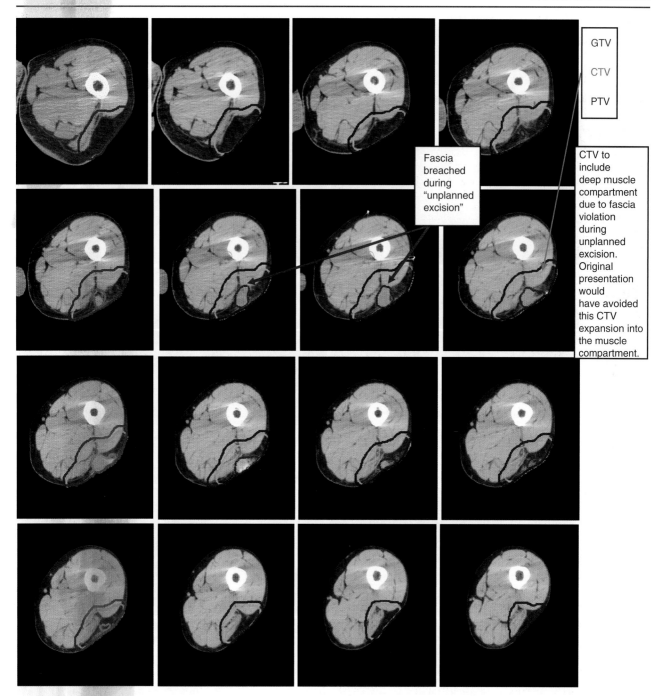

**Fig. 2** T2bN0M0 grade 3 dedifferentiated liposarcoma in the posterolateral thigh treated with preoperative radiotherapy to 50 Gy in 25 fractions. This patient presented with a previous unplanned and incomplete excision of a superficial lesion where the fascia of the vastus lateralis was breached, and the tumor had not involved the deeper compartment originally. CT simulation used 2.0 mm slice thickness. Note the area of violated fascia (*arrows*) due to previous surgical error which now must be included in the CTV with a substantial volume increase (also see Fig. 3). Shown are representative slices

## 4 Target Volume Delineation and Treatment Planning

- For preoperative planning target volume definition, CT simulation imaging fused with MR imaging should be performed, ideally with the patient in the treatment position. These will facilitate delineation of the gross tumor volume (GTV) and clinical target volume (CTV) (see Figs. 2 and 3).

- For postoperative planning target volume definition after presumed complete surgical resection, there is no GTV to delineate. The location of the original GTV following the

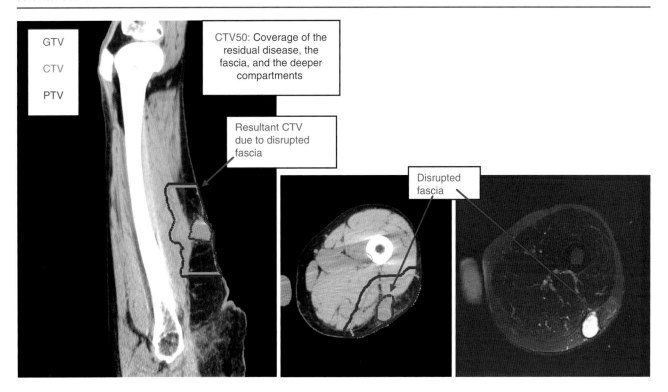

GTV

CTV

PTV

CTV50: Coverage of the residual disease, the fascia, and the deeper compartments

Resultant CTV due to disrupted fascia

Disrupted fascia

**Fig. 3** Example of the GTV, CTV, and PTV for the case in Fig. 2 displayed in the sagittal view as well as an axial MRI view of the disrupted fascia as a result of an unplanned excision with the corresponding planning CT target volumes

operation ($_{postop}$GTV) should be recreated as realistically as possible in the original planning CT dataset using preoperative CT/MR imaging if available (see Figs. 4 and 5).

- For preoperative cases, 50 Gy is ordinarily used and target volumes include the GTV and the CTV$_{50}$ and should be delineated on every slice of the planning CT dataset.
- For postoperative RT delivery, 66 Gy is ordinarily used (60 Gy can be used in surgical margin clear, low-grade cases) and should encompass the prior location of the GTV with an additional peripheral elective subclinical CTV volume for tissues with lesser risk of microscopic tumor infestation, i.e., equivalent to 50 Gy in 25 fractions, e.g., 56 Gy in 33 fractions, or 54 Gy in 30 fractions if a simultaneously integrated boost technique is used (see Table 2 and Fig. 5).

- For unresectable residual gross disease, 70 Gy in 2 Gy/fraction or an equivalent dose fractionation is ordinarily used depending on the tolerance of the anatomic region. This is delivered to the location of any residual GTV with an additional peripheral elective dose CTV volume.
- Suggested target volumes for different treatment settings are as follows:
  - GTV and CTV$_{50}$ for preoperative IMRT of extremity STS are detailed in Table 1. (Figs. 2, 3, 10, 11, 12, 13)
  - $_{postop}$GTV and CTV$_{66}$ for postoperative IMRT of extremity STS are detailed in Table 2. (Figs. 4, 5, 8, 9)
  - GTV and CTV (dose 50–50.4 Gy) for preoperative IMRT of retroperitoneal STS are detailed in Table 3 (Figs. 6, 7).

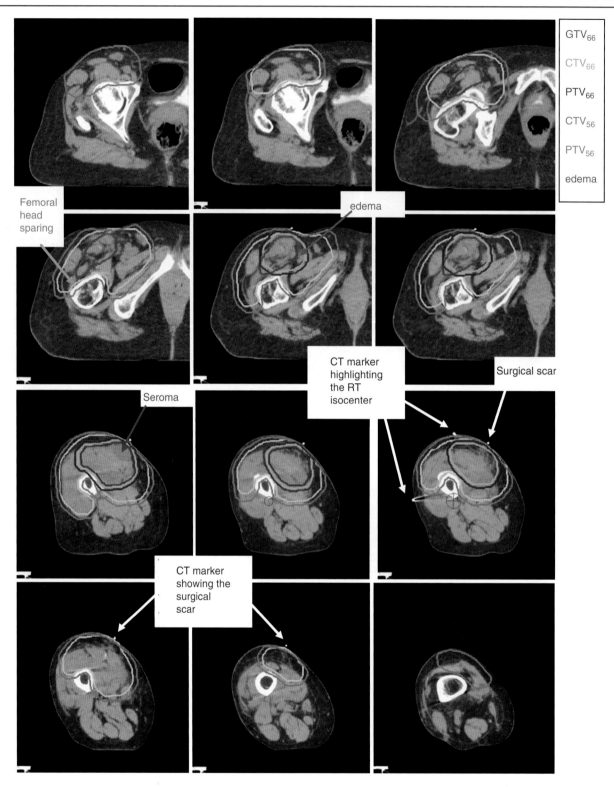

**Fig. 4** T2bN0M0 grade 3 pleomorphic rhabdomyosarcoma in the left anterior thigh treated with postoperative radiotherapy to 66 Gy in 33 fractions. This patient received postoperative RT for negative but close margins. CT simulation used 2.0 mm slice thickness. Edema was contoured in the superior aspect of the $_{postop}$GTV and included in the CTV$_{56}$. Shown are representative slices. CTV$_{56}$ is limited by the femoral head and bone throughout the target. In some cases where the subcutaneous tissues have been contaminated, bolus may be applied to the surgical scar for a component of the treatment (e.g., 50 Gy)

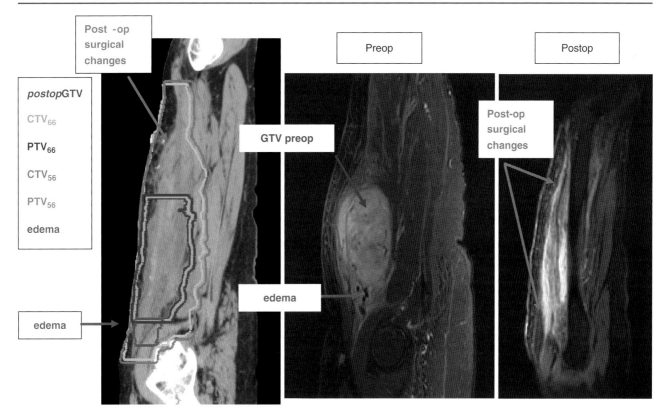

**Fig. 5** Sagittal CT simulation view of the radiotherapy target volumes for the postoperative STS case demonstrated in Fig. 4 with the corresponding preoperative and postoperative MRI. Note the CTV$_{56}$ is defined by edema and the postoperative surgical changes. Where the CTV and PTV target volumes may appear concordant in this scaled anatomic illustration, the usual margins were applied (e.g., 0.5–1 cm PTV expansion). In addition, the preoperative imaging was imported and co-registered with the postoperative RT planning CT dataset in order to appreciate the original tumor extent for delineation of the $_{postop}$GTV

**Table 1** Suggested target volumes for preoperative extremity STS

| Target volumes | Definition and description |
|---|---|
| GTV | Primary: all gross disease on physical examination and imaging. T1-weighted contrast-enhanced MRI preferable (Fig. 2). Co-registration of the MRI and planning CT datasets is facilitated by immobilizing the patient in the treatment position |
| CTV$_{50}$[a] | Includes all areas at risk of subclinical spread defined by the distance from the GTV or edema |
| | Includes the GTV + 4 cm margin in the longitudinal dimensions + 1.5 cm margin in the radial dimension limited to but including any anatomic barrier to tumor spread, such as the bone and fascia (Fig. 2) |
| | Suspicious peritumoral edema, best demonstrated on T2-weighted MRI sequences, may contain microscopic tumor cells and should be contoured separately with an adequate margin (usually 1–2 cm) |
| | For cases of "unplanned excision," margins should include $_{postop}$GTV or any residual GTV and all surgically manipulated and disturbed tissues and violated fascia + 4 cm longitudinally + 1.5 cm radially limited to but including any barrier to tumor spread |
| PTV$_{50}$[a] | CTV$_{50}$ + 0.5 to 1.0 cm, determined by individual institutional protocols and procedure |

[a]The subscript denotes the radiation dose intended. Suggested gross tumor dose is 2.0 Gy/fraction to 50 Gy

**Table 2** Suggested target volumes for postoperative extremity STS

| Target volumes | Definition and description |
|---|---|
| $_{postop}$GTV | $_{postop}$GTV should identify the original site of the tumor |
| | Important to review and import presurgical imaging when contouring on the CT simulation scan for RT planning to ensure adequate coverage of the original tumor extent |
| CTV$_{66}$[a] | CTV$_{66}$ should encompass the entire $_{postop}$GTV and immediate area of surgical disruption + 1 to 2 cm margin in the longitudinal plane + 1.5 cm margin in the transverse plane. This may, but not always, include all surgically disturbed tissues, scars, and drain sites, which may be included in a wider subclinical elective volume (see CTV$_{56}$ volume suggestions) |
| PTV$_{66}$[a] | CTV$_{66}$ + 0.5 to 1.0 cm, determined by individual institutional protocols and procedure (Figs. 4 and 5) |
| CTV$_{56}$[a] | Includes all areas at risk of subclinical spread defined by the distance from the $_{postop}$GTV and additional disturbed tissues |
| | Includes the $_{postop}$GTV + 4 cm margin in the longitudinal dimensions + 1.5 cm margin in the radial dimension limited to but including any anatomic barrier to disease spread (Fig. 5); additional disturbed surgical tissues and any scars or drain sites are ordinarily included + 1 to 2 cm margin if they are not included in the CTV$_{66}$ |
| | Suspicious peritumoral edema should be contoured separately and included with an adequate margin. Like surgically disrupted tissue, it is best identified from a recent postoperative MRI scan |
| | Discussion with the surgeon and review of surgical and pathology reports will facilitate the decision about whether or not any seroma, lymphocele, or hematoma should be included |
| PTV$_{56}$[a] | CTV$_{56}$ + 0.5 to 1.0 cm, determined by individual institutional protocols and procedure |

Table describes single-phase simultaneously integrated boost techniques. An alternative is the more traditional sequentially phased *shrinking field* technique that delivers 50 Gy in 25 fractions to all areas of subclinical disease followed by a boost to deliver the final 16 Gy in 8 fractions or 10 Gy in 5 fractions

[a]The subscript denotes the radiation dose intended. High-risk subclinical dose, 2.0 Gy/fraction to 66 Gy. For lower-risk subclinical regions 1.69 Gy/fraction to 56 Gy delivered to the CTV$_{56.}$ Surgical margin negative low-grade tumors may alternatively receive 60 Gy in 30 fractions with 54 Gy to the subclinical region

**Table 3** Suggested RT target volumes for preoperative retroperitoneal STS

| Target volumes | Definition and description |
|---|---|
| GTV[a] | Primary: all gross disease on physical examination and imaging (Figs. 6 and 7) |
| CTV | Includes all areas at risk of subclinical spread defined by the distance from the GTV |
| | Includes the GTV + 2 cm margin in the longitudinal dimensions + 0.5 – 2.0 cm margin in the radial dimension limited to but including any anatomic barrier to tumor spread and critical anatomy. For example, if the tumor is approximating an intact liver, 0.5 cm of the liver is included |
| | 2 cm margins are usually used posteriorly to include fatty tissues and vessels |
| | Ipsilateral kidney may need to be sacrificed provided the contralateral kidney has acceptable function. In such cases, dose to the uninvolved opposite kidney should be kept as low as reasonably achievable |
| | Other organs at risk include the small bowel, liver, spinal cord, and lung |
| PTV | CTV + 0.5 cm, determined by individual institutional protocols and procedure |

[a]Suggested gross tumor dose range of 50 Gy/25 fractions to 50.4 Gy/28 fractions. The 50.4 Gy dose is chosen to acknowledge the large volumes and tolerance of adjacent structures, especially the bowel

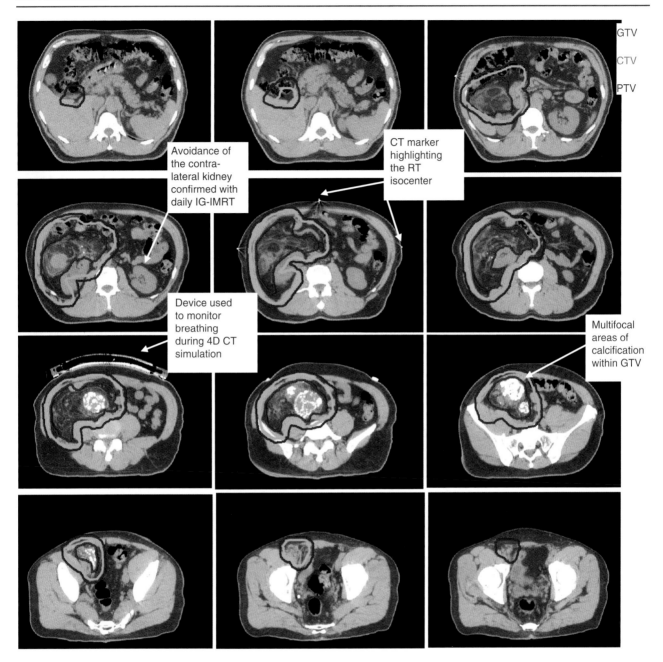

**Fig. 6** A right-sided T2bN0M0 grade 3 undifferentiated pleomorphic retroperitoneal sarcoma juxtaposed to the duodenum, the right kidney, and the iliac vessels. CT simulation used a 2.0 mm slice thickness. Representative slices are shown to illustrate preoperative radiotherapy. Note the small amount of liver that needed to be included in the CTV and PTV in the first three axial slices. Multifocal areas of calcifications within the tumor aided in daily image guidance for targeted IMRT (IG-IMRT). 4D CT simulation is encouraged

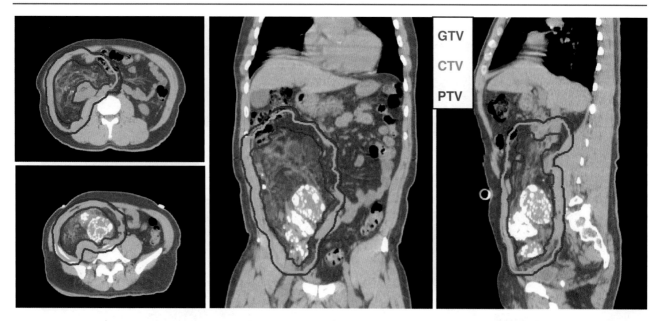

**Fig. 7** An axial, coronal, and sagittal display of the right-sided retroperitoneal sarcoma depicted in Fig. 6, undergoing preoperative radiotherapy. Note the bowel displacement by the tumor, a major advantage of preoperative radiotherapy in this setting. The daily image guidance algorithm prioritized a vertebral bony match but also included user soft tissue and target coverage assessment. In addition, RT avoidance of the functioning kidney on the contralateral side is established on a daily basis using image guidance software. For cases that include a 4D CT simulation, the CTV is contoured on the inhale and exhale CT scans. For the CT planning scan, the inhale and exhale CT is combined to form an internal target volume (ITV)

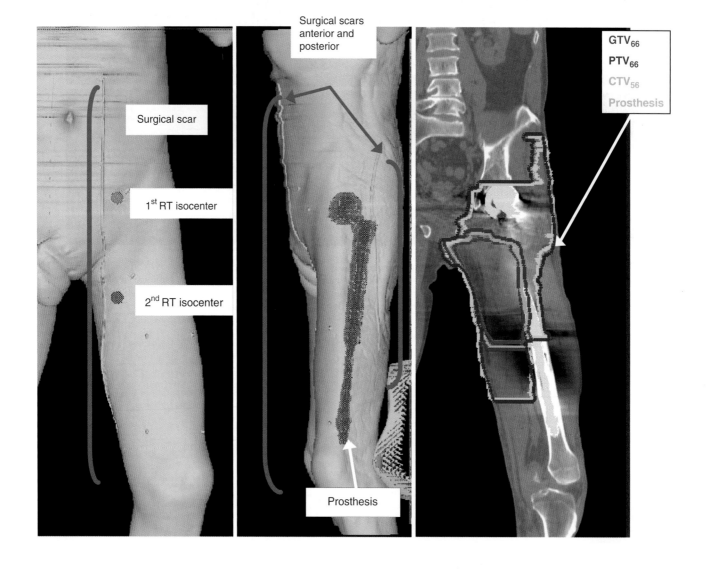

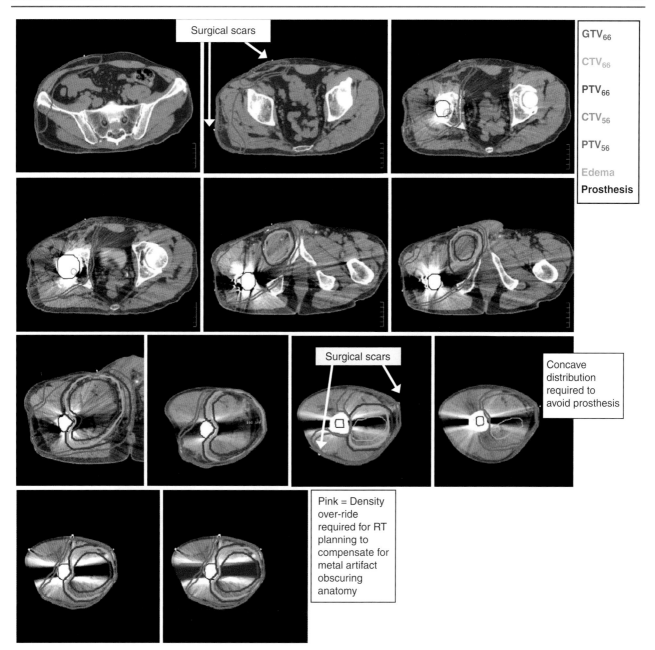

**Fig. 9** Representative axial slices are shown to illustrate the dual isocenter large volume RT technique for the case described in Fig. 8. The final two axial slices demonstrate how the artifact from the metal prosthesis is overcome in RT planning using a density override function. CT simulation used a 2.0 mm slice thickness. Representative slices are shown

**Fig. 8** *Dual isocenter large volume technique*: T2bN0M0 grade 3 undifferentiated sarcoma resected from the left adductor compartment of the thigh with clear surgical margins despite involvement of the femoral cortex. En bloc resection of the proximal femur was required to remove the tumor adequately. Dissection of the femoral neurovasculature anteriorly, and the sciatic nerve posteriorly, was required through separate exposures. Postoperative radiotherapy was chosen to maximize wound closure and fixation of the cemented prosthesis; these goals could have been jeopardized with preoperative radiotherapy. An unconventional postoperative RT target volume was chosen. The entire surgical volume was not included due to its prodigious size, and the cemented tumor endoprosthesis was not irradiated in its entirety to minimize fixation failure. The bone dose in the inferior part of the volume was restricted to <40 Gy. The target volume was so large that it required a dual isocenter technique to deliver a dose of 66 Gy in 33 fractions to the high-risk soft tissue region and 56 Gy to other elective subclinical areas

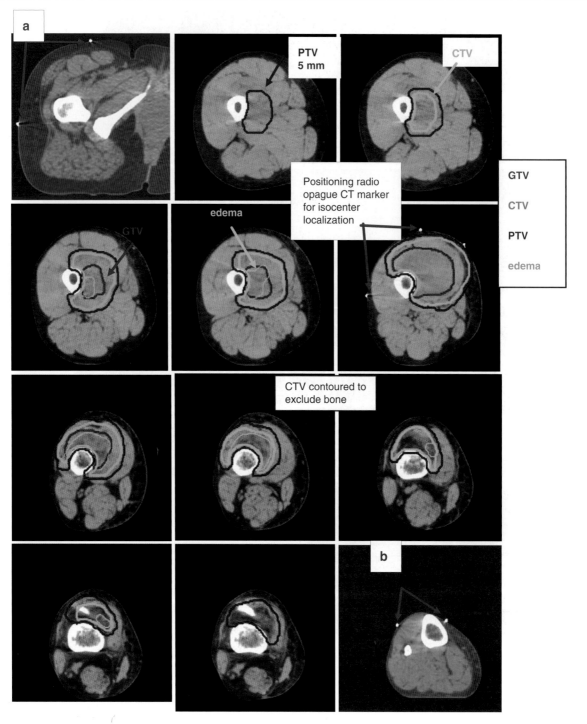

**Fig. 10** Preoperative case with bone stripping: T2bN0M0 grade 3 pleomorphic liposarcoma in the left thigh juxtaposed to the periosteum, which provides a barrier to tumor spread. The periosteum is included but the target volume does not need to extend further into the cortex. Postoperative radiotherapy would have required a significant increase in target volume that would have encompassed the adjacent bone cortex due to the surgically disturbed periosteum that normally acts as a tumor barrier. (**a, b**) Patient positioning CT radioopaque markers placed superior (**a**) and inferior (**b**) along the central axis and sagittal plane approximately 15 cm from the patient set up center (outside of the treatment volume)

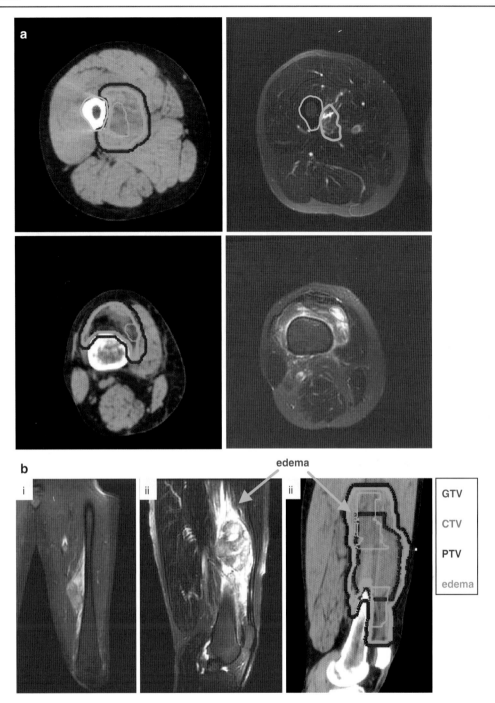

**Fig. 11** Axial, sagittal, and coronal slices demonstrating edematous tissues from the case described in Fig. 10. (**a**) Edema located at the superior CTV and inferior extent of the CTV shown in *light blue* on both the CT and MRI. Bone is outlined in light orange, CTV *light green*, and PTV *royal blue*. (**b**) MRI and CT images: (*i*) coronal view MR, (*ii*) sagittal view MR, and (*iii*) sagittal view CT simulation scan with the target volumes and edema contoured

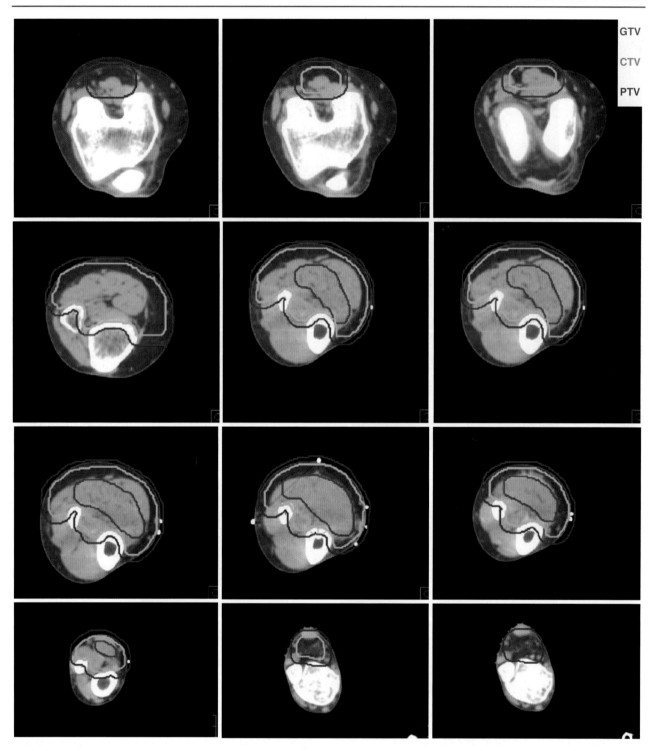

**Fig. 12** Preoperative case: T2bN0M0 pseudomyogenic hemangioendothelioma in the right calf. This uncommon and distinctive type of sarcoma is characterized by multifocality and only rarely metastasizes but has a high risk of multifocal local recurrence within the limb following surgery alone. CT simulation used a 2.0 mm slice thickness. Representative slices are shown (Hornick JL, Fletcher CD (2011) Pseudomyogenic hemangioendothelioma: a distinctive, often multicentric tumor with indolent behavior. Am J Surg Pathol 35(2):190–201)

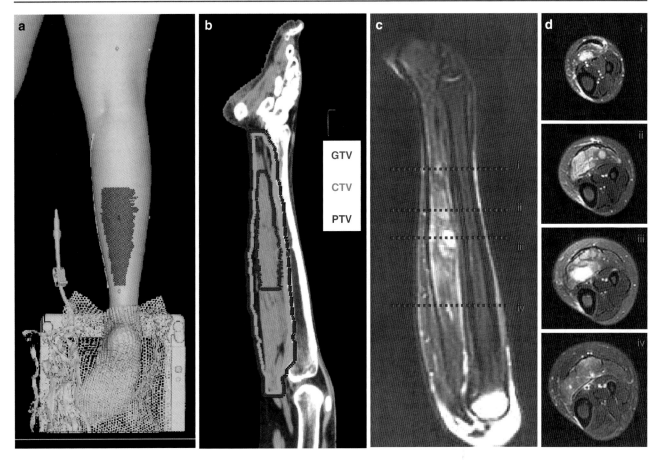

**Fig. 13** Additional depictions of the case shown in Fig. 12. The CTV (shown in *green*) encompasses all suspicious areas, but an unusually large longitudinal distance is required to encompass the extent of potential microscopic disease with an adequate margin beyond the multifocal areas shown (**b**). A reconstructed image of the patient in setup position is shown (**a**). The immobilization device was placed on the foot in the prone position. MRI axial views (**d**, *i–iv*) correspond to the demarcated positions on the adjacent sagittal MRI view (**c**, *i–iv*). Position D still demonstrates edematous tissue which is reflected in the increase in the superior CTV margin shown on the sagittal CT view (**b**)

## 5 Plan Assessment

- In cases with critical structure invasion (e.g., extensive liver involvement in retroperitoneal sarcoma), normal structure constraints are prioritized due to the potentially adverse consequences, including death or permanent avoidable severe functional disability, e.g., renal function eradication or spinal cord damage. In other cases, constraints on normal structures must be balanced within the context of treatment goals (e.g., bone avoidance objectives to minimize the risk of fracture versus risk of local failure).
- Target coverage criteria of greater than 99 % of the PTV should receive >97 % of the prescribed dose have been used in clinical trials, although 95 % coverage of the 95 % isodose volume is also an acceptable goal.
- No more than 20 % of the PTV should receive ≥110 % of the prescription dose, and it is exceptional to require this upper dose range.
- STS organs at risk (OARs) in radiation therapy depend on the site of STS. The bone is the major dose avoidance structure in extremity tumors as well as a longitudinal

limb region (i.e., a "strip") of uninvolved tissue, while additional organs including the small bowel, liver, kidneys, and spinal cord need to be considered in abdominal/retroperitoneal sarcomas.

- Some general site-specific OARs include:

| General site | Organs at risk |
|---|---|
| Retroperitoneal | Bowel, lung, liver, kidneys, heart, spinal cord |
| Upper extremity | Bone, lung, brachial plexus, spinal cord, a longitudinal region/"strip" of tissue/lymphatics in the limb to maintain proper lymph flow |
| Lower extremity | Bone, external genitalia, unaffected contralateral leg, a longitudinal region of uninvolved tissue/lymphatics to maintain proper lymph flow |
| Pelvis | Bowel, rectum, bone, genitalia, kidneys |
| Chest wall | Spinal cord, lung, heart |
| Head and neck | Spinal cord, brain stem, bone, parotids, lung, optic nerves and chiasm, optic globes, pharynx, brachial plexus |

- The chosen technique and the necessary dose/volume parameters depend heavily on tumor location, the goal of treatment, normal tissue preservation, and the availability of delivery and imaging devices/equipment.

- Selected IMRT dose constraints typically employed are as follows:

| Organs at risk | Dose constraints |
|---|---|
| [a]Bone | Mean dose < 37 Gy |
| | Max dose < 59 Gy |
| | [b]V40 < 67 % |
| Spinal cord | Max dose 45 Gy to any point |
| Liver | V30 < 30 % |
| Small intestine | V45 < 10 % |
| Lungs | V20 < 20 % |
| Testis | V3 < 50 % to reserve fertility |
| Kidney | V14 < 50 % for both kidneys |
| | V20 < 1/3 of one kidney |

[a]Dickie CI, Parent AL, Griffin AM et al (2009) Bone fractures following external beam radiotherapy and limb-preservation surgery for lower extremity soft tissue sarcoma: relationship to irradiated bone length, volume, tumor location and dose. Int J Radiat Oncol Biol Phys 75:1119–1124

[b]V__: the volume of tissue receiving the specified dose in Gy. For example, the volume of bone receiving 40 Gy should be kept below 67 %. Other volumes and doses should be correspondingly labeled

## Suggested Reading

Davis AM, O'Sullivan B, Turcotte R et al (2005) Late radiation morbidity following randomization to preoperative versus postoperative radiotherapy in extremity soft tissue sarcoma. Radiother Oncol 75:48–53

Dickie CI, Parent AL, Griffin AM et al (2009) Bone fractures following external beam radiotherapy and limb-preservation surgery for lower extremity soft tissue sarcoma: relationship to irradiated bone length, volume, tumor location and dose. Int J Radiat Oncol Biol Phys 75:1119–1124

Dickie CI, Parent AL, Chung PW et al (2010) Measuring interfractional and intrafractional motion with cone beam computed tomography and an optical localization system for lower extremity soft tissue sarcoma patients treated with preoperative intensity-modulated radiation therapy. Int J Radiat Oncol Biol Phys 78:1437–1444

Haas RL et al (2012) Radiotherapy for management of extremity soft tissue sarcomas: why, when, and where? Int J Radiat Oncol Biol Phys 84(3):572–80

Joensuu H, Fletcher C, Dimitrijevic S et al (2002) Management of malignant gastrointestinal stromal tumours. Lancet Oncol 3:655–664

Kepka L, Delaney TF, Suit HD et al (2005) Results of radiation therapy for unresected soft-tissue sarcomas. Int J Radiat Oncol Biol Phys 63:852–859

O'Sullivan B, Davis AM, Turcotte R et al (2002) Preoperative versus postoperative radiotherapy in soft-tissue sarcoma of the limbs: a randomised trial. Lancet 359:2235–2241

Pawlik TM, Pisters PW, Mikula L et al (2006) Long-term results of two prospective trials of preoperative external beam radiotherapy for localized intermediate- or high-grade retroperitoneal soft tissue sarcoma. Ann Surg Oncol 13:508–517

Pisters PW, Pollock RE, Lewis VO et al (2007) Long-term results of prospective trial of surgery alone with selective use of radiation for patients with T1 extremity and trunk soft tissue sarcomas. Ann Surg 246:675–681; discussion 681–682

Rosenberg SA, Tepper J, Glatstein E et al (1982) The treatment of soft-tissue sarcomas of the extremities: prospective randomized evaluations of (1) limb-sparing surgery plus radiation therapy compared with amputation and (2) the role of adjuvant chemotherapy. Ann Surg 196:305–315

Strander H, Turesson I, Cavallin-Stahl E (2003) A systematic overview of radiation therapy effects in soft tissue sarcomas. Acta Oncol 42:516–531

White LM, Wunder JS, Bell RS et al (2005) Histologic assessment of peritumoral edema in soft tissue sarcoma. Int J Radiat Oncol Biol Phys 61:1439–1445

Yang JC, Chang AE, Baker AR et al (1998) Randomized prospective study of the benefit of adjuvant radiation therapy in the treatment of soft tissue sarcomas of the extremity. J Clin Oncol 16:197–203

# Index

Printing: Ten Brink, Meppel, The Netherlands
Binding: Ten Brink, Meppel, The Netherlands